Progress in
Cancer Research and Therapy
Volume 7

IMMUNE MODULATION AND CONTROL OF NEOPLASIA BY ADJUVANT THERAPY

Progress in
Cancer Research and Therapy

Vol. 1: Control Mechanisms in Cancer
Wayne E. Criss, Tetsuo Ono, and John R. Sabine, editors, 1976

Vol. 2: Control of Neoplasia by Modulation of the Immune System
Michael A. Chirigos, editor, 1977

Vol. 3: Genetics of Human Cancer
John J. Mulvihill, Robert W. Miller, and Joseph F. Fraumeni, Jr., editors, 1977

Vol. 4: Progesterone Receptors in Normal and Neoplastic Tissues
William L. McGuire, Jean-Pierre Raynaud, and Etienne-Emile Baulieu, editors, 1977

Vol. 5: Cancer Invasion and Metastasis: Biologic Mechanisms and Therapy
Stacey B. Day, W. P. Laird Myers, Philip Stansly, Silvio Garattini, and Martin G. Lewis, editors, 1977

Vol. 6: Immunotherapy of Cancer: Present Status of Trials in Man
William D. Terry and Dorothy Windhorst, editors, 1978

Vol. 7: Immune Modulation and Control of Neoplasia by Adjuvant Therapy
Michael A. Chirigos, editor, 1978

Progress in
Cancer Research and Therapy
Volume 7

Immune Modulation and Control of Neoplasia by Adjuvant Therapy

Edited by

Michael A. Chirigos, Ph.D.

Laboratory of RNA Tumor Viruses
National Cancer Institute
National Institutes of Health
Bethesda, Maryland

Raven Press ▪ New York

Raven Press, 1140 Avenue of the Americas, New York, New York 10036

Raven Press, New York 1978
Made in the United States of America

Library of Congress Cataloging in Publication Data

Main entry under title:

Immune modulation and control of neoplasia by
    adjuvant therapy.

    (Progress in cancer research and therapy; v. 7)
    "Sponsored by the National Cancer Institute, U.S.A."
    Includes bibliographical references and index.
    1. Cancer--Immunological aspects. 2. Immunotherapy.
3. Immune response--Regulation. 4. Cancer--Chemotherapy.
I. Chirigos, Michael A. II. United States. National Cancer
Institute. III. Series. [DNLM: 1. Neoplasms--Immunology
--Congresses. 2. Neoplasms--Drug therapy--Congresses.
W1 PR667M / QZ200 I327 1976]
RC271.I45I45   616.9'94'061   76-5665
ISBN 0-89004-220-9

Preface

The immunological surveillance of the cancer patient is suppressed both by the disease itself and the cytoreductive therapy required to manage it. The early return of host immune function is of major importance for the successful control and, hopefully, the cure of cancer, as well as preventing life-threatening secondary infectious diseases resulting from immune suppression. The availability of several chemical and biological agents capable of reconstituting and/or stimulating the cellular components of the immune response provides the cancer therapist greater flexibility in developing different combined modality treatment regimens. The ability to modulate host immunity is today a reality and the rapidly developing field of immunotherapy is becoming an important aspect of cancer therapy.

The second volume of this important series was devoted to experimental and clinical studies with four rapidly emerging agents demonstrating immune-stimulatory activity: levamisole, thymosin, glucan, and pyran copolymer. The present volume contains 45 authoritative chapters by distinguished research specialists reporting the most recent information concerning experimental and clinical findings with these and other new, potentially effective, immunostimulators. In-depth reports are presented, describing clinical findings with levamisole, thymosin, and glucan as well as describing their mechanism(s) of action. The particular cellular components of the immune system affected by these agents when used singly or in combined treatment are described.

This volume will be invaluable to clinical and experimental oncologists, chemotherapists, immunologists, as well as immunochemists.

The editor and contributors of this volume wish to express their gratitude to Dr. J. B. Moloney, Associate Director for Viral Oncology, Division of Cancer Cause and Prevention, National Cancer Institute, National Institutes of Health, and to Dr. Milo D. Leavitt, Jr., Director of The Fogarty International Center, National Institutes of Health, and his staff for their encouragement and invaluable support that made the conference, on which this volume is based, possible.

Michael A. Chirigos,
Editor

Contents

LEVAMISOLE: PRECLINICAL FINDINGS

1   Treatment of the Compromised Host with Levamisole, a Synthetic Immunotherapeutic Agent
J. Symoens

11   Effect of Levamisole in Combination with Radiotherapy in Modifying the Growth of Murine Tumors of Differing Immunogenicity
Carleton C. Stewart, Carlos A. Perez, and Barbara Hente

23   Cyclic Adenosine Monophosphate Levels in Lymphocytes from Patients with Melanoma and Squamous Cell Carcinoma Treated with Levamisole
Zbigniew L. Olkowski

29   Levamisole and Human Monocyte Chemotaxis: Reversal of an Influenzal-Induced Chemotactic Defect
Ralph Snyderman, Marilyn C. Pike, and Charles A. Daniels

39   *In Vitro* Effects of Levamisole on Human Mononuclear Phagocytes
Mohamed S. Al-Ibrahim

49   Chemoimmunotherapy of Human Malignant Lymphoma with Levamisole: Induction of Lymphocytotoxic Antibodies and Differential Effect on Accidental Infections
R. Mertelsmann, S. B. Ellis, R. Schwerdt, and H. Hildebrandt

65   Effects of Levamisole on the E-Rosette Formation of Peripheral Human T Lymphocytes
H. Verhaegen, W. De Cock, J. De Cree, W. Amery, M. L. Verhaegen-Declercq, and F. Verbruggen

75   Effect of Levamisole on Suckling Rat Spleen Cells: Evidence for Macrophage Regulation
Gerald W. Fischer, Martin H. Crumrine, Melvin W. Balk, Sandra P. Chang, Yoshitsugi Hokama, Patricia Heu, and S. C. Chou

85   Effect of Levamisole on an *In Vitro* Model of Cellular Immunity
F. J. Persico and W. A. Potter

LEVAMISOLE: CLINICAL FINDINGS

93   Overview of Levamisole Effectiveness in Experimental and Clinical Cancer Studies
Willem K. Amery

107 Effect of Levamisole on Cell-Mediated Immunity in Patients with Lung Cancer
E. Carmack Holmes and Sidney H. Golub

119 Chemoimmunotherapy of Refractory Malignant Melanoma with Actinomycin D and Levamisole
Stephen W. Hall, Robert S. Benjamin, Lance Heilbrun, Uri Lewinski, Jordan U. Gutterman, and Giora Mavligit

131 Levamisole in the Treatment of Breast Cancer
G. N. Hortobagyi, J. U. Gutterman, G. R. Blumenschein, C. K. Tashima, A. U. Buzdar, and E. M. Hersh

141 Unblocking Effect of Levamisole on a Subpopulation of T Lymphocytes in Hodgkin's Disease Patients
Bracha Ramot, Miriam Biniaminov, and Esther Rosenthal

147 Combination Immunotherapy with Levamisole, BCG, and Tumor Vaccines: Toward a Rationale
L. M. Jerry, M. G. Lewis, H. R. Shibata, P. W. A. Mansell, A. Capek, and G. Marquis

157 Interpretation of Management of Levamisole-Associated Side Effects
R. Douglas Thornes

165 Levamisole Therapy in Congenital Immunodeficiencies
C. Griscelli, A. M. Prieur, and F. DaGuillard

GLUCAN

171 Enhancement of the Inhibitory Effect of Cyclophosphamide on Experimental Acute Myelogenous Leukemia by Glucan Immunopotentiation and Response of Serum Lysozyme
N. R. Di Luzio, J. A. Cook, C. Cohen, J. Rodrigue, P. Kokoshis, and R. B. McNamee

183 Comparative Evaluation of the Role of Macrophages and Lymphocytes in Mediating the Antitumor Action of Glucan
J. A. Cook, D. Taylor, C. Cohen, J. Rodrigue, V. Malshet, and N. R. Di Luzio

195 Increased Granulopoiesis and Macrophage Production in Glucan-Treated Mice
Carmen Burgaleta and David W. Golde

201 Glucan-Activated Macrophages: Functional Properties and Cytotoxicity Against Syngeneic Leukemia Cells
David W. Golde and Carmen Burgaleta

207   Suppression of Hepatic Metastases by Immunization with Glucan
William Browder, Craig Cohen, Rose McNamee, E. O. Hoffmann, and N. R. Di Luzio

221   Comparison of the Antitumor Effects of Glucan, BCG, and Levamisole
J. W. Proctor, B. G. Auclair, L. Stokowski, and P. W. A. Mansell

235   Comparative Evaluation of Tumor-Inhibitory Activity of Glucan and *Corynebacterium parvum* in a Mouse Fibrosarcoma Model
Herman D. Suit, Arthur Elman, Robert Sedlacek, and Vlatko Silobrcic

241   Tumoricidal Effect *In Vitro* of Peritoneal Macrophages from Mice Treated with Glucan
Richard M. Schultz, Joseph D. Papamatheakis, and Michael A. Chirigos

249   Treatment of Cutaneous and Subcutaneous Metastatic Tumors with Intralesional Glucan
Lucien Israel and Richard Edelstein

255   Clinical Experiences with the Use of Glucan
P. W. A. Mansell, G. Rowden, and C. Hammer

THYMOSIN

281   Recent Developments in the Chemistry and Biology of Thymosin
A. L. Goldstein, T. L. K. Low, J. L. Rossio, J. T. Ulrich, P. H. Naylor, and G. B. Thurman

293   Maturation of Thymus-Derived Cells Under the Influence of Thymosin
Aftab Ahmed, Allan H. Smith, and Kenneth W. Sell

305   *In Vitro* and *In Vivo* Studies with Thymosin
Michael A. Chirigos

313   Thymocyte-Mitogen Bioassay for Thymosin
Patrick W. Trown, Carol Lewinski, Phyllis L. Meyer, Alicia V. Palleroni, and Oksana Krochak

319   *In Vitro* Induction of Human T-Cell Differentiation
Sheldon Horowitz

333   *In Vitro* and *In Vivo* Effects of Thymosin on T-Lymphocyte Function in Primary Immunodeficiency Disease
Diane W. Wara, Alan C. Johnson, and Arthur J. Ammann

347   Lymphocyte Response to Thymosin *In Vitro* in Cancer Patients: Correlation with Initial T-Cell Levels
Daniel E. Kenady, Claude Potvin, and Paul B. Chretien

357   Clinical and Immunological Evaluation of the Use of Thymosin Plus
       BCG ± DTIC in the Adjuvant Treatment of Stage 3B Melanoma
       *Yehuda Z. Patt, Evan M. Hersh, Larry A. Schafer, Lance K. Heilbrun,
       Marvette L. Washington, Jordan U. Gutterman, Giora M. Mavligit,
       and Allan L. Goldstein*

373   Thymosin in Patients with Disseminated Solid Tumors: Phase I and
       II Results
       John J. Costanzi, Nick Harris, and Allan Goldstein

PYRAN AND OTHER CHEMICAL ADJUVANTS

381   Immunoadjuvant and Antitumor Properties of Amphotericin B
       J. R. Little, T. J. Blanke, F. Valeriote, and G. Medoff

389   BM 06 002: A New Immunostimulating Compound
       U. Bicker

403   Phase I Study for a New Immunostimulating Drug, BM 06 002, in
       Man
       M. Micksche, E. M. Kokoschka, P. Sagaster, and U. Bicker

415   Immunopotentiation Against the L1210 Leukemia by Pyran Copo-
       lymer and Crude Tumor Antigen
       Stephen J. Mohr and Michael A. Chirigos

427   Effect of Dose, Route, and Timing of Pyran Copolymer Therapy
       Against the Madison Lung Carcinoma
       Joseph D. Papamatheakis, Michael A. Chirigos, and Richard M. Schultz

435   Immunoregulatory Macrophages from Pyran-Treated Mice
       Lynn G. Baird and Alan M. Kaplan

447   Antiviral and Antitumor Functions of Activated Macrophages
       Page S. Morahan and Alan M. Kaplan

459   Correlation Between Antitumor Activity and Macrophage Activation
       by Polyanions
       Richard M. Schultz, Joseph D. Papamatheakis, and M. A. Chirigos

469   Clinical Study of the Synthetic Polyanion Pyran Copolymer (NSC
       46015, Diveema) and Its Role in Future Clinical Trials
       *W. Regelson, B. I. Shnider, J. Colsky, K. B. Olson, J. F. Holland,
       C. L. Johnston, Jr., and L. H. Dennis*

491   *Subject Index*

Contributors

Aftab Ahmed
Cellular Immunology Division
Clinical and Experimental Immunology
   Department
Naval Medical Research Institute
Bethesda, Maryland 20014

Mohamed S. Al-Ibrahim
Department of Medicine
Veterans Administration Hospital
Baltimore, Maryland 21218

Willem K. Amery
Janssen Pharmaceutica
B-2340 Beerse (Antwerp), Belgium

Arthur J. Ammann
Department of Pediatrics
Immunology Section
and
Pediatric Clinical Research Center
University of California
San Francisco, California 94143

B. G. Auclair
McGill University Cancer Research Unit
Montreal, Quebec, Canada

Lynn G. Baird
Departments of Microbiology and Surgery
NCV/VCU Cancer Center
Medical College of Virginia
Virginia Commonwealth University
Richmond, Virginia 23298

Melvin W. Balk
Department of Pediatrics and Clinical
   Investigation Service
Tripler Army Medical Center
Honolulu, Hawaii 96819
and
Departments of Pathology and
   Pharmacology
John A. Burns School of Medicine
University of Hawaii
Honolulu, Hawaii 96822

Robert S. Benjamin
Department of Developmental
   Therapeutics
The University of Texas System Cancer
   Center
M. D. Anderson Hospital and Tumor
   Institute
Houston, Texas 77030

U. Bicker
Medical Research
Boehringer Mannheim GmbH
6800 Mannheim 31, Germany

Miriam Biniaminov
Chaim Sheba Medical Center
Tel-Aviv University
Sackler School of Medicine
Tel-Hashomer, Israel

T. J. Blanke
Department of Surgery
Washington University School of Medicine
St. Louis, Missouri 63110

G. R. Blumenschein
Medical Breast Section
Department of Medicine
University of Texas System Cancer Center
M. D. Anderson Hospital and Tumor
   Institute
Houston, Texas 77030

William Browder
Department of Surgery
Tulane University School of Medicine
New Orleans, Louisiana 70112

Carmen Burgaleta
Division of Hematology–Oncology
Department of Medicine
UCLA School of Medicine
Los Angeles, California 90024

A. U. Buzdar
Medical Breast Section
Department of Medicine
University of Texas System Cancer Center
M. D. Anderson Hospital and Tumor
  Institute
Houston, Texas 77030

A Capek
McGill University Cancer Research Unit
Montreal, Quebec, Canada

Sandra P. Chang
Departments of Pathology and
  Pharmacology
John A. Burns School of Medicine
University of Hawaii
Honolulu, Hawaii 96822

Michael A. Chirigos
Laboratory of RNA Tumor Viruses
National Cancer Institute
National Institutes of Health
Bethesda, Maryland 20014

S. C. Chou
Departments of Pathology and
  Pharmacology
John A. Burns School of Medicine
University of Hawaii
Honolulu, Hawaii 96822

Paul B. Chretien
Surgery Branch
National Cancer Institute
National Institutes of Health
Bethesda, Maryland 20014

Craig Cohen
Department of Physiology
Tulane University School of Medicine
New Orleans, Louisiana 70112

J. Colsky
Cedars of Lebanon Hospital
Miami, Florida 33136

J. A. Cook
Department of Physiology
Tulane University School of Medicine
New Orleans, Louisiana 70112

John J. Costanzi
Department of Medicine
University of Texas Medical Branch
Galveston, Texas 77550

Martin H. Crumrine
Department of Pediatrics and Clinical
  Investigation Service
Tripler Army Medical Center
Honolulu, Hawaii 96819

F. DaGuillard
Groupe de Recherches d'Immunologie et
  de Rhumatologie Pédiatriques
INSERM U 132
Hôpital des Enfants Malades
75015 Paris, France

Charles A. Daniels
Department of Pathology
Duke University Medical Center
Durham, North Carolina 27710

W. De Cock
Clinical Research Unit
St. Bartholomeus
B-2060 Merksem (Antwerp), Belgium

J. De Cree
Clinical Research Unit
St. Bartholomeus
B-2060 Merksem (Antwerp), Belgium

L. H. Dennis
831 University Boulevard
Silver Spring, Maryland 20903

N. R. Di Luzio
Department of Physiology
Tulane University School of Medicine
New Orleans, Louisiana 70112

Richard Edelstein
Centre Hospitalier Universitaire
Université Paris Nord
93000 Bobigny, France

S. B. Ellis
Memorial Sloan-Kettering Cancer Center
New York, New York 10021

Arthur Elman
Edwin L. Steele Laboratory of Radiation Biology
Department of Radiation Medicine
Massachusetts General Hospital
Boston, Massachusetts 02114

Gerald W. Fischer
Department of Pediatrics
School of Medicine
Uniformed Services University of the Health Sciences Center
Bethesda, Maryland 20014

David W. Golde
Division of Hematology–Oncology
Department of Medicine
UCLA School of Medicine
Los Angeles, California 90024

Allan L. Goldstein
Division of Biochemistry
University of Texas Medical Branch
Galveston, Texas 77550

Sidney H. Golub
Division of Surgical Oncology
UCLA School of Medicine
Los Angeles, California 90024

C. Griscelli
Groupe de Recherches d'Immunologie et de Rhumatologie Pédiatriques
INSERM U 132
Hôpital des Enfants Malades
75015 Paris, France

Jordan U. Gutterman
Department of Developmental Therapeutics
The University of Texas System Cancer Center
M. D. Anderson Hospital and Tumor Institute
Houston, Texas 77030

Stephen W. Hall
Department of Developmental Therapeutics
The University of Texas System Cancer Center
M. D. Anderson Hospital and Tumor Institute
Houston, Texas 77030

C. Hammer
McGill University Cancer Research Unit
and
Division of Oncology
Royal Victoria Hospital
Montreal, Quebec, Canada

Nick Harris
Divisions of Biochemistry and Surgery
University of Texas Medical Branch
Galveston, Texas 77550

Lance K. Heilbrun
Department of Developmental Therapeutics
and
Section of Biometrics
Department of Biomathematics
The University of Texas System Cancer Center
M. D. Anderson Hospital and Tumor Institute
Houston, Texas 77030

Barbara Hente
Section of Cancer Biology
Mallinckrodt Institute of Radiology
Washington University School of Medicine
St. Louis, Missouri 63110

Evan M. Hersh
Section of Immunology
Department of Developmental Therapeutics
The University of Texas System Cancer Center
M. D. Anderson Hospital and Tumor Institute
Houston, Texas 77030

Patricia Heu
Departments of Pathology and Pharmacology
John A. Burns School of Medicine
University of Hawaii
Honolulu, Hawaii 96822

H. Hildebrandt
Universitäts-Krankenhaus Eppendorf
Hamburg, Federal Republic of Germany

E. O. Hoffmann
Department of Pathology
Louisiana State University
School of Medicine
New Orleans, Louisiana 70112

Yoshitsugi Hokama
Departments of Pathology and
Pharmacology
John A. Burns School of Medicine
University of Hawaii
Honolulu, Hawaii 96822

J. F. Holland
Mt. Sinai Hospital
New York, New York 10029

E. Carmack Holmes
Division of Surgical Oncology
UCLA School of Medicine
Los Angeles, California 90024

Sheldon Horowitz
Division of Immunology
Department of Pediatrics
University of Wisconsin Center for Health
Sciences
Madison, Wisconsin 53706

G. N. Hortobagyi
Medical Breast Section
Department of Medicine
University of Texas System Cancer Center
M. D. Anderson Hospital and Tumor
Institute
Houston, Texas 77030

Lucien Israel
Centre Hospitalier Universitaire
Université Paris Nord
93000 Bobigny, France

L. M. Jerry
Oncology Research Group
Faculty of Medicine
The University of Calgary
Calgary, Alberta, Canada

Alan C. Johnson
Department of Pediatrics
Immunology Section
and
Pediatric Clinical Research Center
University of California
San Francisco, California 94143

C. L. Johnston, Jr.
Medical College of Virginia
Virginia Commonwealth University
Richmond, Virginia 23298

Alan M. Kaplan
Departments of Microbiology and Surgery
MCV/VCU Cancer Center
Medical College of Virginia
Virginia Commonwealth University
Richmond, Virginia 23298

Daniel E. Kenady
Surgery Branch
National Cancer Institute
National Institutes of Health
Bethesda, Maryland 20014

E. M. Kokoschka
Department of Dermatology
University of Vienna
Vienna, Austria

P. Kokoshis
Department of Physiology
Tulane University School of Medicine
New Orleans, Louisiana 70112

Oksana Krochak
Department of Chemotherapy
Hoffmann-La Roche Inc.
Nutley, New Jersey 07110

Carol Lewinski
Department of Chemotherapy
Hoffmann-La Roche Inc.
Nutley, New Jersey 07110

Uri Lewinski
Department of Developmental
Therapeutics
The University of Texas System Cancer
Center
M. D. Anderson Hospital and Tumor
Institute
Houston, Texas 77030

M. G. Lewis

*McGill University Cancer Research Unit
and
Department of Pathology
Royal Victoria Hospital
Montreal, Quebec, Canada*

J. R. Little

*Departments of Medicine and
Microbiology and Immunology
Washington University School of Medicine
St. Louis, Missouri 63110*

T. L. K. Low

*Division of Biochemistry
University of Texas Medical Branch
Galveston, Texas 77550*

V. Malshet

*Department of Physiology
Tulane University School of Medicine
New Orleans, Louisiana 70112*

P. W. A. Mansell

*Comprehensive Cancer Center for the
State of Florida
P. O. Box 520875
Biscayne Annex
Miami, Florida 33152*

G. Marquis

*Department of Medicine
Royal Victoria Hospital
Montreal, Quebec, Canada*

Giora M. Mavligit

*Section of Immunology
Department of Developmental
Therapeutics
The University of Texas System Cancer
Center
M. D. Anderson Hospital and Tumor
Institute
Houston, Texas 77030*

Rose B. McNamee

*Department of Physiology
Tulane University School of Medicine
New Orleans, Louisiana 70112*

G. Medoff

*Departments of Medicine and
Microbiology and Immunology
Washington University School of Medicine
St. Louis, Missouri 63110*

R. Mertelsmann

*Memorial Sloan-Kettering Cancer Center
New York, New York 10021*

Phyllis L. Meyer

*Department of Chemotherapy
Hoffmann-La Roche Inc.
Nutley, New Jersey 07110*

M. Micksche

*Institute for Cancer Research
University of Vienna
Vienna, Austria*

Stephen J. Mohr

*Division of Urology
University of Colorado Medical Center
Denver, Colorado 80220*

Page S. Morahan

*Departments of Microbiology and Surgery
Medical College of Virginia
Virginia Commonwealth University
Richmond, Virginia 23298*

P. H. Naylor

*Division of Biochemistry
University of Texas Medical Branch
Galveston, Texas 77550*

Zbigniew L. Olkowski

*Laboratory of Tumor Biology and Clinical
Immunology
Winship Clinic for Neoplastic Diseases
Emory University School of Medicine
Atlanta, Georgia 30322*

K. B. Olson

*810 Oak View Drive
New Smyrna Beach, Florida 32069*

Alicia V. Palleroni

*Department of Chemotherapy
Hoffmann-La Roche Inc.
Nutley, New Jersey 07110*

Joseph D. Papamatheakis
Laboratory of RNA Tumor Viruses
National Cancer Institute
National Institutes of Health
Bethesda, Maryland 20014

Yehuda Z. Patt
Section of Immunology
Department of Developmental
  Therapeutics
The University of Texas System Cancer
  Center
M. D. Anderson Hospital and Tumor
  Institute
Houston, Texas 77030

Carlos A. Perez
Section of Cancer Biology
Mallinckrodt Institute of Radiology
Washington University School of Medicine
St. Louis, Missouri 63110

F. J. Persico
Department of Biochemical Research
Ortho Pharmaceutical Corporation
Raritan, New Jersey 08869

Marilyn C. Pike
Department of Microbiology and
  Immunology
Duke University Medical Center
Durham, North Carolina 27710

W. A. Potter
Department of Biochemical Research
Ortho Pharmaceutical Corporation
Raritan, New Jersey 08869

Claude Potvin
Surgery Branch
National Cancer Institute
National Institutes of Health
Bethesda, Maryland 20014

A. M. Prieur
Groupe de Recherches d'Immunologie et
  de Rhumatologie Pédiatriques
INSERM U 132
Hôpital des Enfants Malades
75015 Paris, France

J. W. Proctor
Division of Radiation Oncology
Clinical Radiation Therapy Research
  Center
Allegheny General Hospital
Pittsburgh, Pennsylvania 15212

Bracha Ramot
Chaim Sheba Medical Center
Tel-Aviv University
Sackler School of Medicine
Tel-Hashomer, Israel

W. Regelson
Medical College of Virginia
Virginia Commonwealth University
Richmond, Virginia 23298

J. Rodrigue
Department of Physiology
Tulane University School of Medicine
New Orleans, Louisiana 70112

Esther Rosenthal
Chaim Sheba Medical Center
Tel-Aviv University
Sackler School of Medicine
Tel-Hashomer, Israel

J. L. Rossio
Division of Biochemistry
University of Texas Medical Branch
Galveston, Texas 77550

G. Rowden
McGill University Cancer Research Unit
and
Division of Oncology
Royal Victoria Hospital
Montreal, Quebec, Canada

P. Sagaster
Department of Internal Medicine
Wilhelminenspital Vienna
Vienna, Austria

Larry A. Schafer
Section of Immunology
Department of Developmental
  Therapeutics
The University of Texas System Cancer
  Center

M. D. Anderson Hospital and Tumor
Institute
Houston, Texas 77030

Richard M. Schultz
Laboratory of RNA Tumor Viruses
National Cancer Institute
National Institutes of Health
Bethesda, Maryland 20014

R. Schwerdt
Universitäts-Krankenhaus Eppendorf
Hamburg, Federal Republic of Germany

Robert Sedlacek
Edwin L. Steele Laboratory of Radiation
Biology
Department of Radiation Medicine
Massachusetts General Hospital
Boston, Massachusetts 02114

Kenneth W. Sell
Cellular Immunology Division
Clinical and Experimental Immunology
Department
Naval Medical Research Institute
Bethesda, Maryland 20014

H. R. Shibata
Department of Surgery
Royal Victoria Hospital
Montreal, Quebec, Canada

B. I. Shnider
Georgetown University School of Medicine
Georgetown University Medical Division
D. C. General Hospital
Washington, D.C. 20003

Vlatko Silobrcic
Institute of Immunology
Zagreb, Yugoslavia

Allan H. Smith
Cellular Immunology Division
Clinical and Experimental Immunology
Department
Naval Medical Research Institute
Bethesda, Maryland 20014

Ralph Snyderman
Division of Rheumatic and Genetic
Diseases
Department of Medicine
and
Department of Microbiology and
Immunology
Duke University Medical Center
Durham, North Carolina 27710

Carleton C. Stewart
Section of Cancer Biology
Mallinckrodt Institute of Radiology
Washington University School of Medicine
St. Louis, Missouri 63110

L. Stokowski
McGill University Center Research Unit
Montreal, Quebec, Canada

Herman D. Suit
Edwin L. Steele Laboratory of Radiation
Biology
Department of Radiation Medicine
Massachusetts General Hospital
Boston, Massachusetts 02114

J. Symoens
Department of Clinical Research
Janssen Pharmaceutica
B-2340 Beerse, Belgium

C. K. Tashima
Medical Breast Section
Department of Medicine
University of Texas System Cancer Center
M. D. Anderson Hospital and Tumor
Institute
Houston, Texas 77030

D. Taylor
Department of Physiology
Tulane University School of Medicine
New Orleans, Louisiana 70112

R. Douglas Thornes
Department of Experimental Medicine
Royal College of Surgeons in Ireland
St. Laurence's Hospital
Dublin, Ireland

G. B. Thurman
Division of Biochemistry
University of Texas Medical Branch
Galveston, Texas 77550

Patrick W. Trown
Department of Chemotherapy
Hoffmann-La Roche Inc.
Nutley, New Jersey 07110

J. T. Ulrich
Division of Biochemistry
University of Texas Medical Branch
Galveston, Texas 77550

F. Valeriote
Department of Radiology
Washington University School of Medicine
St. Louis, Missouri 63110

F. Verbruggen
Clinical Research Unit
St. Bartholomeus
B-2060 Merksem (Antwerp), Belgium

H. Verhaegen
Clinical Research Unit
St. Bartholomeus
B-2060 Merksem (Antwerp), Belgium

M. L. Verhaegen-Declercq
Clinical Research Unit
St. Bartholomeus
B-2060 Merksem (Antwerp), Belgium

Diane W. Wara
Department of Pediatrics
Immunology Section
and
Pediatric Clinical Research Center
University of California
San Francisco, California 94143

Marvette L. Washington
Section of Immunology
Department of Developmental
Therapeutics
The University of Texas System Cancer
Center
M. D. Anderson Hospital and Tumor
Institute
Houston, Texas 77030

*Immune Modulation and Control of Neo-
plasia by Adjuvant Therapy,* edited by M. A.
Chirigos. Raven Press, New York, 1978.

Treatment of the Compromised Host with Levamisole, a Synthetic Immunotherapeutic Agent

J. Symoens

Department of Clinical Research, Janssen Pharmaceutica, B-2340 Beerse, Belgium

It is now generally recognized that levamisole influences host defenses by modulating cell-mediated immune mechanisms.

The body of knowledge on the drug is considerable and probably greater than any other immunomodulating agent. It is evident that this knowledge cannot be dealt with in detail in this chapter alone; therefore, I will review briefly the various immunological functions influenced by levamisole, and outline its therapeutic potential and safety. Some thoughts will be developed concerning its possible mode of action.[1]

Studies on isolated phagocytes and lymphocytes show that levamisole influences virtually all cell functions involved in cell-mediated immune responses (Table 1). It restores such functions in compromised hosts but does not stimulate immune responses above the normal physiological level. It does not seem to influence B lymphocytes directly.

In patients or experimental animals with hypofunctional cells, levamisole restores the movement of polymorphonuclear neutrophils or mononuclear phagocytes to the target area and promotes phagocytosis and intracellular killing. Where lymphocytes are concerned, levamisole restores E-rosette formation and reduces excessive B- or null cell numbers. It boosts nucleic acid or protein synthesis by T cells in response to antigenic stimulation, increases antigen-induced lymphokine production, and stimulates suppressor activity, cytotoxicity, lysosomal activity, and plaque cell formation.

Levamisole does not consistently influence antibody production (Table 2). Effects, when observed, are probably secondary to the drug's effects on macrophages or T cells. Levamisole improves delayed skin hypersensitivity, graft-versus-host reaction, blood clearance of colloidal particles, and macrophage migration in skin wounds, all models in which responsiveness depends on intact T cell or macrophage function.

In contrast, levamisole is inactive in models designed to measure immune

---

[1] References of all statements made in this chapter can be found in a recent and extensive review by Symoens and Rosenthal (1).

TABLE 1. *Effect of levamisole on the function of isolated phagocytes and lymphocytes from compromised hosts*

Phagocytes	Lymphocytes
Random migration ↗	E-rosette formation ↗
Chemotaxis ↗	Nucleic acid and protein synthesis ↗
Migration inhibition ↗	Lymphokine production ↗
Phagocytosis ↗	Suppressor activity ↗
Intracellular killing ↗	Killer activity ↗
Cytotoxicity ↗	Lysosomal activity ↗
	Plaque cell formation (Jerne) ↗

↗, increased.

stimulation, such as skin graft rejection time or the induction of experimental allergic encephalomyelitis and adjuvant arthritis in rats.

Levamisole is also devoid of antiinflammatory activity. It does not reduce the primary lesions of adjuvant arthritis or carrageenan-induced pleurisy.

In experimental animals (Table 3), levamisole causes stabilization of tumor remission and increases the protective effect of certain bacterial, protozoal, or tumor vaccines that do not depend on antibodies for protection. Only animals with a weak response to the vaccine appear to benefit. Levamisole also reduces the frequency, duration, and intensity of chronic and recurrent infections caused by bacteria, viruses, protozoa, and fungi. It does not prevent primary invasion by pathogens but restores host defenses so that the course of disease is shortened.

Levamisole has a favorable effect on the course of spontaneous immune deficiency diseases in animals. It tempers the evolution of autoimmune nephritis in NZB/NZW mice and of aleutian disease in mink.

In certain animal species, the *in vivo* effect of levamisole seems to be due to a serum factor, which after treatment appears in responder animals only. This factor mimics the effects of levamisole when injected into untreated animals or into treated nonresponders. The factor restores the sensitivity to azathioprine of rosette-forming splenocytes from thymectomized mice, increases plaque-forming cell production and enhances carbon particle clearance, causes a reduction of tumor load and stabilization of tumor remission, and converts

TABLE 2. In vivo *studies of the effect of levamisole on the immune response*

No effect on humoral immunity	No stimulation above normal level
Antibody production 0	Skin graft rejection 0
	Experimental allergic encephalomyelitis (↗)
Potentiation of cell-mediated immunity	Adjuvant arthritis, secondary response (↗)
Delayed skin hypersensitivity ↗	
Graft-versus-host reaction ↗	No antiinflammatory effect
Blood clearance of colloidal particles ↗	Adjuvant arthritis, primary response 0
Macrophage migration in SC coverslips ↗	Carrageenan-induced pleurisy 0

↗, increased; (↗), increased in the presence of Freund's adjuvant only; 0, not influenced.

TABLE 3. *Animal studies of the effect of levamisole on host resistance*

Primary invasion by infectious agents or tumoral cells	0
Secondary invasion by infectious agents or tumoral cells	
Potentiation of vaccination	↗
Stabilization of tumor remission	↗
NZB/NZW nephritis in mice	↙
Aleutian disease in mink	↙

↗, improved; ↙, tempered; 0, not influenced.

nonresponder mice into responders. Such a factor, contributing to enhanced *in vitro* lymphocyte stimulation, has also been demonstrated in human serum after levamisole treatment.

Levamisole is being tested in most human diseases with suspected imbalance of immune homeostasis, including chronic and recurrent infections, primary immune deficiency syndromes, allergic disorders, and rheumatic, neurological, gastrointestinal, and neoplastic diseases.

So far, evidence of efficacy from controlled trials has been obtained in rheumatoid arthritis, in several recurrent or chronic infections, and in certain malignant diseases (Table 4). Since W. K. Amery *(this volume)* deals with malignant diseases, I will limit the discussion to nononcological indications.

In patients with rheumatoid arthritis, the chronic inflammatory process is tempered. Concomitant improvement of blood sedimentation rate and clinical parameters such as pain, morning stiffness, joint tenderness, and joint size was observed in three double-blind, placebo-controlled studies involving 110 patients. Approximately two-thirds of the patients responded to treatment, sometimes with dramatic improvement.

In recurrent aphthous ulceration, approximately two-thirds of the patients also responded to levamisole. They had prolonged disease-free intervals and the duration and severity of outbreaks were reduced.

A majority of patients with tuberculoid and lepromatous leprosy treated with levamisole improved rapidly by clinical, histological, and bacteriological criteria. Patients showing active lesions of intertrigo inguinalis were clinically cured after 3 months of levamisole monotherapy. Placebo-treated patients did not improve.

TABLE 4. *Human diseases for which efficacy of levamisole was shown in controlled studies*

Rheumatoid arthritis
Recurrent aphthous ulceration
Leprosy
Intertrigo
Recurrent upper respiratory tract infections in children
Postviral anergy: influenza and measles

TABLE 5. *Effect of levamisole on recurrent upper respiratory tract infections in children*

Score as compared with previous winter	Percentage of patients	
	Levamisole group	Placebo group
Markedly better	54	7
Better	35	36
No change	11	50
Worse	0	7

From ref. 2.

In children with recurrent upper respiratory tract infections (winter illness), levamisole was found to reduce considerably the number, duration, and severity of the infections, as compared to placebo-treated patients (Table 5).

Levamisole seems to abolish the anergy that usually follows viral infections like influenza or measles and that is characterized clinically by a slow recovery or by bacterial superinfections. Levamisole counteracted the depression of chemotaxis produced by incubating normal monocytes with influenza *in vitro*. In volunteers, it prevented the decreased delayed skin hypersensitivity to tuberculin induced by the virus. In patients with acute influenza, it significantly shortened the recovery period, as evidenced by the more rapid disappearance of bronchial symptoms and muscular pain, and by the ability of the levamisole-treated patients to return to work sooner than the placebo-treated patients (Table 6).

TABLE 6. *Effect of levamisole on recovery from influenza infection*

	No. of patients					
	1 week		2 weeks		3 weeks	
	Leva	Plac	Leva	Plac	Leva	Plac
Recovered	10	0	23	8	27	16
Improved	9	4	2	8	0	6
Not improved	7	16	2	5	0	0

	Statistical analysis (X^2)		
	1 week	2 weeks	3 weeks
Recovery	0.001	0.003	0.014
Coughing	0.0008	0.005	NS
Mucus	0.02	0.008	NS
Myalgia	0.002	NS	NS
Asthenia	NS	NS	NS
Appetence	NS	NS	NS

From ref. 3.

TABLE 7. *Effect of levamisole on frequency of complications of measles in children*

	No. of patients		
	Without complications	With complications	Dead
Levamisole	19	2	1
Control	7	8	3

From ref. 4.

Similar effects were observed in African children with measles (Table 7). The frequency of complications, such as pneumonia or meningitis, was significantly less in children who received levamisole than in those who received placebo.

Of the many other possible indications for which levamisole was tested, some are particularly promising (Table 8).

In recurrent herpes infections, levamisole reduced the duration and the severity of outbreaks and prolonged the disease-free intervals.

Patients with chronic pyogenic and mycotic skin infections or with acne conglobata had their lesions cleared during levamisole treatment.

In children with primary immune deficiency syndromes or with selective immune deficits, levamisole reduced the incidence and severity of skin and respiratory tract infections.

In patients with severe pulmonary insufficiency due to chronic bronchiectasis or asthma and *Pseudomonas* superinfection, pulmonary function markedly improved during levamisole treatment and *Pseudomonas* disappeared from the sputum.

Patients with chronic brucellosis, mononucleosis, toxoplasmosis, and paracoccidioidomycosis improved or recovered clinically and had their anergy restored after levamisole treatment.

TABLE 8. *Evidence of efficacy of levamisole in various diseases in open pilot studies*

Chronic and recurrent infections
    Recurrent herpes labialis, genitalis, and corneae
    Pyogenic and mycotic skin infections, acne conglobata
    Pulmonary superinfections *(Pseudomonas)*
    Chronic brucellosis, chronic toxoplasmosis
    Primary immune deficiency diseases
Other chronic diseases
    Reiter's disease
    Systemic lupus erythematosus
    Ankylosing spondylitis
    Crohns' disease

Finally, some very encouraging results have been obtained in patients with Reiter's syndrome, systemic lupus erythematosus, ankylosing spondylitis, and Crohns' disease.

Immunological deficiency was recognized in many patients who responded favorably to levamisole treatment. Some patients had a reduced cellular immune responsiveness and an increased B cell activity. Some were anergic to several antigens; others had a reduced response to the invading antigen only. Sometimes, one single immunological parameter was disturbed, all others being within normal range.

During levamisole treatment, T cell and phagocyte functions were very often restored, and B cell hyperactivity was reduced. As a rule, however, there was no good correlation between immunological and therapeutic effects. None of the variables of cellular immunity represents a reliable means of predicting therapeutic response to levamisole treatment.

The clinical effects of levamisole cannot be explained by a direct effect on invading organisms or cells or by an antiinflammatory effect of the drug. Many of the responding diseases are characterized by a reduced cellular immune responsiveness, antigenic persistence, chronic inflammation, and B cell hyperactivity (Fig. 1). It is likely that levamisole, by improving cellular immune functions such as chemotaxis, migration inhibition, phagocytosis, cytotoxicity, T suppressor activity, etc., stimulates early inflammatory events, removes the persisting antigen, and controls B cell hyperactivity. This would explain why exacerbations sometimes occur during the first 2 months of treatment and why many of the diseases in which levamisole is effective are currently being treated with corticosteroids and antiinflammatory and immunosuppressive drugs. These drugs reduce the chronic inflammation but they do not seem to influence the basic course of the disease. An immediate flare-up is usually seen after cessation of therapy. In contrast, the prolonged effect that is generally seen after cessation of levamisole therapy indicates that levamisole acts on the disease process itself.

So far, experience with approximately 3,000 patients has been reported (1). Half of the patients have been treated for more than 3 months. Treatment has been predominantly intermittent, that is, on 2 to 4 days every week or every other week. The daily dose was approximately 2.5 mg/kg.

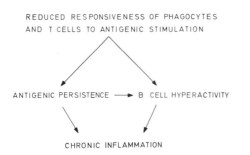

REDUCED RESPONSIVENESS OF PHAGOCYTES
AND T CELLS TO ANTIGENIC STIMULATION

ANTIGENIC PERSISTENCE ⟶ B CELL HYPERACTIVITY

CHRONIC INFLAMMATION

FIG. 1. Possible pathogenesis of chronic inflammatory diseases.

TABLE 9. *Side effects of levamisole*[a]

	No. of patients	No. stopped
Gastrointestinal complaints	<5%	15
CNS stimulation	<5%	0
Flu-like syndrome[b]	<5%	18
Skin rash	64 (33 in RA[c])	17
Transient granulocytopenia	23 (16 in RA)	23
Transient thrombocytopenia	1	1

[a]3,046 patients treated and reported until November 1976.
[b]Fatigue, headache, dizziness, excessive perspiration, shivering and chills, fever, myalgia, and arthralgia.
[c]RA, rheumatoid arthritis.
From ref. 1.

Significant adverse reactions were transient granulocytopenia and allergic skin reactions (Table 9). Other side effects, such as nausea, abdominal pain, anorexia, nervousness, insomnia, sensory stimulation, or a flu-like syndrome, were generally mild and rarely required interruption of drug intake. Skin rash could be severe and necessitate arrest of treatment. The majority of rashes, however, were mild and also occurred with placebo.

Of 23 cases with transient granulocytopenia reported so far, 16 occurred in patients with rheumatoid arthritis, although less than 10% of all patients treated with levamisole had rheumatic disease. The granulocytopenia is most probably caused by a peripheral immunological mechanism, without bone marrow involvement. Granulocyte antibodies causing agglutination in the presence of levamisole have been demonstrated in the serum of three patients, and three patients relapsed when challenged with levamisole. Bone marrow contained only a few cells during granulocytopenia and contained predominantly promyelocytes during recovery.

Twenty of the 23 patients with granulocytopenia recovered spontaneously on discontinuation of treatment. Three children, who had debilitating disease, died. These children had received high doses of corticosteroids for long periods of time, and it is likely that reduced host defenses resulting from corticosteroid treatment were responsible for the rapid and fatal evolution in these children.

The variety of cells and the multitude of functions that are affected make it likely that levamisole influences a basic mechanism common to these cells. The major functions of the immune system respond to manipulations of intracellular concentrations of the cyclic nucleotides cyclic AMP and cyclic GMP (Table 10). Drugs that elevate intracellular levels of cyclic GMP in leukocytes, such as cholinergic agents, exert a general stimulatory action on the effector functions of these cells. Drugs that elevate intracellular levels of cyclic AMP, such as the β-adrenergic agents histamine and theophylline, have the opposite effect and decrease effector leukocyte functions. These same agents however induce T and B cell differentiation.

Levamisole increases intracellular levels of cyclic GMP in peripheral leukocytes and mimics the effects of agents that elevate cyclic GMP levels in these

TABLE 10. *Effects of cyclic nucleotide manipulations on leukocyte functions*

	cyclic GMP inducers	cyclic AMP inducers	Levamisole
Effector functions			
E-rosette formation	↗	↙	↗
Lymphocyte proliferation	↗	↙	↗
Plaque cell formation	↗	↙	↗
Cytotoxicity	↗	↙	↗
Phagocyte motility	↗	↙	↗
Chemotaxis	↗	↙	↗
Migration inhibition	↗	↙	↗
Phagocytosis	↗	↙	↗
Lysosomal enzyme release	↗	↙	↗
Intracellular killing	↗	↙	↗
T and B cell differentiation			
Appearance of differentiation antigens		↗	↗ (T)
Acquisition of functional activity		↗	↗ (T)

↗, increased; ↙, reduced.

cells. It reverses the inhibitory effects of cyclic AMP-inducing agents such as histamine, dibutyryl cyclic AMP, and theophylline in peripheral leukocytes.

On the other hand, levamisole induces T cell differentiation: Lymphocytes from levamisole-treated thymectomized mice were rendered sensitive to azathioprine, and nude mice spleen cells acquired characteristic thymic differentiation antigens after levamisole treatment.

Levamisole thus seems to exert a dual effect, inducing T cell differentiation—an apparently central, cyclic AMP-mediated process—and increasing effector leukocyte function—a cyclic GMP-mediated process.

A similar dual mechanism has been suggested for thymopoietin, a potent, selective T cell differentiator that also seems to modulate peripheral leukocyte functions (Fig. 2).

It is possible that levamisole modulates leukocyte functions by virtue of its effect on cyclic nucleotide accumulation. It may influence cyclic nucleotide production directly or by interaction with leukocyte receptors for autonomic neurohormones or thymic hormone. Due to the striking similarity between the effects of levamisole and thymic hormone, the latter effect seems most probable. If this is true, levamisole may be called a thymomimetic compound.

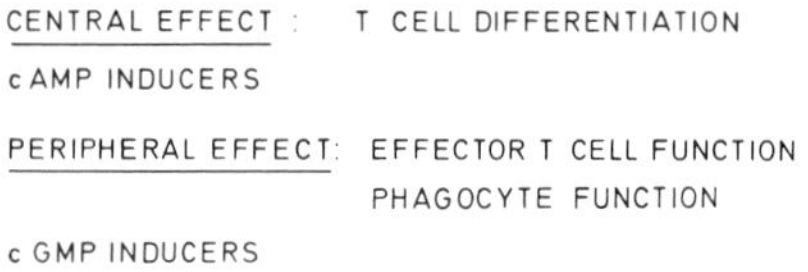

CENTRAL EFFECT :   T CELL DIFFERENTIATION

c AMP INDUCERS

PERIPHERAL EFFECT: EFFECTOR T CELL FUNCTION
                    PHAGOCYTE FUNCTION

c GMP INDUCERS

FIG. 2. Possible dual effect of levamisole and thymopoietin.

In conclusion, it seems that levamisole is the first member of a new series of simple chemical agents that mimic hormonal regulation of the immune system. Further experimental work with levamisole should aim at its basic biological activities to allow a better understanding of its mode of action and should refrain from pure descriptive observations. Future clinical work with this drug should essentially involve controlled studies to prove or disprove efficacy in each of its potential indications.

Levamisole is not the "all-around drug" that should be tested in any clinical condition. It might, however, represent the first agent to be of great benefit in several, yet poorly controlled, diseases by restoring a common basic deficiency.

REFERENCES

1. Symoens, J., and Rosenthal, M. (1977): A review. Levamisole in the modulation of the immune response: The current experimental and clinical state. *J. Reticuloendothel. Soc.,* 21:175.
2. Van Eygen, M., Znamensky, P. Y., Heck, E., and Raymaekers, I. (1976): Levamisole in prevention of recurrent upper-respiratory-tract infections in children. *Lancet,* 1:382.
3. Krömer, K. (March 1977): Doppelblindstudie Levamisole gegen Placebo bei 50 Patienten mit sogenannten grippalen Infekten *(unpublished data).*
4. Barbaix, E. (July 1976): Effectiveness of levamisole in preventing complications of measles in high-risk infants and children. Unpublished Clinical Research Report on Levamisole, No. 53.

Immune Modulation and Control of Neoplasia by Adjuvant Therapy, edited by M. A. Chirigos. Raven Press, New York, 1978.

Effect of Levamisole in Combination with Radiotherapy in Modifying the Growth of Murine Tumors of Differing Immunogenicity

Carleton C. Stewart, Carlos A. Perez, and Barbara Hente

Section of Cancer Biology, Mallinckrodt Institute of Radiology, Washington University School of Medicine, St. Louis, Missouri 63110

The antihelminthic agent levamisole has recently been shown to have some efficacy in the treatment of both laboratory animal (3,4,8,11,14) and human neoplasias (13). Its mode of action is thought to be mediated by a general stimulation of the host defense mechanism. Several studies have shown that animals treated with the agent have increased resistance to infection (7), enhanced cell-mediated (1,2,5,6,17,19,21,22) and antibody-mediated immunity (9,12), and augmented reticuloendothelial function (18,20).

In this study, we investigated the efficacy of levamisole in combination with local single-dose radiotherapy in the treatment of three murine tumors that vary in their ability to elicit a host defense. The dose (100 mg/m^2) and administration schedule of levamisole were chosen to approximate its use in the treatment of human cancer.

MATERIAL AND METHODS

Tumors

Three tumor cell systems have been selected for this study on the basis of their relative abilities to produce a measurable host response; the criteria used are summarized in Table 1. The tumors chosen were the EMT6 tumor, which is syngeneic with BALB/cK mice, and the Gardner 6C$_3$HED lymphosarcoma and the KHT fibrosarcoma, both of which are syngeneic with C$_3$H/He mice.

Tumor Cell Preparation

The tumors were maintained by biweekly subcutaneous injection of 10^6 viable cells in 0.1 ml into the flank of mice syngeneic with the tumor. Mice used for the experiments were similarly injected.

To prepare the tumor cell suspensions, tumors were dissected from the flanks of mice, minced in medium [α-minimum essential medium (α-MEM), 20%

TABLE 1. *Comparison of host antitumor reactivity*

Defense parameter	Tumor		
	EMT6	6C$_3$HED	KHT
Immunized with killed cells	Yes	No	No
Concomitant immunity	Yes	Yes	No
Cured mice resist challenge	Yes	Yes	No
Tumor takes in substrains[a]	No	Yes	Yes
Lymphocyte and macrophage infiltration	Yes	Yes	Yes
TD$_{50}$ (number of viable cells)	10^2–10^3	10^1–10^2	10^1–10^2
In vitro plating efficiency[b]	20–40%	0%	<10%

[a] Same mouse strain but from a breeding colony different from the one of origin.

[b] Number of tumor colonies/100 cells resulting from a direct explant of recovered viable tumor cells.

fetal calf serum], and, except for the EMT6, passed through a fine (120-mesh) stainless steel screen. The EMT6 tumor was trypsinized in 10 ml 0.05% trypsin for 1 hr before passage through the screen. Cell suspensions were centrifuged at 200 Xg for 10 min, counted, and adjusted to 10^7 viable cells per ml.

Local Irradiation

The tumor-bearing flank was locally irradiated when the tumors became palpable (2 to 4 mm in diameter). Animals were shielded with a special lead block as previously described (10) to limit the whole body exposure to 1 to 2% of the tumor dose. Irradiation was given with 220 kvp X-rays, 15 ma, 2mm copper half value layer, at approximately 400 rads per minute.

Levamisole

The drug was kindly supplied from Janssen Pharmaceutical Co., New Brunswick, N.J. The powder was dissolved in saline at a concentration of 600 μg/ml.

RESULTS

Growth of Tumors

To determine the growth kinetics, groups of 20 mice were injected with 0.1 ml serial 10-fold dilutions ranging from 10^7 to 10^2 tumor cells into the flank. The time required for palpable tumors to develop in 50% of mice is shown in Fig. 1. The ordinate intercept gives an estimate of the number of tumor cells required for the mass to be palpable, while the slope gives an estimate of the tumor-doubling time; these data are shown in the figure inset. Once the tumor

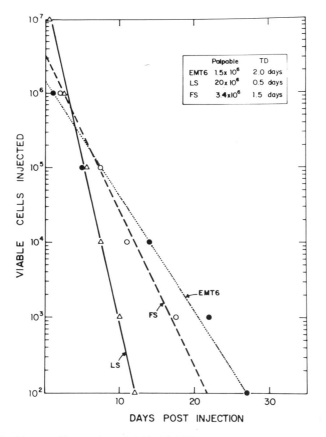

	Palpable	TD
EMT6	1.5×10^6	2.0 days
LS	20×10^6	0.5 days
FS	3.4×10^6	1.5 days

FIG. 1 Growth of tumors. The number of viable 6C₃HED lymphosarcoma (△, LS), KHT fibrosar-coma (○, FS), or EMT6 (●) tumor cells injected is plotted as a function of the time 50% of mice had a palpable tumor. The inset shows the number of tumor cells required for a tumor to be palpable (col 1) and the tumor-doubling (TD) time (col 2).

is palpable, 50% of untreated animals are dead 18 days later for the lymphosar-coma, 24 days later for the KHT, and 40 days later for the EMT6.

Tumor Curability

In these experiments, a dose of radiation was selected to produce a small percentage of tumor-free mice so that the effect of levamisole could be clearly demonstrated. Thus, groups of 20 mice were injected with 10^6 viable tumor cells and locally irradiated with various single doses of 220 kvp radiation when their tumors were palpable. The results are shown in Fig. 2. Doses of 6,000 rads and above cured all mice having the EMT6 tumor and 6C₃HED lymphosar-coma, but only 80 to 85% of mice having the KHT fibrosarcoma could be cured. Whereas 3,000 rads produced no complete regressions of the KHT fibro-

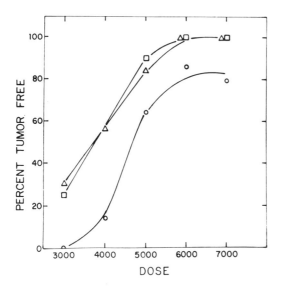

FIG. 2. Radiation dose to cure mouse tumors. The percent of tumor-free mice is plotted as a function of the total local dose delivered to the tumor volume. The time after irradiation that mice were evaluated to be tumor free for the data plotted was 70 days for the EMT6 (□), 45 days for the 6C₃HED (△), and 70 days for the KHT (o).

sarcoma, it caused cures in about 30% of mice bearing the EMT6 and the 6C₃HED lymphosarcoma and was chosen for these experiments in order to maintain uniformity in the biological effect on normal host function (e.g. immunosuppression).

Effect of Levamisole in Combination with Radiotherapy

The experimental schema for these studies is shown in Fig. 3. From the human levamisole dose of 100 mg/m² (150 mg/day maximum) used by the Southeastern Cancer Study Group, the equivalent dose for mice was calculated to be 600 µg/mouse, assuming the standard man to be 1.5 m² at 70 kg and the standard 8-week-old mouse to be 20 to 25 g, and using a surface area conversion from man to mouse of 13 (F. Valeriote, *personal communication*). Mice were injected with the appropriate tumors and palpated daily until all had palpable tumors. The tumors were then locally irradiated to 3,000 rads

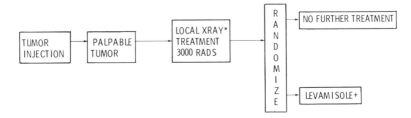

FIG. 3. Levamisole combined with radio therapy—treatment schema. *, A control group received no X-ray treatment or levamisole injection; †, i.p. injections of 600 µg each were given twice per week for eight injections. The first injection was 4 hr following radiation.

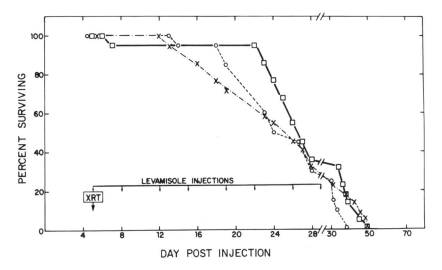

FIG. 4. Survival of mice bearing the KHT fibrosarcoma treated with levamisole in combination with radiation. The time of irradiation (XRT) and levamisole injection are shown by the appropriate arrows. Mice received 3,000 rads to the tumor-bearing flank. ○, control; X, XRT alone; □, XRT + levamisole.

and randomized to receive either no further treatment or two intraperitoneal injections of 600 μg levamisole twice per week for a total of eight injections. The first injection was given approximately 4 hr after completion of the radiation treatments. A third group of tumor-bearing animals received no therapy and served as controls. Tumors in these control animals never regressed.

For the KHT fibrosarcoma a total of 22 mice in each group was evaluated in two separate experiments. In both groups of irradiated animals, tumor growth was retarded, and this retardation was qualitatively greater in the group receiving levamisole; however, no tumors ever completely regressed. As shown in Fig. 4, all animals were dead from their disease by day 50. However, those animals treated with radiation and levamisole began to die later than those treated with radiation alone. Even the untreated control animals had a longer initial survival than did those given radiation alone.

For the 6C₃HED lymphosarcoma, a total of 24 mice in each group was evaluated in two separate experiments; the results are shown in Fig. 5. In Fig. 5A, the percentage of mice with palpable tumors is plotted as a function of time. Unlike the KHT fibrosarcoma, the 6C₃HED lymphosarcoma often regresses shortly after radiation; by day 6 nearly all animals had no palpable tumors. These tumors then recurred over the next 2 weeks. Animals treated with radiation alone had a recurrence rate of 70% with no further recurrences observed after day 18. Levamisole showed no further effect in changing the course of this tumor.

In Fig. 5B, the survival of animals bearing the lymphosarcoma is shown.

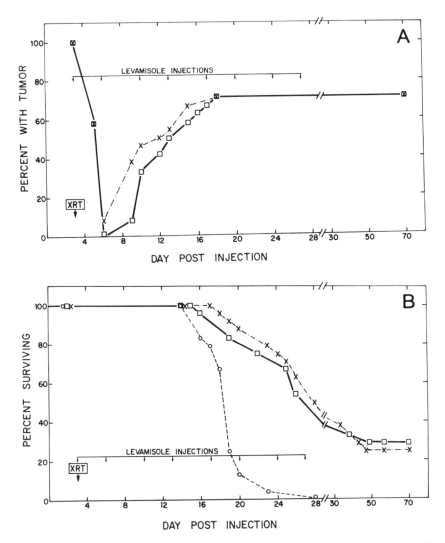

FIG. 5. Treatment of mice bearing the 6C$_3$HED lymphosarcoma with levamisole in combination with radiation. The time of irradiation (XRT) and levamisole injection are shown by the appropriate arrows. Mice received 3,000 rads to the tumor-bearing flank. A: Mice bearing palpable tumors. B: Mouse survival. ○, Control; X, XRT alone; □, XRT + levamisole.

Untreated control mice were all dead by 28 days. Radiation prolonged the life of all animals relative to the untreated controls and resulted in a long-term survival in 27% of mice. Treatment with levamisole combined with radiation had no effect on survival.

Levamisole was most effective when used on the EMT6 tumor in combination with radiation (Fig. 6). A total of 70 mice in each group was evaluated in three separate experiments. Control animals receiving no treatment all developed

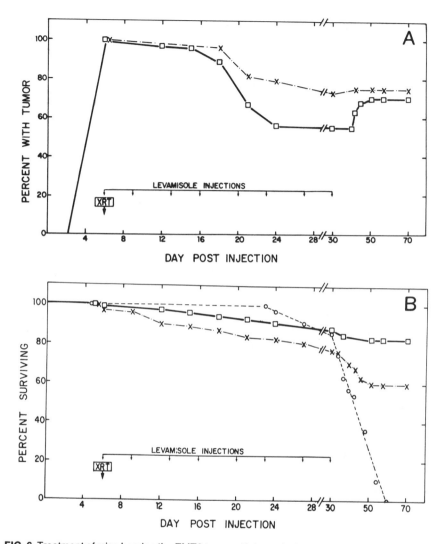

FIG. 6. Treatment of mice bearing the EMT6 tumor with levamisole in combination with radiation. The time of irradiation (XRT) and levamisole injection are shown by the appropriate arrows. A: Mice bearing palpable tumors. B: Mouse survival. o, Control; X, XRT alone; □, XRT + levamisole.

tumors that never regressed. The percentage of mice with palpable tumors is shown as a function of time in Fig. 6A. By day 30, both treatment groups reached a nadir in the percentage of mice tumor bearing. At this time, there was a significant difference between the group receiving both levamisole and radiation and that group receiving radiation alone (Table 2). The time course of regressions was also slightly enhanced in the group treated with levamisole. However, the tumor-free status in the levamisole-treated group was not perma-

TABLE 2. *Relative proportion of mice with no evidence of tumor on day 30 for three different experiments using the EMT6 tumor*

Experiment no.	Radiation[a]	Radiation plus levamisole
1	4/10 (40%)	7/10 (70%)
2	4/30 (13%)	10/30 (33%)
3	11/30 (36%)	17/30 (56%)
Total	19/70 (27%)	34/70 (48%)

[a]3,000 rads to the tumor-bearing flank.

nent, and by day 42 tumors began to recur. By day 50 this recurrence rate approached the failure rate of the radiation alone group.

The survival of mice bearing the EMT6 tumor is shown in Fig. 6B. By day 60, all untreated mice were dead, whereas 83% of mice treated with both radiation and levamisole were still surviving. At this time only 60% of mice treated with radiation alone were still surviving. The prolonged life-span for the levamisole-treated mice is a reflection of the greater fraction whose tumors initially regressed but later recurred.

Figure 6 shows the combined results from three separate experiments. As an indication of the reproducibility among these experiments, Table 2 gives the percentages of tumor-free mice on day 30. Note that a 20 to 30% difference is maintained between the group treated with both radiation and levamisole and the group treated with radiation alone, regardless of the absolute proportion of tumor-free mice. Thus, in experiment 1 where 40% of mice were tumor free on day 30 in the radiation alone group, 70% were tumor free in the levamisole group; in experiment 2 where only 13% were tumor free in the radiation alone group, 33% were tumor free in the levamisole group; and in experiment 3 36% and 56% were tumor free in the two respective groups.

DISCUSSION

The design of these experiments and the tumor models employed have several features relevant to human cancer. First, an attempt has been made to use a dose and administration schedule comparable to that used for human treatment. Second, the tumors employed have widely varying abilities to elicit host defense (Table 1). Third, by using different tumors, the general efficacy of the agent can be determined. In these experiments, however, mice were treated with single rather than fractionated doses of radiation, and levamisole was administered intraperitoneally rather than orally; these procedures deviate from human treatment protocols. Experiments are in progress to determine the significance of these differences.

The survival of animals bearing the KHT fibrosarcoma is poorest among those given radiation alone during the first 3 weeks (Fig. 4). The addition of levamisole considerably improved survival even though all tumors continued to progress. A similar profile, but to a much lesser extent, was observed in animals bearing the EMT6 tumor (Fig. 6B) but not in those with the lymphosarcoma (Fig. 5B). One possible explanation of this observation is that the local radiation has a detrimental effect including the antitumor host defense, resulting in early deaths of some animals (not necessarily due directly to the tumor). We have previously shown that the host defense begins during the first week after tumor cell inoculation (16), which is the time these animals were locally irradiated. This is likely to be the time when the immunosuppressive effects of radiation are at their maximum because immunity in its developmental stage is much more sensitive to radiation than established immunity (15). Levamisole might act to promote a more rapid recovery (i.e., it has a restorative effect) from the detrimental effects of radiation; in the case of animals bearing the KHT fibrosarcoma, this results in significantly longer survival than either the untreated control animals or those receiving radiation alone. This possibility is presently being investigated using these model tumor systems in a protocol in which levamisole is given before, during, or after local fractionated irradiation.

One reason levamisole was without effect on animals bearing the KHT fibrosarcoma could be that the radiation dose employed was too low to sufficiently reduce the tumor cell burden to a level where levamisole might have been effective. Further studies are in progress using higher doses of local irradiation.

When mice bearing the EMT6 tumor were treated with both radiation and levamisole, there was a significantly greater fraction of mice whose tumor initially regressed. The tumor-free interval for these mice lasted from day 24 to day 40 at which time tumors recurred over the next week. By day 50, there was no difference between those receiving radiation alone or in combination with levamisole. This suggests that the duration of the tumor-free interval may be related to the length of time levamisole is injected; had the injection schedule for levamisole been prolonged past day 27, these later recurrences might have been delayed even longer or even prevented. Thus, the ability to prolong the disease-free interval or to produce cures may result from the duration of host defense stimulation, from the total cumulative dose of adjuvant injected, or both. This possibility is presently being studied, since it is very important to know how long immune adjuvant therapy ought to be given.

Levamisole appears to be capable of enhancing the host defense by only a fixed amount that is dependent on the tumor burden left after radiation (Table 2). These data would support the concept that the host defense is capable of eliminating a finite number of tumor cells. As has been previously proposed (16), different animals display different degrees of immunoreactivity, i.e., some are able to eliminate greater tumor cell burdens than others. Levamisole might act to improve immunoreactivity, allowing a greater proportion of the lower immunoreactive animals to cope effectively with a greater tumor cell burden.

These results suggest that not all tumors are responsive to levamisole. Whether this is related to the ability of the animal to develop a response to the tumor or to the degree to which the response is developed still needs to be determined. There is, however, no prior reason to believe an immunoadjuvant shows efficacy against every tumor system. The results do suggest, however, that levamisole in combination with radiation either mobilizes or restores the host defense to a level capable of coping with a relatively higher cell burden than radiation alone.

We believe these murine models more closely resemble human studies and can be exploited to study dose and time schedules of immunotherapy in combination with other therapeutic modalities. In addition, the murine models employed will be useful in studying basic factors involved in the host defense, such as the effect of tumor cell burden, the degree of macrophage-lymphocyte infiltration into the tumor, and the cytotoxic efficiencies of these two cell types.

SUMMARY

In this study three murine tumors varying in their ability to elicit a host response were used to study the efficacy of levamisole combined with X-ray therapy. The KHT fibrosarcoma induces a negligible host defense, the $6C_3HED$ lymphosarcoma induces a moderate defense, and the EMT6 tumor induces the greatest defense. The dose of levamisole used in these studies was 600 μg per injection; two injections were given per week for a total of eight injections. This regimen is approximately similar to that used in humans. Tumors were treated with a local tumor dose of 3,000 rads.

Levamisole in combination with local tumor radiation caused a significantly greater tumor regression rate in animals bearing the EMT6 tumor; a nadir was reached 18 days after radiation with 48% of the experimental animals free of tumor. However, these regressions were not all permanent, and tumors began to recur 2 weeks after levamisole treatment (day 42) was terminated; by day 50 these recurrences had reduced the levamisole cure rate to the same level (27%) as that achieved with radiation alone.

At the radiation dose employed, no regressions occurred when the least immunogeneic tumor, the KHT fibrosarcoma, was treated either with radiation alone or in combination with levamisole. However, levamisole significantly improved the survival of some tumor-bearing mice. Levamisole treatment showed no effect on animals bearing the mildly immunogeneic $6C_3HED$ lymphosarcoma.

These results suggest that levamisole improves both the disease-free interval and survival of mice harboring some, but not all, tumor types. The degree of levamisole's effectiveness may be related to the tumor cell burden, the host's ability to respond to the tumor, and the agent's ability to enhance the host defense. This last ability appears to be dependent on the presence of the adjuvant in the host, and thus, the length of time of administration is important. These studies have shown that levamisole in combination with radiotherapy to reduce the tumor mass may prove effective for the treatment of some types of human cancer.

ACKNOWLEDGMENT

This investigation was supported by grant no. 5P01CA13053–05, awarded by the National Cancer Institute, DHEW.

REFERENCES

1. Binaminov, M., and Ramot, B. (1975): Letter: *In vitro* restoration by levamisole of thymus-derived lymphocyte function in Hodgkin's disease. *Lancet,* 1:464–465.
2. Chan, S. H., and Simons, M. J. (1975): Letter: Levamisole and lymphocyte responsiveness. *Lancet,* 1:1246–1247.
3. Chirigos, M. A., Fuhrman, F., and Pryor, J. (1975): Prolongation of chemotherapeutically induced remission of a syngeneic murine leukemia by 1–2,3,4,6–tetrahydro-6-phenylimidazo 2,1-beta thiazole hydrochloride. *Cancer Res.,* 35:927–931.
4. Chirigos, M. A., Pearson, J. W., and Pryor, J. (1973): Augmentation of chemotherapeutically induced remission of a murine leukemia by a chemical immunoadjuvant. *Cancer Res.,* 33:2615–2618.
5. Churchill, W. H., and David, J. R. (1973): Levamisole and cell mediated immunity. *N. Engl. J. Med.,* 289:375–376.
6. Copeland, D., Stewart, T., and Harris, J. (1974): Effect of levamisole (NSC-177023) on *in vitro* human lymphocyte transformation. *Cancer Chemother. Rep.,* 58:167–170.
2. Fischer, G. W., Pedgore, J. F., Bass, J. W., Kelley, J. L., and Kobayaski, G. Y. (1975): Enhanced host defense mechanisms with levamisole in suckling rats. *J. Infect. Dis.,* 132:578–581.
8. Johnson, K. K., Houchens, D. P., Gaston, M. R., and Goldin, A. (1975): Effects of levamisole (NSC-177023) and tetramisole (NSC-1020631) in experimental tumor systems. *Cancer Chemother. Rep.,* 59:697–705.
9. Lods, J. C., Dujardin, P., and Halpern, G. (1975): Action of levamisole on antibody protection after vaccination with anti-typhoid and para-typoid A and B. *Ann. Allergy,* 34:210–212.
10. Perez, C. A., Stewart, C. C., Palmer-Hanes, L. A., and Powers, W. E. (1973): Role of the regional lymph nodes in the cure of a murine lymphosarcoma. *Cancer,* 32:562–572.
11. Perk, K., Chirigos, M. A., Fuhrman, F., and Pettigrew, H. (1975): Some aspects of host response to levamisole after chemotherapy in a murine leukemia. *J. Natl. Cancer Inst.,* 54:253–256.
12. Renoux, G., and Renoux, M. (1974): Modulation of immune reactivity by phenylimidothiazole salts in mice immunized by sheep red blood cells. *J. Immunol.,* 113:779–790.
13. Rojas, A. F., Feierstein, J. N., Nickiewicz, E., Glait, H., and Olivari, A. J. (1976): Levamisole in advanced human breast cancer. *Lancet,* 1:211–215.
14. Sadow, J. M., and Rapp, F. (1975): Inhibition by levamisole of metastases by cells transformed by herpes simplex virus type I. *Proc. Soc. Exp. Biol. Med.,* 149:219–222.
15. Stewart, C. C., and Perez, C. A. (1976): Effect of irradiation on immune responses. *Radiology,* 118:201–210.
16. Stewart, C. C., Perez, C. A., and Wagner, B. N. (1976): Initiation and evolution of antitumor immunity to a transplanted murine lymphosarcoma. *Int. J. Radiat. Oncol. Biol. Phys.,* 1:439–445.
17. Tripodi, D., Parks, L. C., and Brugmans, J. (1973): Drug-induced restoration of cutaneous delayed-hypersensitivity in anergic patients with candida. *N. Engl. J. Med.,* 289:354–357.
18. Van Ginckel, R. F., and Hoebeke, J. (1975): Carbon clearance enhancing factor in serum from levamisole treated mice. *J. Reticuloendothel. Soc.,* 17:65–72.
19. Verhaegen, H., De Cock, W., De Cree, J., Verbruggen, F., Verhaegen-Declercq, M., and Brugmans, J. (1975): Letter: *In vitro* restoration by levamisole of thymus-derived lymphocyte functions in Hodgkin's disease. *Lancet,* 1:978.
20. Versijp, G., van Zwet, T. L., and van Furth, R. (1975): Letter: Levamisole and functions of peritoneal macrophages. *Lancet,* 1:798.
21. Woods, W. A., Fliegleman, M. J., and Chirigos, M. A. (1975): Effect of levamisole on the *in vitro* immune response of spleen lymphocytes. *Proc. Soc. Exp. Biol. Med.,* 148:1048–1050.
22. Woods, W. A., Siegel, M. J., and Chirigos, M. A. (1974): *In vitro* stimulation of spleen cells cultures by poly I:poly C and levamisole. *Cell. Immunol.,* 14:327–331.

Immune Modulation and Control of Neoplasia by Adjuvant Therapy, edited by M. A. Chirigos. Raven Press, New York, 1978.

Cyclic Adenosine Monophosphate Levels in Lymphocytes from Patients with Melanoma and Squamous Cell Carcinoma Treated with Levamisole

Zbigniew L. Olkowski

Laboratory of Tumor Biology and Clinical Immunology, Winship Clinic for Neoplastic Diseases, Emory University School of Medicine, Atlanta, Georgia 30322

Patients with malignant melanoma and squamous cell carcinoma (SCC) of the head and neck present with impaired immunocompetence (3,4,9,10,11,15). Since activation of the immune response genes is likely necessary in order to elicit an immune response in the lymphocytes (5,8,13) and since cyclic nucleotides are very likely to be involved in this process (for reviews see 12, 14), we determined the levels of cyclic adenosine monophosphate (cyclic AMP) in lymphocytes from melanoma and SCC patients before treatment, following surgical excision of the lesion, and during immunotherapy with levamisole.

MATERIALS AND METHODS

A total of 46 patients with malignant melanoma, 35 patients with SCC of the head and neck, and 13 healthy, age-matched controls were studied.

In the melanoma group there were 14 patients with metastatic disease who received no treatment during the testing period, 18 patients who had curative surgery and no further treatment, and 14 patients who continued to demonstrate impaired cellular immunity following curative surgery and were treated with levamisole (150 mg p.o., twice a week).

In the SCC group there were 10 patients with metastatic disease, 11 patients who were evaluated before surgery, seven patients who had curative surgery and no further therapy, and seven patients who were treated with levamisole (150 mg p.o., twice a week) following curative surgery.

Lymphocytes were isolated from peripheral blood samples on a Ficoll-Hypaque gradient as described previously (11). Following a final centrifugation, the cell pellet was treated with cold 5% trichloroacetic acid, sonicated, and the precipitate and neutralized supernatant frozen separately until time of analysis. Cyclic AMP was evaluated using Kuo and Greengard's (7) method. Portions of some samples were analyzed for prostaglandins (PG) using a commercially available radioimmunoassay kit.

STATISTICAL ANALYSES

To determine whether a healthy control group had significantly different average values for cyclic AMP and prostaglandin $F_{2\alpha}$ ($PGF_{2\alpha}$) when compared with values obtained from various groups of cancer patients, preliminary one-way analyses of variance were performed for each variable. Scheffe's method of multiple comparison was then used to test hypotheses on mean differences (2).

RESULTS

Results of cyclic AMP levels in lymphocytes from healthy, age-matched controls and from cancer patients are presented in Tables 1 and 2 and Fig. 1. Results of $PGF_{2\alpha}$ levels are presented in Table 3. The mean cyclic AMP level in lymphocytes of healthy controls was 38.5 pmoles/mg protein. Mean level of this nucleotide in lymphocytes from patients with metastatic melanoma was 10.7 pmoles/mg protein (Table 1), and from patients with metastatic SCC of head and neck, 13.7 pmoles/mg protein (Table 2), both values significantly lower than controls. Mean cyclic AMP level in lymphocytes isolated from SCC patients before surgery was 13.3 pmoles/mg protein, also significantly lower than controls (Table 2). Melanoma patients with no evidence of clinical disease (NED) tested approximately 3 weeks following surgery had mean cyclic AMP levels of 21.8 pmoles/mg protein (Table 1) and corresponding SCC patients had a mean of 18.1 pmoles/mg protein of cyclic AMP (Table 2) in isolated lymphocytes. In melanoma patients remaining free of disease following surgery and 8 to 16 weeks of levamisole therapy, cyclic AMP levels increased significantly to a mean of 43.1 pmoles/mg protein. In contrast, in the one patient who developed a recurrence after 8 weeks of levamisole therapy, cyclic AMP in lymphocytes isolated at the time of recurrence was only 12.0 pmoles/mg protein (Table 1).

Lymphocytes isolated from three melanoma patients (C.T., C.A., and L.R.M.) treated with surgery followed by levamisole therapy for 32 to 60 weeks revealed

TABLE 1. *Cyclic AMP levels in lymphocytes of patients with melanoma*

Subjects		Number of cases	Cyclic AMP pmoles/mg protein		
			Mean	SD	—
Healthy controls		13	38.5	9.9	—
Metastatic melanoma		14	10.7	3.6	$p < 0.01$
After surgery, NED, no immunotherapy		18	21.8	7.9	$p < 0.01$
After surgery 8–16 weeks on levamisole	Responders, NED	13	43.1	13.3	NS
	Nonresponders	1	12.0	—	—

TABLE 2. *Cyclic AMP levels in lymphocytes of patients with SCC of head and neck*

Subjects		Number of cases	Cyclic AMP pmoles/mg protein		
			Mean	SD	—
Healthy controls		13	38.5	9.9	—
Metastatic SCC		10	13.7	4.3	$p < 0.01$
Before surgery		11	13.3	6.6	$p < 0.01$
After surgery, NED, no immunotherapy		7	18.1	4.5	$p < 0.01$
After surgical excision, NED	Responders, NED	2	30.7	—	—
8–16 weeks on immunotherapy	Non-responders	5	9.9	4.1	$p < 0.01$

very low levels of this nucleotide (18.1, 8.8, and 1.1 pmoles/mg protein). All three patients remained clinically free of disease, and all had cyclic AMP levels similar to control values (Table 1) when tested 8 to 16 weeks after immunotherapy. Correspondingly we found that *in vitro* lymphocyte cytotoxicity to a melanoma cell line decreased in these three patients as treatment with levamisole progressed (see Fig. 1).

In the SCC group two patients remained free of disease following 6 months of levamisole therapy and had a mean cyclic AMP level of 30.7 pmoles/mg protein, which is significantly higher than the pretreatment value of 13.3 pmoles/mg protein. Five patients who recurred within the 6 months of levamisole immunotherapy had a mean cyclic AMP level of 9.9 pmoles/mg protein, which is significantly lower than the control values (Table 2) and similar to pretreatment levels.

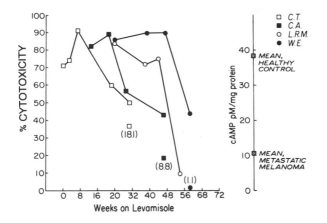

FIG. 1. *In vitro* lymphocyte cytotoxicity to cultured malignant melanoma (BMCL cell line).

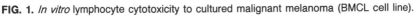

TABLE 3. *Prostaglandin $F_{2\alpha}$ levels in lymphocytes from patients with melanoma and SCC (ng/10^6 cells)*

Subjects		Number of cases	PGF$_{2\alpha}$		
			Mean	SD	
Healthy controls		6	0.42	0.42	
Metastatic melanoma		5	4.27	0.43	$p < 0.01$
Metastatic cancer, breasts		5	6.48	2.69	$p < 0.01$
SCC head and neck	Before surgery	6	5.01	2.25	$p < 0.01$
	After surgery NED	6	1.36	0.59	$p < 0.01$

PGF$_{2\alpha}$

The mean value of PGF$_{2\alpha}$ in six healthy controls was 0.42 ng/10^6 lymphocytes (Table 3). The mean value of this prostaglandin in lymphocytes from patients with metastatic breast cancer was 6.48 ng/10^6 cells and those with metastatic melanoma 4.27 ng/10^6 cells, respectively. Six patients with SCC of head and neck tested before surgery showed a mean PGF$_{2\alpha}$ level in the peripheral lymphocytes of 5.01 ng/10^6 cells. These same patients tested 3 weeks following surgery with no clinical evidence of disease had mean 1.36 ng/10^6 cells.

COMMENTS

Results from these experiments indicate that there are significant differences in cyclic AMP levels in lymphocytes isolated from healthy controls, from patients with metastatic melanoma or SCC of head and neck, and from patients undergoing immunotherapy with levamisole. The tendency of cyclic AMP levels in lymphocytes of levamisole-treated patients to return to control levels suggests a mechanism of action of levamisole *in vivo* in cancer patients. It is conceivable that this drug affects some of the metabolic pathways of cyclic nucleotides, as suggested earlier by Hadden (6), resulting in the increase in levels of cyclic AMP observed in the lymphocytes isolated from responders who remained clinically free of disease. The observation that patients surgically cured had significantly lower cyclic AMP levels in peripheral lymphocytes when compared to the group treated with levamisole is consistent with this hypothesis. Further interpretation of these results must await the separation of the accidental population of lymphocytes into T cells, B cells, null cells, and possibly other subclasses, and evaluations of cyclic guanosine monophosphate, guanyl cyclase, adenyl cyclase, and phosphodiesterase activities in these types of cells.

Decreased lymphocyte cyclic AMP in three melanoma patients treated with levamisole for 32 to 60 weeks and the concomitant decrease of their lymphocytotoxicity to a malignant melanoma cell line *in vitro* suggested either an overdose of levamisole or the imminent recurrence of disease. Further observations of these patients revealed the recurrence of melanoma in one patient (L.R.M.) 3 months following the sudden drop in cyclic AMP level and the decrease in lymphocyte cytotoxicity. The other two patients had increased immunocompetence and remained clinically free of disease for 8 months after the initial drop in their immunity. The elevated levels of $PGF_{2\alpha}$ found in lymphocytes isolated from patients with metastatic breast carcinoma, melanoma, and operable SCC of the head and neck are very interesting, especially since earlier information suggests that prostaglandins of the E and F series may be involved in regulating cyclic nucleotide metabolism (1). It is well established that prostaglandins of the E series are more efficient in the stimulation of cyclic AMP synthesis than $PGF_{2\alpha}$ in human lymphocytes (1). Elevated $PGF_{2\alpha}$ levels may be mechanistically related to the significantly decreased levels of cyclic AMP found in peripheral lymphocytes from patients with metastatic disease. Pair analysis of patients with SCC of the head and neck before and after surgery revealed a significant decrease in $PGF_{2\alpha}$ levels in lymphocytes 3 weeks following surgery (Table 3). These patients also had a slight increase in lymphocyte cyclic AMP levels (from 13.3 to 18.1 pmoles/mg protein). If these trends continue to be found in a larger number of cancer patients, we may hypothesize about the possible role of prostaglandins in the response of lymphocytes to antigenic stimulation.

SUMMARY

Cyclic AMP and $PGF_{2\alpha}$ levels were evaluated in peripheral lymphocytes from 81 patients with malignant melanoma and SCC of head and neck, who had surgical resection for complete removal of the tumor, and patients with metastatic disease. Groups of patients with no clinical evidence of the disease were given levamisole (150 mg/day, p.o., 2 days a week) and maintained on this dose for up to 60 weeks. Decreased cyclic AMP levels and increased $PGF_{2\alpha}$ levels in lymphocytes from patients with metastatic disease were observed. Patients with NED maintained on levamisole for 8 to 16 weeks showed cyclic AMP levels similar to control values.

ACKNOWLEDGMENTS

Many thanks are due to Drs. J. R. McLaren, Samuel A. Wilkins Jr., and D. R. Murray, for referring their patients to our laboratory and for valuable discussions on the subject.

Many thanks are also due to Dr. J. F. Kuo for his invaluable expertise and cyclic AMP techniques, including isolation of cyclic AMP protein kinase and to Dr. Michael Kutner for statistical analysis of data. I wish to express great thanks to my associates Kristina Wright, M. J. Skeen, R. Y. Boswell, and Wendy Hsiao for invaluable technical help and to Peggy Firth for art work. Levamisol was obtained from Janssen R & D, Inc., and the collaboration of S. Schlossberg in this matter is acknowledged.

This work was supported by a grant from Winship Clinic for Neoplastic Diseases, Emory University School of Medicine.

REFERENCES

1. Bach, M., and Bach, J. F. (1974): Effects of prostaglandins and indomethacin on rosette-forming lymphocytes: Interactions with thymic hormone. In: *Prostaglandin Synthetase Inhibitors,* edited by H. J. Robinson and J. R. Vane, pp. 241–248. Raven Press, New York.
2. Bahn, A. E. (1972): *Basic Medical Statistics,* 5th ed. Grune & Stratton, New York.
3. Cassel, W. A., Murray, D. R., Torbin, A. H., Olkowski, Z. L., and Moore, M. F. (1977): Viral oncolysate in the management of malignant melanoma. *Cancer,* 40:672–679.
4. Cheney, P., Kuo, J. R., McLaren, J. R., Wilkins, S. A., and Olkowski, Z. L. (1976): Cyclic nucleotide levels in the lymphocytes of carcinoma patients (abstract). *Proc. Annu. Mtg. Radiation Research Society, San Francisco.* Academic Press, New York.
5. Greaves, M. F., Owen, J. J. T., and Raff, M. C. (1973): *T and B Lymphocytes. Origins, Properties and Roles in Immune Responses.* American Elsevier, New York.
6. Hadden, J. W., Coffey, R. G., Hadden, E. M., Lopez-Corrales, E., and Sunshine, G. M. (1975): Effects of levamisole and imidazole on lymphocyte proliferation and cyclic nucleotide levels. *Cell. Immunol.,* 20:92–103.
7. Kuo, J. F., and Greengard, P. (1970): Cyclic nucleotide dependent protein kinases. VIII. An assay method for the measurement of adenosine 3' 5' monophosphate in various tissues in the study of agents influencing its level in adipose cells. *J. Biol. Chem.,* 245:8067–8074.
8. McDevitt, H. O., and Landy, M. (editors) (1972): *Genetic Control of the Immune Response: Brook Lodge Symposium.* Academic Press, New York.
9. Olkowski, Z. L., and Nixon, D. W. (1976): Immunological evaluation of breast cancer patients during chemotherapy. *Proc. 3rd Int. Symp. Cancer Prevention and Detection, New York, April 26–May 1, 1976.* Marcel Dekker, New York.
10. Olkowski, Z. L., Murray, D. R., and McLaren, J. R. (1975): Whither immunocompetence? *J. Med. Assoc. Ga.,* June 1975: 246–247.
11. Olkowski, Z. L., and Wilkins, S. A. (1975): T-lymphocyte levels in the peripheral blood of patients with cancer of the head and neck. *Am. J. Surg.,* 130:440–446.
12. Oppenheim, J. J., and Rosenstreich, D. L. (1976): Signals regulating *in vitro* activation of lymphocytes. *Prog. Allergy,* 20:65–194.
13. Walford, R. L., Smith, G. S., and Waters, H. (1971): Histocompatibility systems and disease status with particular reference to cancer. *Transplant Rev.,* 7:78.
14. Wedner, J. H., and Parker, C. W. (1976): Lymphocyte activation. *Prog. Allergy,* 20:195–300.
15. Wilkins, S. A., and Olkowski, Z. L. (1977): Immunocompetence of patients treated with levamisole. *Cancer,* 39:487–493.

Immune Modulation and Control of Neoplasia by Adjuvant Therapy, edited by M. A. Chirigos. Raven Press, New York, 1978.

Levamisole and Human Monocyte Chemotaxis: Reversal of an Influenzal-Induced Chemotactic Defect

*Ralph Snyderman, **Marilyn C. Pike, and †Charles A. Daniels

*Division of Rheumatic and Genetic Diseases, Department of Medicine, and Departments of †Pathology and ** Microbiology and Immunology, Duke University Medical Center, Durham, North Carolina 27710*

The central importance of normal macrophage function for immunologically mediated defense against microbial invasion and neoplasia is becoming increasingly well recognized. Macrophages are phagocytic, wandering cells with intracellular microbiocidal properties. They also possess cytotoxic potential for neoplastic cells *in vitro* (2,5). Blood monocytes and tissue macrophages are able to detect and migrate in response to chemical gradients of chemotactic factors (15), and their rapid accumulation at sites of microbial invasion or neoplastic transformation would appear to be vital to normal immune function. Over the past several years, our laboratory has developed quantitative *in vitro* methods that allow the study of monocyte and macrophage chemotactic responsiveness in health and in various disease states (13). It is now clear that abnormalities of macrophage locomotion can be reproducibly found in certain human diseases characterized by increased susceptibility to infection or neoplasia (1,3,4,6,16–18). The contribution of abnormalities of monocyte chemotaxis to actual disease expression can only be surmised at present; however, it seems reasonable to conclude that pharmacological agents that enhance monocyte or macrophage chemotactic responsiveness could be important therapeutic agents in certain immune deficiency or neoplastic diseases.

The following data demonstrate that levamisole enhances the directed migratory response of human monocytes. In addition, this drug can reverse or prevent the depressed chemotaxis produced by influenza.

MATERIALS AND METHODS

Pharmacological Agents

Levamisole [(−) tetramisole], 1,2,3,5,6-tetrahydro-6-phenyl-imidazo-[2,lb]-thiazole hydrochloride, its stereoisomer (+) tetramisole, and *p*-Br-(−) tetrami-

---

* Dr. Snyderman is also the Director of the Howard Hughes Medical Institute, Laboratory of Immune Effector Functions at Duke University Medical Center.

sole, the parabromo derivative of levamisole, were kindly provided by Janssen R&D, Inc., New Brunswick, New Jersey.

Chemotaxis Assays

Human monocyte chemotaxis was assayed *in vitro* by a minor modification of a previously described technique (4). Briefly, peripheral blood monocytes were isolated on Ficoll-Hypaque gradients, washed extensively, and resuspended to contain 1.5×10^6 monocytes per ml in medium RPMI 1640 (Grand Island Biological Company, Grand Island, New York). The cell suspension was placed in the upper compartment of a modified Boyden chamber and separated from the chemotactic stimulant or control in the lower compartment by a 5.0-μm polycarbonate (Nuclepore) filter. After incubation for various lengths of time at 37°C in humidified air, the chambers were emptied, and the filters were removed, fixed in ethanol, and stained with hematoxylin (13).

Human polymorphonuclear leukocyte (PMN) chemotaxis was quantified similarly (14). PMNs were isolated from whole blood by sedimentation with 3% Dextran T500 (Pharmacia, Upsala, Sweden) in saline, washed extensively, and resuspended to contain 2.2×10^6 PMN per ml in Gey's balanced salt solution (BSS) containing 2% bovalbumin (Flow Laboratories, Rockville, Maryland), pH 7.2. A 5.0-μm nitrocellulose filter (Millipore Filter Corp., New Bedford, Mass.) was used to separate the upper and lower compartments of the chemotaxis chambers. Following incubation for 3 hr at 37°C, the filters were processed as described previously (14).

In the quantification of PMN and monocyte chemotaxis, all assays were performed in triplicate, and the chemotactic response was assessed by counting and averaging the number of cells that migrated completely through the filter per microscopic field in 20 fields (×1540 for monocytes, ×780 for PMNs).

Virus Preparation

Influenza A, PR8 strain (A/PR/8/34 [HON 1]) was prepared as described previously (8) and assayed as hemagglutination units (HAU) using chick erythrocytes.

Patients and Controls

Patients were four previously healthy students, aged 18 to 20, who were admitted to the Duke University Infirmary with an acute, febrile upper respiratory illness diagnosed as influenza. Blood was obtained from all patients within 48 hr of admission. Serum samples were obtained at the time of initial testing and 3 weeks after discharge and were stored at −70°C until delivered to the North Carolina State Laboratory for quantification of influenza-antibody titers. The diagnosis of a current or recent infection with Influenza A/England/864/ 75 or A/Port Chalmers/1/73 was established by finding a fourfold or greater increase in antiinfluenza antibody as measured by either the hemagglutination inhibition (HAI) or the complement fixation tests (7,11,12). Controls consisted of normal healthy volunteers.

RESULTS

Effect of Levamisole and Its Isomers on Monocyte Chemotactic Responsiveness

To determine the effect of (−) tetramisole, (+) tetramisole, and p-Br-(−) tetramisole on monocyte chemotaxis, isolated cells were incubated with various doses of the drugs contained in RPMI 1640 or with medium alone and tested for chemotactic responsiveness to lymphocyte-derived chemotactic factor (LDCF), endotoxin activated human serum (AHS), or the chemotactically active peptide N-formyl-methionyl-phenylalanine (f-met-phe) (9). Doses of levamisole ranging from 10^{-5} to 10^{-3} M enhanced the chemotactic responsiveness of monocytes to the three chemotactic factors by 20 to 148% (Table 1). Similar doses

TABLE 1. *Effect of isomers of tetramisole on human monocyte chemotactic responsiveness*

Monocytes incubated with[a]	Chemotactic activity[b] of monocytes in response to:		
	LDCF[c]	AHS[d]	f-met-phe[e]
Medium alone	43.9 ± 3.6	79.5 ± 6.3	36.0 ± 3.0
(−) Tetramisole			
1 × 10^{-3} M	98.0 ± 1.0	114.8 ± 7.3	89.4 ± 1.7
1 × 10^{-4} M	73.9 ± 6.9	107.6 ± 10.2	53.1 ± 4.3
1 × 10^{-5} M	59.1 ± 0.3	95.4 ± 1.3	44.9 ± 5.5
p-Br-(−) tetramisole			
5 × 10^{-5} M	82.5 ± 6.8		
1 × 10^{-5} M	61.7 ± 3.5		
1 × 10^{-6} M	49.8 ± 2.1		
(+) Tetramisole			
1 × 10^{-3} M	49.8 ± 5.3		
1 × 10^{-4} M	49.2 ± 2.0		
1 × 10^{-5} M	45.5 ± 5.6		

[a] Human monocytes were isolated on Ficoll-Hypaque gradients, washed extensively, and resuspended (1.5 × 10^6/ml) in medium containing various molar concentrations of the indicated isomers of tetramisole or in medium alone. Following incubation (37°C for 30 min) the monocytes were placed in the upper compartment of a modified Boyden chamber and tested for chemotactic responsiveness.

[b] Chemotactic activity is expressed as the average number of monocytes in triplicate samples migrating completely through a 5.0-μm-polycarbonate filter per oil immersion field (×1540) ± SEM.

[c] LDCF was obtained from supernatants of concanavalin A-stimulated lymphocyte cultures. LDCF was diluted to 15% vol/vol in RPMI 1640 for use as a chemotactic stimulant.

[d] AHS was prepared by incubation of normal serum with *S. typhosa* endotoxin (1 mg/ml serum) for 60 min at 37°C followed by 56° for 30 min. AHS was then diluted to 0.5% vol/vol in RPMI 1640 for use as a chemotactic stimulant.

[e] F-met-phe was diluted to 10^{-6} M in RPMI 1640 for use as a chemotactic stimulant. Adapted from ref. 9.

of (+) tetramisole had no significant ($p > 0.2$) effect on monocyte chemotactic responsiveness to LDCF. Increased chemotaxis to LDCF was also noted when monocytes were incubated with doses of p-Br-($-$) tetramisole ranging from 10^{-6} to 5×10^{-5} M; however, at doses higher than 5×10^{-4} M, p-Br-($-$) tetramisole was toxic to the monocytes, as judged by trypan blue dye uptake, and also depressed chemotactic responsiveness. Enhanced monocyte chemotaxis was not seen when levamisole was placed in the lower compartment of the chemotaxis chamber and incubated with the chemotactic factor rather than with the cells. In addition, the enhancing effect of levamisole was removed by washing the cells extensively after a 30-min incubation with the drug. These data indicated that enhancement of monocyte chemotaxis is stereospecific and that the drug exerts its effect on the monocyte.

To ascertain whether levamisole increased the rate of cell migration or the total number of cells capable of responding chemotactically, monocytes were incubated with RPMI 1640 alone or with the medium containing 10^{-3} M levamisole, and the number of cells responding to LDCF after various times of incubation in the chemotaxis chambers was determined (9). Figure 1 illustrates that levamisole increased both the rate of monocyte chemotactic responsiveness and the maximum number of cells capable of responding chemotactically. To determine whether enhancement of monocyte chemotaxis by levamisole required binding of the drug to the monocytes, cells were incubated with medium containing various doses of levamisole alone or with medium containing levamisole plus (+) tetramisole and tested for chemotactic responsiveness to LDCF. Figure 2 demonstrates that doses of 10^{-4} and 10^{-3} M (+) tetramisole reduced the

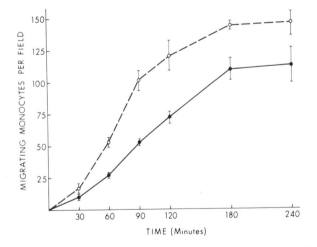

FIG. 1. Kinetics of enhancement of monocyte chemotactic responsiveness by ($-$) tetramisole. Isolated monocytes were incubated (37°C for 30 min) with medium alone or containing 10^{-3} M ($-$) tetramisole and tested for chemotactic responsiveness to LDCF (15% v/v) after the indicated incubation time in the chemotaxis chamber. ○———○, 10^{-3} M ($-$) tetramisole; ●———●, medium alone. (From ref. 9.)

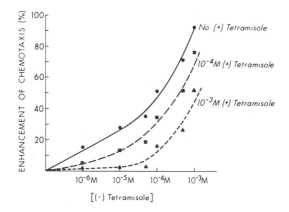

FIG. 2. Competitive inhibition of (−) tetramisole-enhancing effect on monocyte chemotactic responsiveness by (+) tetramisole. Isolated monocytes were incubated (37°C for 30 min) with medium containing 10^{-3} M (−) tetramisole alone, or with 10^{-3} M (−) tetramisole plus 10^{-3} M or 10^{-4} M (+) tetramisole and tested for chemotactic responsiveness to LDCF (15% v/v). K_D (−) tetramisole $= 10^{-4}$; K_D (+) tetramisole $= 0.8 \times 10^{-4}$.

$$\text{Percent enhancement} = \left(\frac{\begin{array}{c}\text{chemotactic responsiveness of cells} \\ \text{incubated with drugs}\end{array}}{\begin{array}{c}\text{chemotactic responsiveness of cells} \\ \text{incubated with medium alone}\end{array}} - 1 \right) \times 100$$

(From ref. 9.)

enhancing effect of levamisole. Moreover, the parallel nature of the curves suggests that (+) tetramisole inhibited the enhancing activity of levamisole by competitive binding (K_D for levamisole $= 1 \times 10^{-4}$; K_D for (+) tetramisole $= 0.8 \times 10^{-4}$) (9).

To determine if levamisole could likewise affect the chemotaxis of PMNs, isolated cells were incubated with Gey's BSS containing doses of the drug ranging from 10^{-6} to 10^{-3} M or with medium alone and tested for response to various dilutions of AHS or f-met-phe. At the doses of levamisole tested, there was no effect on the chemotactic response of PMNs, indicating a differential effectiveness of the drug for monocytes.

Reversal of Influenza-Induced Depression of Monocyte Chemotaxis by Levamisole

To ascertain whether levamisole could reverse the depression of monocyte chemotactic responsiveness produced by influenza, isolated normal monocytes were suspended in medium RPMI 1640 alone or with medium containing various concentrations of influenza, incubated for 15 min at 37°C, centrifuged, resuspended in medium alone or in medium containing 10^{-3} M levamisole, incubated an additional 30 min at 37°C, and then tested for chemotactic responsiveness to LDCF (10). The chemotactic responsiveness of monocytes treated with levamisole after incubation with influenza was markedly enhanced when compared to monocytes exposed to the virus but not incubated with levamisole (Table 2). In fact, the chemotactic responsiveness of virally exposed cells treated with levamisole was restored to that of cells not exposed to virus when a maximal dose of LDCF was used. It can also be seen that levamisole improved the responsiveness of virally treated cells to the lower dose of chemotactic factor, but did not completely reverse the defect produced by the virus.

To determine whether levamisole could likewise counteract the depression of monocyte chemotactic responsiveness in patients with acute influenza, isolated monocytes from four patients with serologically proved influenza were incubated with medium alone or with medium containing levamisole and then tested for chemotactic responsiveness to a maximal and less than maximal dose of LDCF (10). Table 3 indicates that the chemotactic responsiveness of monocytes from three of four patients with influenza was significantly ($p < 0.0025$) depressed. The response of the patients' monocytes to a maximal dose of chemotactic factor was restored to normal by 10^{-3} M levamisole and to just below normal when incubated with 10^{-4} M levamisole. The response of the patients' monocytes to less than a maximal dose of chemotactic factor also was markedly improved by levamisole treatment.

TABLE 2. *Effect of levamisole on depressed monocyte chemotaxis produced by* in vitro *treatment of MNL with influenza*

Cells treated with:[a]	Dose of chemotactic factor[b] (%)	Concentration of influenza (HAU/ml) exposed to MNL[c]			
		0	10^3	10^2	10^1
			(Chemotactic response)[d]		
Medium alone	15	41.9 ± 2.0	7.6 ± 2.6	15.2 ± 4.6	30.0 ± 5.9
Levamisole		89.8 ± 4.6	34.7 ± 5.6	51.2 ± 2.3	79.5 ± 2.6
Medium alone	30	80.9 ± 2.0	38.0 ± 4.6	59.1 ± 7.6	70.3 ± 9.2
Levamisole		78.2 ± 1.3	82.2 ± 3.0	84.5 ± 4.0	86.8 ± 4.0

MNL, mononuclear leukocytes.

[a] Following exposure to PR8 virus (15 min at 37°C), the monocytes were centrifuged, resuspended in medium alone or containing 10^{-3} M levamisole, and incubated for 30 min at 37°C prior to quantification of monocyte chemotaxis.

[b] LDCF was diluted in medium RPMI to contain an amount sufficient to produce either a maximal response (30% LDCF vol/vol) or a less than maximal response (15% LDCF vol/vol) using normal human monocytes as responder cells.

[c] Isolated human MNL (1.5×10^6 monocytes/ml) were suspended in medium alone or containing the indicated amount of PR8 and incubated for 15 min at 37°C.

[d] Chemotactic activity is expressed as the average number of monocytes per oil immersion field ($\times 1540$) migrating completely through the filter for triplicate samples $\pm$ SEM. The response of uninfected cells to medium alone (no chemotactic factor) was 3.4 ± 0.3.

Adapted from ref. 10.

TABLE 3. *Effect of levamisole on the monocyte chemotaxis of patients with acute influenza*

Monocytes isolated from:	Clinical and laboratory diagnosis[a]	Dose of chemotactic factor (%)[b]	Chemotactic activity[c] of cells incubated with:[d]		
			Medium alone	10^{-4} M levamisole	10^{-3} M levamisole
M.P.	Healthy	15	67.3 ± 5.0	80.9 ± 5.6	91.1 ± 1.0
		30	96.7 ± 3.0	92.4 ± 5.6	91.1 ± 2.0
M.N.	Healthy	15	60.4 ± 2.0	—	86.5 ± 3.3
		30	92.7 ± 1.3	90.8 ± 4.0	91.1 ± 5.6
K.H.	Influenza	15	41.3 ± 7.9	61.7 ± 7.9	67.7 ± 7.3
		30	57.1 ± 5.0	81.2 ± 1.0	93.4 ± 2.6
T.W.	Influenza	15	37.6 ± 1.3	65.0 ± 7.9	63.4 ± 9.6
		30	52.8 ± 5.9	83.2 ± 4.3	94.7 ± 3.6
W.R.	Influenza	15	39.9 ± 3.3	55.4 ± 0.7	64.4 ± 1.0
		30	75.2 ± 2.0	85.8 ± 2.0	95.4 ± 3.6
G.P.	Influenza	15	60.1 ± 2.6	66.3 ± 2.0	84.2 ± 7.9
		30	86.5 ± 5.3	87.8 ± 2.6	91.7 ± 2.3

[a] All patients had a fourfold or greater increase in complement fixation or HAI titer to influenza A/England/864/75 or A/Port Chalmers/1/73.

[b] LDCF was diluted to be a maximal (30% vol/vol) or less than maximal (15% vol/vol) chemotactic stimulus.

[c] Chemotactic activity is expressed as the average number of cells per oil immersion field (×1540) of triplicate samples ± SEM migrating completely through the filter in a 90-min incubation period.

[d] The isolated mononuclear leukocytes from patients and normals were incubated with either medium alone or medium containing 10^{-3} or 10^{-4} M levamisole and tested for chemotactic responsiveness.

Adapted from ref. 10.

DISCUSSION

The preceding results demonstrate that levamisole and p-Br-($-$) tetramisole enhance monocyte chemotaxis by increasing both the rate of cell migration and the number of cells capable of responding chemotactically. The enhancing effect is stereospecific, and the drug must bind to the monocytes since addition of the dextroisomer competitively inhibited the stimulating effect of levamisole. Both isomers have approximately the same dissociation constant for monocyte binding ($K_D \simeq 10^{-4}$) (9).

The potential clinical usefulness of levamisole in augmenting the depressed delayed hypersensitivity seen in patients with viral illnesses is suggested by the finding that the drug can reverse both *in vivo* and *in vitro* influenza-induced depression of monocyte chemotactic responsiveness (10). Incubation of normal monocytes with levamisole following *in vitro* exposure to influenza reversed much of the depression of chemotaxis produced by this virus.

Little information is available concerning the mechanisms by which chemotactically active cells translate the information contained in a gradient of a chemotactic factor into directed cell movement. Data now available suggest that chemotaxis requires recognition of the chemotactic molecule by membrane binding sites, alterations in transmembrane ion flux, contraction of actin-like proteins, and utilization of metabolic pathways to produce the energy required for the above processes. It is not known at this time at which step the monocyte is affected in patients with influenza, or how levamisole enhances the directed cell migration of monocytes. The study of levamisole's effects on normal and abnormal monocyte function may contribute to the elucidation of cellular mechanisms of chemotaxis. In addition, the ability of levamisole to enhance monocyte chemotactic function in the presence of viruses that depress chemotaxis suggests that this drug may be useful in reversing depressed cellular immunity in patients who contract influenza.

ACKNOWLEDGMENT

This work was supported in part by the National Institute of Dental Research, NIH, Research Grant No. 5R01 DE03738–05.

REFERENCES

1. Boetcher, D. A., and Leonard, E. (1974): Abnormal monocyte chemotaxis in cancer patients. *J. Natl. Cancer Inst.,* 52:1091–1099.
2. Evans, R., and Alexander, P. (1972): Mechanisms of immunologically specific killing of tumor cells by macrophages. *Nature,* 236:168–170.
3. Gallin, J. I. (1975): Abnormal chemotaxis: Cellular and humoral components. In: *The Phagocytic Cell in Host Resistance,* edited by J. A. Bellanti and D. H. Dayton, pp. 227–243. Raven Press, New York.
4. Hausman, M. S., Brosman, S., Snyderman, R., Mickey, M. R., and Fahey, J. (1975): Defective monocyte function in patients with genitourinary carcinoma. *J. Natl. Cancer Inst.,* 55:1047–1054.
5. Hibbs, J. B., Lambert, L. H., and Remington, J. S. (1972): Possible role of macrophage mediated nonspecific cytotoxicity tumor cell killing. *Nature,* 235:48–50.
6. Kleinerman, E. S., Snyderman, R., and Daniels, C. A. (1975): Depression of human monocyte chemotaxis during acute influenza infection. *Lancet,* ii:1063–1064.
7. Lennette, E. H. (1969): General principle underlying laboratory diagnoses of viral and rickettsial infection. In: *Diagnostic Procedures for Viral and Rickettsial Infections,* 4th ed., edited by E. H. Lennette and N. J. Schmidt, pp. 52–58. American Public Health Association, New York.
8. Lief, F. S., and Henle, W. (1956): Studies on the soluble antigen of influenza virus I. The release of S antigen from elementary bodies by treatment with ether. *Virology,* 2:752–771.
9. Pike, M. C., and Snyderman, R. (1976): Augmentation of human monocyte chemotactic response by levamisole. *Nature,* 261:136–137.
10. Pike, M. C., Daniels, C. A., and Snyderman, R. (1976): Influenza induced depression of monocyte chemotaxis: Reversal by levamisole. *Cell Immunol.,* 32:234–238.
11. Robinson, R. Q., and Dowdle, W. R. (1969): Influenza viruses. In: *Diagnostic Procedures for Viral and Rickettsial Infections,* 4th ed., edited by E. H. Lennette and N. J. Schmidt, pp. 428–430. American Public Health Association, New York.
12. Sever, J. L. (1962): Application of a microtechnique to viral serological investigations. *J. Immunol.,* 88:320–329.
13. Snyderman, R., Altman, L. C., Hausman, M., and Mergenhagen, S. E. (1972): Human mononuclear leukocyte chemotaxis: A quantitative assay for humoral and cellular chemotactic factors. *J. Immunol.,* 108:857–860.

14. Snyderman, R., and Mergenhagen, S. E. (1972): Characterization of polymorphonuclear leuko-cyte chemotactic activity in serums activated by various inflammatory agents. In: *Biological Activities of Complement,* edited by D. G. Ingram, pp. 117–132. Karger, Basel.
15. Snyderman, R., and Mergenhagen, S. E. (1976): Chemotaxis of macrophages. In: *Immunobiology of the Macrophage,* edited by D. S. Nelson, pp. 323–348. Academic Press, New York.
16. Snyderman, R., Pike, M. C., and Altman, L. C. (1975): Abnormalities of leukocyte chemotaxis in human disease. *Ann. NY Acad. Sci.,* 256:386–401.
17. Snyderman, R., Seigler, H. F., and Meadows, L. (1977): Abnormalities of monocyte chemotaxis in patients with melanoma: Effects of immunotherapy and tumor removal. *J. Natl. Cancer Inst.,* 58:37–41.
18. Snyderman, R., and Stahl, C. (1975): Defective immune effector function in patients with neoplas-tic and immune deficiency diseases. In: *The Phagocytic Cell in Host Resistance,* edited by J. A. Bellanti and D. H. Dayton, pp. 267–281. Raven Press, New York.

Immune Modulation and Control of Neoplasia by Adjuvant Therapy, edited by M. A. Chirigos. Raven Press, New York, 1978.

In Vitro Effects of Levamisole on Human Mononuclear Phagocytes

Mohamed S. Al-Ibrahim

Department of Medicine, Veterans Administration Hospital, Baltimore, Maryland 21218

Immunotherapy of patients with cancer is currently of widespread interest. Although augmentation of humoral and cellular immune responses has been described with a variety of agents, the exact mechanisms by which this effect is produced are not well understood. In addition, there is little certainty regarding optimal dosages of immunopotentiating agents, the type of immune-reactive cell influenced, and the likelihood of benefit for a given tumor.

These studies report the *in vitro* effects of levamisole (LMS) on human mononuclear glass-adherent phagocytes. Much of this work was done in collaboration with Robert Holzman and H. Sherwood Lawrence at New York University School of Medicine. Recent preliminary data are presented suggesting a possible mechanism of action of LMS on these cells.

METHODS AND MATERIALS

Blood

Leukocytes were obtained from healthy volunteers none of whom had taken any medication for at least 3 weeks prior to the study. Mononuclear cells were separated after centrifugation on a Ficoll-Hypaque column (4). The cell population obtained usually contained less than 5% polymorphonuclear leukocytes; of the mononuclear cells, approximately 15% were monocytes. For the phagocytosis experiments the cell concentration was adjusted to give 1×10^6 mononuclear cells (macrophages and lymphocytes) per ml of Eagle's Minimum essential medium (MEMS; Flow Laboratories, Rockville, Md.) containing 15% autologous platelet-free plasma. Monocyte monolayers were then prepared by placing 1-ml aliquots of this cell suspension into plastic wells (Linbro Chemicals Co., Inc., New Haven, Conn.), each containing a 12-mm-diameter cleaned and sterilized glass coverslip. After allowing the cells to settle, nonadherent cells were washed off. Of the glass adherent population, more than 95% were mononuclear phagocytic cells.

Preparation of Labeled Polystyrene Particles

The labeling procedure has been described in detail elsewhere (2). Briefly, latex particles (Dow Chemical Co., Indianapolis, Ind.) of diameter 1.09 μm[1] were incubated with sodium pertechnetate. After mixing, a solution of 0.1% stannous chloride was added. The latex particles (LP) were then washed free of unbound isotope, counted by nephelometry, and adjusted to the desired concentration in culture medium with 15% pooled human serum.

Incubation of Macrophage Monolayers with LMS

Preservative-free LMS (kindly supplied by Janssen, Inc.) was dissolved in MEMS and sterilized by filtration. Final concentrations of LMS were made in MEMS containing 15% autologous plasma. Monolayers were then incubated with and without LMS in a 5% CO_2-air atmosphere at 37°C.

Assay of Phagocytosis

Following incubation with LMS, latex particles were added to the monolayers and 30 min were allowed for phagocytosis. This period was determined to be optimal for this system by previous experiments and allowed for the ingestion of 5 to 15 LP per macrophage. Coverslips were allowed to air dry, and radioactivity was determined in a gamma counter.

Expression of Phagocytosis Data

Each coverslip was incubated overnight in 0.1 ml IN NaOH, and the protein content of the monolayers was assayed by the method of Lowry et al. (18). For each coverslip the radioactive cpm/μg protein were obtained, and the mean for each triplicate sample was calculated. Results were also expressed as ratio of cpm/μg protein in the presence of LMS to cpm/μg protein in the absence of LMS. As a control for adherence of LP to glass and cells, comparably treated monolayers were incubated at 4°C. The counts obtained from these coverslips were taken as background and subtracted.

Leukocyte Cultures

Leukocyte cultures were performed according to standard methods in flatbottomed microtiter plates (Linbro), each well containing 0.1×10^6 lymphocytes. Final LMS concentrations varied from 0.08 to 20 μg/ml. In some experiments tuberculin [purified protein derivative (PPD), preservative free; Connaught Laboratories, Toronto, Canada] was added to a final concentration of 10, 1.0, 0.1,

---

[1] In some experiments latex particles of 2.0-μm diameter were used.

and 0.01 µg/ml, whereas in others, phytohemagglutinin (PHA-P, Difco) was added. These experiments have been described in detail elsewhere (3).

RESULTS

Effect of Levamisole on Phagocytosis

Optimal LMS Dose

In the initial experiments macrophages were incubated for 72 hr with LMS at a concentration range of 0.08 to 50 µg/ml after which phagocytosis was assessed. Enhancement of phagocytosis was evident at the 2.5 to 10 µg/ml LMS dose range. Figure 1 shows the results of such an experiment using macrophage populations obtained from four donors. Maximal phagocytic uptake was seen in the presence of LMS at a concentration of 5 µg/ml, and this dose of LMS was used for most subsequent experiments. Phagocytic enhancement could not be related to the presence or absence of LMS during the period of phagocytosis.

In these experiments significant depression of phagocytosis was not detected at any of the LMS doses used.

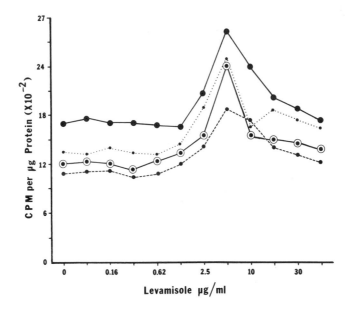

FIG. 1. Effect of increasing doses of LMS on phagocytosis by macrophages obtained from four donors after 72-hr incubation. (From ref. 4, with permission of the University of Chicago Press.)

Duration of LMS Treatment and Phagocytic Enhancement

The effect of varying the period of incubation with LMS was examined. Phago-cytosis of macrophages cultured with and without LMS was assessed at 24-hr intervals for 4 days. Although some phagocytic enhancement was noted after 48 hr of incubation with LMS, significant enhancement was seen only after 72 hr. Further prolongation of the incubation time did not result in greater phagocytic stimulation.

Effect of LMS on Cell Adherence and Macrophage Morphology

No significant differences could be detected in the protein content of coverslips incubated with and without LMS. Similarly, no differences could be found when control or LMS-treated monolayers were subjected to light and phase micro-scopic examination.

Extent of LMS-Induced Phagocytic Enhancement

The results of experiments using macrophages obtained from 17 normal donors and incubated for 72 hr at a LMS concentration of 5 μg/ml are shown in Fig. 2. In this series of experiments, macrophages obtained from 12 donors

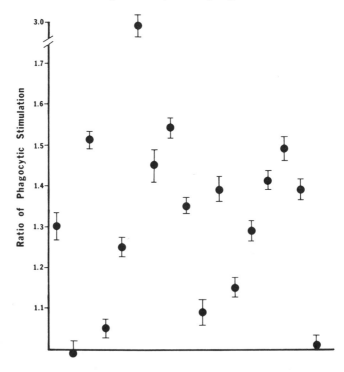

FIG. 2. Stimulation of phagocytosis after 72-hr incubation with LMS (5 μg/ml). Each point represents a different macrophage donor.

showed phagocytic stimulation following LMS treatment. With rare exception the degree of enhancement was modest, generally being in the range of 130 to 150% that of control cells.

LMS and Lymphocyte Proliferation

Sensitive lymphocytes were cultured with various concentrations of both PPD and levamisole in checkerboard fashion (3). A highly significant interaction between LMS concentration and PPD response was found. This could be summarized as follows (Fig. 3):

1. At all concentrations, LMS depressed thymidine incorporation by unstimulated lymphocytes. Since the level of this spontaneous incorporation is so low (average 90 cpm/well), it is of questionable importance.

2. When PPD-stimulated lymphocytes were cultured in LMS concentrations of 5 µg/ml or higher, inhibition of thymidine uptake was uniformly observed.

3. At low levels of LMS (0.08 to 1.25 µg/ml) antigen-dependent lymphocyte stimulation was observed. Enhancement was observed at suboptimal levels of antigen (in this system 0.1 and 1.0 µg/ml PPD); peak enhancement, 185% ± 22 (SD), occurred at 0.1 µg/ml PPD and 0.08 µg/ml LMS. Cells stimulated by optimal doses of antigen (10 µg/ml PPD) were not significantly affected by LMS presence. Similar results were noted for PHA-induced lymphocyte stimulation.

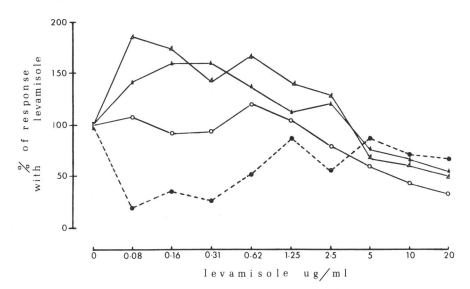

FIG. 3. ^{14}C-thymidine incorporation by sensitive lymphocytes cultured with PPD and LMS. ○——○, 10 µg/ml PPD, 100% = 2,452 cpm; ▲——▲, 1 µg/ml PPD, 100% = 1,367 cpm; △——△, 0.1 µg/ml PPD, 100% = 712 cpm; ●······●, 0 PPD, 100% = 90 cpm. (Adapted from ref. 3.)

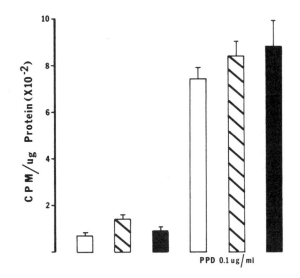

FIG. 4. Effect of LMS on incorporation of ^{14}C-glucosamine by activated macrophages. LMS (μg/ml): □, 0; ▨, 4.5; ■, 9.0.

Effect of LMS on Incorporation of ^{14}C-Glucosamine

The uptake of ^{14}C-glucosamine by activated macrophages has been described by Hammond et al. (12,13). We have adapted this method for measurement of the immunologic activation of human monocytes in the presence of antigen-stimulated lymphocytes (16). Preliminary results (Fig. 4) show that LMS, at a concentration of 4.5 μg/ml, augmented glucosamine incorporation by resting macrophages (i.e., macrophages cultured with lymphocytes but without antigen). Interestingly, this concentration did not enhance glucosamine incorporation in fully activated macrophages cultured in the presence of sensitive lymphocytes and tuberculin. It should be pointed out, however, that the dose of PPD used in these experiments (0.1 μg/ml) was close to that producing maximal macrophage activation.

DISCUSSION

Recently, studies describing stimulation of the immune response by diverse biologic (1,11,19,21) and chemical (5,7,14) means have been reported. Agents capable of enhancing host defense mechanisms would be a valuable adjunct to the management of an increasing population of immunologically compromised individuals.

LMS has received considerable attention in this regard particularly as its use in man has been associated with only minor toxicity. Many studies related to the immunostimulatory effects of this compound have been conducted in animal models (8,9,22). Clinical studies in man (10,23) have shown some immune enhancement by LMS in patients with cancer. Most of the *in vitro* studies with human cells have utilized lymphocyte proliferation. In this regard, some workers have reported augmentation of lymphocyte proliferation (3,17), whereas others have found no such effect with LMS (6). Although some data suggest that LMS enhances phagocytic cell function in animal cells (15), little information is available regarding the effect of this drug on human mononuclear phagocytes.

Our investigation into the effects of LMS on human lymphocyte proliferation confirms augmentation with suboptimal antigen or mitogen concentration but only with low doses of LMS. It is possible that a biphasic-dose response to LMS could have been elicited if concentrations higher than 20 μg/ml were used.

Our findings also indicate that LMS directly enhances phagocytosis of latex particles by normal human macrophages. In our lymphocyte-free system phagocytosis was stimulated optimally at a LMS dose of 5 μg/ml, a concentration that inhibited lymphocyte proliferation. Interestingly, similar doses of LMS enhanced glucosamine uptake by macrophages cultured in the presence of unstimulated lymphocytes but did not affect macrophages fully activated by antigen-stimulated lymphocytes.

These studies do not establish the mechanism of LMS-mediated immunopotentiation in man. As has been previously noted, morphologic changes in LMS-treated macrophages were not detected in these experiments. It is of interest to note, however, that the 48- to 72-hr lag period required for phagocytic enhancement is similar to that required for the activation of macrophages by immunologic means (20). Our preliminary studies, as well as those of Hammond et al., suggest that glucosamine is incorporated into macrophage membrane. This would suggest that phagocytic enhancement induced by LMS was brought about by membrane activation and that this can be produced directly and independently of lymphokines. Whether LMS-induced changes in lymphokine production affected glucosamine uptake in some of our experiments is uncertain and is under study in our laboratory.

These studies do demonstrate that LMS may act on more than one point in the immune response. They also suggest that the optimal dose of drug required for enhancement may depend on the cell system under investigation. The fact that enhancement was detected in only a proportion of our healthy donors raises questions about whether immune reactive cells of suppressed individuals can be similarly stimulated; it is indeed possible that the optimal dose of drug for this group may differ significantly from that required for normal persons. Careful *in vitro* observation may aid in the elucidation of the mechanism of action of this agent.

ACKNOWLEDGMENT

The technical assistance of V. Currid is gratefully acknowledged. Most of the studies reported here were supported by the United States Public Health

Services Research Grant AI-01254–18 and Training Grant AI-00005–15. Part of these studies were supported by the Medical Research Service of the Veterans Administration.

REFERENCES

1. Adlam, C., and Scott, M. T. (1973): Lymphoreticular stimulatory properties of *Corynebacterium parvum* and related bacteria. *J. Med. Microbiol.,* 6:261–274.
2. Al-Ibrahim, M. S., Chandra, R., Kishore, R., Valentine, F. T., and Lawrence, H. S. (1976): A micro-method for evaluating the phagocytic activity of human macrophages by ingestion of radio-labelled polystyrene particles. *J. Immunol. Methods,* 10:207–218.
3. Al-Ibrahim, M. S., Holzman, R. S., and Lawrence, H. S. (1977): Concentrations required for enhanced proliferation of human lymphocytes and phagocytosis by macrophages. *J. Infect. Dis.,* 135:517–523.
4. Boyum, A. (1968): Separation of leukocytes from blood and bone marrow. *Scand. J. Clin. Lab. Invest.,* 21 (Suppl. 97): 77–89.
5. Collavo, D., Finco, B., and Chiecco-Bianchi, L. (1972): Immune reactivity following poly I-poly C treatment in mice. *Nature (New Biol.),* 237:154–155.
6. Copeland, D., Stewart, T., and Harris, J. (1974): Effect of levamisole (NSC—177023) on *in vitro* human lymphocyte transformation. *Career Chemother. Rep.,* 58:167–170.
7. Diamantstein, T., and Wagner, B. (1973): The use of polyanions to break immunological tolerance. *Nature (New Biol.),* 241:117.
8. Fischer, G. W., Oi, V. T., Kelly, J. L., Podgore, J. K., Bass, J. W., Wagner, F. S., and Gordon, B. L. II (1974): Enhancement of host defense mechanisms against gram-positive pyogenic ioccal infections with levo-tetramisole (levamisole) in neonatal rats. *Ann. Allergy,* 33:193–198.
9. Fischer, G. W., Podgore, J. K., Bass, J. W., Kelly, J. L., and Kobayashi, G. Y. (1975): Enhanced host defense mechanisms with levamisole in suckling rats. *J. Infect. Dis.,* 132:578–581.
10. Glogau, R., Spitler, L., Helms, D., O'Connor, R., Olsen, J., Ostler, J., Silverman, S., and Smolin, G. (1975): Clinical and immunologic effects of levamisole. *Clin. Res.,* 23:291 A.
11. Gutterman, J. U., Mavligit, G., Reed, R., Richman, S., McBride, C. E., and Hersh, E. M. (1975): Immunology and immunotherapy of human-malignant melanoma: Historical review and perspectives for the future. *Semin. Oncol.,* 2:155–174.
12. Hammond, M. E., and Dvorak, H. F. (1972): Antigen-induced stimulation of glucosamine incorporation by guinea-pig peritoneal macrophages in delayed hypersensitivity. *J. Exp. Med.,* 136:1518–1532.
13. Hammond, M., Selvaggio, S. S., and Dvorak, H. E. (1975): Antigen-enhanced glucosamine incorporation by peritoneal macrophages in cell-mediated hypersensitivity. *J. Immunol.,* 115:914–921.
14. Hirsch, M. S., Black, P. H., Wood, M. L., and Monaco, A. P. (1972): Effects of pyrancopolymer on oncogenic virus infections in immunosuppressed hosts. *J. Immunol.,* 108:1312-1318.
15. Hoebeke, J., and Franchi, G. (1973): Influence of tetramisole and its optical isomers on the mononuclear phagocytic system. *J. Reticuloendothel. Soc.,* 14:317–323.
16. Hoover, D. L., and Al-Ibrahim, M. S. (1976): Measurement and clinical correlation of immunologic activation of human macrophages *in vitro (manuscript in preparation).*
17. Lichtenfeld, J. L., Desner, M., Mardinery, M., and Wiernik, P. H. (1974): Augmentation of lymphocyte transformation with levamisole. *Fed. Proc.,* 33:790.
18. Lowry, O. H., Rosebrough, N. J., Farr, A. L., and Randall, R. J. (1951): Protein measurement with the folin-phenol reagent. *J. Biol. Chem.,* 193:265–275.
19. Meltzer, M. S., Tucker, R. W., Sanford, K. K., and Leonard, E. J. (1975): Interaction of BCG-activated macrophages with neoplastic and non-neoplastic cell lines *in vitro:* Quantitation of the cytotoxic reaction by release of tritiated thymidine from prelabeled layer cells. *J. Natl. Cancer Inst.,* 54:1177–1184.
20. Nathan, C. F., Remold, H. G., and David, J. R. (1971): Alterations of macrophage functions by mediators from lymphocytes. *J. Exp. Med.,* 133:1356–1376.

21. O'Neill, G., Henderson, D. C., and White, R. G. (1973): The role of anerobic coryneforms on specific and nonspecific immunological responses. *Immunology,* 24:977–995.
22. Renoux, G., and Renoux, M. (1974): Modulation of immune reactivity by phenylimidathiazole salts in mice immunized with sheep red blood cells. *J. Immunol.,* 113:779–790.
23. Tripodi, D., Parks, L. C., and Brugmans, J. N. (1973): Drug-induced restoration of cutaneous delayed hypersensitivity in anergic patients with cancer. *N. Engl. J. Med.,* 289:354–357.

Immune Modulation and Control of Neoplasia by Adjuvant Therapy, edited by M. A. Chirigos. Raven Press, New York, 1978.

Chemoimmunotherapy of Human Malignant Lymphoma with Levamisole: Induction of Lymphocytotoxic Antibodies and Differential Effect on Accidental Infections

R. Mertelsmann, S. B. Ellis, *R. Schwerdt, and *H. Hildebrandt

*Memorial Sloan-Kettering Cancer Center, New York, New York 10021; and * Universitäts-Krankenhaus Eppendorf, Hamburg, Federal Republic of Germany*

Levamisole, a low-molecular-weight synthetic antihelminthic used in many countries for both humans and animals (61) with few untoward side effects (8,30) was later shown to enhance immune responses in laboratory animals to bacterial (49,52), xenogeneic erythrocyte (53,54), and histocompatibility (50,54) antigens. Although the exact mechanism of action still remains unknown (58), the available data suggest that the amplification of immune responsiveness by levamisole is based on T cell activation (54). As a result, levamisole has attracted widespread interest as an agent that may stimulate cell-mediated immune responses to tumors without severe and dangerous side effects. Promising observations regarding remission induction and survival have been made in laboratory animals with both solid tumors (19,51) and leukemia (13,43). In clinical trials, the drug has been shown to increase cutaneous delayed hypersensitivity (29,63) and to enhance E-rosette formation *in vivo* and *in vitro* (36,48) in anergic patients with cancer. Moreover, levamisole has been reported to prolong the disease-free interval and to increase survival time after radiotherapy in patients with stage III carcinoma of the breast (55). In chemoimmunotherapy of disseminated breast cancer, levamisole has been shown to be as effective as BCG with prolongation of the disease-free interval and survival time (23). After primary resection of bronchiogenic carcinomas, a favorable influence of levamisole has been reported regarding disease-free interval and distant recurrences (4).

Clinical improvement after levamisole has also been observed in a variety of nonneoplastic conditions with proved or suspected suppression of the cell-mediated immune response, such as recurrent aphthous ulceration and rheumatic diseases (62).

However, there are some conflicting reports that show that the drug has no effect on *in vitro* lymphocyte responses (14) and no effect on some animal tumor models (44). Also, in human malignancies several of the reported findings regarding cutaneous delayed hypersensitivity and other immune parameters have not been confirmed by other investigators (17,22,33,69).

Untoward effects of levamisole appear to be rare in cancer patients (3), but a number of recent reports about severe, in some cases lethal, granulocytopenias associated with levamisole (6,56,57) do stress the importance of a careful multi-parameter analysis to reveal unexpected (65) and potentially harmful side effects in patients receiving levamisole. In view of the subjectiveness of many of the immunological and clinical parameters, a double-blind trial is, in our opinion, essential for the further clinical evaluation of this drug.

We report in this chapter the results of double-blind evaluation of levamisole in chemoimmunotherapy of human malignant lymphomas. The lymphoprolifera-tive disorders appeared to us most suitable for a clinical evaluation because of:

1. The promising results reported in Hodgkin's disease (29,48) and in immu-noblastic lymphadenopathy (7,18);
2. The standardized chemotherapeutic regimens used in most centers allowing direct comparison with future observations by other investigators;
3. An average survival of more than 6 months to allow the evaluation of possible long-term effects of levamisole.

Furthermore, the study of levamisole in malignant lymphomas, which are associated with certain deficiencies of the immune response, might contribute to our understanding of the mode of action of this drug.

In view of recent reports of a favorable effect of levamisole on bone marrow restoration after chemotherapy (31), this study was also carried out to evaluate levamisole regarding a possible reduction of the myelosuppression and immuno-suppression associated with intensive chemotherapy (21).

PATIENTS AND METHODS

Patients and Clinical Evaluation

Consecutive patients with Hodgkin's disease (HD), non-Hodgkin's malignant lymphomas (NHL), chronic lymphocytic leukemia (CLL), and multiple mye-loma (MM), scheduled to receive chemotherapy at the I. Medizinische Universi-tätsklinik, Hamburg, Germany, were entered into the study. In addition, four patients with soft tissue sarcomas (STS), receiving the same chemotherapy as patients with NHL, were included, assuming that this chemotherapy (see below) would dominate the clinical picture for the 6-month period of study. Standard informed consent was obtained from all patients. Patents were asked to keep a daily record of body temperature, infections, and other observations possibly related to levamisole. Patients were seen at 4-week intervals by the investigators for physical examination, assessment of quality of life (Karnofsky scale), and routine laboratory investigations (complete blood count, bone marrow aspiration when necessary, ESR, serum protein and electrophoresis, serum iron and copper, alkaline phosphatase, γ-glutamyl transferase, SGOT, SGPT, LDH, and other studies as required).

Chemotherapy and Levamisole

Levamisole or placebo was given under strict double-blind conditions. Patients received levamisole (or placebo) at a dose of 3×50 mg on 2 consecutive days each week (4) for 6 months.

Cyclic chemotherapy for HD stage III, IV was as described by DeVita et al. (COPP; 16). Patients with HD refractory to COPP and patients with NHL stage III, IV and with STS stage II, III (45) received a combination of adriamycin (60 mg/m^2, day 1, 8), cyclophosphamide (650 mg/m^2, day 1, 8), oncovin (1.4 mg/m^2, day 1, 8) and prednisone (40 mg/m^2, day 1 to 14)(CHOP) applied in 4-week cycles $\times$ 6, similar to the COPP regimen.

CLL stage 0 (47) received no chemotherapy; stages I to III were treated with chlorambucil (0.6 mg/kg, every 4 weeks) and prednisone (0.8 mg/kg day 1 to 14, 0.4 mg/kg day 15 to 28 of each cycle with subsequent reductions if possible). Patients with MM were treated with melphalan (0.15 mg/kg, day 1 to 7) and prednisone (1.2 mg/kg, day 1 to 14, 0.8 mg/kg day 15 to 28). Low-dose melphalan (0.05 mg/kg) and prednisone (0.2 mg/kg) were continued after 4 to 6 weeks and doses subsequently adjusted as necessary.

Some patients also received local radiotherapy during the study period.

Skin Tests

Cutaneous delayed hypersensitivity (25) was studied at 0, 3, and 6 months by intradermal injection of 0.05 ml *Candida* vaccine (Behringwerke) and 35 units of streptokinase-streptodornase (SKSD, "Varidase®," Lederle) and by use of the Tine Test (Behringwerke). The skin was assessed at 24 and 48 hr and rated as follows 0 = no induration (IND), $\leq$ 0.5 cm inflammation (INF); 1+ = 0.5 cm IND, 0.6 to 2 cm INF; 2+ = 0.6 to 2 cm IND, 2 to 4 cm INF; 3+ = > 2 cm IND, > 4 cm INF; 4+ = vesicle formation.

E-Rosettes

All patients were studied for E-rosette-forming cells prior to receiving levamisole or placebo, and after 3 and 6 months. In addition, patients receiving chemotherapy according to the COPP or CHOP regimen were studied weekly during one 4-week cycle. Lymphocytes were separated on a Ficoll-Hypaque gradient (10); 10^6 isolated and washed mononuclear cells in 0.5 ml of 5% human albumin—50 mM Tris-HCl pH 7.4—0.9% NaCl were added to 0.3 ml of twice washed, pelleted sheep red blood cells (SRBC), centrifuged for 5 min at 50 *g*, and subsequently incubated for 12 hr at 0°C (24). After gentle resuspension, E-rosette-forming cells were counted using an interference phase contrast microscope (Nomarksi optics, Leitz). Cells with 1 to 2 SRBC and $\geq$ 3 SRBC attached were counted separately. Viability of lymphocytes was determined by trypan blue exclusion. Monocytes were defined by ingestion of latex particles. Calculations of absolute numbers of E-rosette-forming cells were based on lymphocyte percentages of differential counts of stained blood smears.

Lymphocytotoxic Antibodies

Sera were studied for the presence of lymphocytotoxic antibodies using the two-step microlymphocytotoxicity assay described for HLA-tissue typing (35). This technique allows demonstration of complement-activated antibodies. The assay for lymphocytotoxic autoantibodies was essentially the same, using autologous lymphocytes in place of the donor panel.

Statistical Methods

Computer-assisted data analysis was performed using an online version of the Statistical Package for the Social Sciences (39). Relationships between categorical variables (sex, diagnosis, etc.) were explored using a crosstabulation technique that employs either the chi-square statistic or Fisher's exact probability ratio as the test of significance (5). Possible differences between the levamisole and control groups in continuous variables (age, survival times, etc.) were examined using the F ratio to check for different variances and the two-tailed Student's t statistic (5) to check for different sample means.

RESULTS

Group Composition

A total of 43 patients were entered into the study. One patient with STS had to be excluded because of a rapidly fatal course. One patient was lost to follow-up. Twenty-one patients (nine male, 12 female) received levamisole, 20 patients (11 male, nine female) placebo. Mean age for the placebo group was 54.8, and for the levamisole group, 56.0 years. Statistical analysis did not show any significant differences between groups regarding diagnosis, year of first diagnosis, stage, therapy, number of this remission-inducing therapy, age, sex, and weight. Diagnoses and chemotherapeutic regimens were equally distributed between groups.

Response to Therapy

Up to now (14 to 19 months of observation after start of levamisole or placebo), five deaths have occurred in each group. Analysis of the clinical course, cause of death, and other parameters has not revealed any significant differences between groups. Detailed statistical analysis of all 41 patients and separate analysis of those still alive have not revealed differences regarding: (a) remission status achieved, (b) survival time from diagnosis, (c) survival time from the beginning of this remission-inducing therapy, (d) Karnofsky index and weight at 0, 3, and 6 months, and (e) changes in the Karnofsky index and weight between 0 to 3, 3 to 6, and 0 to 6 months of levamisole or placebo therapy. Separate analysis of subgroups according to chemotherapeutic regimen, diagnosis, and sex has also failed to reveal significant differences between patients receiving levamisole or placebo regarding the above-mentioned parameters.

Accidental Infections

Infections were defined as 3 days with temperature $> 38.5°C$, plus clinical or bacteriological evidence, or both, of infection. Table 1 shows the number of infections per month according to therapy and diagnosis. Patients receiving combination chemotherapy according to the COPP or CHOP regimen tended to have a lower infection rate in the levamisole group, whereas the opposite observation was made in patients receiving alkylating agents and prednisone.

TABLE 1. *Number of infections per month by therapy and diagnosis*

	Levamisole		Placebo		Total	
	N	mean	*N*	mean	*N*	mean
Therapy						
COPP	5	1.3	2	1.7	7	1.4
CHOP	6	1.3	4	2.1	10	1.6
Alkylating agents	6	1.0	5	0.47	11	0.77
Radiotherapy	1	1.0	7	1.2	8	1.1
Diagnosis						
HD	5	1.3	5	1.8	10	1.6
NHL	5	1.1	5	1.2	10	1.1
HD + NL						
All	10	1.2	10	1.5	20	1.4
Chemotherapy	9	1.2	5	2.1	14	1.5[a]
STS	2	1.7	1	1.2	3	1.5
MM	4	0.9	3	0.51	7	0.73
CLL						
All	5	1.4	6	0.88	11	1.1
Chemotherapy	2	1.2	1	0.67	3	1.0
Radiotherapy	1	1.0	3	1.2	4	1.2
No therapy	2	1.9	2	0.46	4	1.2
CLL + MM						
All	9	1.2	9	0.75	18	0.97
Without radiotherapy	8	1.2	6	0.52	14	0.91[b]

[a] $p = 0.056$.
[b] $p = 0.050$.

When patients are grouped according to diagnosis, patients with HD and NHL have a lower infection rate in the levamisole group. This finding approaches statistical significance at the 0.05 level if only those patients with HD or NHL who received combination chemotherapy (COPP + CHOP) during the study period are considered. On the other hand, patients with CLL and MM tend to have a higher infection rate in the levamisole group. Combined analysis of both diagnostic groups after exclusion of patients receiving radiotherapy demonstrates this difference to be statistically significant ($p = 0.050$). The trend to more frequent infections in the levamisole group does seem to be similar for patients with CLL or MM who received chemotherapy or no therapy other than levamisole or placebo.

Cutaneous Delayed Hypersensitivity

Cutaneous delayed hypersensitivity before and after 3 to 6 months of levamisole or placebo was compared in 39 patients. The findings are summarized in Table 2, which shows the percentages of patients with: (a) an increased reaction, (b) no change—showing the same positive reaction as initially, (c) no change—remaining negative, and (d) a decreased reaction against the antigens used. Comparing all patients, no difference is seen between the levamisole and placebo group. Five of nine patients with HD or NHL receiving combination chemotherapy and levamisole showed an increased hypersensitivity reaction as compared to one of five in the placebo group whereas levamisole does not seem to affect cutaneous delayed hypersensitivity in patients with CLL or MM.

Analysis of skin test reactivity according to cycle day in patients receiving COPP or CHOP showed a marked decrease until the 26th day (data not shown). No differences were found between levamisole and placebo.

Separate analysis of each antigen does not give additional information. In one patient, a flare-up phenomenon was observed after ingestion of levamisole at the site of a previously performed, then negative, Tine Test.

TABLE 2. *Comparison of delayed cutaneous hypersensitivity before and after 3 to 6 months of levamisole or placebo*

Diagnosis N	Levamisole			Placebo		
	All 20	HD + NHL[a] 9	CLL + MM[b] 7	All 18	HD + NHL[a] 5	CLL + MM[b] 5
Percent						
Increased	50	56	57	44	20	50
No change, pos.	15	0	14	33	0	50
No change, neg.	10	33	29	11	40	0
Decreased	25	11	0	11	40	0

[a]CHOP + COPP, only.
[b]Without radiotherapy.

E-Rosettes, Leukocyte and Lymphocyte Counts

Combined analysis of all patients does not show any significant differences between the levamisole and placebo groups regarding leukocytes, lymphocytes, E-rosettes with 1 to 2 SRBC or with $\geq$ 3 SRBC, and avital lymphocytes (absolute numbers and percentages). Table 3 shows the counts of total leukocytes (WBC), lymphocytes, and E-rosette-forming cells (with $\geq$ 3 SRBC attached), before and while receiving (3 to 6 months) levamisole/placebo, according to diagnosis. The only significant difference found between the levamisole and placebo group is the percentage of E-rosette-forming cells in patients with CLL after initiation of chemoimmunotherapy ($p = 0.017$). In MM, HD, and NHL, no obvious differences are visible between the levamisole and placebo groups regarding percentages and absolute counts of lymphocytes and E-rosette-forming cells. However, there tends to be a more pronounced fall of the WBC counts following chemotherapy in patients with CLL, HD, and NHL in the levamisole group.

Analysis of data according to cycle day for HD and NHL receiving COPP or CHOP demonstrates a more profound and longer depression of the WBC count in patients receiving levamisole (data not shown). Between days 15 and 26 of the cycle, the WBC count in the placebo group has recovered (7,000/mm^3), whereas it reaches its lowest value (3,800/mm^3, $p = 0.035$) in the levamisole group at this point. This is, however, followed by a fast recovery, reaching 12,300 WBC/mm^3 in the levamisole group before the next cycle of chemotherapy

TABLE 3. *E-rosettes, leukocyte and lymphocyte counts (mean values)*

	Levamisole		Placebo	
	0 mo	1–6 mo	0 mo	1–6 mo
CLL				
WBC/mm³ (X10⁻³)	21.0	9.5	28.9	20.5
Lymphocytes (%)	72	74	71	76
E-rosettes (%)	31	34[a]	26	15[a]
Lymph./mm³ (X10⁻³)	17.4	7.8	24.4	17.2
E-ros./mm³ (X10⁻³)	2.3	1.7	3.2	1.5
MM				
WBC/mm³ (X10⁻³)	4.5	4.7	4.6	5.0
Lymphocytes (%)	23	16	23	23
E-rosettes (%)	37	36	32	41
Lymph./mm³ (X10⁻³)	1.0	0.7	1.1	1.1
E-ros./mm³ (X10⁻³)	0.4	0.3	0.3	0.4
HD + NHL[b]				
WBC/mm³ (X10⁻³)	12.6	5.0	8.0	5.6
Lymphocytes (%)	26	26	24	23
E-rosettes (%)	31	37	50	47
Lymph./mm³ (X10⁻³)	3.4	1.8	1.6	1.3
E-ros./mm³ (X10⁻³)	1.1	0.4	0.7	0.6

[a] $p = 0.017$; p for all other values > 0.1.
[b] Receiving CHOP or COPP.

as compared to 9,600 WBC/mm³ in the placebo group (not significant). Separate analyses of the percentages and absolute numbers of avital lymphocytes and E-rosettes with 1 to 2 SRBC reveal, as the only difference, a higher number (absolute and percent) of avital lymphocytes in the second 2 weeks of each cycle in the levamisole group (10 as compared to 5%, $p = 0.030$).

Lymphocytotoxic Antibodies

No differences between the placebo and levamisole group were found regarding Coombs' test and agglutinating thrombocyte and lymphocyte antibodies. However, a striking increase in the number of patients developing lymphocytotoxic antibodies was observed in the levamisole group (Fig. 1). If all patients (with > 2 determinations) who developed antibodies for the first time or showed an

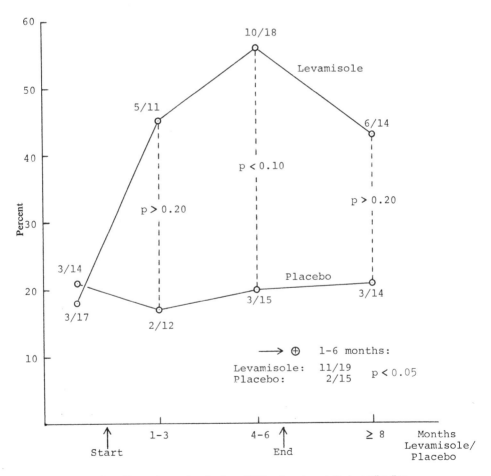

FIG. 1. Percentage of patients exhibiting lymphocytotoxic antibodies.

increase in titer while receiving levamisole (11/19) or placebo (2/15) are considered together, this difference is significant ($p < 0.05$).

The new antibodies appeared after approximately 3 months of levamisole therapy and were no longer detected 4 months after discontinuation of the drug in most patients. After discontinuation of levamisole, no new antibodies were detected in this group, whereas two additional patients in the placebo group developed antibodies after 8 months. Differences in the number of transfusions between groups do not explain the increased presence of lymphocytotoxic antibodies in the levamisole group. Lymphocytotoxic autoantibodies were detected in only two patients in the placebo group who also showed antibodies cytotoxic for heterologous lymphocytes. Antierythrocyte antibodies were not detected in these patients. A lymphocytotoxic activity of autoanti-I or anti-Le^a can therefore be excluded.

Analysis of antibody induction by diagnosis and therapy did not reveal any statistically significant relationships. Patients receiving combination chemotherapy, however, appear to have a higher tendency to develop lymphocytotoxic antibodies in the levamisole group (8/11) compared to the placebo group (2/6).

Clinical Side Effects

The pattern of side effects observed (Table 4) is similar to that described by others (3). Side effects that appear to be more common in the levamisole group

TABLE 4. *Side effects in patients on levamisole and patients on placebo*

Side effect	No. of patients on levamisole	No. of patients on placebo
Gastrointestinal		
Nausea	5	2
Lack of appetite	2	3
Increased appetite	0	1
Vomiting	1	2
Diarrhea	0	1
Aversion to meat	1	0
CNS phenomena		
Fatigue	3	3
Inertia	3	3
Dizziness	1	1
Headache	1	1
Nervousness	3	0
Miscellaneous		
Epigastric pain	1	0
Excessive perspiration	0	1
Prolonged leukopenia	4	2
Severe Coombs'-positive hemolytic anemia	1	0
Interstitial pneumonitis	1	0
Healing of a chronic herpes labialis/genitalis	2	0

include nausea, severe nervousness, and prolonged leukopenia. In one patient each with chronic herpes labialis and genitalis receiving levamisole, healing of long-standing ulcerations was observed after 4 weeks of therapy. Possibly levamisole-related severe side effects included an interstitial pneumonitis (cleared after discontinuation of levamisole) in a patient with CLL needing repeated blood transfusions (see below) and a severe, eventually lethal, therapy-resistant Coombs' positive hemolytic anemia, which developed in this patient 6 weeks after discontinuation of levamisole. No significant differences between groups were observed in all routine laboratory parameters followed.

DISCUSSION

Detailed analysis of both groups has confirmed their random composition and, as a result, their overall comparability. Comparison of all patients in the levamisole group to those receiving placebo did not show any significant differences regarding the parameters tested (clinical and laboratory) apart from the much higher frequency of lymphocytotoxic antibodies in patients receiving levamisole. Since only a few patients received blood transfusions in either group, the possibility of an endogenous sensitization has to be considered, possibly via altered antigenicity of cell structures as a result of cytotoxic therapy or the subsequent degradation of cellular materials, or both. Although it is a rare phenomenon under normal conditions to find leukocyte antibodies in patients without a history of transfusions (9,26,42), patients with hematopoietic tumors in general (42) and especially with malignant lymphoproliferative diseases receiving cytoreductive therapy (32), do show a higher frequency of autoimmune complications directed against blood cells. Leukocyte-agglutinating antibodies (38,67) were not observed with higher frequency in the levamisole group suggesting that the antibodies induced by chemoimmunotherapy with levamisole were lymphocyte specific.

The titers of lymphocytotoxic antibodies observed were low in all our patients, and no clinical side effects could be attributed to these antibodies. The observation of pulmonary infiltrates in one patient on levamisole after blood transfusions, which cleared after discontinuation of levamisole, might have been caused by a leukoagglutinin transfusion reaction (68).

Analysis of the incidence of lymphocytotoxic antibodies by subgroups (therapy, diagnosis) demonstrated the highest incidence in patients receiving combination chemotherapy and levamisole. Since this group showed a lower incidence of infections compared to the placebo group, a negative effect on the immune response exerted by these lymphocytotoxic antibodies does not appear probable. Although a clinical relevance of these lymphocytotoxic antibodies still has not been demonstrated, caution seems necessary when giving levamisole to patients where lymphocyte or leukocyte antibodies might have a harmful effect on the clinical course, such as in patients with repeated transfusion requirements (11) and in bone marrow transplantation candidates (34, 59).

The general observations by other investigators regarding increased cutaneous delayed hypersensitivity (29,63) and increased rosette formation (29,36,48) in most patients with various malignant diseases receiving levamisole have not been confirmed under the conditions of our study. A significantly higher percentage of E-rosette-forming cells was observed in patients with CLL only. A positive, although not significant, effect on skin test reactivity was only detected in patients with HD and NHL.

One of the unexpected findings of our study was the differential effect of levamisole on the infection rate in HD and NHL, on the one hand, and on CLL and MM, on the other hand. HD and NHL patients receiving combination chemotherapy and levamisole exhibited a lower infection rate compared to patients receiving chemotherapy and placebo, whereas CLL and MM showed a higher infection rate in the levamisole group. In these comparisons the more mature B cell lymphomas (CLL + MM; 1,20,46,60) being treated with alkylating agents were considered together. Similarly, HD and NHL, comprising more immature cell proliferations of B cell or of so far undetermined lineage (2,12, 27,40) and treated with comparable chemotherapeutic regimens, were grouped together.

Since patients with STS receiving the same chemotherapeutic regimen as patients with NHL and with HD resistant to COPP did not show this trend, whereas patients with CLL receiving chemotherapy or no cytoreductive therapy behaved similarly regarding infection rates, the diagnosis appears to be a more important factor than therapy in determining the effect of levamisole on infection rate. Even though the small number of patients does not allow any further analysis, the significant increase in infection rate in the CLL + MM group warrants careful multiparameter controls when evaluating levamisole in these patients. Our data strongly suggest that levamisole is a useful adjunct to intensive chemotherapy in HD and NHL to reduce the incidence of the sometimes life-threatening accidental infections caused by bone marrow or immunosuppression, or both.

No definite explanation for this differential effect of levamisole on infection rates can be given so far. The fact that levamisole is effective in patients severely immunosuppressed by intensive chemotherapy (21) suggests that this effect is mediated via macrophages, which are much more resistant than lymphocytes to chemotherapeutic agents. The enhancement of phagocytosis by macrophages (41) and granulocytes (15) is a well-documented effect of levamisole. Since macrophages do exert an important regulatory role in hematopoiesis (37) and are an integral part of the immune system (64), increased phagocytosis most probably reflects only one effect of levamisole on macrophages. The more pronounced bone marrow depression followed by a more rapid recovery in patients receiving COPP or CHOP and levamisole as compared to the placebo group, suggests a more actively proliferating bone marrow that, as a result, is more sensitive to chemotherapy, but also recovers more quickly. Similar clinical observations have been reported (31). Since infection rate in these patients is mainly a result of bone marrow depression, this explanation might be pertinent to the reduced infection rate observed in patients receiving levamisole and intensive chemotherapy. In agreement with this interpretation are the observations by Verhaegen et al. (66) about the effect of levamisole in cyclic neutropenia.

The preferential induction of lymphocytotoxic antibodies in patients receiving COPP or CHOP and levamisole, suggests an additional effect on antibody production, possibly by affecting antigen processing by macrophages. The abundant quantity of antigens derived from destroyed normal and malignant lymphocytes in these patients receiving intensive chemotherapy in addition to an activation of the macrophage system could be responsible for the induction of lymphocytotoxic antibodies. Since the antibody response is severely impaired in CLL and MM and leukocytopenia does not dominate the clinical course using the therapy described, this could be one of the reasons why levamisole does not exert a favorable influence on infection rates in patients with CLL and MM. It can only be speculated why levamisole increases infection rates under these circumstances. One explanation could be that macrophages needed for other functions in hematopoiesis or the immune system, or both, are diverted to activities for which functioning responder cells are not present.

No influence of levamisole on the response to therapy, remission duration, or survival, could be demonstrated in our study for any subgroup. After further follow-up the data will be repeatedly analyzed. Serious clinical side effects to be unequivocally attributed to levamisole were not observed.

Although our observations do need confirmation in a larger trial, our study has demonstrated: (a) a significantly increased incidence of lymphocytotoxic antibodies, (b) an increased incidence of accidental infections in CLL and MM, and (c) a decreased incidence of accidental infections in HD and NHL in patients receiving chemoimmunotherapy with levamisole. In our opinion, more phase I-type double-blind studies with multiparameter analysis including clinical parameters in addition to immunological parameters are necessary before entering larger trials. In this way a faster and more accurate definition of the indications and, possibly, unexpected contraindications for levamisole in human malignant diseases will be achieved.

REFERENCES

1. Aisenberg, A. C., and Block, K. J. (1972): Immunoglobulins on the surface of neoplastic lymphocytes. *N. Engl. J. Med.,* 287:272–276.
2. Aisenberg, A. C., and Long, J. C. (1975): Lymphocyte characteristics in malignant lymphoma. *Am. J. Med.,* 58:300–306.
3. Amery, W. (1975): Levamisole. *Lancet,* 1:574.
4. Amery, W. K. (1976): Double-blind levamisole trial in resectable lung cancer. *Ann. NY Acad. Sci.,* 277:260–268.
5. Armitage, P. (1974): *Statistical Methods in Medical Research.* Wiley, New York.
6. Benoist, M., Pollak, Y., and Bloch-Michel, H. (1976): A new case of agranulocytosis in association with rheumatoid arthritis treated with levamisole. *Nouv. Press Med.,* 5:2474–2475.
7. Bensa, J. C., Faure J., Martin, H., Sotto, J.-J., and Schaerer, R. (1976): Levamisole in angio-immunoblastic lymphadenopathy. *Lancet,* 1:1081.

8. Bouyer, C. (1970): Traitement des parasitoses intestinales par le levamisole. *Bull. Soc. Pathol. Exot.,* 63:255–260.
9. Boxer, L. A., Greenberg, M. S., Boxer, G. J., and Stossel, T. P. (1975): Autoimmune neutropenia. *N. Engl. J. Med.,* 293:748–753.
10. Böyum, A. (1968): Isolation of mononuclear cells and granulocytes from human blood. *Scand. J. Lab. Clin. Invest.,* Suppl. 21:77–89.
11. Brittingham, T. E., and Chaplin, H. (1975): Febrile transfusion reactions caused by sensitivity to donor leukocytes and platelets. *JAMA,* 165:819–825.
12. Bukowski, R. M., Noguchi, S., Hewlett, J. S., and Deodhar, S. (1976): Lymphocyte subpopulations in Hodgkin's disease. *Am. J. Clin. Pathol.,* 65:31–39.
13. Chirigos, M. A., Pearson, J. W., and Pryor, J. (1973): Augmentation of chemotherapeutically induced remission of a murine leukemia by a chemical immunoadjuvant. *Cancer Res.,* 33:2615–2618.
14. Copeland, D., Stewart, T., and Harris, J. (1974): Effect of levamisole (NSC-177023) on *in vitro* human lymphocyte transformation. *Cancer Chemother. Rep.,* 58:(Part 1): 167–170.
15. De Crée, J., Verhaegen, H., De Cock, W., Van Huele, R., Brugmans, J., and Schuerman, V. (1974): Impaired neutrophil phagocytosis. *Lancet,* 2:294–295.
16. DeVita, V. T., Serpick, A. A., and Carbone, P. P. (1970): Combination chemotherapy in the treatment of advanced Hodgkin's disease. *Ann. Intern. Med.,* 73:881–896.
17. Drochmans, A. (1973): *Levamisole in Anergic Patients with Hodgkin's Disease.* Janssen Clinical Research Report, Serial No. R 12564/13. Janssen Pharmaceutica, Beerse.
18. Ellegaard, J., and Boesen, A. M. (1976): Restoration of defective cellular immunity by levamisole in a patient with immunoblastic lymphadenopathy. *Scand. J. Haematol.,* 17:36–43.
19. Gordon, D. S., Hall, L. S., and McDougal, J. S. (1977): Levamisole and cytoxan in a murine tumor model: *In vivo* and *in vitro* studies. In: *Control of Neoplasia by Modulation of the Immune System. (Progress in Cancer Research and Therapy, Volume 2.),* edited by M.A. Chirigos, pp. 121–133. Raven Press, New York.
20. Hämmerling, U., Chin, A. F., and Abbott, J. (1976): Ontogeny of murine B-lymphocytes: Sequence of B-cell differentiation from surface-immunoglobulin-negative precursors to plasma cells. *Proc. Natl. Acad. Sci. USA,* 73:2008–2012.
21. Harris, J., Sengar, D., Stewart, T., and Hyslop, D. (1976): The effect of immunosuppressive chemotherapy on immune function in patients with malignant disease. *Cancer,* 37:1058–1069.
22. Hirshaut, Y., Pinsky, C. M., Wanebo, H. J., and Oettgen, H. F. (1976): Design of Phase-I trials of immunopotentiators for cancer therapy: Levamisole and Corynebacterium parvum. *Ann. NY Acad. Sci.,* 277:252–259.
23. Hortobagyi, G. N., Gutterman, J. U., Blumenschein, G. R., Tashima, C. K., Buzdar, A.U., and Hersh, E. M. (1978): *This volume.*
24. International Union of Immunological Societies (IUIS), Report—July, 1974 (1975): Identification, enumeration and isolation of B and T lymphocytes from human peripheral blood. *Clin. Immunol. Immunopathol.,* 3:584–597.
25. Kopersztych, S., Rezkallah, M. T., Miki, S. S., Naspitz, C. K., and Mendes, N. F. (1976): Cell-mediated immunity in patients with carcinoma. Correlation between clinical stage and immunocompetence. *Cancer,* 38:1149–1154.
26. Lalezari, P., Jiang, A.-F., Yegen, L., and Santorineou, M. (1975): Chronic autoimmune neutropenia due to anti-NA2 antibody. *N. Engl. J. Med.,* 293:744–747.
27. Leech, J. H., Glick, A. D., Waldron, J. A., Flexner, J. M., Horn, R. G., and Collins, R. D. (1975): Malignant lymphoma of follicular center origin in man. I. Immunologic studies. *J. Natl. Cancer Inst.,* 54:11–21.
28. Lehner, T., Wilton, J. M. A., and Ivany, L. (1976): Double blind cross-over trial of levamisole in recurrent aphthous ulceration. *Lancet,* 2:926–929.
29. Levo, Y., Rotter, V., and Ramot, B. (1975): Restoration of cellular immune response by levamisole in patients with Hodgkin's disease. *Biomedicine,* 23:198–200.
30. Lionel, N. D. N., Mirando, E. H., Nanayakkara, J., and Soysa, P. E. (1969): Levamisole in the treatment of ascariasis in children. *Br. Med. J.,* 4:340–341.
31. Lods, J. C., Dujardin, P., and Halpern, G. M. (1976): Levamisole and bone marrow restoration after chemotherapy. *Lancet,* 1:548.
32. Ludwin, D., Sacks, P., Lynch, S., Jacobs, P., Bezwoda, W., and Bothwell, T. H. (1974): Autoimmune complications occurring during the treatment of malignant lymphoproliferative diseases. *South Africa Med. J.,* 48:2143–2145.

33. Marx, J. L. (1976): Cancer immunotherapy: Focus on the drug levamisole. *Science,* 192:57.
34. Mathe, G., Schwarzenberg, L., Amiel, J. L., Schneider, M., Cattan, A., Schlumberger, J. R., Tubiana, M., and Lalanne, Cl. (1967): Immunogenetic and immunological problems of allogeneic haematopoietic radio-chimaeras in man. *Scand. J. Haematol.,* 4:193–216.
35. Mittal, K. K., Mickey, M. R., Singal, D. P., and Terasaki, P. I. (1968): Serotyping for homotransplantation. 18. Refinement of microdroplet lymphocyte cytotoxicity test. *Transplantation,* 6:913–927.
36. Moncada-Gonzalez, B., Rodriguez-Escobedo, M. L., and Castanedo de Alba, J. P. (1976): Effect of levamisole on E rosettes. *N. Engl. J. Med.,* 295:230.
37. Moore, M. A. S. (1976): Regulatory role of macrophages in haemopoiesis. *J. Reticuloendothel. Soc.,* 20:89–91.
38. Neop, A. G., Gunay, U., Boxer, L. A., and Honig, G. R. (1975): Autoimmune neutropenia in an infant. *J. Pediatr.,* 87:251–254.
39. Nie, N., Hull, C., Jenkins, J., Steinbrenner, K., and Bent, D. (1975): *Statistical Package for the Social Sciences,* 2nd ed. McGraw-Hill, New York.
40. Noguchi, S., Bukowski, R., Deodhar, S., and Hewlett, J. S. (1976): T and B lymphocytes in non-Hodgkin's lymphoma. *Cancer,* 37:2247–2254.
41. Oliveira, L. A., Javierre, M. Q., Dias da Silva, W., and Sette Camara, D. (1974): Immunological phagocytosis: Effects of drugs on phosphodiesterase activity. *Experientia,* 30:945–946.
42. Payne, R. (1957): Leukocyte agglutinins in human sera. *Arch. Intern. Med.,* 99:587–606.
43. Perk, K., Chirigos, M. A., Fuhrman, F., and Pettigrew, H. (1975): Some aspects of host response to levamisole after chemotherapy in a murine leukemia. *J. Natl. Cancer Inst.,* 54:253–256.
44. Potter, C. W., Carr, I., Jennings, R., Rees, R. C., McGinty, F., and Richardson, V. M. (1974): Levamisole inactive in the treatment of four animal tumors. *Nature,* 249:567–569.
45. Pratt, C. B., Hustu, H. O., Fleming, I. D., and Pinkel, D. (1972): Coordinated treatment of childhood rhabdomyosarcoma with surgery, radiotherapy, and combination chemotherapy. *Cancer Res.,* 32:606–610.
46. Preud'homme, J. L., and Seligmann, M. (1972): Surface bound immunoglobulins as a cell marker in human lymphoproliferative diseases. *Blood,* 40:777–794.
47. Roi, K. R., Sawitsky, A., Cronkite, E. P., Chanana, A. D., Levy, R. N., and Pasternack, B. S. (1975): Clinical staging of chronic lymphocytic leukemia. *Blood,* 46:219–234.
48. Ramot, B., Bimiaminov, M., Shoham, Ch., and Rosenthal, E. (1976): Effect of levamisole on E-rosette-forming cells *in vivo* and *in vitro* in Hodgkin's disease. *N. Engl. J. Med.,* 294:809–811.
49. Renoux, G., and Renoux, M. (1971): Effet immunostimulant d'un imidothiazole dans l'immunisation des souris contre l'infection par Brucella abortus. *CR Acad. Sci.,* 272D:349–350.
50. Renoux, G., and Renoux, M. (1972): Action du phenylimidothiazole (tetramisole) sus la réaction du greffon contre l'hôte. *CR Acad. Sci.,* 274D:3320–3323.
51. Renoux, G., and Renoux, M. (1972): Levamisole inhibits and cures a solid malignant tumor and its pulmonary metastases in mice. *Nature* [New Biol.], 240:217–218.
52. Renoux, G., and Renoux, M. (1973): Stimulation of anti-Brucella vaccination in mice by tetramisole, a phenylimidothiazole salt. *Infect. Immun.,* 8:544–548.
53. Renoux, G., and Renoux, M. (1974): Modulation of immune reactivity by phenylimidothiazole salts in mice immunized by sheep red blood cells. *J. Immunol.,* 113:779–790.
54. Renoux, G., Renoux, M., Teller, M. N., McMahon, S., and Guillaumin, J. M. (1976): Potentiation of T-cell mediated immunity by levamisole. *Clin. Exp. Immunol.,* 25:288–296.
55. Rojas, A. F., Mickiewicz, E., Feierstein, J. N., Glait, H., and Olivari, A. J. (1976): Levamisole in advanced human breast cancer. *Lancet,* 1:211–215.
56. Rosenthal, M., Trabert, U., and Müller, W. (1976): Leucocytotoxic effect of levamisole. *Lancet,* 1:369.
57. Ruuskanen, O., Remes, M., Mäkelä, A.-L., Isomäki, H., and Toivanen, A. (1976): Levamisole and agranulocytosis. *Lancet,* 2:958–959.
58. Sampson, D., and Lui, A. (1976): The effect of levamisole on cell-mediated immunity and suppressor cell function. *Cancer Res.,* 36:952–955.
59. Storb, R., Thomas, E. D., Buckner, C. D., Clift, R. A., Johnson, F.-L., Fefer, A., Glucksberg, H., Giblett, E. R., Lerner, K. G., and Neiman, P. (1974): Allogeneic marrow grafting for treatment of aplastic anemia. *Blood,* 43:157–180.
60. Takamashi, J., Old, L. J., and Boyse, E. A. (1970): Surface alloantigens of plasma cells. *J. Exp. Med.,* 131:1325–1341.

61. Thienpoint, D., Vanparijs, O. F. J., Raeymaekers, A. H. M., Vandenberk, J., Demoen, P. J. A., Allewijn, F. T. N., Marsboom, R. P. H., Niemegeers, C. J. E., Schellekens, K. H. L., and Janssen, P. A. J. (1966): Tetramisole, a new potent broad spectrum antihelminthic. *Nature,* 209:1084–1086.

62. Trabert, U., Rosenthal, M., and Müller, W. (1976): The treatment of rheumatic diseases with levamisole, an immunomodulatory agent. *Schweiz. Med. Wochenschr.,* 106:1293–1300.

63. Tripodi, D., Parks, L. C., and Brugmans, J. (1973): Drug induced restoration of cutaneous delayed hypersensitivity in anergic patients with cancer. *N. Engl. J. Med.,* 289:354–357.

64. Turk, J. L. (1975): The role of macrophages—in vitro correlates of delayed hypersensitivity. In: *Delayed Hypersensitivity,* pp. 235–261. American Elsevier, New York.

65. Van Belle, H. (1976): Alkaline phosphatase. 1. Kinetics and inhibition by levamisole of purified isoenzymes from humans. *Clin. Chem.,* 22:972–976.

66. Verhaegen, H., De Crée, J., De Cock, W., and Brugmans, J. (1976): Levamisole treatment of a child with severe aphthous stomatitis and neutropenia. *Postgrad. Med. J.,* 52:511–514.

67. Walford, R. L. (1960): *Leukocyte Antigens and Antibodies,* pp. 20, 24, 56, 66, 135. Grune & Stratton, New York.

68. Ward, H. (1970): Pulmonary infiltrates associated with leuko-agglutinin transfusion reactions. *Ann. Intern. Med.,* 73:689–694.

69. Webster, D. J. T., and Hughes, L. E. (1976): Levamisole-double blind immunological study. *Br. J. Cancer,* 34:319–320.

Immune Modulation and Control of Neoplasia by Adjuvant Therapy, edited by M. A. Chirigos. Raven Press, New York, 1978.

Effects of Levamisole on the E-Rosette Formation of Peripheral Human T Lymphocytes

H. Verhaegen, W. De Cock, J. De Cree, *W. Amery, M. L. Verhaegen-Declercq, and F. Verbruggen

*Clinical Research Unit, St. Bartholomeus, B-2060 Merksem (Antwerp), Belgium; and *Janssen Pharmaceutica, B-2340 Beerse (Antwerp), Belgium*

The sheep red blood cell (SRBC) rosette formation is a convenient technique for detecting T lymphocytes. These E-rosettes are formed by light centrifugation of a mixture of lymphocytes and SRBC after a short incubation at 37°C, followed by an incubation at a low temperature. Using this method the relative number of rosette-forming cells (RFC) is significantly lower in cancer patients with advanced disease than in healthy subjects (5,15,18,26). In a study of 173 cancer patients and 80 healthy subjects we found that the decrease in RFC in cancer patients was stage dependent (42). Levamisole, an antianergic chemotherapeutic agent (33), has been reported to enhance low RFC of patients with immunologic disorders (41) and is currently being investigated for its immunomodulating properties in cancer patients (2,3,30). This study was undertaken to evaluate the *in vivo* and *in vitro* effects of levamisole on RFC of cancer patients and to investigate some possible mechanisms of action of levamisole.

MATERIAL AND METHODS

E-Rosette Test

Mononuclear cells were isolated from heparinized blood on a Ficoll-Isopaque mixture as previously described (41). A 0.25-ml aliquot cell suspension ($2 \cdot 10^6$ cells/ml) was mixed with 0.25 ml of 1% SRBC suspension, incubated for 5 min at 37°C, centrifuged at 700 rpm for 5 min, and then incubated for 1 hr at 0°C. After gentle resuspension RFC were counted in a hemocytometer. Two hundred cells were counted, and lymphocytes binding three or more SRBC were considered positive.

In Vivo Effects of Levamisole on RFC of Cancer Patients

Sixty-two patients with various malignant diseases entered the study. Thirty-four patients received a single dose of 150 mg of levamisole daily for 1 week, and 28 patients were similarly treated with a placebo. The E-rosette test was performed before and after 1 week of treatment.

In Vitro Effects of Levamisole on RFC of Healthy Subjects and Cancer Patients

Mononuclear cells ($2 \cdot 10^6$ cells/ml) of 57 healthy subjects and 62 cancer patients were preincubated for 1 hr at 37°C with hanks' balanced salt solution (HBSS, control cells) or a levamisole solution (endconcentration $3 \cdot 10^{-7}$ M). After this incubation the E-rosette test was performed.

In Vitro Effects of Azathioprine and Levamisole on RFC of Healthy Subjects and Cancer Patients

Peripheral blood was obtained from 15 healthy subjects, 20 cancer patients in remission after surgery, and 21 patients with extended localized or metastatic tumors.

A 0.2-ml aliquot mononuclear cell suspension ($2 \cdot 10^6$ cells/ml) was mixed with (a) 0.4 ml HBSS, (b) 0.2 ml HBSS and 0.2 ml azathioprine (Wellcome, Kent, England, 150 μg/ml), (c) 0.2 ml azathioprine and 0.2 ml levamisole (0.24 μg/ml, 10^{-6} M) and (d) 0.2 ml HBSS and 0.2 ml levamisole. These four mixtures were incubated for 1 hr at 37°C, and the E-rosette test was performed.

In Vitro Effects of Dibutyryl-cyclic AMP and Levamisole on RFC of Healthy Subjects.

Peripheral blood was obtained from 12 healthy subjects. A 0.2-ml aliquot mononuclear cell suspension ($2 \cdot 10^6$ cells/ml) was mixed with (a) 0.4 ml HBSS, (b) 0.2 ml HBSS and 0.2 ml 10^{-3} M dibutyryl-cyclic AMP (db-cAMP) (Sigma, St. Louis, Mo.), (c) 0.2 ml 10^{-3} M db-cAMP and 0.2 ml 10^{-6} M levamisole, and (d) 0.2 ml HBSS and 0.2 ml 10^{-6} M levamisole. After incubation at 37°C for 30 min, the E-rosette test was performed.

In Vitro Effects of Adenosine and Levamisole on RFC of Healthy Subjects

Peripheral blood was obtained from nine healthy subjects. The experimental design was the same as for the db-cAMP experiments. db-cAMP was replaced by 10^{-4} M adenosine (Serra, Heidelberg, Germany).

In Vitro Effects of db-cAMP and Levamisole on the Reappearance of SRBC Receptors on Trypsinized Lymphocytes by Culture

Mononuclear cells of five healthy subjects were treated with 0.05% trypsine (Serra, Heidelberg, Germany) for 30 min. Trypsinization completely abolished the E-rosette formation of T lymphocytes.

After washing with Eagle's medium (MEM, Wellcome Laboratories, Kent, England) supplemented with 10% normal AB serum inactivated at 56°C and absorbed with SRBC (MEMS), trypsinized lymphocytes were resuspended in MEMS to a concentration of $2 \cdot 10^6$ cells/ml. A 0.2-ml aliquot cell suspension was mixed with (a) 0.4 ml MEMS, (b) 0.2 ml MEMS and 0.2 ml 10^{-3} M db-cAMP, (c) 0.2 ml 10^{-3} M db-cAMP and 0.2 ml 10^{-6} M levamisole, and (d) 0.2 ml MEMS and 0.2 ml levamisole. After 12 hr of culture at 37°C the E-rosette test was performed.

STATISTICAL ANALYSIS

Intergroup differences were analyzed by the Mann-Whitney U test (two-tailed) (32).

Intragroup differences were analyzed by the Wilcoxon matched-pairs signed-ranks test (two-tailed) (32).

RESULTS

One week of levamisole therapy did not significantly enhance RFC of the total group of cancer patients. In the control group the mean percentage of RFC was 57.2% in the first test and 58.1% in the second test. In the levamisole-treated group the mean percentage of RFC was 56.5% before treatment and 57.2% after treatment. However when only the patients with low E-rosettes (<50%, being 2 SD lower than the mean percentage RFC of healthy subjects) were considered, levamisole significantly enhanced low E-rosette formation ($p = 0.01$), whereas in the control group the RFC remained low (Fig. 1).

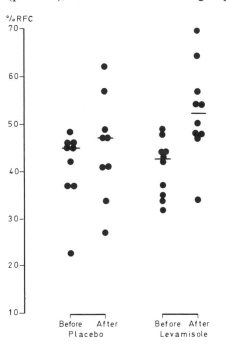

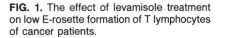

FIG. 1. The effect of levamisole treatment on low E-rosette formation of T lymphocytes of cancer patients.

In vitro treatment of mononuclear cells with 10^{-6} M levamisole significantly enhanced rosette formation of T lymphocytes of both healthy subjects ($p < 0.01$) and cancer patients ($p < 0.05$).

The capacity of T lymphocytes to form rosettes with SRBC was significantly inhibited by azathioprine treatment in healthy subjects ($p < 0.001$) and cancer patients in remission ($p = 0.001$). In contrast, RFC of cancer patients with advanced disease were not inhibited by azathioprine. Intergroup statistical analysis showed that cancer patients with advanced disease significantly differed from healthy subjects ($p = 0.001$) and patients in remission ($p = 0.001$) regarding the azathioprine sensitivity of their T lymphocytes. In Fig. 2 the effect of levamisole on azathioprine-treated T lymphocytes of healthy subjects and cancer patients is represented. The azathioprine-inhibited RFC of healthy subjects could be restored ($p < 0.001$) in all subjects by levamisole. The effects of azathioprine and levamisole on RFC of cancer patients led to three different responses. In 15 patients azathioprine inhibited RFC, and this inhibition could be offset by

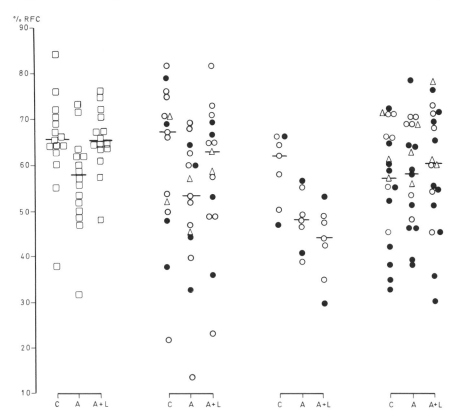

FIG. 2. *In vitro* effects of azathioprine (A) and levamisole (L) on control RFC (C) in 16 healthy subjects and 41 cancer patients, divided into three groups of different response. □, Healthy subjects; ○, cancer patients in remission; △, cancer patients with local tumor; ●, cancer patients with metastatic tumor.

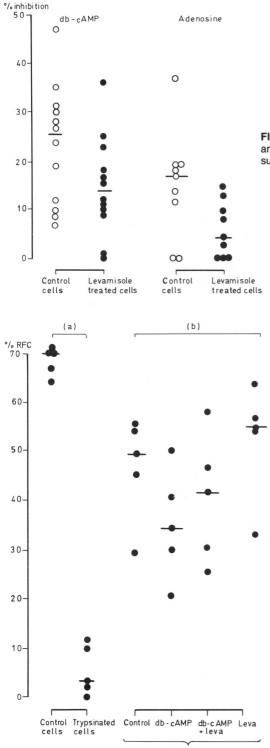

FIG. 3. The inhibition of control RFC and levamisole-treated RFC of healthy subjects by db-cAMP and adenosine.

FIG. 4. a: The effect of trypsine on the RFC of healthy subjects. **b:** The effect of db-cAMP (10^{-3} M) and/or levamisole (10^{-6} M) on the appearance of SRBC receptors on trypsinated T lymphocytes induced by culture conditions.

levamisole, and in seven patients the azathioprine-inhibited RFC could not be restored by levamisole; the other 19 patients had no azathioprine-sensitive RFC. The distribution of patients according to the three different responses and arranged according to the stage of the disease is shown in the same figure.

RFC of healthy subjects were significantly inhibited by 10^{-3} M db-cAMP ($p < 0.001$) and 10^{-4} M adenosine ($p = 0.001$). Levamisole significantly restored db-cAMP-inhibited RFC ($p = 0.001$) and also adenosine-inhibited RFC ($p < 0.001$). The difference between the effect of db-cAMP or adenosine on control RFC and on levamisole-treated RFC was compared in order to evaluate whether levamisole could interfere with the effects of db-cAMP or adenosine. As shown in Fig. 3, levamisole-treated RFC were significantly less sensitive to inhibition by db-cAMP ($p < 0.05$) and by adenosine ($p < 0.05$) than control cells.

SRBC receptors partly reappeared on the surface of trypsinated T lymphocytes after a 12-hr culture. db-cAMP inhibited, whereas levamisole stimulated, the reappearance of SRBC receptors on T lymphocytes during culture (Fig. 4).

DISCUSSION

Encouraging results have been obtained with levamisole in the treatment of recurrent aphthous stomatitis (16,21,24,34,38), rheumatoid arthritis (20,29,-31,43), Crohn's disease (9), recurrent infections (36,39), systemic lupus erythematosus (17), and HBAg chronic persistent hepatitis (14), all of them diseases with underlying immunologic abnormalities and with low E-rosette formation a common feature. In some of these diseases we could demonstrate that levamisole enhanced low RFC (41). Available reports (2,3,30) in cancer patients also show promising results of levamisole therapy on the course of the disease. It is of interest that we found low RFC in cancer patients with advanced disease (42), that levamisole ameliorated rosette formation in such patients, and that the better clinical results with levamisole treatment in cancer seemed to occur particularly in those patients who had larger tumor masses before their primary treatment (3). The increase of low RFC by levamisole treatment has also been demonstrated in patients with Hodgkin's disease (10,28).

The mechanism by which levamisole enhances RFC and relieves symptoms of a variety of diseases with underlying immunologic abnormalities is still unknown, but some suggestions based on animal and human experiments can be made. Van Ginckel and Hoebeke (37) showed that levamisole *in vivo* could depress the azathioprine sensitivity of spleen RFC of normal mice and could induce azathioprine sensitivity in spleen RFC of athymic mice. Similar effects have been reported with thymic extracts (13) and drugs that elevate intracellular cAMP levels (6). Our results also showed that levamisole *in vitro* could depress the azathioprine-inhibited peripheral RFC of healthy subjects and cancer patients in remission. The inhibition of RFC by azathioprine is thought to be a measure of the θ-antigenicity of T lymphocytes (7,27); the less T cells are differentiated, the more sensitive they are to azathioprine inhibition. Therefore our results and those of Van Ginckel and Hoebeke (37) suggest that levamisole mimics thymic extracts and drugs that elevate intracellular cAMP levels in inducing T-cell changes that may be a prerequisite for T cell maturation.

On the other hand, the stimulatory effects of levamisole on different immunologic cell functions (4,11,12,22,23,25,35,39,40,44) are opposed to the inhibitory effects of drugs that elevate intracellular cAMP levels, and levamisole has been reported to decrease cAMP levels in mouse lymphocytes (19), human lymphocytes (28), and polymorphonuclear cells (1). Our results, too, clearly showed that levamisole could reverse db-cAMP or adenosine-inhibited RFC of healthy subjects. It seems possible that the influence of levamisole on the cyclic nucleotide metabolism has a dual character dependent on the maturation stage of the cell, increasing intracellular cAMP levels in immature cells and decreasing cAMP levels in fully differentiated cells. A similar dual mechanism has been proposed for the thymic hormone (8) being a potent T cell differentiator that also seems to stimulate peripheral leukocyte functions (G. Goldstein and J. Hadden, *personal communication*).

ACKNOWLEDGMENTS

We are indebted to Drs. A. de Beukelaar and F. Krug, St. Bartholomeus Hospital, Merksem, Antwerp, and to Dr. Ceulemans, H. Familie Hospital, Antwerp, for sending us the patients, to O. Vogels and L. Van der Veken for technical assistance, to J. Dony for statistical analysis, and to H. Vanhove for reviewing the manuscript.

REFERENCES

1. Al-Ibrahim, M. S., Holzman, R. S., and Lawrence, H. S. (1977): Concentrations of levamisole required for enhanced proliferation of human lymphocytes and phagocytosis by macrophages. *J. Infect. Dis.,* 735:517.
2. Amery, W. K. (1975): Immunopotentiation with levamisole in resectable bronchogenic carcinoma: A double-blind controlled trial. *Br. Med. J.,* 3:461.
3. Amery, W. K. (1976): A placebo-controlled levamisole study in resectable lung cancer. *Presented at Int. Mtg. Immunotherapy of Cancer: Present Status of Trials in Man, NIH, Bethesda, Md.*
4. Anderson, R., Glover, A., Koornhof, H. J., and Rabson, P. (1976); *In vitro* stimulation of neutrophil motility by levamisole. Maintenance of cGMP levels in chemotactically stimulated levamisole treated neutrophils. *J. Immunol.,* 117:428.
5. Anthony, H. M., Kirk, J. A., Madsen, K. E., Mason, M. K., and Templeman, G. H. (1975): E and EAC rosetting lymphocytes in patients with carcinoma of bronchus. *Clin. Exp. Immunol.,* 20:29.
6. Bach, M. A., and Bach, J. F. (1973): Studies on thymus products. VI. The effects of cyclic nucleotides and prostaglandins on rosette forming cells. Interactions with thymic factor. *Eur. J. Immunol.,* 3:778.
7. Bach, J. F., Dardenne, M., and Fournier, C. (1969): *In vitro* evaluation of immunosuppressive drugs. *Nature,* 222:998.
8. Basch, R. S., and Goldstein, G. (1975): Antigenic and functional evidence for the *in vitro* inductive activity of thymopoetin (thymin) on thymocyte precursors. *Ann. NY Acad. Sci.,* 244:290.

9. Bertrand, J., Renoux, G., Renoux, M., and Palat, A. (1974): Maladie de Crohn et lévamisole. *Nouv. Presse Med.,* 3:2265.
10. Biniaminov, M., and Ramot, B. (1975): *In vitro* restoration by levamisole of thymus-derived lymphocyte function in Hodgkin's disease. *Lancet,* i:464.
11. Chan, S. H., Lee, S. N., and Simons, M. J. (1976): Levamisole augmentation of lymphocyte hyporesponsiveness to phytohaemagglutinin in patients with pulmonary tuberculosis (39292). *Proc. Soc. Exp. Biol. Med.,* 151:716.
12. Chan, S. H., and Simons, M. J. (1975): Levamisole and lymphocyte responsiveness. *Lancet* i:1246.
13. Dardenne, M., and Bach, J. F. (1973): Studies on thymus products. I. Modification of rosette forming cells by thymic extracts. Determination of the target RFC subpopulation. *Immunology,* 25:343.
14. De Cree, J., Verhaegen, H., De Cock, W., and Brugmans, J. (1974): The effect of levamisole on the immunologic response of HBAg-positive patients. *Digestion,* 10:306.
15. Dellon, A. C., Potvin, C., and Chretien, P. B. (1975): Thymus-dependent lymphocyte levels in bronchogenic carcinoma: Correlations with histology, clinical stage and clinical course after surgical treatment. *Cancer,* 35:687.
16. De Meyer, J., Degraeve, M., Clarysse, J., Deloose, F., and Peremans, W. (1977): Levamisole (R 12564) in aphthous stomatitis: Evaluation of three regimens. *Br. Med. J.,* 1:671.
17. Gordon, B. L., and Keenan, J. P. (1975): The treatment of systemic lupus erythematosus (SLE) with the T-cell immunostimulant drug levamisole: A case report. *Ann. Allergy,* 35:343.
18. Gross, R. L., Latty, A., Williams, E. A., and Newberne, P. M. (1975): Abnormal spontaneous rosette formation and rosette inhibition in lung carcinoma. *N. Engl. J. Med.,* 292:439.
19. Hadden, J. W., Coffey, R. G., Hadden, E. M., Lopez-Corrales, E., and Sunshine, G. H. (1975): Effects of levamisole and imidazole on lymphocyte proliferation and cyclic nucleotide levels. *Cell. Immunol.* 20:98.
20. Huskisson, E. C., Dieppe, P. A., Scott, J., Trapnell, G., Balma, H. W., and Willoughby, D. A. (1976): Immunostimulant therapy with levamisole for RA. *Lancet,* i:393.
21. Lehner, T., Wilton, J. M. A., and Ivanyi, L. (1976): Double-blind cross-over trial of levamisole in recurrent aphthous ulceration. *Lancet,* ii:926.
22. Lichtenfeld, J. J., Desner, M. J., Wiernik, P. H., and Mardiney, M. R. (1976): The modulating effects of levamisole on human lymphocyte response *in vitro. Cancer Treat. Rep.,* 60:571.
23. Lieberman, R., and Hsu, M. (1976): Levamisole-mediated restoration of cellular immunity in peripheral blood lymphocytes of patients with immunodeficiency diseases. *Clin. Immunol. Immunopathol.,* 5:142.
24. Olson, J. A., Nelms, D. A., Silverman, S., and Spitler, L. E. (1976): Levamisole: A new treatment for recurrent aphthous stomatitis. *Oral Surg.,* 41:588.
25. Pike, M. C., and Snyderman, R. (1976): Augmentation of human monocyte chemotactic response by levamisole. *Nature,* 261:136.
26. Potvin, C., Tarpley, J. C., and Chretien, B. (1975): Thymus-derived lymphocytes in patients with solid malignancies. *Clin. Immunol. Immunopathol.,* 3:476.
27. Poulter, L. W., Bradley, N. J., and Turk, J. L. (1974): Differential effect of azathioprine on θ-antigenicity of mouse lymphocytes. *Immunology,* 26:777.
28. Ramot, B., Biniaminov, M., Shoham, Ch., and Rosenthal, E. (1976): The effect of levamisole on E-rosette forming cells *in vivo* and *in vitro* in Hodgkin's disease patients. *N. Engl. J. Med.,* 294:809.
29. Rosenthal, M., Trabert, U., and Müller, W. (1976): The effect of levamisole on peripheral blood lymphocyte subpopulations in patients with rheumatoid arthritis and ankylosing spondylitis. *Clin. Exp. Immunol.,* 25:493.
30. Rojas, A. F., Feierstein, J. N., Mickiewicz, B., Glait, H., and Olivari, A. J. (1976): Levamisole in advanced human breast cancer. *Lancet,* i:211.
31. Schuermans, Y., De Cree, J., Symoens, J., and Verhaegen, H. (1976): Le traitement de la polyarthrite rhumatoide par le levamisole. *Rev. Rhum.,* 43:437.
32. Seigel, S. (1956): *Nonparametric Statistics,* pp. 75–83, 116–127. McGraw-Hill, New York.
33. Symoens, J. (1977): Levamisole, an antianergic chemotherapeutic agent: An overview. In: *Control of Neoplasia by Modulation of the Immune System* edited by M. A. Chirigos, pp. 1–24. Raven Press, New York.
34. Symoens, J., and Brugmans, J. (1974): Treatment of recurrent aphthous stomatitis and herpes with levamisole. *Br. Med. J.,* 4:592.

35. Tripodi, D., Parks, L. C., and Brugmans, J. (1973): Drug-induced restoration of cutaneous delayed hypersensitivity in anergic patients with cancer. *N. Engl. J. Med.,* 289:354.
36. Van Eygen, M., Znamensky, P. Y., Heck, E., and Raeymaekers, I. (1976): Levamisole in prevention of recurrent upper-respiratory-tract infections in children. *Lancet,* i:382.
37. Van Ginckel, R. F., and Hoebeke, J. (1976): Effects of levamisole on spontaneous rosette forming cells in murine spleen. *Eur. J. Immunol.,* 6:305.
38. Verhaegen, H., De Cree, J., and Brugmans, J. (1973): Treatment of aphthous stomatitis. *Lancet,* ii:842.
39. Verhaegen, H., De Cock, W., and De Cree, J. (1976): *In vitro* phagocytosis of *Candida albicans* by peripheral polymorphonuclear neutrophils of patients with recurrent infections. Case reports of serum-dependent abnormalities. *Biomedicine,* 24:164.
40. Verhaegen, H., De Cree, J., De Cock, W., and Verbruggen, F. (1973): Levamisole and the immune response. *N. Engl. J. Med.,* 289:1148.
41. Verhaegen, H., De Cree, J., De Cock, W., and Verbruggen, F. (1977): Restoration by levamisole of low E-rosette forming cells in patients suffering from various diseases. *Clin. Exp. Immunol.,* 27:313.
42. Verhaegen, H., De Cree, J., De Cock, W., and Verbruggen, F. (1977): Total and high affinity rosette forming cells in cancer patients. *(in manuscript).*
43. Veys, E. M., Mielants, H., De Bussere, A., Decrans, L., and Gabriel, P. (1976): Levamisole in rheumatoid arthritis. *Lancet,* i:808.
44. Whitcomb, M. E., Merluzzi, V. J., and Cooperband, S. R. (1976): The effect of levamisole on human lymphocyte mediator production *in vitro. Cell. Immunol.,* 21:272.

Immune Modulation and Control of Neoplasia by Adjuvant Therapy, edited by M. A.
Chirigos. Raven Press, New York, 1978.

Effect of Levamisole on Suckling Rat Spleen Cells: Evidence for Macrophage Regulation

*Gerald W. Fischer, Martin H. Crumrine, Melvin W. Balk, Sandra P. Chang, Yoshitsugi Hokama, Patricia Heu, and S. C. Chou

Department of Pediatrics and Clinical Investigation Service, Tripler Army Medical Center, Honolulu, Hawaii 96819; and Departments of Pathology and Pharmacology, John A. Burns School of Medicine, University of Hawaii, Honolulu, Hawaii 96822

Although levamisole (LMS) has been shown to enhance immunologic re-sponses, little is known about the mechanism by which this is accomplished. Studies in suckling rats have demonstrated that LMS provides protection from lethal challenge with bacterial or viral pathogens (2,4). When LMS was given to animals challenged with *Staphylococcus aureus,* increased neutrophil chemo-taxis and phagocytosis was observed (4), whereas in herpesvirus encephalitis it appeared that cellular immunity was enhanced (2,3). Furthermore, splenec-tomy studies in the herpesvirus model determined that LMS was ineffective in splenectomized animals and demonstrated that spleen cells were necessary for effective LMS therapy (3). The purpose of these studies was to analyze the effect of LMS on suckling rat spleen cells.

MATERIALS AND METHODS

Animals

Ten-day-old Wistar rats were used throughout these studies. The animals were housed in polycarbonate, solid-bottom cages, and the mothers were fed standard laboratory food and water *ad libitum.*

LMS and DNA Synthesis

Levamisole (3.0 mg/kg/dose) was given subcutaneously on days 9 and 10 of life. Two hours after the second LMS dose spleens were removed aseptically and minced in Eagle's Minimum Essential Medium (MEM) with 1 mM glutamine, 10% fetal calf serum, penicillin (100 U/ml), streptomycin (100 µg/

---

* *Present address:* Department of Pediatrics, Uniformed Services University of the Health Sciences Center, Walter Reed Army Medical Center, Washington, D.C. 20012

ml), and buffered to pH 7.4 with NaHCO$_3$. The cell-enriched suspension was washed twice with Hanks balanced salt solution (HBSS). The final cell pellet was suspended in MEM medium and adjusted to a concentration of 2.5 × 10^6 viable mononuclear cells per ml. Culture conditions in sterile 5-ml plastic culture tubes were as follows:

0.2 ml MEM medium
0.1 ml normal adult rat serum
0.05 ml radioisotope:
    DNA studies—2 μCi ^{3}H-thymidine/0.05 ml
    RNA studies—2 μCi ^{3}H-uridine/0.05 ml
0.01 ml cells (2.5 × 10^5 cells/0.1 ml)

Duplicate sets of culture tubes for each spleen cell suspension were tightly capped and incubated at 37°C. After incubation for 30 min, 4, 24, 36, 48, and 72 hr, radioactive uridine or thymidine (1,000 ×) was added to the appropriate tubes. Aliquots of 0.1 ml were pipetted in duplicate onto Whatman filter paper disks and prepared for liquid scintillation counting. Cells from thymus, liver, and peripheral blood were analyzed for tritiated thymidine incorporation in a similar fashion.

In Vitro DNA Studies

Spleens were removed from normal 10-day-old rats, and cell suspensions were prepared as described above. Cultures were incubated with LMS 10.0 μg/ml. Tritiated thymidine incorporation was then analyzed as described for the *in vivo* studies.

Distribution Studies

Pregnant Wistar rats were given a subcutaneous injection of tritiated levamisole (^{3}H-LMS) (10 μCi) approximately 24 hr prior to delivery. One litter was removed prior to delivery for analysis, and one litter delivered spontaneously and was allowed to suckle for 6 to 8 hr. The animals were killed, and tissues were removed immediately after death and analyzed for tissue radioactivity in a liquid scintillation counter.

Tritiated Levamisole

Spleens from 10-day-old suckling rats were removed aseptically and minced in MEM suspension culture medium with 1 mM glutamine, 10% fetal calf serum, penicillin (100 U/ml), and streptomycin (100 μg/ml), and buffered to pH 7.4 with NaHCO$_3$. The cell-enriched suspension was washed twice with HBSS. The final cell pellet was suspended in MEM medium and adjusted to a concentration of 2.5 × 10^6 viable mononuclear cells per ml. A portion of the spleen cells were further fractionated into adherent and nonadherent cells by incubation with glass beads for 10 min with gentle agitation. This separation was carried out before incubation with ^{3}H-LMS for one set of cultures and after incubation with ^{3}H-LMS for another set of cultures. Culture conditions in sterile 5-ml plastic culture tubes were as follows:

0.2 ml MEM medium
0.1 ml normal adult rat serum
0.5 ml radioisotope:
    ^{3}H-LMS—1.0 µCi ^{3}H-LMS (specific activity
        10.7 µCi/mM) 0.05 ml
0.1 ml cells (2.5 × 10⁵ cells/0.1 ml)

Duplicate sets of culture tubes for each spleen cell suspension were tightly capped and incubated at 37°C for the following time periods—10 and 30 min, 1, 6, 16, and 24 hr. After the required incubation period, 1 ml of cold phosphate-buffered saline (PBS) was added to each tube, and the suspensions were immediately centrifuged. The cell pellet was washed in PBS, resuspended in 0.5 ml PBS, and 4 ml Aquasol® (diluting fluid; New England Nuclear, Boston), placed in plastic vials, and counted in the liquid scintillation counter.

RESULTS

Spleen cells from suckling rats treated with LMS had significantly increased incorporation of tritiated thymidine, but tritiated uridine incorporation was not increased (Table 1). Addition of 10 µg/ml of LMS *in vitro* significantly increased DNA synthesis over control values and reached maximal values by 24 hr incubation (Table 1). Thymus, liver, and peripheral blood cells did not show increased DNA synthesis when exposed to LMS (Fig. 1).

Distribution studies with tritiated LMS demonstrated that LMS crossed the placenta and that ^{3}H-LMS was present in the milk in stomachs of suckling rats. Highest levels of ^{3}H-LMS were observed in amniotic fluid, spleen, and brain (Table 2).

Tritiated LMS was associated with both adherent cells[1] (considered macrophages) and nonadherent cells (considered lymphocytes). At 60 min incubation, only 25% of the ^{3}H-LMS was in the lymphocyte cultures, whereas after 6 hr proportionately more lymphocytes had taken up the ^{3}H-LMS, but 64% was still associated with the adherent cells (Fig. 2).

Different patterns of ^{3}H-LMS incorporation were observed when total spleen cell cultures were compared to macrophage-depleted cultures (Fig. 3). The rate of ^{3}H-LMS uptake by lymphocytes in total spleen cell cultures was less than

---

[1] The adherent cells were morphologically macrophages and exhibited phagocytic capabilities. We recognize that small numbers of other cell types such as B lymphocytes may also demonstrate adherence.

TABLE 1. *Effect of levamisole on tritiated thymidine and uridine incorporation in suckling rat spleen cells*

Incorporation (cpm)	Treatment	Animals	Incubation time in hr				
			½	4	24	48	72
Tritiated thymidine	*In Vivo* LMS	7	2,421 ± 415	9,092 ± 1,670	11,356 ± 2,826	9,098 ± 2,324	8,674 ± 1,837[a]
	Control	6	ND	1,201 ± 424	1,752 ± 557	1,623 ± 720	1,780 ± 678
Tritiated uridine	*In Vivo* LMS	9	1,721 ± 413	ND	2,406 ± 732	2,076 ± 871	1,779 ± 108[b]
	Control	6	1,928 ± 283	1,909 ± 322	1,716 ± 376	1,588 ± 406	1,541 ± 245
Tritiated thymidine	*In Vitro* LMS	—	957 ± 46	6,718 ± 203	9,965 ± 680	8,966 ± 705[a]	—
	Control	—	1,144 ± 83	5,191 ± 312	6,145 ± 1,407	7,439 ± 577	—

ND, no data.
[a] Statistically significant differences between LMS and control samples at all time periods.
[b] No significant difference between LMS or control samples.

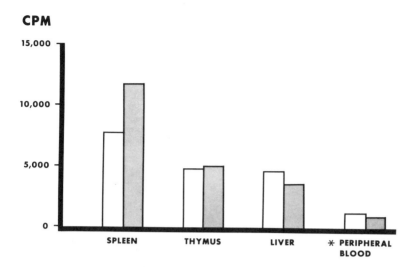

FIG. 1. The effect of levamisole on tritiated thymidine incorporation in suckling rat spleen, thymus, liver, and peripheral blood cells. *, Five-day-old animals; □ control; ■, LMS.

TABLE 2. *Distribution of ³H-LMS in suckling rat and fetal tissues*

Organ	Cmp/mg tissue
Spleen	2.7
Brain	2.0[a]
Kidney	1.5
Milk (stomach)	1.2
Liver	0.002[a]
Lung	0
Amniotic fluid	600[a]

[a]Fetus removed prior to birth.

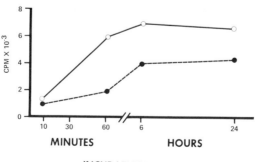

FIG. 2. ³H-LMS labeling of spleen cells from 10-day-old rats demonstrating increased association of LMS with adherent cell population. ○——○, Adherent cells; ●——●, nonadherent cells.

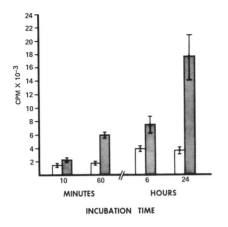

FIG. 3. ^{3}H-LMS uptake by splenic lymphocytes incubated in the presence or absence of macrophages. □, Total spleen cells; ■, macrophage depleted; ⌶, standard error of the mean.

the uptake in macrophage-depleted cultures. When macrophages were removed prior to incubation with ^{3}H-LMS, lymphocytes were rapidly labeled and continued to increase their count to greater than 17,000 cpm. In the presence of macrophages, lymphocyte labeling did not exceed 4,000 cpm.

DISCUSSION

LMS is currently being used to treat patients with a variety of diseases including cancer (11), systemic lupus erythematosus (5), and herpesvirus infections (1). The mechanism of action of LMS, however, remains unknown. Some studies have suggested that LMS primarily affects T lymphocytes in both rodents and man (7,10–12), whereas others propose that the macrophage is of primary importance (6).

Using suckling rats, we have demonstrated that LMS provides protection from both viral and bacterial infections. The present studies indicate that ^{3}H-LMS can be found in the spleen after transplacental and oral acquisition and that spleen cells increase DNA synthesis in the presence of LMS. Although both macrophages and lymphocytes are associated with ^{3}H-LMS, the macrophage appears to become labeled more rapidly and is consistently associated with the majority of the drug. The presence of an excess of ^{3}H-LMS suggests that LMS was available, but that the lymphocyte was regulated by the macrophage in its rate and total amount of LMS incorporation. In macrophage-depleted cultures, ^{3}H-LMS uptake by lymphocytes was significantly increased when compared to lymphocytes incubated with macrophages. These studies strongly suggest that although both lymphocytes and macrophages are associated with LMS, the macrophage is the cell that modulates the ability of LMS to interact with lymphocytes.

Recently we have been studying the effect of LMS on intracellular enzyme systems using *Tetrahymena pyriformis* (a ciliated protozoan) as a potential phagocytic cell model. They have enzyme systems characteristic of most eukaryotic

TABLE 3. *Effect of LMS on DNA and RNA synthesis in* T. pyriformis *nuclei*

Drug inhibitor	Concentration (μg/ml)	Synthesis[a]	
		DNA	RNA
LMS	2	+ 4.5	+216
	10	+ 8.1	+218
	20	+25.8	+200
	50	−19.1	+157
	100	−54.1	+64
DNAase	0.1 (mg/ml)	−70.1	−10
RNAase	0.1 (mg/ml)	− 4.7	−75.9
Actinomycin D	20	—	−39.1

[a]Percent stimulation (+) or inhibitor (−) synthesis when compared to simultaneously evaluated controls.

cells and were initially used to study the effect of LMS on enzyme systems. First, to determine if LMS increased DNA synthesis in these cells as it did in rat spleen cells, isolated *Tetrahymena* nuclei were incubated with various concentrations of LMS (Table 3). Both tritiated uridine and thymidine incorporation were increased with 2, 10, and 20 μg/ml LMS. These data suggested that the action of LMS on *Tetrahymena* nuclei might be comparable to that observed in suckling rat spleen cells and that this might be a suitable cell model for study. In a second study using isolated *Tetrahymena* mitochondria, both inhibition and stimulation of the citric acid cycle were observed with various concentrations of LMS (Table 4). At all levels studied, LMS stimulated the formation of malate and oxaloacetate whereas most other enzymes were inhibited. The citric acid cycle under these circumstances would be nonfunctional, and cellular metabolism would have to proceed via another route. If the effect of LMS resulted in increased efficiency and activity of the hexose monophosphate shunt (HMPS) and the production of hydrogen peroxide, the effect of LMS on phagocytes might be explained since this process is linked to increased neutrophil

TABLE 4. *Effect of levamisole on oxidation of trichloroacetic acid cycle intermediates in* T. pyriformis *mitochondria*[a]

Substrate	LMS (μg/ml)[b]		
	25	50	100
Citrate	− 12	− 12	−19
Isocitrate	− 29	− 27	−62
α-Keto glutarate	+2.8	− 22	+0.9
Succinate	− 16	− 39	−59
Fumarate	+ 72	+ 65	+60
Malate	+136	+103	+82
Oxaloacetate + Acetyl Co-A	−9.4	− 33	−65

[a]Expressed as percent of control value.
[b](+), Stimulation; (−), inhibition.

and macrophage metabolic activity (8) and killing of both microbial agents and tumor cells (9). To determine if the enhanced maturational effect of LMS previously seen in suckling rats was due to stimulation of the HMPS, the effect of LMS on enzymes in immature spleen cells was evaluated. Two- and 5-day-old rats were utilized because a marked increase in protective immunity to bacterial invasion is noted over the first 5 days of life. Two-day-old control rats had low levels of peroxidase activity, whereas 5-day-old controls had increased levels suggesting that with maturation these enzymes do in fact increase (Fig. 4). Levamisole increased the spleen cell peroxidase activity in 2-day-old animals to approximately the level of activity in spleen cells from 5-day-old animals. Levamisole did not further increase peroxidase activity in spleen cells from 5-day-old animals over controls. These *in vitro* observations correlate well with previous *in vivo* studies that showed that 5-day-old animals survived serious bacterial infections, whereas 2-day-old rats could not. These data suggest that at least in part LMS may enhance maturation of phagocytes by stimulating enzyme activity.

In summary, studies in suckling rats suggest that LMS may protect immature animals from viral and bacterial infection by enhancing phagocyte activity. *In vitro* LMS is primarily associated with adherent spleen cells, most probably macrophages, and the macrophage appears to regulate the association of LMS with lymphocytes. Evidence in *Tetrahymena* and suckling rats both suggest that LMS alters cellular metabolism by enzymatic inhibition or stimulation, or both. Stimulation of the HMP shunt with increased peroxidase activity could account for increased phagocyte activity and would allow a single mechanism to explain protection from both bacterial and viral pathogens. Furthermore, these metabolic processes for killing invading microbes have also been shown to be important in killing tumor cells. Future studies are necessary to establish the role of the macrophage in regulating the activity of LMS and to further document the mechanism of action of this drug, but at present it seems quite clear that augmentation of phagocytes is an important effect of LMS therapy.

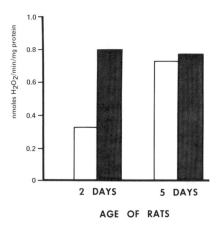

FIG. 4. The effect of LMS on spleen cell peroxidase activity from 2- and 5-day-old rats. □, Control; ■, LMS.

Finally, LMS unquestionably produces effects on lymphocytes, but our studies would suggest that the macrophage is the cell that controls this interaction and may modulate the association of LMS with other cell types as well.

REFERENCES

1. Allen, E. A., Pinnell, S. R., and Tindall, J. P. (1975): Levamisole therapy for recurrent herpes simplex and aphthous stomatitis. *Presented at Am. Acad. Derm., 1975.*
2. Fischer, G. W., Balk, M. W., Crumrine, M. H., and Bass, J. W. (1976): Immunopotentiation and antiviral chemotherapy in a suckling rat model of herpesvirus encephalitis. *J. Infect. Dis.,* Suppl. 133:A217–A220.
3. Fischer, G. W., Crumrine, M. H., Balk, M. W., Chang, S. P., and Hokama, Y. (1976): Immunopotentiation in a herpesvirus model: An overview *(in press).*
4. Fischer, G. W., Podgore, J. K., Bass, J. W., Kelley, J. L., and Kobayashi, G. Y. (1975): Enhanced host defense mechanisms with levamisole in suckling rats. *J. Infect. Dis.,* 132:578–581.
5. Gordon, B. L., and Keenan, J. P. (1975): The treatment of lupus erythematosus with the T-cell immunostimulant drug levamisole: Case report. *Ann. Allergy,* 35:343–355.
6. Larson, J. L. (1975): Levamisole. *Cutis.,* 16:928–930.
7. Lichtenfeld, J. L., Desner, M., Mardineg, M., Fischer, G. W., Crumrine, M. H., Balk, M. W., and Bass, J. W. (1974): Amplification of immunologically induced lymphocyte ^{3}H-thymidine incorporation by levamisole. *Fed. Proc.,* 58:790.
8. Karnovsky, M. L. (1968): Metabolism of leukocytes. *Semin. Hematol.,* 5:156–165.
9. Philpott, G. W., Bower, R. J., and Parker, C. W. (1973): Selective iodination and cytotoxicity of tumor cells with an antibody-enzyme conjugate. *Surgery,* 74:51–58.
10. Ramot, B., Biniaminov, M., Shoham, Ch., and Rosenthal, E. (1976): Effect of levamisole on E-rosette-forming cells *in vivo* and *in vitro* in Hodgkin's disease. *N. Engl. J. Med.,* 294:809–811.
11. Rojas, A. F., Mickiewicz, E., Feierstein, J. N., Glait, H., and Olivari, A. J. (1976): Levamisole in advanced human breast cancer. *Lancet,* 1:211–215.
12. Woods, W. A., Siegal, M. J., and Chirigos, M. A. (1974): *In vitro* stimulation of spleen cells cultures by poly I, poly C, and levamisole. *Cell. Immunol.,* 14:327–331.

Immune Modulation and Control of Neoplasia by Adjuvant Therapy, edited by M. A. Chirigos. Raven Press, New York, 1978.

Effect of Levamisole on an *In Vitro* Model of Cellular Immunity

F. J. Persico and W. A. Potter

Department of Biochemical Research, Ortho Pharmaceutical Corporation, Raritan, New Jersey 08869

The anthelminthic drug tetramisole (13) and its L-isomer levamisole (LMS) have been reported to possess the capacity to stimulate a variety of reactions of an immunological nature (for a review, see ref. 5). Tripodi et al. (14) and Brugmans et al. (6) demonstrated that LMS could restore cutaneous delayed hypersensitivity to dinitrochlorobenzene in cancer patients initially anergic to that agent, suggesting a potential for this drug in the treatment of neoplastic disease. Clinical trials of this agent are in progress (5). It was, therefore, of interest to study the effect of LMS on the lymphocyte-mediated cytotoxic response.

We report herewith a preliminary study demonstrating that LMS can enhance the sensitization of lymphocytes as evidenced by an increased capacity on their part to effect target cell destruction in the efferent phase of an *in vitro* model of cell-mediated immunity.

METHODS AND MATERIALS

The system studied was a modification of the *in vitro* model of cellular immunity described by Feldman et al. (8). Basically, this model involved the sensitization of lymphocytes from the lymph nodes of normal rats to the transplantation antigens of mouse embryo fibroblasts.

Embryo fibroblast cultures were prepared by tryptic digestions of 16- to 19-day-old decapitated, minced embryos of C3HeB/FeJ mice. Primaries were prepared in Waymouth's medium (all media and supplements were obtained from Grand Island Biological Company) supplemented with 20% heat-inactivated calf serum, 20 mM L-glutamine, 100 units/ml penicillin, and 100 μg/ml streptomycin, but all further passages were made in lactalbumin hydrolysate medium [ELH-0.5% lactalbumin hydrolysate in Earle's balanced salt solution, buffered with sodium bicarbonate (pH ~7.5) and with 0.5% phenol red indicator added, supplemented with 5% heat-inactivated calf serum and penicillin-streptomycin solution as above]. In our experience, the fibroblasts should be maintained in ELH for 2 weeks prior to their use in sensitizing lymphocytes.

Fibroblasts destined to be employed for sensitization were treated with mitomycin C (25 μg/ml for 20 min at 37°C) prior to being seeded (8 × 10⁵) in 25 cm² flasks under conditions such that a gradient of cell density was formed in the flask. Since the condition of the monolayers was of primary importance in achieving sensitization (10), the preparation of such a gradient insured that at least some area of the monolayer was appropriate for supporting sensitization.

Lymphocyte suspensions were obtained by expressing the pooled lymph nodes, excised from male Wistar rats, through stainless steel screens into Dulbecco's modified Eagle's medium (EM) supplemented with 20% heat-inactivated horse serum plus penicillin-streptomycin, as above. The lymph node cells were washed and seeded onto the fibroblast monolayers at a concentration of 3.3 × 10⁷ cells per flask. The fibroblast monolayer was then employed as an immunoabsorbent by incubating at 37°C with 10% CO_2 in humidified air for 1 hr in the presence of the lymphocytes. During this period, those lymph node cells that have receptors enabling them to interact with the fibroblast antigens adhere to the monolayer. At the end of the hour period, lymphocytes that had not absorbed to the monolayer were removed and discarded. Altman et al. (1) reported that good separation was achieved at 1 hr, and thus absorption enriched the adherent lymphocyte population with cells that had the capacity to react with the fibroblasts. The flasks were incubated as above for a period of 5 days, with a medium change on the third day as described by Berke et al. (3). It was during this period that the lymphocytes became sensitized and multiplied.

Lymphocyte-mediated cytotoxic effects were assessed by the release of ⁵¹Cr or ³H-proline from appropriately labeled C3HeB/FeJ target fibroblasts in Microtest II plates (Falcon #3040). Labeling with ⁵¹Cr was as described by Berke et al. (3). Labeling with ³H-proline (2) was achieved by growing the cells overnight in the presence of 20 μCi/ml ³H-proline (New England Nuclear) in Eagle's minimal medium supplemented with 15% calf serum, L-glutamine, and penicillin-streptomycin solution as above. After labeling, the fibroblasts were treated with 0.5% trypsin and transferred to the Microtest II plates at a concentration of 10⁴ cells per well per 0.2 ml EM. The cells were incubated overnight to allow for attachment, and then washed three times with fresh EM before use as target cells. The *in vitro* sensitized lymphocytes were removed from the originator monolayers, counted, and their viability (trypan blue exclusion) determined. If good sensitization had been achieved, viability should be in excess of 70%. The lymphocytes were placed in the Microtest II wells at various concentrations to provide a variety of effector-to-target-cell combinations. Cytotoxic effects were assessed after 30 to 48 hr of incubation. Maximum release was determined for each well as the sum of the radioactivity released into the medium plus the bound counts released by treatment with IN NH_4OH. In our hands, in addition to increased convenience, hydrolysis with alkali released more bound counts than three cycles of freezing-thawing. The percent cytotoxicity was calculated as follows:

$$\% \text{ cytotoxicity} = \frac{\text{cytotoxic release-average spontaneous release}}{\text{maximum release-average spontaneous release}} \times 100$$

RESULTS

Figure 1 demonstrated the specificity achieved with this *in vitro* model of cell-mediated immunity. Rat lymphocytes sensitized to C3HeB/FeJ mouse fibro-blast monolayers bearing the H-2^k histocompatibility antigen were capable of producing a significant cytotoxic response when presented with syngeneic target fibroblasts. Thus, a 60% cytotoxic effect was achieved with C3HeB/FeJ target fibroblasts, whereas there was virtually no cytotoxic effect exerted against C57 fibroblasts bearing the H-2^b transplantation antigen. This demonstrated that the *in vitro* reaction was not merely the result of the fact that the mouse fibroblasts were recognized as foreign by rat lymphocytes, but rather that the reaction had the capacity to distinguish between mouse strains. This was in agreement with the results of Berke et al. (4) and was the result of recognition of, and reaction to, the H-2 antigen of the fibroblasts.

The cytotoxic response exerted by the rat lymphocytes was a consequence of their *in vitro* sensitization and was dependent on the effector-to-target-cell

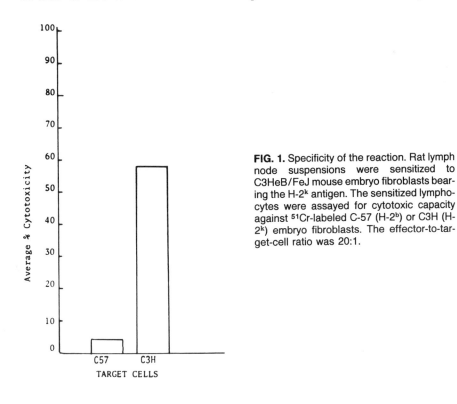

FIG. 1. Specificity of the reaction. Rat lymph node suspensions were sensitized to C3HeB/FeJ mouse embryo fibroblasts bearing the H-2^k antigen. The sensitized lymphocytes were assayed for cytotoxic capacity against ^{51}Cr-labeled C-57 (H-2^b) or C3H (H-2^k) embryo fibroblasts. The effector-to-target-cell ratio was 20:1.

ratio. In the experiment shown in Fig. 2, the cytotoxic effect varied directly with the lymphocyte-to-target-cell ratio. Within the range tested, lymphocyte-mediated cytotoxicity decreased as the ratio of effector to target cells decreased. Furthermore, Fig. 2 demonstrates that lymphocytes must be sensitized to exert significant cytotoxic responses when exposed to labeled target cells at the same ratios that resulted in extensive destruction of target cell monolayers when mediated by *in vitro* sensitized lymphocytes. The slight killing visited by the normal lymphocyte suspensions was most likely the result of sensitization of some of these cells during the 2-day effector phase.

Figure 2 also compared the effectiveness of two types of radioactive labeling

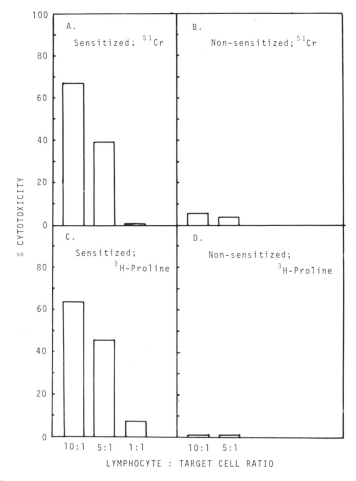

FIG. 2. The requirements for lymphocyte sensitization to achieve target cell destruction. Normal, freshly excised lymphocytes (**B** and **D**) or lymphocytes sensitized *in vitro* to mouse fibroblast antigens (**A** and **C**) were tested at the effector-to-target-cell ratios shown for cytotoxic capacity against embryo fibroblast target cells labeled with either ^{51}Cr (**A** and **B**) or ^{3}H-proline (**C** and **D**).

in this system. ^{3}H-Proline has become the label of choice in this system for two reasons. For one thing, in our hands, it seemed to do better at detecting cytotoxicity at low lymphocyte:target cell ratios, as evidenced by the fact that some radioactive release was detected at the 1:1 ratio with ^{3}H-proline, but none was seen with [51]Cr. Furthermore, nonspecific release, or "noise" seemed to be greater with ^{51}Cr, as shown by greater radioactivity being released when normal lymphocytes were employed in conjunction with this label than when ^{3}H-proline was utilized.

LMS was able to enhance the sensitization of lymphocytes to mouse fibroblasts in this *in vitro* system. As shown in Fig. 3, lymphocytes exposed to LMS in conjunction with the process of their sensitization to fibroblast antigens were able to exert a significantly enhanced killing effect compared to lymphocytes sensitized in the absence of the drug. The enhanced cytotoxic response was evident at all lymphocyte-to-target-cell combinations tested in this experiment, although this was not always so. Our first observations of LMS's ability to enhance the *in vitro* sensitization phase were made when LMS was present

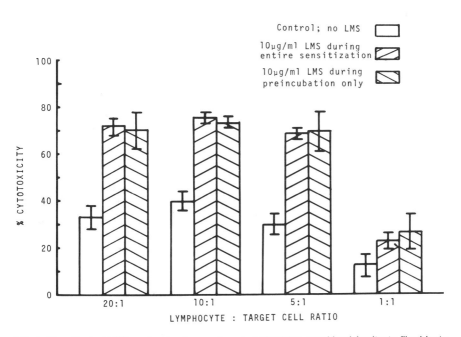

FIG. 3. The effect of LMS on the *in vitro* reaction. Lymphocytes sensitized *in vitro* to fibroblasts either in conjunction with or in the absence of LMS treatment were tested for their ability to mediate target cell destruction at the effector-to-target-cell ratios shown. The lymph node cells were exposed to LMS at a concentration of 10 μg/ml either during a 25-min preincubation or throughout the entire sensitization phase. In the case of preincubation, the cells were washed two times with fresh medium to free them of residual LMS before being seeded on fibroblast monolayers for absorption and sensitization in the absence of drug. The standard deviations are shown.

throughout the 5-day period required for sensitization. Later studies demonstrated that this was not necessary. Thus, in the experiment shown in Fig. 3, treatment of unsensitized lymphocytes with LMS for a brief period (25 min) prior to their exposure to the sensitizing antigens was just as effective in the eventual production of a population of killer lymphocytes as was exposure to the drug during the entire sensitization period. This indicated that, at least in this *in vitro* situation, LMS exerted an effect on the lymphocyte very quickly and without concomitant presence of the antigen.

Figure 4 shows that the effect of LMS on the *in vitro* sensitization of lymph node cells to xenogeneic antigens was dose responsive at a variety of lymphocyte-to-target-cell ratios. The optimal dose appeared to be between 10 and 100 μg/ml. The dose-response curve was bell-shaped, and because of the greater cytotoxic effects achieved at the higher effector-to-target-cell ratios by lymphocytes sensitized in the absence of LMS, the most effective stimulation (approximately fourfold) achieved with LMS in this experiment was seen at the lowest lymphocyte-

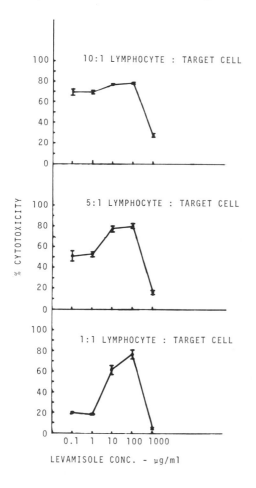

FIG. 4. Dose-response curve. Lymph node cells were preincubated with levamisole at the concentration shown for 25 min before sensitization was initiated. Following sensitization the lymphocytes were tested at various effector:target cell ratios for their ability to lyse ^{3}H-proline-labeled target fibroblasts. Effector cells sensitized in the absence of the drug produced, respectively, 19.1 ± 2.8% and 74.4 ± 3.5% cytotoxicities at 1:1 and 10:1 lymphocyte:target cell ratios, respectively. The standard deviations are shown.

to-target-cell ratio. It is also worth noting that the 1 mg/ml concentration of LMS inhibited sensitization, as evidenced by decreased cytotoxicity in the effector phase. The reason for this is as yet unknown, but the observation was consistent and not a function of decreased viability.

DISCUSSION

Reports of LMS's capacity to restore or augment cell-mediated cytotoxic response have been mixed (e.g., 7, 9, 11, and 12). The present study demonstrates that in a completely *in vitro* model, LMS can enhance the sensitization of suspensions of lymph node cells from normal rats to antigens present on embryo fibroblasts of murine origin. The enhanced sensitization was reflected in the increased destruction of target cells by lymphocytes exposed to the compound either shortly before or during sensitization, compared to that by cells sensitized in its absence. LMS's augmentation of cytotoxicity was most evident when the lymphocyte-to-target-cell ratio was suboptimal; increasing the number of effector cells often resulted in excessive target cell destruction that was not influenced by LMS. Since comparisons of cytotoxic effects by cells sensitized in the presence and absence of LMS were based on the response of equal numbers of effector cells, the augmentation seen in this system appeared to reflect a real increase in killing capacity on the part of the lymphocyte population sensitized in the presence of the drug rather than simply an increase in the number of reactive lymphocytes due to an effect of LMS on lymphoid DNA synthesis (15). Thus, sensitization in the presence of LMS resulted in a greater number of target cells killed per lymphocyte during the effector phase. However, a number of questions remain to be answered.

For one, although this *in vitro* reaction appears to be T cell mediated (1), it has not been demonstrated that such lymphocytes are the direct target for LMS in the augmented reaction. It could be envisioned that the primary effect of LMS is on some auxiliary cell in the system that in turn interacts with the T lymphocyte in some way as to eventually confer on the latter an amplified cytotoxic capacity. Although such a possibility is considered unlikely, it cannot as yet be eliminated.

Furthermore, although it has been demonstrated that this *in vitro* reaction is specific in the absence of the drug, it has not been shown that specificity is retained in the LMS-augmented reaction. Indeed, the possibility exists that the augmented reaction is the result of a drug-induced activation of a population (or subpopulation) of lymph node cells, potentially nonspecific in their cytotoxic capacity, that are quiescent during sensitization in the absence of LMS. The specificity of the reaction in the presence of LMS has to be examined.

Despite the existence of these and other questions, the observation that sensitization to cellular antigens can be augmented by a chemically defined agent is significant in that cytotoxic effects mediated by lymphocytes sensitized to tumor-associated antigens undoubtedly play at least some role in tumor rejection *in vivo*.

SUMMARY

LMS enhances lymph node-derived immunocytes' sensitization to cellular antigens in an *in vitro* system of cell-mediated immunity. The augmentation of sensitization is dose responsive, does not require the concomitant presence of antigen, and is reflected in an increase in lymphocyte-rendered destruction of appropriate target cells.

REFERENCES

1. Altman, A., Cohen, I. R., and Feldman, M. (1973): Normal T-cell receptors for alloantigens. *Cell. Immunol.,* 7:134.
2. Bean, M. A., Pees, H., Rosen, G., and Oettgen, H. F. (1973): Prelabelling target cells with ³H-proline as a method for studying lymphocyte cytotoxicity. *Natl. Cancer Inst. Monogr.,* 23:527.
3. Berke, G., Ax, W., Ginsburg, H., and Feldman, M. (1969): Graft reaction in tissue culture. II. Quantification of the lytic action on mouse fibroblasts by rat lymphocytes sensitized on mouse embryo monolayers. *Immunology,* 16:643.
4. Berke, G., Clark, W. R., and Feldman, M. (1971): *In vitro* induction of a heterograft reaction. Immunological parameters of the sensitization of rat lymphocytes against mouse cells *in vitro.* *Transplantation,* 12:237.
5. Brugmans, J. (1977): The effects of levamisole on host defense mechanisms: A review. *Fogarty Int. Ctr. Proc.,* No. 28:3.
6. Brugmans, J., Schuermans, V., De Cock, W., Thienpont, D., Janssen, P., Verhagen, H., Van Nimmen, L., Louwagie, A. C., and Stevens, E. (1974): Restoration of host defense mechanisms in man by levamisole. *Life Sci.,* 18:1499.
7. Cappel, R., Henry, C., and Thiry, L. (1975): Experimental immunosuppression induced by herpes simplex virus. *Arch. Virol.,* 49:67.
8. Feldman, M., Cohen, I. R., and Wekerle, H. (1972): T-cell mediated immunity *in vitro:* An analysis of antigen recognition and target cell lysis. *Transplant. Rev.,* 12:57.
9. Fidler, I. J., and Spitler, L. E. (1975): Effects of levamisole on *in vivo* and *in vitro* murine host response to syngeneic transplantable tumor. *J. Natl. Cancer Inst.,* 55:1107.
10. Ginsburg, H. (1965): Growth and differentiation of cells of lymphoid origin on embryo cell monolayers. *Wistar Inst. Symp. Monogr.,* 4:21.
11. Montovani, A., and Spreafico, F. (1975): Allogeneic tumor enhancement by levamisole, a new immunostimulatory compound: Studies on cell-mediated immunity and humoral antibody response. *Eur. J. Cancer,* 11:537.
12. Shibata, H. R., Jerry, L. M., Lewis, M. G., Mansell, P. W. A., Cupek, A., and Marquis, G. (1976): Immunotherapy of human malignant melanoma with irradiated tumor cells, oral bacillus calmette-guérin and levamisole. *Ann. NY Acad. Sci.,* 177:355.
13. Thienpont, D., Vanparijs, O. F. J., Raetmaekers, A. H. M., Vanderberk, J., Demoen, P. J. A., Allewijn, F. T. N., Marsboom, R. P. H., Niemegeers, C. J. E., Schellekens, K. H. L., and Janssen, P. A. J. (1966): Tetramisole (R 8299), a new, potent broad spectrum anthelminthic. *Nature,* 209:1084.
14. Tripodi, D., Parks, L.C., Brugmans, J. (1973): Drug induced restoration of cutaneous delayed hypersensitivity in anergic patients with cancer. *N. Engl. J. Med.,* 289:354.
15. Woods, W. A., Siegel, M. J., and Chirigos, M. A. (1974): *In vitro* stimulation of spleen cell cultures by Poly I:Poly C and levamisole. *Cell. Immunol.,* 14:327.

Immune Modulation and Control of Neoplasia by Adjuvant Therapy, edited by M. A. Chirigos. Raven Press, New York, 1978.

Overview of Levamisole Effectiveness in Experimental and Clinical Cancer Studies

Willem K. Amery

Janssen Pharmaceutica, B-2340 Beerse, Belgium

More than 5 years have past since levamisole was first reported to have immunotropic properties (31). During these 5 years, an enormous amount of information has been made available concerning the immunotropic effects both *in vitro* and *in vivo* and concerning the use of this new immunomodulating substance in experimental models of human diseases and in their clinical counterpart. This overview is confined to the *in vivo* use of levamisole in both experimental and clinical cancer. Immunological effects of levamisole treatment in cancer-bearing subjects are beyond the scope of this chapter and are considered only in as far as the available data have been related to the eventual outcome of the disease. It suffices here to call to mind that levamisole behaves as an anti-anergic chemotherapeutic agent that seems to restore the function of mobile cells involved in the host defense mechanisms.

The bulk of material covered in this chapter has been covered at length elsewhere (5), and, therefore, only the main points are expounded here.

LEVAMISOLE IN EXPERIMENTAL CANCERS

No well-established and commonly accepted animal models for cancer immunotherapy are available (8). Also, most investigators who are familiar with this type of research are well aware of the fact that it is often extremely difficult to design a carefully standardized model that yields reproducible results. Some of the reasons for this lack of reproducibility are quite obvious, whereas others are less well known, although not less important. Table 1 is an attempt to summarize the most pertinent variables that may influence the result of cancer immunotherapy models. Although this list is already impressive, it should not be considered to be complete—quite the contrary. In addition, factors related to the investigator may be quite important as well. It is, for example, understandable that most investigators try to cut down expenses by limiting the number of animals used for an experiment, but this usually leads to one of the two following inadequate experimental designs:

1. All animals are treated with the new immunotherapeutic agent, and the results are compared with those of previous experiments. These "historical con-

TABLE 1. *Variables that may affect the outcome of immunotherapy studies in experimental cancer models (as they have been reported to affect the immunity/or the biological behavior, or both, of experimental tumors)*

Factors related to the tumor
  1. Growth rate
  2. Superinfection of inoculate, particularly by viruses (ref. 14)
  3. Macrophage content of inoculate (refs. 15,41)
Factors related to the host
  1. Sex and age (ref. 24)
  2. Intercurrent infections (ref. 21)
  3. Factors related to chronobiological phenomena
      Circadian rhythms may be important relative to the timing (i.e., hour of the day) of tumor inoculation, of first cytoreductive therapy (ref. 19), and of administration of immunotherapy
      Season of the year (ref. 20).
Environmental factors
  1. Stress (refs. 17,20,29,30, and 36)
  2. Room temperature (ref. 20)
  3. Room illumination (ref. 20)
  4. Food composition (refs. 9,23, and 28)
  5. Composition of the room atmosphere (ref. 20)

trols" are inadequate, among other reasons because the factors listed in Table 1 are hardly comparable.

2. Contemporary controls are used, but the number of animals in each treatment group is so low that statistically significant differences can only be expected if dramatic results are produced by the immunotherapy. This, in turn, creates situations in which the same results are considered positive by some (optimistic investigators) and negative by others (pessimistic ones).

To avoid these pitfalls, we decided to separately consider each experiment and label it "positive" as soon as an even small trend in favor of levamisole was found. The rationale and the criticism of this method are discussed elsewhere (5). It is obvious that this optimistic approach overestimates the actual number of positive experiments, but, on the other hand, this would level off existing trends rather than accentuate them.

Figure 1 summarizes the most important findings from our analysis of the data in mice (5). In summary, levamisole appears to be most effective when it is used in a dosage exceeding 2.5 but lower than 10 mg/kg, when slow-growing tumors are studied, when the effect on metastasis formation is chiefly evaluated, and when the drug is used as an adjunct to classic anticancer treatment. Although data from studies in other animal species are scarcer, they tend to confirm the fact that levamisole behaves as an antimetastatic drug and that it is more effective if used in an adjuvant therapeutic setting. In none of these studies was there any evidence that levamisole, if properly used, could enhance tumor growth instead of inhibiting it (5).

One particular experiment (22) may bear special relevance to the clinical treatment of cancer when levamisole is used as an adjunct to the first effective

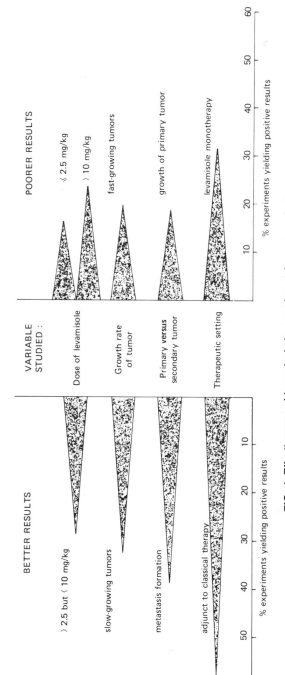

FIG. 1. Effectiveness of levamisole in experimental cancers of mice.

cytoreductive therapy (usually surgery or radiation treatment). Although levamisole monotherapy produced only a marginal prolongation of survival in the slightly allogeneic Fortner's melanotic melanoma no. 1 of Syrian golden hamsters, it induced tumor regression when given to animals showing early local melanoma recurrence following surgical excision; such regressions were observed in two-thirds of the treated animals, and about one-half of these even proved to be tumor free at autopsy. These data, observed in a slightly allogeneic model, suggest that the antimetastatic effects of levamisole reported in syngeneic models are, at least in part, due to the regression of microscopic foci of the disseminated tumor. Extrapolating to the clinic, this would mean that levamisole may be expected to eliminate existing (but clinically undetectable) micrometastases if it is used in combination with the eradication of the primary tumor.

LEVAMISOLE IN CLINICAL CANCERS

Immunology-Prognosis Link-Up

Although several investigators have confirmed the fact that levamisole may restore different aspects of the cellular host defense mechanisms, if these are deficient, in cancer-bearing patients, the effects are usually limited to a certain percentage of the levamisole-treated patients and are not always reproducible (5). There is, however, every reason to continue research in this field in order to delineate the subgroup of patients susceptible to the levamisole effect, and to search for better, i.e., more reliable and reproducible, immunological tests for doing this type of work.

However, in performing immunological evaluations of cancer patients before and after levamisole treatment, we ought not to forget that all of this is meaningless as long as we do not know how these measures correlate with the prognosis of such patients. In other words, inducing immunological changes should not be the goal of levamisole treatment. The goal should be to change the patient's prognosis (through a manipulation of the immunity). If we forget about this aspect, we may be doing nothing more than exercising immunological cosmetics.

Therefore, it is sad to say that so far, only very few investigators have been looking at the prognostic impact of levamisole-induced immunological changes in cancer patients. On the other hand, these small-scale experiences look promising enough to advocate a more thorough exploration of this field. The available experiences are as follows:

1. In a placebo-controlled study (40) on patients with advanced solid cancers, the 2,4-dinitrochlorobenzene (DNCB) reactivity appeared to increase in the group of patients treated with levamisole. There was a parallel improvement of the survival time.

2. In another study (34,35) an increase in reactivity to DNCB and to *Candida albicans* extract was primarily seen in irradiated stage III breast cancer patients who remained free of disease during levamisole maintenance treatment.

3. Also, in patients with intractable cancer, who had been submitted to levamisole therapy, restored lymphocyte reactivity to phytohemagglutinin appeared to be associated with prolonged survival (32,33).

Apart from these reports on clinical cancers, findings in two patients with (angio-) immunoblastic lymphadenopathy—a disease that is on the borderline of the cancer area—have confirmed that immunological amelioration may accompany and even precede clinical amelioration if the patient is treated with levamisole (6,16).

Controlled Clinical Evaluations of the Prognosis of Cancer Patients

Studies Confined to a Single Type of Cancer

So far, four consecutive interim reports (1–3,39) are available concerning the results of an unfinished multicenter study in resectable lung cancer. This is a randomized placebo-controlled double-blind study in which the treatment (levamisole 50 mg or a placebo t.i.d.) is given for 3 consecutive days every fortnight, starting 3 days before surgery and continuing for 2 years or until relapse is documented. The most important and provisional findings from this investigation have been that:

1. The fixed dose of levamisole used in this study is probably not adequate for all patients, as the beneficial effects seem confined to the patients who received a daily dose of 2.1 to 2.8 (median, 2.4) mg/kg, whereas no effect at all is observed in those who have been taking 1.3 to 2.1 (median, 1.9) mg/kg/day. The difference regarding recurrence rates and disease mortality is very significantly in favor of levamisole in the patients who received the higher doses of the drug.

2. The drug proves to be particularly effective in those patients who had a heavier tumor load at the time of surgery.

3. Levamisole seems to be more effective in controlling blood-borne secondary tumors than in affecting intrathoracic relapses. This is illustrated in Fig. 2.

In another double-blind study, still under progress, 132 patients with primary or recurrent malignant melanoma have been randomized to receive placebo or levamisole (a single 150-mg dose for 3 consecutive days every 2 weeks) after surgery. The first interim analysis of the data (37) did not produce any difference between the two treatment groups. However, the patient material breaks up into six clinically and prognostically distinct subgroups, and the investigators insist that this is only a preliminary report that does not allow final conclusions to be drawn as the number of patients followed for a prolonged time is rather low.

One controlled study in irradiated stage III breast cancer has been reported (34,35). After completion of the radiation treatment, the 48 patients were alter-

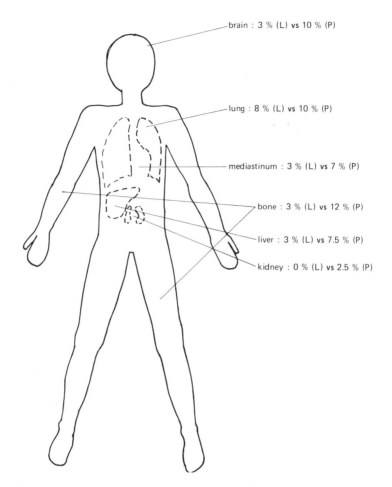

FIG. 2. Sites of first recurrence in adequately dosed patients with resectable lung cancer. L, levamisole-treated patients; P, placebo controls.

nately assigned to either the control group or the levamisole-treated group. The dose of levamisole was 150 mg/day given orally during 3 successive days every fortnight. Forty-three patients (20 treated with levamisole and 23 controls) were evaluable and had been followed for at least 21 months after termination of the radiotherapy. A statistically significant increase of the disease-free interval and of the survival time was associated with levamisole treatment, and this was not due to a bad performance of the controls as the median disease-free interval among the latter (9 months, in contrast to 25 months with levamisole) proved to be very comparable with that of historical controls treated in the same institution. These investigators also evaluated the site and frequency of all metastases in their patients and found an increased incidence of lung metastases in the levamisole-treated patients who had shown a relapse. However, if the incidences of metastatic sites are recalculated and related to the total number of patients studied (instead of to the number of patients showing relapse, as was done by the investigators), a decrease of metastasis formation seems associated with levamisole treatment. This is summarized in Table 2. Lung metastases, however, remain an exception to this rule, but this might be explained by the fact that levamisole should not be expected to antagonize the increased metastasis formation occurring after radiation damage to the lung, as explained elsewhere (4). Recently, the authors made a second analysis of their data after 1 more year of follow-up and found (27) essentially the same type and degree of differences except for local recurrences that had increased more in frequency in the levamisole group than in the controls during the same observation period. Finally, as discussed above, these authors also found that skin test conversion to DNCB and to *C. albicans* during levamisole treatment appeared to be associated with an increased chance of disease-free survival.

Information about the use of levamisole as an adjunct to cytostatic chemotherapy is still scarce, and this for understandable reasons (5). Nevertheless, at least one study has been initiated, and a preliminary interim report is available. This is a double-blind placebo-controlled and randomized study in adult acute myeloid leukemia. After consolidation chemotherapy (given to stabilize the first clinical remission obtained with cytostatic drugs), the patients are maintained on an intermittent cytostatic program (1 week per month). In addition, they are randomized to receive either a placebo or levamisole (2.5 mg/kg daily for 3 consecutive days every other week), but the synchronous use of the double-blind treatment and the cytostatic courses is avoided. When the first interim analysis was performed (7), 24 patients had been randomized and followed for at least 6 months in this study. The median duration of the first complete remission in the placebo-treated group was 10 months, and the percentage of patients still in remission during follow-up, as assessed by the actuarial method, was completely comparable to that of a similar but larger group of patients treated with an almost identical type of cytostatic maintenance therapy (10).

TABLE 2. *Sites of all observed metastases in a stage III breast cancer study*

Site of recurrence[a]	Control group (N = 23)		Levamisole group (N = 20)	
	Actual No.	Percent	Actual No.	Percent
Local relapses	6	26	2	10
Skin	3	13	1	5
Nodes	5	22	2	10
Lungs	4	17	8	40
Bones	8	35	3	15
Liver	4	17	0	0
Other	3	13	1	5
Total[b]	21	91	11	55

[a]Data reported originally by Rojas et al. (34).
[b]Several patients had recurrences in more than one site.

The median duration of the first complete remission in levamisole-treated patients, on the other hand, was 16 months. The difference between placebo and
levamisole was, however, not statistically significant as could be expected in
view of the low number of patients in each group.

Studies Involving Several Malignancies

Levamisole treatment (150 mg daily for 3 successive days every other week)
or no immunotherapy was given in addition to appropriate irradiation to 375
cancer patients referred to a radiotherapy department for an initial treatment
of their disease. The patients are being followed up, regardless of the effect of
the radiation treatment, and mortality is registered. These patients have now
been followed for a maximum period of 4 years (median, 3 years) from the
day of admission to the study. The data obtained during the last analysis (13)
are as follows. A slight difference is found in favor of levamisole as 55% of
the levamisole-treated patients were still alive after 42 months, in contrast to
36% of the controls (percentages calculated by the actuarial method). Also,
the median survival time was not yet reached with levamisole by the 42nd
month and was approximately 33 months in the control population. Moreover,
a favorable trend was consistently present in all types of cancer, except for
lung carcinoma, as shown in Table 3. This may be related to the fact that
lung cancer was, perhaps, the most radioresistant malignancy studied in this
trial as, in animal models, levamisole only helps in stabilizing remission but
not in inducing regression. On the other hand, the most promising results were
obtained in two radiosensitive cancers, i.e., cancer of the breast and head and
neck cancers. Finally, it was found in this study that (Fig. 3) levamisole did
not improve the survival in stages I to III breast cancer patients within the

TABLE 3. *Death rates in a controlled levamisole study*

| | No. of patients included in study | | Percentage of deaths (actuarial method) | | | | | | | |
| | | | ≤6 months | | ≤12 months | | ≤24 months | | ≤36 months | |
Tumor site	R	L	R	L	R	L	R	L	R	L
Breast	62	58	11	3	18	5	24	20	37	25
Head and neck	27	37	7	3	19	17	31	23	82	40
Lung	24	21	42	48	75	76	88	95	92	95
Ovaries and corpus uteri	22	19	14	15	28	26	48	37	48	43
Skin, rectosigmoid, G. U.	22	17	32	30	61	51	71	72	86	79
Blood-forming organs	6	11	17	19	38	27	38	45	79	64
Cervix uteri	16	20	13	5	31	21	38	27	69	27
Musculoskeletal	10	3	10	33	30	33	40	33	50	33
Total	189	186	18	13	34	25	44	38	60	45

R, reference group; L, levamisole.

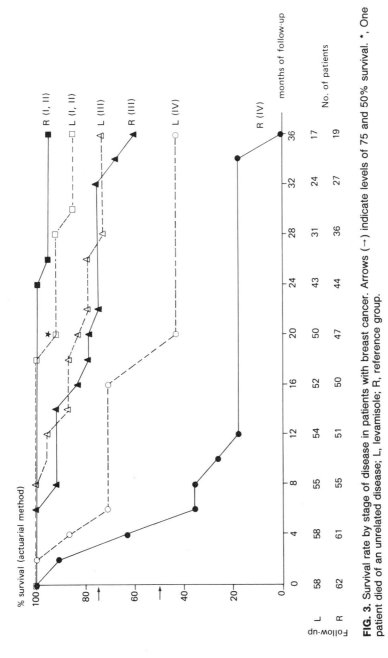

FIG. 3. Survival rate by stage of disease in patients with breast cancer. Arrows (→) indicate levels of 75 and 50% survival. *, One patient died of an unrelated disease; L, levamisole; R, reference group.

first 3 years of the study but that it substantially prolonged survival in stage IV patients.

Lastly, in another multicenter study, all cancer patients, who have just received full remission-inducing cytoreductive therapy, are included without further pre-selection. These patients are then randomized into levamisole therapy (50 mg t.i.d. for 2 consecutive days every week) or placebo treatment, and this double-blind treatment is started as early as possible after the completion of the primary anticancer treatment. At the time of the first analysis (18) 246 patients had been included in the study, but the median duration of follow-up was only 5 months. Nevertheless, more patients (20%) had already died in the placebo group than in the levamisole group (13%), and this trend was present in all five centers where mortality had already occurred. A breakdown of the data according to the tumor type was not (yet) available, however.

CONCLUSIONS

Several clinical data appear to line up with the animal findings:

1. A certain threshold dose of levamisole should probably be exceeded in order to obtain benefit from this type of treatment. This threshold dose in the human being seems to be approximately 2 mg/kg/day (on the treatment days), and, therefore, in future trials, it seems wise to pursue a daily dose of 2.5 mg/kg or about 100 mg/m^2 of body surface.

2. Levamisole seems to inhibit hematogenous dissemination. Therefore, it is recommendable to have the site of the first recurrence carefully registered in future trials; this will probably prove more indicative of a preferential effect on metastasis formation than the total percentage of new foci during the entire course of the disease. On the other hand, an effect of levamisole on local recurrence still seems to be possible, although if there is any, it will probably be less marked.

3. Although the use of levamisole as a monotherapy in clinical cancer has not been discussed in this overview, the bulk of clinical data (5) seem to confirm the animal findings that levamisole should be used as an adjunct to classic anticancer treatment.

On the other hand, the importance of the growth rate of the tumor, discovered through the animal data, has not yet been confirmed in the clinic. However, clinical data may still be too scarce to allow a thorough search into this aspect, and these animal findings are certainly to be kept in mind in discussing future clinical results.

Finally, the clinical experience seems to have added a new hint to our knowledge as it was already found in two independent controlled studies that the better results are obtained in those patients who have a heavier tumor load before eradication of their primary tumor. This may indicate that such patients are better immunized against their tumor or that their immunity is more suppressed by the presence of a more extended cancer.

It now seems appropriate to make a few recommendations for further clinical studies. It is my feeling that the main emphasis should now be put on trials intended to find out whether the apparent trends can be confirmed or not. Therefore, I see every reason to advocate large-scale trials in those clinical cancers that, although still potentially curable at the time of the first treatment, carry a bad prognosis because of their known marked tendency to metastasize and that are, preferably, already locally advanced. The latter would also imply that small skin tumors, such as malignant melanoma, may prove to be a wrong choice, although this cancer is known to readily disseminate. In such conditions, the available information seems to suggest that the levamisole treatment preferably be started before tumor eradication, if surgery is used, but after completion of it when cytostatic drugs are given. The optimal timing for the combination with radiotherapy is not clear, and, perhaps, it may be prudent to start after irradiation has been completed as long as we have no straightforward comparison between the synchronous and the sequential use of radiotherapy and levamisole. The dose of levamisole to be used in such trials has previously been discussed; this daily dose (divided into two to three intakes) is given for either 2 consecutive days every week or 3 successive days every fortnight.

Recommendations for the evaluation of levamisole treatment in other clinical settings are naturally more speculative. It may suffice here to list several possibilities and add a few remarks:

1. There is still a substantial need for a reliable immunological test that can indicate whether the patient is receiving an adequate dose or not and a test that is helpful in defining the categories of patients susceptible to the beneficial effects of the drug. Perhaps, in the latter context, too little attention has been paid to the possibility that levamisole may counteract the effects of immunosuppressive factors such as the immunoregulatory α-globulin or IRA (11,12), the pregnancy-associated α-macroglobulin or PAM (38), and several others. Also, it seems worthwhile to initiate more research on the possible effects of levamisole on the motility of lymphocytes and monocytes in cancer patients.

2. Therapeutic studies in more advanced cancer may also be of interest. However, one should keep in mind the animal data when such studies are designed and analyzed. Indeed, these animal data tend to indicate that levamisole only stabilizes remissions, perhaps also partial remissions, for some time, but that it does not increase the number of responders to cytostatic chemotherapy or irradiation nor the degree of such responses.

On the other hand, some of these studies may provide an opportunity to evaluate the sometimes controversial aspect of the theoretical risk of tumor enhancement by immunotherapy. However, this ought to be studied by reliable measures (as clinical impressions are both unreliable and subject to major doubt).

As far as I know the only reliable measure is the assessment of the doubling time of the tumor.

3. Other studies in advanced cancer may provide an answer to the following questions:

> Does levamisole decrease the incidence of intercurrent infections, and, in that way, perhaps increase survival time?
>
> Do levamisole-treated patients feel subjectively better and can this be measured by, e.g., the Karnofsky scale?
>
> Does levamisole treatment promote bone marrow reconstitution after cytostatic treatment as it has already been claimed (25,26)?

One final remark regarding the dose to be used in studies with levamisole in advanced cancer. The same dose as the one we recommended for "minimal tumor residue" settings may be used. However, higher doses might be necessary if levamisole proves to antagonize, in a competitive way, immunosuppressive serum factors. As this last possibility has not yet been ruled out, there may perhaps be room for initiating a few controlled studies comparing the effects of the usual daily dose, i.e., 100 mg/m^2, with a dose that is somewhat higher, e.g., 150 mg/m^2.

SUMMARY

An overview is given of the available data from experimental and clinical studies with levamisole in cancer. These data indicate that levamisole may prolong life-span and disease-free interval if it is used as an adjunct to tumor eradication by classic anticancer treatment and if its daily dose is adjusted to the weight of the patient or to his body surface. Levamisole may be particularly effective in controlling hematogenous dissemination and will probably prove to be especially useful in those patients who had a heavy tumor load before eradication of their cancer. Finally, recommendations are given for the future studies of levamisole treatment in clinical cancer.

REFERENCES

1. Amery, W. K. (1976): Double-blind levamisole trial in resectable lung cancer. *Ann. NY Acad. Sci.,* 277:260–268.
2. Amery, W. K. (1976): Double-blind trial with levamisole in resectable lung cancer. In: *Proc. 9th Int. Cong. Chemotherapy.* Plenum Publ. New York *(in press).*
3. Amery, W. K. (1976): A placebo-controlled levamisole study in resectable lung cancer. *Presented at the Int. Mtg. Immunotherapy of Cancer: Present Status of Trials in Man, NIH, Bethesda, Md., October 27–29.*
4. Amery, W. K. (1977): Levamisole as an immunotherapeutic agent. *World J. Surg. (in press).*
5. Amery, W. K., Spreafico, F., Rojas, A. F., Denissen, E., and Chirigos, M. A. (1976): Adjuvant treatment with levamisole in cancer. A review of experimental and clinical data. *(in manuscript).*
6. Bensa, J. C., Faure, J., Martin, H., Sotto, J. J., and Schaerer, R. (1976): Levamisole in angio-immunoblastic lymphadenopathy. *Lancet,* i:1081.

7. Brincker, H., Thorling, K., and Jensen, K. B. (1976): Prolongation of the duration of remission in acute myeloid leukaemia (AML) with levamisole. *Presented at the Spring Meeting of Scandinavian Haematologists, Aarhus, June 5.*

8. Carter, S. K. (1976): Immunotherapy in the strategy of cancer treatment. *Cancer Immunol. Immunother.,* 1:115–118.

9. Chandra, R. K. (1975): Antibody formation in first and second generation offspring of nutritionally deprived rats. *Science,* 190:289–290.

10. Clarkson, B. D. (1972): Acute myelocytic leukemia in adults. *Cancer,* 30:1572–1582.

11. Cooperband, S. R., Nimberg, R., Schmid, K., and Mannick, J. A. (1976): Humoral immunosuppressive factors. *Transplant. Proc.,* 8:225–242.

12. Cooperband, S. R., Badger, A. M., and Mannick, J. A. (1976): Nonhormonal serum suppressive factors. In: *Mitogens in Immunobiology,* edited by J. J. Oppenheim & D. L. Rosenstreich, p. 555. Academic Press, New York.

13. Debois, J. M. (1976): *Four-Year Experience with Levamisole in Cancer Patients. Second Interim Report.* Clinical Research Report No. R 12 564/55. Janssen Research Products Information Service.

14. Eaton, M. D., Heller, J. A., and Scala, A. R. (1973): Enhancement of lymphoma cell immunogenicity by infection with nononcogenic virus. *Cancer Res.,* 33:3293–3298.

15. Eccles, S. A., and Alexander, P. (1974): Macrophage content of tumours in relation to metastatic spread and host immune reaction. *Nature,* 250:667–669.

16. Ellegaard, J., and Boesen, A. M. (1976): Restoration of defective cellular immunity by levamisole in a patient with immunoblastic lymphadenopathy. *Scand. J. Haematol.,* 17:36–43.

17. Friedman, S. B., Glasgow, L. A., and Ader, R. (1969): Psychosocial factors modifying host resistance to experimental infections. *Ann. N.Y. Acad. Sci.,* 164:381–392.

18. Grandval, C. M., Bugnard, E., Cardama, E., Estevez, R., Paraskevas, G., Angelakis, Ph., and Thornes, R. D. (1976): *Interim Analysis of Patient Data from Protocol No. R 12 564/066.* Clinical Research Report No. 12 564/47. Janssen Research Products Information Service.

19. Halberg, F., Haus, E., Cardoso, S. S., Scheving, L. E., Kühl, J. F. W., Shiotsuka, R., Rosene, G., Pauly, J. E., Runge, W., Spalding, J. F., Lee, J. K., and Good, R. A. (1973): Toward a chronotherapy of neoplasia: Tolerance of treatment depends upon host rhythms. *Experientia,* 29:909–934.

20. Halle-Pannenko, O., Bourut, C., Martin, M., Stupfel, M., and Moutet, J. P. (1975): L'influence de certains facteurs de l'environnement sur l'état immunitaire de la souris. *J. Physiol. (Paris),* 70:671–672.

21. Hanna, M. G., Jr., Nettesheim, P., Richter, C. B., and Tennant, R. W. (1973): The variable influence of host microflora and intercurrent infection on immunological competence and carcinogenesis. *Isr. J. Med. Sci.,* 9:229–238.

22. Ibrahim, A. B., Triglia, R., Dau, P. C., and Spitler, L. E. (1977): The anti-tumor effects of levamisole on allogeneic hamster melanoma and a syngeneic rat hepatoma. In: *Control of Neoplasia by Modulation of the Immune System,* edited by M. A. Chirigos. Raven Press, New York *(in press).*

23. Jose, D. G., and Good, R. A. (1973): Quantitative effects of nutritional essential amino acid deficiency upon immune responses to tumors in mice. *J. Exp. Med.,* 137:1–9.

24. Lemonde, P. (1974): Ambivalent influence of BCG in malignant conditions. *Presented at the XIth Int. Cancer Congr., Florence, October 20–26.*

25. Lods, J. C., Dujardin, P., and Halpern, G. M. (1976): Levamisole and bone-marrow restoration after chemotherapy. *Lancet,* i:548.

26. Lods, J. C., and Dujardin, P. (1976): Etude clinique expérimentale d'un immunostimulant: Le lévamisole. *Med. Hyg.,* 34:53–55.

27. Olivari, A. J., Rojas, A. F., Feierstein, J. N., and Glait, H. M. (1976): Levamisole action in breast cancer stage III. *Presented at the Int. Mtg. Immunotherapy of Cancer: Present Status of Trials in Man, NIH, Bethesda, Md., October 27–29.*

28. Perper, R. J., Oronsky, A. L., Sanda, M., and Stecher, V. J. (1975): *In vivo* chemotaxis of rat leukocytes in the presence of circulating chylomicrons. *Atherosclerosis,* 22:257–269.

29. Pradhan, S. N., and Ray, P. (1974): Effects of stress on growth of transplanted and induced tumors and their modification by psychotropic drugs. *J. Natl. Cancer Inst.,* 53:1241–1245.

30. Rasmussen, A. F., Jr. (1969): Emotions and immunity. *Ann. NY Acad. Sci.,* 164:458–461.

31. Renoux, G., and Renoux, M. (1971): Effet immunostimulant d'un imidothiazole dans l'immunisation. Des souris contre l'infection par Brucella abortus. *CR Acad. Sci. (Paris),* 272:349–350.

32. Renoux, G., Renoux, M., and Palat, A. (1974): Influences of levamisole on T-cell reactivity and on survival of untractable cancer patients. *Presented at the 1st Conf. Modulation of Host Resistance in the Prevention or Treatment of Induced Neoplasias, NIH, Bethesda, Md., December 9–11.*

33. Renoux, G., and Renoux, M. (1976): Influence de l'administration de lévamisole sur la reactivité des lymphocytes T de cancéreux avancés. *Nouv. Presse Med.,* 5:67–70.

34. Rojas, A. F., Feierstein, J. N., Mickiewicz, E., Glait, H., and Olivari, A. J. (1976): Levamisole in advanced human breast cancer. *Lancet,* i:211–215.

35. Rojas, A. F., Feierstein, J. N., Glait, H. N., Varela, O. A., Pradier, R., and Olivari, A. J. (1976): Clinical action of levamisole and effects of radiotherapy on immune response. In: *Control of Neoplasia by Modulation of the Immune System,* edited by M. A. Chirigos. Raven Press, New York *(in press).*

36. Solomon, G. F. (1969): Emotions, stress, the central nervous system, and immunity. *Ann. NY Acad. Sci.,* 164:335–343.

37. Spitler, L. E., Sagebiel, R. W., Glogau, R. G., Wong, P. P., Malm, T. M., Chase, R. H., and Gonzalez, R. L. (1976): A randomized double-blind trial of adjuvant therapy with levamisole versus placebo in patients with malignant melanoma. *Presented at the Int. Mtg. Immunotherapy of Cancer: Present Status of Trials in Man, NIH, Bethesda, Md., October 27–29.*

38. Stimson, W. (1976): Studies on the immunosuppressive properties of a pregnancy-associated α-macroglobulin. *Clin. Exp. Immunol. (in press).*

39. Study Group for Bronchogenic Carcinoma (1975): Immunopotentiation with levamisole in resectable bronchogenic carcinoma: A double-blind controlled trial. *Br. Med. J.,* 3:461–464.

40. Vandercammen, R., and Bollen, J. (1975): *DNCB-Reactivity, as Related to Survival, in Patients with Advanced Solid Cancers. A Double-Blind Placebo-Controlled Pilot Study with Levamisole.* Clinical Research Report No. R 12 564/24. Janssen Research Products Information Service.

41. Wood, G. W., and Gillespie, G. Y. (1975): Studies on the role of macrophages in regulation of growth and metastasis of murine chemically induced fibrosarcomas. *Int. J. Cancer,* 16:1022–1029.

Immune Modulation and Control of Neoplasia by Adjuvant Therapy, edited by M. A. Chirigos. Raven Press, New York, 1978.

Effect of Levamisole on Cell-Mediated Immunity in Patients with Lung Cancer

E. Carmack Holmes and Sidney H. Golub

Division of Surgical Oncology, UCLA School of Medicine, Los Angeles, California 90024

Defects in cell-mediated immunity have been demonstrated in a variety of cancer patients (2,5,8,10). The degree of impairment appears to be associated with the stage of the disease or the tumor burden. All solid neoplasms are capable of suppressing the immune response to some extent when the tumor burden becomes sufficiently large. However, patients with lung cancer become immunosuppressed earlier in the course of their disease when compared to patients with other solid neoplasms (8). Several studies of lung cancer patients have pointed out that the immunosuppression associated with lung cancer is related to the stage of the disease as well as to resectability and survival (4,8,15). It has been postulated that this immunosuppression associated with lung cancer is related to the highly lethal nature of this disease. Perhaps the correction of these defects in cell-mediated immunity would be associated with an improvement in survival. At least two recent studies have indicated that immunotherapy may, indeed, result in a prolongation of the disease-free interval in patients with resected lung cancer (1,12). In one of these studies levamisole, a new synthetic chemical that can be taken orally, was used. Since the side effects are minimal and it can be taken orally, levamisole is an attractive agent to evaluate as an immunostimulator. For these reasons levamisole has received a great deal of attention in the recent years. Levamisole appears to be capable of increasing antibody production in mice (11). It does prolong chemotherapy-induced remission and overall survival in animal tumor models and is capable of restoring increased T cell levels to normal in patients with Hodgkin's disease (3,13). In addition, previous studies have indicated that levamisole may be effective in increasing delayed cutaneous hypersensitivity reactions in patients with suppressed DCH reactions (14).

In view of the seemingly beneficial effects of levamisole on the disease-free interval in patients with resected lung cancer and of the apparent ability of this agent to augment cell-mediated immunity in certain situations, we designed the present study to evaluate the effects of levamisole on sequentially tested *in vitro* and *in vivo* cell-mediated immunity in lung cancer patients.

MATERIALS AND METHODS

Patients

Patients with all stages of lung cancer were eligible for this study. The only study requirements were that the patients had not received previous immunotherapy or cortisone therapy and they had not received radiation therapy or chemotherapy within 6 weeks of the study. Fifty-six patients were entered into the study, but only 32 were available for evaluation. Some patients chose to withdraw from the study, and the attrition rate of the disease was responsible for the remainder of unevaluable patients. Patients were categorized by the stage of the disease into three categories:

1. Resected patients who were clinically free of disease,
2. Unresectable patients with persistent disease, and
3. Patients with rapidly progressive disease.

Patients were randomized to receive either placebo or levamisole therapy. The levamisole (kindly supplied by Janssen Pharmaceuticals R & D, New Brunswick, New Jersey) was administered daily for 3 days every 2 weeks for a period of 3 months. The daily dosage was 2.5 mg/kg, which was then rounded off to the nearest 50 mg since the tablets were prepared in 50-mg quantities. The patients underwent initial 2,4-dinitrochlorobenzene (DNCB) sensitization and challenge, and lymphocytes were obtained prior to initiation of therapy for base-line *in vitro* lymphocyte studies.

Measurement of Cell-Mediated Immunity

Patients were sensitized to DNCB, and challenged 2 weeks later. After an initial level of reactivity was determined, the patients were then begun on levamisole and were skin tested with DNCB every 2 weeks for a minimum of 90 days. Patients were always skin tested during the 3 day period in which they were receiving oral levamisole.

Patients were tested with DNCB as previously described. First, 2,000 μg of DNCB dissolved in acetone was placed on the medial aspect of the arm. Patients were subsequently challenged with 100, 50, 25, and 12.5 μg of DNCB 14 days later. Reactions were recorded at 48 hr, and at each testing the smallest amount of DNCB that elicited a positive delayed cutaneous hypersensitivity reaction was determined.

In Vitro Lymphocyte Function

Lymphocytes were obtained from the patients prior to treatment at 15, 30, 60, and 90 days. Lymphocytes were then cryopreserved by a technique previously described, and the *in vitro* blastogenesis and mixed lymphocyte culture (MLC) reactions could then be performed on all lymphocyte samples obtained from a single patient on 1 day (7). Twenty-two patients were evaluated with sequential *in vitro* data—eight patients on placebo, and 14 patients receiving levamisole.

Lymphocyte blastogenesis was carried out with freeze-preserved lymphocytes according to the technique previously described (8). The microblastogenesis assay was employed, and all tests were routinely performed in quadruplicate. Lymphocytes from the lung cancer patients were evaluated for the incorporation of tritiated thymidine (blastogenesis) in the presence of the mitogens—phytohemagglutinin, 0.1% (PHA); pokeweed mitogen, 0.1% (PWM); Concanavalin A, 1 μg (Con A); and the recall antigen purified protein derivative (PPD), 1 mg. The lymphocytes were also stimulated with pooled mitomycin C-treated allogeneic lymphocytes in MLC. The lymphocytes from cancer patients were incubated with each of these various stimulators for 5 days, pulsed with 0.5 μCi of tritiated thymidine for 18 hr, and collected on fiberglass filter paper strips with the MASH-1 collecting apparatus. The extent of incorporation of the isotope tritiated thymidine into the lymphocytes was then determined by counting in a Beckman liquid scintillation counter. The counts per minute (cpm) were then determined, and the average cpm for each quadruplicate sample were determined. The magnitude of the cpm was directly related to the ability of the lymphocytes to be stimulated by the various stimulating agents. The cpm were converted to average $\log_{10}$ cpm for the purpose of statistical analysis as previously reported (8). The data were analyzed via the two-tailed *t*-test corrected for unequal variance.

Four patients who initially received placebo for a 90-day period were then treated with levamisole for an additional 90-day period, and the studies of cell-mediated immunity during the placebo period were compared to the evaluation of the cell-mediated immunity during the levamisole treatment.

RESULTS

With the doses of levamisole employed in this study there were no untoward side effects. We were not able to discern between those receiving levamisole and placebo. Specifically, there were no instances of identifiable anorexia or nausea, no instances of leukopenia or rash.

Sequential DNCB Skin Tests

As we have previously reported, patients with resectable disease who are clinically free of disease at the time of skin testing have a higher level of DNCB reactivity *initially* than patients who are unresectable. This observation was corroborated in the present study. Patients with resectable disease who showed no evidence of the disease at the time of skin testing had a significantly higher base-line skin test reactivity to DNCB than those patients who were unresectable and had persistent disease (Fig. 1).

In the disease-free group there was no statistically significant difference in

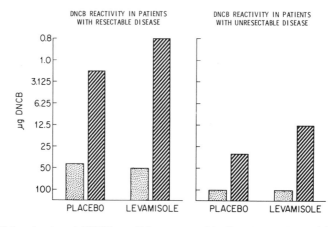

FIG. 1. Initial pretreatment DNCB reactivity compared to the strongest reactivity during the study. The vertical axis represents the average minimum amount of DNCB to which each group reacted. ▨, Pre Rx; ▨, Rx.

the change in DNCB reactivity between the placebo group and the levamisole-treated group. However, the patients receiving levamisole, as a group, had a greater increase than the placebo group. In the group of patients with unresectable disease, whereas both the placebo group and the levamisole group increased their skin test reactivity, patients receiving levamisole had a more striking increase in their levamisole reactivity, but the differences did not reach statistical significance (Fig. 1). It is clear from these studies that even in patients with unresectable disease and suppressed initial DNCB reactivity, sequential repeated skin testing with DNCB every 2 weeks consistently augments the reactivity to DNCB.

Therefore, sequential DNCB skin testing every 2 weeks is not an ideal assay for the evaluation of the effects of levamisole on cell-mediated immunity. Since repeated skin testing with DNCB causes an augmentation of DNCB reactivity, this stimulation may mask any effect of levamisole on cell-mediated immunity. Repeated DNCB skin testing was capable of stimulating the response to DNCB in all patients studied with the exception of those patients with rapidly progressive disease. Patients who have significant tumor burden and rapidly progressive disease usually have a very suppressed initial reactivity to DNCB, and repeated DNCB challenges do not augment this reactivity. In addition, the administration of levamisole to these patients does not reverse this progressive decline in DNCB reactivity (Fig. 2).

In Vitro Lymphocyte Studies

Lung cancer patients in this study and in previous studies almost always had suppressed *in vitro* lymphocyte reactivity when compared to age-matched controls. Patients will significant tumor burden consistently had suppressed *in*

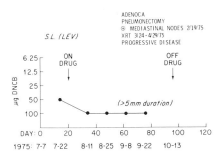

FIG. 2. Progressive decline in DNCB reactivity despite repeated DNCB testing and levamisole treatment in a patient with rapidly progressive disease.

vitro reactivity when compared to patients who were resected and had no evidence of disease. Both groups consistently have depressed reactivity when compared to normal controls with the exception of PHA and PPD reactivity (Fig. 3). Therefore, these data confirm our previous observations that lung cancer is an immunosuppressive disease and that the degree of immunosuppression is related to the tumor burden. These data also indicate that patients with residual tumor burden who were unresectable had initially lower *in vitro* lymphocyte responses than patients with resectable disease.

Figure 4 represents the sequential MLC reactivity in patients receiving placebo and those receiving levamisole. This sequential reactivity represents the average reactivity of all treatment groups including those with resectable disease and those with unresectable persistent disease at each point in time. The *in vitro* lymphocyte reactivity is represented on the vertical axis, and the cpm are expressed in $\log_{10}$ cpm. The elevation of the *in vitro* reactivity in the levamisole-treated group at 30 days compared to the placebo-treated group at 30 days was a consistent observation in all the *in vitro* tests (Fig. 4). This difference disappeared consistently by day 60. The data were therefore analyzed on the basis of the reactivity on treatment day 30 and also the average reactivity during

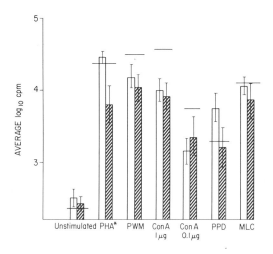

FIG. 3. *In vitro* lymphocyte blastogenesis in lung cancer patients who are free of disease and those who have significant tumor burden compared to healthy age-matched controls. Vertical axis represents $\log_{10}$ cpm, and $3 = 1,000$ cpm, $4 = 10,000$ cpm, and $5 = 100,000$ cpm. □, NED ($N = 12$); ▨, significant tumor burden ($N = 11$); ———, healthy controls ($N = 30$).

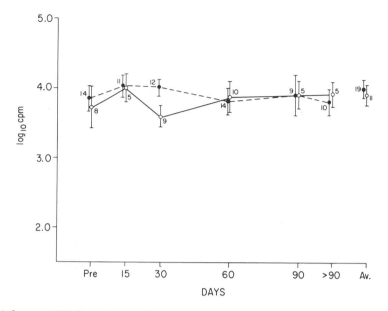

FIG. 4. Sequential MLC reactivity in all patients. On the vertical axis 3 = 1,000 cpm, 4 = 10,000 cpm, and 5 = 100,000 cpm. o———o, Placebo; ●‑‑‑●, levamisole.

the 90 days of treatment. In other words, the pretreatment reactivity was compared to that after 30 days of treatment and to the average reactivity during the 90 days of therapy.

Evaluation of Difference Between Pretreatment Reactivity and Average Reactivity During Treatment

Figure 5 represents the reactivity of the placebo group and the levamisole group to PHA and PWM both pretherapy and during therapy. There is an increase in reactivity in both the placebo and the levamisole groups. Figure 6 demonstrates in a similar fashion *in vitro* reactivity to Con A, 1 μg and 0.1 μg, to PPD, and to MLC. Again, there is a consistent increase in reactivity in both the placebo and levamisole group. The only statistically significant increase in reactivity, however, was the increase in the levamisole group's response to Con A, 0.1 μg. The other increase during treatment with placebo and levamisole did not reach statistical significance. However, in general the magnitude of the increase in levamisole-treated patients was greater than the placebo group.

Evaluation of Pretreatment Reactivity with Reactivity on Day 30 of Study

When the 30-day reactivity was compared to the base-line pretreatment reactivity, there were statistically significant differences in favor of the levamisole

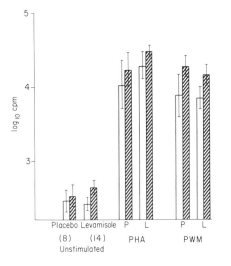

FIG. 5. Lymphocyte blastogenesis to PHA and PWM. Pretherapy cpm compared to the average cpm obtained during treatment with placebo or levamisole. □, Pretherapy; ▨, on drug.

group. Figure 7 reveals an increase in the unstimulated cpm in the levamisole group at 30 days and a decrease in the placebo group. In addition, the response to PHA was significantly increased in the levamisole-treated group, but not in the placebo-treated group ($p < 0.02$). The response to PWM at 30 days was increased in the levamisole-treated group and essentially unchanged in the placebo-treated group. However, the increase in the response to PWM in the levamisole-treated group from pretreatment levels to the 30-day treatment level was not statistically significant.

Figure 8 compared the pretherapy response and the 30-day-treatment response to Con A, 1 μg, Con A, 0.1 μg, PPD, and MLC in the placebo and levamisole-

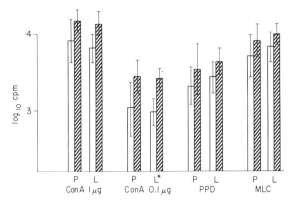

FIG. 6. Lymphocyte blastogenesis: Con A, PPD, and MLC reaction. Pretherapy cpm compared to the average cpm obtained during treatment with placebo or levamisole. *The difference between the pretherapy response to Con A 0.1 μg and the response during levamisole treatment was statistically significant ($p < 0.02$). The difference for the placebo response was not significant. P, placebo; L, levamisole; □, pretherapy; ▨, on drug.

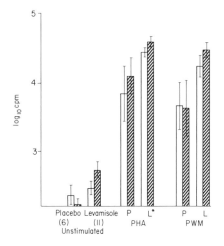

FIG. 7. Pretherapy cpm compared to the response after 30 days of treatment with placebo or levamisole. *The difference between the pretherapy response to PHA and the response during levamisole treatment is statistically significant ($p < 0.05$). The difference for the placebo response was not significant. □, Pretherapy; ▨, 30-day response.

treated group. There was a statistically significant increase in the response to Con A, 0.1 μg, in the levamisole-treated group. The change in the placebo-treated group was not statistically significant. There was actually a decrease in the response to PPD and MLC in the placebo group, however, there was an increase in the levamisole-treated group in both of these categories.

Interestingly, there was a general rise in the *in vitro* lymphocyte response in both the placebo- and levamisole-treated groups. This increase never reached statistical significance in the placebo-treated group, however, it did in the levamisole-treated group in several categories. This suggests that DNCB skin testing every 2 weeks has an adjuvant effect on the *in vitro* lymphocyte reactivity.

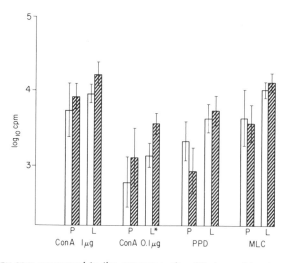

FIG. 8. Pretherapy cpm compared to the response after 30 days of treatment with placebo or levamisole. *Difference between the pretherapy response to Con A 0.1 μg is statistically significant ($p < 0.02$). □, Pretherapy; ▨, 30-day response.

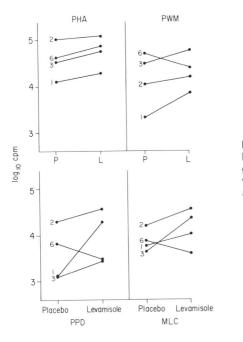

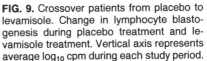

FIG. 9. Crossover patients from placebo to levamisole. Change in lymphocyte blastogenesis during placebo treatment and levamisole treatment. Vertical axis represents average $\log_{10}$ cpm during each study period.

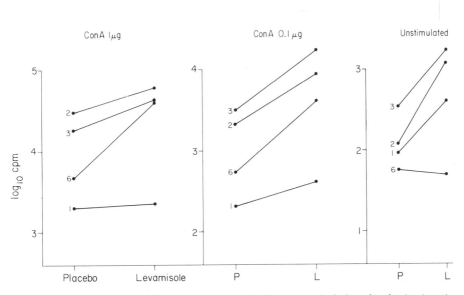

FIG. 10. Cross-over patients. Change in lymphocyte blastogenesis during placebo treatment and levamisole treatment. Vertical axis represents average $\log_{10}$ cpm during each study period.

Four patients were treated with placebo for 3 months and then with levamisole for the ensuing 3 months, and their *in vitro* lymphocyte studies while on placebo and levamisole were compared. The average reactivity during placebo therapy was compared to the average reactivity during levamisole therapy. All four patients increased their reactivity to PHA during levamisole treatment (Fig. 9). Three of the four patients increased their reactivity to PWM, and three of the four patients increased their reactivity to PPD and in the mixed lymphocyte reaction (Fig. 9). All patients increased their reactivity to Con A, 1 and 0.1 μg during levamisole therapy (Fig. 10). Three of four patients increased their unstimulated counts during levamisole therapy, and one patient had a diminution (Fig. 10). The same patient (no. 6) was responsible for the decline in reactivity in those tests in which there was a decline, and was the only patient who did not have an increase in reactivity in every category during levamisole therapy. This patient had a considerable tumor burden and had been treated with radiation therapy prior to this study.

DISCUSSION

Previous studies have indicated that under certain conditions levamisole is capable of augmenting depressed cell-mediated immunity (9,10). These studies have also indicated that levamisole is not capable of augmenting a normal cell-mediated immune response. Since our own studies have shown that a single DNCB skin test in patients with lung cancer correlates very closely with tumor burden and prognosis, we felt that the suppressed DNCB reactivity in these patients would offer a convenient parameter for measuring the effect of levamisole on cell-mediated immunity. We did not anticipate that the repeated DNCB skin testing every 2 weeks would provide a sufficient antigenic stimulus to markedly increase the previously suppressed DNCB reactivity in these patients. It became clear from these studies that sequential DNCB skin testing provided sufficient antigenic stimulation to overcome the suppressive effects of the disease on delayed cutaneous hypersensitivity to this antigen. Even patients with severely suppressed initial DNCB reactivity with significant tumor burden were capable of increasing their reactivity to DNCB during repetitive sequential challenges with this antigen. In similar studies evaluating sequential DNCB reactivity in a group of 140 melanoma patients, we have also noted that repeated sequential DNCB skin testing consistently causes a rise in the magnitude of the reactivity. The only patients who did not develop an augmented response to DNCB during this study were those who had rapidly progressive disease, and who expired during the study. In these patients repeated DNCB skin testing did not increase their level of reactivity, nor did the administration of levamisole reverse this regressive decline in their reactivity.

Sequential frequent DNCB skin testing, therefore, is not an ideal assay for the purpose of determining the effects of levamisole or any other immunopotentiator on cell-mediated immunity. Previous studies have correctly pointed out

that the level of response to DNCB does reflect the stage of the disease (5,6,8).
A patient who has resected lung cancer and who is free of disease when tested
has a higher level of DNCB reactivity than that same individual tested subsequently when recurrent disease has developed. However, in any given patient
the effects of sequential DNCB testing provide sufficient antigenic stimulus to
overcome the immunosuppressive effect of the disease. We have seen this in
patients who were initially free of disease, who were sequentially skin tested
every 2 weeks for several months, and who then developed recurrent disease
while maintaining a vigorous DNCB response in spite of the recurrent disease.
However, if these patients are not sequentially skin tested, but are only tested
at the time of their recurrence, they are almost always anergic or severely
suppressed.

The *in vitro* lymphocyte function studies should provide an assay that is
not influenced by repeated antigenic stimulation. Certainly, previous studies
have indicated that the systemic administration of levamisole or the placement
of levamisole *in vitro* is capable of augmenting *in vitro* lymphocyte functions
in patients with suppressed parameters. This has been especially noticeable in
patients with suppressed T cells whose suppression has been completely or partially corrected with the administration of levamisole (13). In our studies, we
did not find consistently suppressed T-cell levels in patients with lung cancer,
and the administration of levamisole did not significantly elevate the T-cell
level in these patients. One would not expect levamisole to elevate an already
normal T-cell level.

Interestingly, many patients in the placebo group as well as in the levamisole
group showed a tendency to increase their *in vitro* lymphocyte reactivity during
the study. In no instance was there a statistically significant increase in *in vitro*
lymphocyte reactivity in the placebo group. However, there was a rather interesting tendency for these patients to increase their *in vitro* reactivity. This suggests
that repeated DNCB skin testing serves as a nonspecific stimulus to *in vitro*
lymphocyte blastogenesis in these patients. The patients receiving levamisole
had a consistent increase in their *in vitro* lymphocyte reactivity. The most striking
and the most consistent increase in the entire study was noted in the levamisole
group approximately 1 month after initiation of therapy. All assays increased
in the levamisole group with PHA and 0.1 μg of Con A, and the increase
was statistically significant. Only three assays—PHA, Con A 1 μg, and Con
A 0.1 μg—increased in the placebo group at 30 days, and none of these increases
reached statistical significance. Four patients were crossed over from placebo to
levamisole treatment following completion of a course of placebo treatment.
Three of these four individuals showed a consistent increase in mitogenic activity
during levamisole therapy.

These *in vitro* studies are consistent with previous claims that levamisole
augments *in vitro* mitogenic reactivity among individuals with severely depressed
immunologic function. These studies also emphasize the need for comparison
placebo groups. Many of the apparent increases that might be attributed to

levamisole were also noted among the placebo recipients in both the *in vitro* and the delayed cutaneous hypersensitivity studies. Although these studies and others indicate that levamisole may well have an immunorestorative ability under certain circumstances, many questions, such as optimum dose, frequency of administration, and others, remain unanswered.

ACKNOWLEDGMENTS

We wish to acknowledge support by Janssen R & D, Inc., New Brunswick, New Jersey, and USPHS grant no CA12582.

REFERENCES

1. Amery, W. (1975): Immunopotentiation with resectable bronchogenic carcinoma: A double blind controlled trial. *Br. Med. J.,* 3:461–464.
2. Catalona, W. J., and Chretien, P. B. (1973): Abnormalities of quantitative dinitrochlorobenzene sensitization in cancer patients: Correlation with tumor stage and histology. *Cancer,* 31:353–355.
3. Chirigos, M. A., Pearson, J. W., and Pryor, J. (1975): Augmentation of chemotherapeutically induced remission of a murine leukemia by a chemical immunoadjuvant. *Cancer Res.,* 33:2615.
4. Dellon, A. L., Potoin, C., and Chretien, P. B. (1975): Thymus-dependent lymphocyte levels in bronchogenic carcinoma: Correlations with histology, clinical stage, and clinical course after surgical treatment. *Cancer,* 35:687.
5. Eilber, F. R., and Morton, D. L. (1970): Impaired immunological reactivity and recurrence following cancer surgery. *Cancer,* 25:362.
6. Eilber, F. R., Nizze, J. A., and Morton, D. L. (1975): Sequential evaluation of general immune competence in cancer patients: Correlations with clinical course. *Cancer,* 35:660–665.
7. Golub, S. H., Sulit, H. L., and Morton, D. L. (1975): The use of viable frozen lymphocytes for studies in human tumor immunology. *Transplantation,* 19:195–202.
5. Holmes, E. C., and Golub, S. H. (1976): Immunologic defects in lung cancer patients. *J. Thorac. Cardiovasc. Surg.,* 71:161–167.
9. Levo, Y., Rotter, Y., and Ramot, B. (1975): Restoration of cellular immune response by Levamisole in patients with Hodgkin's disease. *Biomedicine,* 23:198–200.
10. Lieberman, R., and Hsu, M. (1976): Levamisole-mediated restoration of cellular immunity in peripheral blood lymphocytes of patients with immunodeficiency diseases. *Clin. Immunol. Immunopathol.,* 5:142–146.
11. Lock, J. C., Dujardin, P., and Holpren, G. (1974): Action of Levamisole on antibody protection after vaccination with anti-thyroid and paratyphoid A and B. *Ann. Allergy,* 34:210–212.
12. McKneally, M. F., Maver, C., Kansel, H. W., and Alley, R. (1976): Regional immunotherapy with intrapleural BCG for lung cancer. *J. Thorac. Cardiovasc. Surg.,* 72:333–338.
13. Ramot, B., Biniaminov, M., Shoham, C., and Rosenthal, E. (1976): Effect of Levamisole on E-rosette-forming cells *in vitro* and *in vivo* in Hodgkin's disease. *N. Engl. J. Med.,* 294:809–811.
14. Tripodi, D., Parks, L. C., and Brugmans, J. (1973): Drug-induced restoration of cutaneous delayed hypersensitivity in anergic patients with cancer. *N. Engl. J. Med.,* 289:354.
15. Wells, S. A. Jr., Burdick, J. F., Joseph, W. L., Christiansen, C. L., Wolfe, W., and Adkins, P. C. (1973): Delayed cutaneous hypersensitivity reactions to tumor cell antigens and nonspecific antigens. *J. Thorac. Cardiovasc. Surg.,* 66:557.

Immune Modulation and Control of Neoplasia by Adjuvant Therapy, edited by M. A.
Chirigos. Raven Press, New York, 1978.

Chemoimmunotherapy of Refractory Malignant Melanoma with Actinomycin D and Levamisole

Stephen W. Hall, Robert S. Benjamin, Lance Heilbrun, Uri
Lewinski, Jordan U. Gutterman, and Giora Mavligit

*Department of Developmental Therapeutics, The University of Texas System Cancer Center,
M.D. Anderson Hospital and Tumor Institute, Houston, Texas 77030*

Dimethyl triazeno imidazole carboxamide (DTIC) is the most effective single chemotherapeutic agent for disseminated melanoma with an overall remission rate of about 20% and complete remission (CR) rate of approximately 5% as determined in several large studies (1,3). The addition of immunotherapy with Bacillus Calmette-Guérin (BCG) has increased remission duration and survival in those patients responding to DTIC therapy (7). Patients failing to respond to DTIC or developing new or progressive tumor on treatment have a dismal prognosis. These patients, refractory to initial DTIC therapy (alone or in combination regimens), have a median survival of 2 to 4 months and a very low response rate to subsequent second-line drug therapy (1,5). We recently reported the results of a study in 22 evaluable patients with refractory melanoma employing high single-dose intermittent actinomycin D (2). There was an overall response rate of 9% [CR + partial remission (PR)], with an additional 27% of the patients obtaining stabilization of previously progressive disease. These data along with those from other studies (1,11) suggested to us that actinomycin D has activity in metastatic melanoma. In an attempt to confirm this activity in a larger number of patients and in hope of increasing remission rate, duration, and survival, we added the immunopotentiating agent levamisole to the treatment regimen. Levamisole was selected because most patients had relapsed on regimens containing immunotherapy with BCG or BCG-related products and because levamisole had shown promise as an immunopotentiating agent *in vitro* and *in vivo* (8). There was also clinical evidence of prolongation of disease-free interval in patients with breast (12) and bronchogenic (13) carcinoma given levamisole as adjuvant therapy after surgical resection of tumor.

METHODS

Sixty adult patients with disseminated melanoma were evaluable in the study. All patients had progressive disease refractory to prior chemotherapy or chemoimmunotherapy regimens that included DTIC. Patients were evaluated in pretreatment with regard to tumor measurements and hematologic, metabolic, and immunologic parameters. Hematologic parameters were followed one to two times weekly with chemistries and tumor measurements repeated before every course of therapy. Informed consent was obtained from all patients before therapy according to institutional policy. The starting dose of actinomycin D in most patients was 2.0 mg/m² with some receiving 1.5 mg/m² because of compromised bone marrow reserve. The drug was given in 100 to 250 cc of 5% dextrose and water, repeated at 4-week intervals with the dose adjusted depending on myelosuppressive and gastrointestinal toxicity. Levamisole was given at a dose of 50 mg orally three times a day on 2 consecutive days each week in 50 patients. Ten patients received intensive levamisole as part of a phase 1 study of this compound. The dosage was 200 mg orally every other day with the dose subsequently decreased for excessive toxicity.

CR was defined as disappearance of all clinical evidence of active tumor and tumor-related symptoms for a minimum of 4 weeks. PR was defined as a ≥ 50% decrease in the sum of the products of the longest perpendicular diameters of all measurable lesions lasting at least 4 weeks without the appearance of new lesions. Stable disease (S) included all patients with a steady state of response less than PR for at least 4 weeks or with no evidence of progressive disease for at least 8 weeks. Progressive disease was defined as an increase of any measured lesion by > 25% or the appearance of any lesions. Survival was calculated according to the method of Kaplan and Meier (6) and compared in a one-tailed test by the Gehan modification of the generalized Wilcoxan test (9). Where possible clinical parameters were compared by the chi-square evaluation.

RESULTS

Response

Sixty patients were evaluable for response (Table 1). There was one CR (2%) in a male patient with soft tissue and nodal disease who remains in remission and on therapy at 10 months. One PR (2%) was seen of short duration (4 weeks) in a patient also with soft tissue disease. There were 18 patients (30%) with stable disease for a median 4 to 5 months (range 3 to 9 months). Three of these 18 patients had definite tumor regression less than PR; two of these involved soft tissue or nodal disease and one liver and lung metastatic deposits. One of the stable patients remains on treatment, whereas 17 have relapsed and have subsequently received different therapy. To date five of these patients are alive on their subsequent therapy. Forty patients (67%) had definite evidence of progressive disease. In 22 of the cases it occurred after one course of therapy and in 18 after two courses. There was an overall response rate (CR + PR) of 3% with 33% of patients at least achieving stable disease (CR + PR + S).

TABLE 1. *Patients evaluable for response*

	Actinomycin D + levamisole	Actinomycin D
No. evaluable patients	60	29
Males (%)	50	62
Females (%)	50	38
Age [a] (yr)	48 (22–75)	41 (28–68)
Metastasis		
Visceral (%)	58	45
Nonvisceral (%)	42	55
CR (%)	2	3
PR (%)	2	3
S (%)	30	28
Progressive disease (%)	66	66
Prior immunotherapy (%)	100	100
Prior chemotherapy (%)	100	100
Prior radiation therapy (%)	17	14

[a] Values are medians with range in parentheses.

Toxicity

Nonhematologic toxicity was evaluable in 50 patients. Forty of these received levamisole 2 days of every week, and 10 received intensive alternate day levamisole. Table 2 shows the incidence of the nonhematologic toxicities in both patient groups. In most instances toxicity was more frequent and severe with the alternate day levamisole with actinomycin D when compared to that with weekly levamisole and actinomycin D. High drug fever, nausea, vomiting, and skin rash were the most common side effects from the alternate day levamisole regimen and

TABLE 2. *Nonhematologic toxicity*

	Actinomycin D + weekly levamisole	Actinomycin D + alternate-day levamisole	All courses actinomycin D + levamisole
No. of patients evaluable	40	10	50
No. of courses evaluable	77	28	105
Mucositis	12	20	10
Nausea, vomiting >3 days	17	50	14
Rash	5	30	6
Fever	2	60	9
Bleeding	7	0	4
Diarrhea	5	0	3
CNS Abnormalities	0	10	1
Hospitalization	2	30	4

Incidence of toxicity is in % of patients, except hospitalization, which is in % of courses.

TABLE 3. *Hematologic toxicity*

Initial course at actinomycin dose	No. courses evaluable	Lowest granulocyte count $\times 10^3/mm^3$	Day lowest	Lowest platelet count $\times 10^3/mm^3$	Day lowest
Actinomycin D + weekly levamisole					
2.0 mg/m²	25	1.6 (0–9.8)	15 (5–28)	134 (20–511)	9 (7–27)
1.5 mg/m²	9	1.5 (0.4–2.4)	17 (7–36)	131 (18–199)	10 (7–27)
Actinomycin D + alternate-day levamisole					
2.0 mg/m²	7	1.4 (0–3.3)	12 (9–25)	110 (20–176)	8 (6–9)

All values are in medians with ranges in parentheses.

could be attributed in large part to the intensive levamisole therapy. Although some of these side effects were seen in patients given actinomycin D alone, the incidence was much higher in patients given the actinomycin D + intensive levamisole therapy than in those given actinomycin D alone or in combination with levamisole 2 days a week. One patient of particular interest developed a headache and seizures culminating in coma, from which he recovered, after receiving the intensive levamisole regimen with actinomycin D. Nausea, vomiting, and mucositis were most common in patients receiving actinomycin with weekly levamisole; however, the frequency of these side effects did not differ substantially from those in our previous study with actinomycin D alone. Levamisole given two consecutive days per week at a dose of 50 mg, p.o., T.I.D. did not appear to give additive toxicity to actinomycin D, but when given at 200 mg on alternate days, there was a substantial increase in toxicity and morbidity, which was unacceptable.

Hematologic toxicity was evaluable in 34 courses of therapy in patients receiving weekly levamisole. Twenty-five of the courses were at the 2.0 mg/m² dose of actinomycin and nine at 1.5 mg/m². The lowest recorded points of myelosuppression on this regimen are shown in Table 3 and compared to seven courses of intensive alternate-day levamisole with 2.0 mg/m² actinomycin D. The extent and duration of granulocytopenia and thrombocytopenia were similar in both groups and comparable to that seen in our previous study of actinomycin D alone. No cumulative myelosuppression was seen. Of 40 patients started at a dose of 2.0 mg/m² of actinomycin, nine (22%) required dose reduction to 1.5 mg/m² and three (8%) were escalated to 2.5 mg/m² based on drug effects. Of nine patients started at 1.5 mg/m², five were escalated to 1.75 or 2.0 mg/m².

Survival

Survival data were obtained on 60 patients receiving actinomycin D + levamisole and on 29 patients who received actinomycin D alone at compa-

TABLE 4. *Clinical and prognostic parameters*

Therapy	Actinomycin D	Actinomycin D + levamisole	p value
No. of patients	29	60	
Males (%)	62	50	
			0.28
Females (%)	38	50	
Age (yr)[a]	41 (28–68)	48 (22–75)	0.9
Primary site (% of patients)			
Head and neck	24	17	
Trunk	38	42	0.63
Extremities	31	39	
Unknown	7	3	
Time to metastasis (mo)[a] (% of patients with occurrence)	12 (0–168)	8 (0–180)	
0–6 mo.	31	43	
7–12 mo	24	23	0.68
13–24 mo	24	17	
>24 mo	21	17	
Site of metastasis (% of patients)			
Lymph nodes	66	59	
Skin, subcutaneous soft tissue	66	57	
CNS	14	15	
Bone	10	10	
Pulmonary	34	43	
Mediastinal	3	5	
Intestine	7	2	
Liver	3	22	
Genitourinary, bone marrow	0	7	
Prior XRT (includes CNS) (% of patients)	21	18	
Prior chemotherapy (% of patients)	100	100	
1 regimen	52	72	0.05
2 regimens	28	23	
3 regimens	10	5	
4 regimens	7	0	
>4 regimens	3	0	
Prior immunotherapy (% of patients)	79	80	
1 regimen	69	56	
2 regimens	7	20	0.4
3 regimens	3	2	
>3 regimens	0	2	
% Patients responding to prior chemotherapy (CR + PR + S)	41	41	
Time from diagnosis of primary to chemotherapy of metastatic disease[a]	14 mo (<1 mo–15 yr)	14 mo (<1 mo–14 yr)	
Time from metastatic disease to chemotherapy with actinomycin D[a]	9 mo (<2 mo–7 yr)	9 mo (<2 mo–4 yr)	
Time from diagnosis of primary to chemotherapy with actinomycin D[a]	20 mo (9 mo–15 yr)	21 mo (2 mo–13 yr)	

[a] Value is median with range in parentheses.

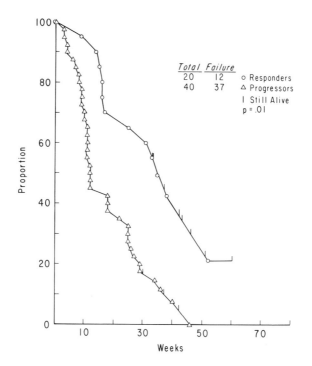

FIG. 1. Survival of actinomycin D + levamisole responders versus nonresponders.

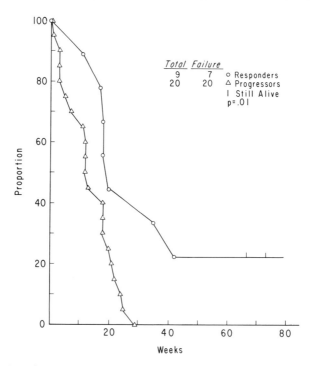

FIG. 2. Survival of actinomycin D responders versus nonresponders.

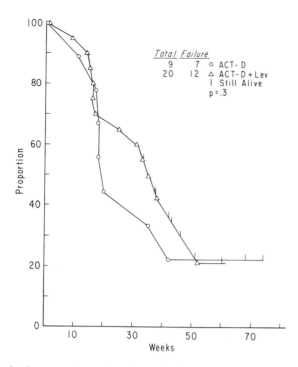

FIG. 3. Survival of responders of actinomycin D versus responders of actinomycin D + levamisole.

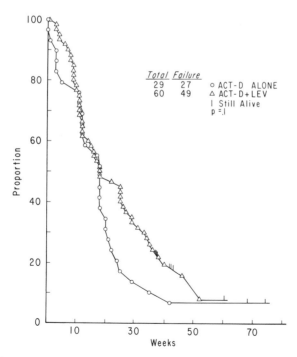

FIG. 4. Survival of all patients treated with actinomycin D versus actinomycin D + levamisole.

rable doses in the study immediately preceding this one. The clinical and prognostic factors for both groups are shown in Table 4.

As has been shown in previous studies of melanoma those patients who respond to therapy have a longer survival than those who do not. The actinomycin D + levamisole responders (CR + PR + S) had a median survival of 35 weeks compared to the nonresponders' 12 weeks ($p = 0.01$) (Fig. 1). In our previous study of actinomycin alone there was also an increased median survival for the responders (19 weeks) as compared with patients with progressive disease (12 weeks) ($p = 0.01$) (Fig. 2). The most important category of patients to examine is that of responders (CR + PR + S) to actinomycin D + levamisole as compared to the responders (CR + PR + S) to actinomycin D alone in order to determine if levamisole increased survival in these patients. Although the number of responders is small in both categories, the median survival of the actinomycin D + levamisole responders was 35 weeks versus 19 weeks for the responders to actinomycin D alone ($p = 0.3$) (Fig. 3). The overall survival of both groups of patients is seen in Fig. 4.

DISCUSSION

This study of actinomycin D + levamisole in DTIC refractory patients with disseminated melanoma when combined with our previous study in a similar population gives a CR rate of 2%, a PR rate of 2%, and a disease stabilization rate of 34%. The duration of response (CR + PR + S) was slightly longer in those patients receiving actinomycin D + levamisole (median 4 months) as compared to those getting actinomycin D alone (median 2 months); however, it was not statistically compared. These response data are usually indicative of drug effect and in conjunction with the survival data suggest use of intermittent single-dose actinomycin D + levamisole in patients with earlier disease in conjunction with DTIC or perhaps other chemoimmunotherapy regimens.

The toxicity of the drug with or without levamisole administered 2 days per week is tolerable without major morbidity and with myelosuppression, nausea, vomiting, and mucositis the major toxicities. There is no question that intensive alternate-day levamisole, as given in this study, had major unacceptable morbidity manifested by excessive gastrointestinal and skin toxicity that was additive or synergistic with that from actinomycin D. In addition, the occurrence of fever and central nervous system abnormalities seen in this study was severe and related to intensive high-dose alternate-day levamisole therapy.

The myelosuppression seen with the combination of actinomycin D and weekly levamisole was comparable to that of actinomycin D alone. There were six episodes of fever unrelated to drug administration in the patients receiving actinomycin with levamisole. These occurred in patients with less than 500 absolute granulocytes/mm^3. There were no documented infections, and all patients with fever responded to antibiotics or granulocyte recovery without difficulty. There were three episodes of bleeding encountered in the patients, all of whom had platelet counts greater than 143,000/μl. These included one patient on warfarin (Coumadin®) who had hematuria; one with upper gastrointestinal bleeding, the source of which was not determined but which responded to conservative treatment, and one with a mild episode of epistaxis. None of these events could therefore be attributed to therapy. Of all the courses evaluable in patients receiving actinomycin D with weekly levamisole, 5% had lowest platelet counts less than 50,000/mm^3 and 17% below 100,000/mm^3. Fourteen percent of the courses of intensive alternate-day levamisole with actinomycin D had platelet counts less than 50,000/mm^3 and 42% less than 100,000/mm^3. Comparison of absolute granulocyte levels showed 14% of the courses of actinomycin D with weekly levamisole had counts less than 1,000/mm^3, whereas 43% of the courses of intensive levamisole with actinomycin fell below this level. Only four patients (5%) required hospitalization for fever or bleeding. Actinomycin D was discontinued in two patients because of unacceptable gastrointestinal toxicity. There were no drug-related deaths.

The comparison of prognostic factors in the groups of patients receiving and not receiving levamisole is important (Table 4). The actinomycin D + levamisole group had a greater number of female patients and a slightly smaller percentage of head and neck primary lesions, neither of which was statistically significant. It had a shorter interval from time of primary diagnosis to metastatic disease (median of 8 months versus 12.0 months) and a greater proportion of patients with visceral metastasis (59 versus 45%). There was one area statistically important and that was the number of prior chemotherapy regimens. The actinomycin D group had significantly ($p = 0.05$) more prior chemotherapy regimens than the actinomycin D + levamisole group. Of the actinomycin D group, 48% had received at least two prior chemotherapy regimens, whereas only 28% of the actinomycin D + levamisole patients had received this much. However, survival curves comparing only those patients having received one and/or two prior chemotherapy regimens on both the actinomycin D and actinomycin D + levamisole study are not statistically significant. Certainly, overall, the two groups are comparable for most important clinical parameters.

Survival data showed as expected that responding patients live longer than patients with progressive disease. The number of CRs and PRs was too small to compare with patients obtaining disease stabilization. The significant prolongation of median survival in the responders (CR + PR + S) of 35 weeks compares favorably with survival in previously untreated patients responding (CR + PR) to DTIC alone (6 to 11 months, median 9) (4,7,10). It appears that adding levamisole immunotherapy to second-line chemotherapy with actinomycin D prolonged survival in responding patients to the equivalent of that seen in previously untreated patients responding to DTIC. Previously untreated patients achieving remission (CR or PR) or stability on DTIC + BCG (7) had median survival of 13 months and approximately 9 months, respectively, which was superior to that of patients treated with DTIC alone (7) or to that of our previously treated patients. The survival of patients with progressive disease in our study was dismal (median 12.0 weeks) and similar to that reported for patients failing first-line therapy with DTIC (10). This poor median survival was the same for progressors on actinomycin with or without levamisole.

The survival for all patients on actinomycin D + levamisole was slightly longer than that of all patients on actinomycin D (Fig. 4). Although median survivals of 18 weeks were the same, the 25th percentile survival was 36 weeks for the levamisole group compared with 22 weeks for the actinomycin D alone group ($p = 0.1$). In addition 11 patients who were entered on the levamisole study are alive compared with only two on the study without levamisole, so there is some opportunity for a greater difference between the groups to become evident.

The survival difference between patients responding (CR + PR + S) to actinomycin D + levamisole and those responding (CR + PR + S) to actinomycin D alone (35 weeks versus 19 weeks) is not statistically significant ($p = 0.03$). Eight of the 20 responding patients are still alive on the actinomycin D + levamisole study, and two of nine patients on the actinomycin D alone study are still alive. Both of these latter patients have been rendered free of disease by surgery, whereas all eight of the actinomycin D + levamisole patients have recurrent active melanoma. The difference between these two patient groups would be slightly greater if the two survivors without evidence of disease on actinomycin D alone were eliminated and may also be greater with continued survival of the eight remaining patients who responded to actinomycin D + levamisole.

The statistical difference between actinomycin D + levamisole and Actinomycin D alone responders (CR + PR + S) ($p = 0.3$) was not changed by repeating both survival curves after eliminating patients whose survival could clinically not be related to the actinomycin D + levamisole therapy. There is a suggestion, however, that patients who responded to actinomycin D + levamisole therapy and then progressed had a better chance of responding to subsequent therapy. They had not received quite as much prior chemotherapy as the actinomycin D group (Table 4), and this might be the explanation. However, it is also possible that the actinomycin D + levamisole patients had significant improvement in their immunocompetence or a smaller decrease in immunosuppression from disease or chemotherapy attributable to levamisole and that this accounted for their improved response to subsequent chemo- or chemoimmunotherapy.

Our data confirm the modest activity of single-dose actinomycin D in previously treated patients with melanoma and suggest that levamisole, like BCG, contributes to prolonged survival of patients with melanoma when given together with chemotherapy, although it does not increase the remission rate. Further investigations of levamisole in combination with DTIC in previously untreated patients might result in much more substantial improvement and are required to define the role of these agents.

ACKNOWLEDGMENTS

We wish to thank Denise Thornton for her technical assistance.
This work was supported in part by grant no. CA-05831 from the National

Cancer Institute, National Institutes of Health, United States Public Health Service, Bethesda, Md., and a grant from Janssen R and D, Inc., New Brunswick, New Jersey.

Robert S. Benjamin is a Junior Faculty Fellow of the American Cancer Society and Jordan U. Gutterman and Giora Mavligit are recipients of the PHS Career Development Award, Nos. 1-KO4-CA-71007 and 1-KO4-CA-00130, respectively. Lance Heilbrun is from the Southwest Oncology Group Statistical Office.

REFERENCES

1. Benjamin, R. S., Gutterman, J. U., McKelvey, E. M., Einhorn, L. M., Livingston, R. B., and Gottlieb, J. A. (1976): Systemic chemotherapy for melanoma. In: *Neoplasms of the Skin and Malignant Melanoma:* Proc. Univ. of Texas System Cancer Center, M.D. Anderson Hospital and Tumor Institute 20th Annu. Clin. Conf., pp. 461–469. Yearbook Med. Publ., Chicago.
2. Benjamin, R. S., Hall, S. W., Burgess, M. A., Wheeler, W. L., Murphy, W. K., Blumenschein, G. R., and Gottlieb, J. A. (1976): A pharmacokinetically based phase I–II study of single-dose Actinomycin-D (NSC-3053). *Cancer Treat. Rep.,* 60:289–291.
3. Comis, R. L., and Carter, S. K. (1974): Integration of chemotherapy into combined modality therapy of solid tumors. IV: Malignant melanoma. *Cancer Treat. Rev.,* 1:285–304.
4. Costanza, M. E., Nathanson, L., Lenhard, R., Walter, J., Colsky, J., Oberfield, R. A., and Shilling, A. (1972): Therapy of malignant melanoma with an imidazole carboxamide and bis-chlorethyl nitrosourea. *Cancer,* 30:1457–1461.
5. Einhorn, J. H., Burgess, M. A., Vallejos, C., Bodey, G. P., Gutterman, J. U., Mavligit, G., Hersh, E. M., Luce, J. K., Frei, E., Freireich, E. J., and Gottlieb, J. A. (1974): Prognostic correlations and response to treatment in advanced malignant melanoma. *Cancer Res.,* 34:1995–2004.
6. Gehan, E. A. (1965): A generalized Wilcoxon test for comparing arbitrarily singly-censored samples. *Biometrika,* 52:203–223.
7. Gutterman, J. U., Mavligit, G., Gottlieb, J. A., Burgess, M. A., McBride, C. E., Einhorn, L., Freireich, E. J., and Hersh, E. M. (1974): Chemoimmunotherapy of disseminated malignant melanoma with dimethyl triazeno imidazole carboxamide and Bacillus Calmette-Guérin. *N. Engl. J. Med.,* 291:592–297.
8. Hokama, Y., Kimura, L., Perreira, S., and Palumbo, N. (1974): Effects of Levamisole and C-reactive protein on mitogen stimulated lymphocytes *in vitro* and on the C-reactive protein response *in vivo. Fed. Proc.,* 33:650.
9. Kaplan, E. L., and Meier, P. (1958): Nonparametric estimation from incomplete observations. *J. Am. Stat. Assoc.,* 53:457–481.
10. Luce, J. K. (1972): Chemotherapy of malignant melanoma. *Cancer,* 30:1604–1615.
11. Molander, D. W., and Oropeza, R. (1969): Management of metastatic malignant melanoma with Actinomycin-D. *Proc. Am. Assoc. Cancer Res.,* 10:60, #237.
12. Rojas, A. F., Mickiewicz, E., Feierstein, J. N., Glait, H., and Olivaric, A. J. (1976): Levamisole in advanced human breast cancer. *Lancet,* 1:211–215.
13. Study Group for Bronchogenic Carcinoma: Immunopotentiation with Levamisole in resectable bronchogenic carcinoma: A double-blind controlled trial. *Br. Med. J.,* 3:461–463.

Immune Modulation and Control of Neoplasia by Adjuvant Therapy, edited by M. A.
Chirigos. Raven Press, New York, 1978.

Levamisole in the Treatment of Breast Cancer

*G. N. Hortobagyi, **J. U. Gutterman, *G. R. Blumenschein,
*C. K. Tashima, A. U. Buzdar, and **E. M. Hersh

*Medical Breast Section, Department of Medicine, and **Department of Developmental
Therapeutics, University of Texas System Cancer Center, M. D. Anderson Hospital and
Tumor Institute, Houston, Texas 77030

Combination chemotherapy with 5-fluorouracil, adriamycin, and cyclophosphamide (FAC therapy) consistently produces objective responses in over 70%
of patients with disseminated breast cancer (4,16). The use of nonspecific immunotherapy combined with optimal cytoreductive chemotherapy in the experimental model produces results that are superior to either modality of treatment
alone (1,22,23). It was recently reported that nonspecific immunotherapy with
Bacillus Calmette-Guérin (BCG) or *Corynebacterium parvum* prolongs the duration of remission and survival of patients with breast cancer responding to
chemotherapy (10,24).

Levamisole is a new synthetic substance that has shown immunorestorative
properties (12,21,32). It affects mainly the cell-mediated arm of the immune
system, and its effects are most noticeable in immunosuppressed subjects (3,
26,27). Amery et al., using levamisole as surgical adjuvant in the treatment of
resectable lung cancer, demonstrated a significant increase in disease-free interval
and survival (29). Similarly, Rojas and collaborators obtained a significant prolongation of the disease-free interval and survival on patients who had stage
III breast cancer (technically inoperable) treated with radical radiation therapy
followed by levamisole (28).

Multiple studies of immunocompetence of advanced breast cancer patients
have appeared in the literature over the last few years. Most report immunosuppression in a sizable percentage of patients, the degree of impairment being
dependent on the stage of disease (8,9,18,25,36,37). This group of immunosuppressed patients would theoretically derive maximum benefit from an immunorestorative agent like levamisole. In the therapeutic program described here, we
combined our previous best combination chemotherapy of 5-fluorouracil, adriamycin, and cyclophosphamide with levamisole. The purpose of this study was
to test if this combination was able to improve the response rate and prolong
the duration of remission and survival of patients with metastatic breast cancer.

MATERIALS AND METHODS

One hundred and twenty-seven patients with metastatic breast cancer were treated with a combination of 5-fluorouracil (500 mg/m^2 i.v. on days 1 and 8 of each chemotherapy course), adriamycin (50 mg/m^2 i.v. on day 1), and cyclophosphamide (500 mg/m^2 i.v. on day 1). Levamisole in a dose of 100 mg/m^2 p.o. in three divided doses a day was given on days 5, 6, 11, 12, 17, and 18 of each course of chemotherapy. Courses of treatment were repeated every 21 days if hematologic recovery permitted. After reaching a cumulative dose of 450 mg/m^2 of adriamycin, maintenance therapy consisting of cyclophosphamide (500 mg/m^2 p.o. on day 2), methotrexate (30 mg/m^2 i.m. on days 1 and 8), and 5-fluorouracil (500 mg/m^2 p.o. on days 1 and 8) was started. Levamisole was continued at the dose and schedule described for the induction part. Dosage modification of all three chemotherapeutic agents was planned so as to keep the lowest absolute granulocyte count between 1,000 and 2,000 and the lowest platelet count over 50,000. In case of documented infection or hemorrhage, or both, the dose of all three myelosuppressive agents was decreased by 25% regardless of change in blood count. Initial evaluation consisted of a history and physical exam, CBC, differential and platelet count, urinalysis, SMA-100, CEA, EKG, chest X-ray, bone survey, bone scan, liver scan, skin tests to a battery of six antigens (dermatophytin, varidase, *Candida,* mumps, KLH, PPD). Follow-up studies included weekly blood counts, SMA-100 before each course of treatment, EKG before each dose of adriamycin, and a complete reevaluation every 3 months.

Evidence of congestive heart failure prompted discontinuation of adriamycin. Severe gastrointestinal toxicity required withholding of 5-fluorouracil until resolution of these symptoms, whereas the appearance of hemorrhagic cystitis required discontinuation of cyclophosphamide. Severe gastrointestinal or neurologic side effects attributable to levamisole required reduction of the dose, and if persistent, discontinuation of this agent.

Criteria for evaluation of response to treatment were as follows: complete

TABLE 1. *Chemoimmunotherapy of stage IV breast cancer—population characteristics by treatment program*

	FAC-BCG	FAC-levamisole
No. of patients	105	110
Age (range)	53 (25–72)	53 (23–76)
Race (%) White	90	88
Black	7	5
Latin	3	7
Premenopausal (%)	23	17
Postmenopausal (%)	77	83
Prior hormonal therapy (%)	65	64
Prior chemotherapy (%)	14	10
Disease-free interval (mo)	15 (0–140)	15 (0–186)

TABLE 2. *Metastatic sites by treatment program*

Metastatic site	FAC-BCG (%)	FAC-levamisole (%)
Soft tissue	33	38
Lymph nodes	28	29
Bone	61	73
Lung	33	36
Pleura	24	32
Liver	22	20

remission—complete disappearance of all objective and subjective manifestations of tumor including recalcification of all osteolytic lesions; partial remission—50% or greater reduction in the areas of all measurable tumor including partial recalcification of osteolytic lesions; stable disease—less than 50% reduction or less than 25% increase in tumor mass; progression—more than 25% increase in tumor mass or the appearance of any new lesions.

The results of this clinical trial were compared to the results of a series of 105 patients treated in an identical fashion with FAC chemotherapy and BCG from April of 1974 through April of 1975 and 44 patients treated with FAC chemotherapy alone from May of 1973 through March of 1974. Criteria for admission to those studies were identical to the present.

Of the one hundred and twenty-seven patients entered, 17 (14%) were considered inevaluable for the following reasons—two patients died before day 14 of the first course of therapy, 11 patients had major protocol violations in their treatment (seven did not receive levamisole), and four patients were considered too early to evaluate at the time of this analysis.

Table 1 shows that the FAC-BCG and FAC-levamisole were comparable in the major features of prognostic significance in breast cancer. Table 2 shows the distribution of metastatic lesions in both groups, which again was identical. A comparability of the FAC and FAC-BCG patient population has been shown before (10).

Remission duration was determined from the date of achieving a partial or complete remission. Duration of stability was measured from the date chemotherapy was started. Survival was measured from the start of treatment to date of death or date of last follow-up examination.

The statistical methods used included the chi-square test for differences in remission rate, a generalized Wilcoxon test with a one-tailed analysis for testing differences in survival curves (7), and the method of Kaplan and Meier for calculating and plotting remission and survival curves (17).

RESULTS

One hundred and ten evaluable patients received an adequate trial with one or more courses of chemoimmunotherapy with FAC and levamisole. Sixty-six patients (50%) achieved a partial or complete remission. Of these, 10 patients

TABLE 3. *Chemoimmunotherapy of stage IV breast cancer—overall response rate by treatment program*

	FAC-BCG	FAC-levamisole
Total evaluable	105	110
Complete remission	20 (19%)	10 (9.2%)
Partial remission	58 (55%)	56 (51%)
Stable	21 (20%)	39 (35.8%)
Progression	6 (6%)	5 (4.6%)

(9.2%) achieved a complete remission and 56 (51%) achieved a partial remission. Stable disease was observed in 39 patients (35.8%), and five patients exhibited progressive disease from the start of chemotherapy (Table 3). When response was analyzed according to distribution of metastatic sites, results were very similar to our previous chemoimmunotherapy studies; response in soft tissues, including lymph nodes, was observed in over 80% of the patients, response in lung, pleura, and liver between 70 and 80%, and response in bone around 60%. These results are similar to those previously reported (14). At a median follow-up of 10 months, only nine out of 66 responding patients have relapsed. The 75th percentile has not been reached yet. At this same point in time only three out of 66 responding patients have died. The duration of remission in this study appears to be identical to that observed in the FAC-BCG study ($p = 0.47$) and significantly better than seen on the FAC chemotherapy alone program ($p = 0.01$). The duration of survival is also similar to that seen on the FAC-BCG study ($p = 0.42$) and significantly superior to the FAC chemotherapy alone study ($p = 0.03$) (Figs. 1 and 2).

This chemoimmunotherapy program has been well tolerated. Table 4 shows the hemotologic toxicity encountered. Leukopenia and especially neutropenia

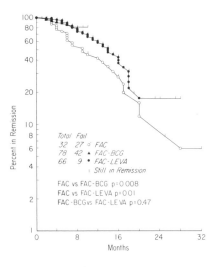

FIG. 1. Chemoimmunotherapy of stage IV breast cancer—duration of response.

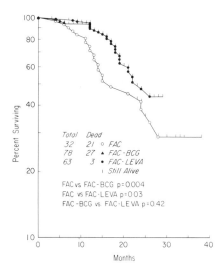

FIG. 2. Chemoimmunotherapy of stage IV breast cancer—survival of responders.

Total Dead
32 21 ○ FAC
78 27 ▲ FAC-BCG
63 3 ● FAC-LEVA
ı Still Alive

FAC vs FAC-BCG p=0.004
FAC vs FAC-LEVA p=0.03
FAC-BCG vs FAC-LEVA p=0.42

TABLE 4. *Chemoimmunotherapy of stage IV breast cancer—FAC-levamisole, hematologic toxicity*

	1st Course	3rd Course	6th Course
Lowest WBC[a]	2.0	2.2	2.2
(range)	(0.4–5.2)	(0.8–7.6)	(1.0–6.1)
Lowest PMN[a]	0.8	1.2	1.0
(range)	(0.–3.4)	(0.2–4.9)	(0.–3.1)
Lowest platelets[a]	209	180	160
(range)	(10–574)	(41–379)	(55–356)
% Dose[a]	100%	90%	80%
(range)	(75–100)	(50–120)	(28–100)
	74 → 100%	45 → 100%	28 → 100%

[a]Median.

TABLE 5. *Chemoimmunotherapy of stage IV breast cancer—FAC-levamisole, nonhematologic toxicity*

Side effects	No./total patients		Percent of patients
Nausea	70/91		77
Vomiting	67/91		74
Diarrhea	6/91		7
Mucositis	13/91		14
Anorexia	7/91		8
Weight Loss (>5 lbs)	7/91		8
Alopecia	27/91	(?)	30
Skin pigmentation	2/91		
Phlebitis	5/91		
Adriamycin infiltration	2/91		
Weakness	9/91		

have been the most consistent manifestations of toxicity. Neutropenia was of short duration, and its timing and recovery from it were very predictable. There was a slight indication of cumulative toxicity, since by the sixth course 50% of the patients were able to receive only 80% of the protocol drug dosage. Nonhemotologic toxicity is described in Table 5 where nausea, vomiting, and alopecia were the most common side effects attributable to the program. Up to this point, cardiac toxicity attributable to adriamycin treatment has not been observed in this program. Table 6 describes the toxicity attributable to levamisole. The drug was very well tolerated, and only a minority of patients had toxic manifestations. Nausea, vomiting, and a low-grade fever were the most common.

TABLE 6. *Chemoimmunotherapy of stage IV breast cancer—FAC-levamisole, levamisole toxicity*

Side effects	No./total patients (%)
Gastrointestinal	
Nausea	19/90 (21)
Vomiting	11/90 (12)
Diarrhea	1/90 (1)
Anorexia	3/90 (3)
Hunger	1/90
Bitter taste	5/90
Halitosis	1/90
Fever	12/90 (13)
Chills	3/90
Autonomic	
Hot flashes	1/90
Facial puffiness	1/90
Chest tightness	1/90
Tachycardia	1/90
Diaphoresis	2/90
Urinary frequency	1/90
Neurologic	
Hyperosmia	4/90
Hyperacusia	1/90
Headache	4/90
Blurry vision	1/90
Red and green lights	1/90
Dizziness	1/90
Syncope	2/90
Lethargy	2/90
Depersonalization	2/90
Nightmares	1/90
Irritability	1/90
Emotional lability	3/90
Depression	2/90
Miscellaneous	
Weakness	3/90
Malaise	6/90
Skin rash	2/90

Dose decreased in 9/90 (10%) patients.
Drug discontinued in 4/90 (5%) patients.

Administering levamisole in divided doses decreased the gastrointestinal toxicity in most cases. A maculopapular, morbilliform rash was observed in two patients, but it disappeared promptly on discontinuation of the drug. Of 90 patients who had adequate information for toxicity of levamisole, only nine (10%) had to have the dose of levamisole decreased, and of these only four (5%) had the drug discontinued because of excessive toxicity.

When comparing this program to the FAC and FAC-BCG regimens, there was no significant difference in the amount of myelosuppression observed or the incidence of minor or major infections.

DISCUSSION

The results described in this chapter suggest that patients with metastatic breast cancer treated with combination chemotherapy and levamisole have remission rates identical to previous studies with chemotherapy alone and chemotherapy with BCG or MER (10,30). Thus far, the durations of remission and survival of responders are identical to previous studies with the same chemotherapy plus BCG. It is also seen, at this time, that patients treated with FAC-levamisole have had a significant prolongation of remission compared to previous studies with chemotherapy alone. However, the follow-up of this study is too short to make any definitive conclusions about the comparability of levamisole and BCG.

Previous reports indicating that levamisole is able to decrease the incidence of infection (33) or the degree of myelosuppression in patients treated with myelotoxic chemotherapy (20) were not confirmed in our study. However, minor differences may have gone undetected. Levamisole, which is a synthetic substance, appears to activate the T-cell system probably by increasing intracellular content of cyclic GMP (2,21). In addition, it does have known effects on the RES system and macrophages (13,34). Although, under certain circumstances, it increases antibody levels, this effect appears to be mediated by T-cell priming of the antibody-producing cells (15,19). The drug is known to act primarily on immunosuppressed subjects (35), whereas its effect on immunocompetent patients is negligible (31). Thus, the immunomodulating action appears to be different from that attributed to the bacterial adjuvants.

Levamisole alone, when used as an adjuvant, following primary treatment for resectable lung cancer appeared to prolong the disease-free interval and survival of treated patients as compared to simultaneous controls (29). Similarly in the study published by Rojas and collaborators, levamisole appeared to prolong the disease-free interval and survival in patients with locally advanced breast cancer treated with radical radiotherapy (28).

It is generally accepted that patients with advanced breast cancer have a deficient immune response. Although the studies published vary in methodology and the parameters measured, it can be safely stated that one or more parameters of cell-mediated immunity are impaired in patients with advanced metastatic disease (8,9,18,25,36,37). A number of investigators have reported that immuno-competence is a favorable prognostic factor in the treatment of cancer patients. Thus, patients who are immunocompetent prior to starting therapy or whose immune response improves during therapy have a higher probability of obtaining a response and of maintaining such response for a longer period of time (5,6,11). Since one of the actions of levamisole is to restore immunocompetence to normal levels, the prognosis of immunosuppressed patients could be improved by the addition of this drug to their therapy. In addition, reactivation of the RES system by levamisole could further favor the clinical course of these patients. An additional advantage of levamisole is the ease of its administration and relative lack of serious toxic reactions.

Based on the differences in mechanism of action between microbial adjuvants and levamisole, approaches to combination immunotherapy to achieve additive or synergistic effect should be explored. Combination chemotherapy with the addition of BCG and levamisole is currently being tested at our institution in a similar group of patients. The combination of *C. parvum* and levamisole added to combination chemotherapy is also an attractive possibility and should be explored in the search for more effective modalities of treatment in breast cancer.

SUMMARY

One hundred and twenty-seven patients with metastatic breast cancer were treated with a combination of 5-fluorouracil, adriamycin, cyclophosphamide, and levamisole. The results were compared to two comparable groups of patients treated with FAC chemotherapy alone and FAC + BCG. Preliminary results suggest that the response rate and the duration of remission are identical to those observed with the FAC-BCG program and significantly better than those observed with the FAC chemotherapy alone. Levamisole appears to be an active immunotherapeutic agent in the treatment of metastatic breast cancer, and, although acting with a different mechanism of action, it appears to achieve clinical results similar to those seen with BCG.

ACKNOWLEDGMENT

We would like to acknowledge the excellent secretarial help of Kathy Calahan in the preparation of this manuscript.

This work was supported by a grant from the Cancer Research Institute, New York, New York, a contract (N01-CB-33888) from the National Cancer Institute, Bethesda, Maryland, and grant no. 167786 of Janssen R&D, Inc.

We would like to acknowledge the assistance of Robert Legendre and Ken Cleaver.

Levamisole was provided by Janssen R&D, Inc., New Brunswick, New Jersey 08903.

REFERENCES

1. Amiel, J. L., and Bernardet, M. (1970): An experiment model of active immunotherapy preceded by cyto-reductive chemotherapy. *Eur. J. Cancer,* 6:557–559.
2. Anderson, R., Glover, A., Koornhof, H. J., and Rabson, A. R. (1976): *In vitro* stimulation of neutrophil motility of levamisole: Maintenance of cGMP Levels in chemotactically stimulated levamisole treated neutrofils. *J. Immunol.,* 117(2):428–432.
3. Biniaminov, M., and Ramot, R. (1975): *In vitro* restoration by levamisole of thymus-derived lymphocyte function in Hodgkin's disease. *Lancet,* 1:464.
4. Blumenschein, G. R., Cardenas, J. O., Freireich, E. J., and Gottlieb, J. A. (1974): FAC-chemotherapy for breast cancer. *Proc. Am. Soc. Clin. Oncol.,* 15:193.
5. Cheema, A. R., and Hersh, E. M. (1971): Patient survival after chemotherapy and its relationship to *in vitro* lymphocyte blastogenesis. *Cancer,* 28:851–855.
6. Eilber, F. R., and Morton, D. L. (1970): Impaired immunologic reactivity and recurrence following cancer surgery. *Cancer,* 25:362–367.
7. Gehan, E. A. (1965): A generalized Wilcoxon test for comparing arbitrarily single censored samples. *Biometrika,* 52:203–223.
8. Glass, U., Wasserman, J., Blomgren, H., and DeSchryver, A. (1976): Lymphopenia in metastatic breast cancer patients with and without radiation therapy. *Int. J. Rad. Oncol. Biol. Phys.,* 1:189–195.
9. Graser, N., and Thompson, D. N. P. (1975): Cell-mediated antitumor immunity in breast cancer patients evaluated by antigen induced leukocyte adherence inhibition in test tubes. *Cancer Res.,* 35:2571–2579.
10. Gutterman, G. U., Cardenas, J. O., Blumenschein, G. R., Hortobagyi, G. N., Burgess, M. A., Livingston, R. B., Mavligit, G. N., Freireich, E. J., Gottlieb, J. A., and Hersh, E. M. (1976): Chemoimmunotherapy of advanced breast cancer: Prolongation of remission and survival with BCG. *Br. Med. J.,* 2:1222–1225.
11. Hersh, E. M., Whitecar, J. P., McCredie, K. B., Bodey, G. P., and Freireich, E. J., (1971): Chemotherapy, immunocompetence, immunosuppression and prognosis in acute leukemia. *N. Engl. J. Med.,* 285:1211–1216.
12. Hirshaut, Y., Pinsky, C., Marquardt, H., and Oettgen, H. F. (1973): Effects of levamisole in delayed hypersensitivity reactions in cancer patients. *Proc. Am. Assoc. Cancer Res.,* 14:109.
13. Hoebeke, J., and Franchi, G. (1973): Influence of tetramizole and its optical isomers on the mononuclear phagocytic system—Effect on carbon clearance in mice. *J. Reticuloendothel. Soc.,* 14:317–323.
14. Hortobagyi, G. N., Gutterman, J. U., Blumenschein, G. R., Mavligit, G. N., and Hersh, E. M. (1976): Chemoimmunotherapy of metastatic breast cancer: Prolongation of remission and survival with BCG. *Am. Soc. Clin. Oncol.,* 17:275 #C-155 (Abstr.).
15. Irwin, M. R., Holmberg, C. A., Knight, H. D., and Hjerpe, C. A. (1976): Effects of vaccination against infectious bovine rhinotracheitis and simultaneous administration of levamisole on primary humoral responses in calves. *Am. J. Vet. Res.,* 37(2):223–226.
16. Jones, S. E., Durie, B. C. and Salmon, S. E. (1975): Combination chemotherapy with adriamycin and cyclophosphamide for advanced breast cancer. *Cancer,* 36:90–97.
17. Kaplan, E. L., and Meier, P. (1958): Non-parametric estimation from incomplete observations. *J. Am. Stat. Assoc.,* 53:457–481.
18. Knight, L. A., and Davidson, W. M. (1975): Reduced lymphocyte transformation in early cancer of the breast. *J. Clin. Pathol.,* 28:372–376.
19. Lods, J. C., Dujardin, P., and Halpern, G. N. (1975): Action of levamisole on antibody protection after vaccination with anti-typhoid and para-typhoid A and B. *Ann. Allergy,* 34:210–212.
20. Lods, J. C., Dujardin, P., and Halpern, G. N. (1976): Levamisole and bone marrow restoration after chemotherapy. *Lancet,* 1:548.
21. Mantovani, A., and Spreafico, S. (1974): Characterization of the immunostimulatory activity of levamisole. *Boll. Ist. Sieroter. Milan.,* 53:302.
22. Pearson, J. W., Chaparas, S. D., and Chirigos, M. A. (1973): Effect of dose and route of Bacillus Calmette-Guerin in chemoimmuno-stimulation therapy of murine leukemia. *Cancer Res.,* 33:1845–1848.
23. Pearson, J. W., Pearson, G. R., Gibson, W. T., Chermann, J. C., and Chirigos, M. A. (1972):

Combined chemoimmunostimulation therapy against murine leukemia. *Cancer Res.,* 32:904–907.

24. Pinsky, C. M., DeJager, R. L., Kaufman, R. J., Mike, V., Hansen, J. A., Oettgen, H. F., and Krakoff, I. H. (1978): Corynebacterium parvum as adjuvant to combination chemotherapy in patients with advanced breast cancer. Preliminary results of a prospective randomized trial. In: *Immunotherapy of Cancer: Present Status of Trials in Man,* edited by W. D. Terry and D. Windhorst. Raven Press, New York. *(in press).*

25. Pinsky, C. M., Domeiri, A., Caron, A. S., Knapper, W. H., and Oettgen, H. F. (1974): Delayed hypersensitivity reactions in patients with cancer. Investigations and stimulation of immunity in cancer patients, p. 37. Springer-Verlag, Berlin.

26. Ramot, B., Biniaminov, M., Shohan, C. H., and Rosenthal, E. (1976): Effect of levamisole on E. rosette-forming cells *in vivo* and *in vitro,* in Hodgkin's disease. *N. Engl. J. Med.,* 294:809–811.

27. Renoux, X. G., Renoux, M., and Palat, A. (1975): Influence of levamisole on T-cell reactivity and in survival of untractable cancer patients. Fogarty Int. Center Proc., #28. U.S. Govt. Printing Office, Washington D.C. *(in press).*

28. Rojas, A. F., Michiewicz, E., Feierstein, J. N., Glatt, H., and Olivari, A. J. (1976): Levamisole in advanced human breast cancer. *Lancet,* 1:211–215.

29. Study Group for Bronchogenic Carcinoma (1975): Immunopotentiation with levamisole in resectable bronchogenic carcinoma: A double blind controlled trial. *Br. Med. J.,* 3:461–464.

30. Tashima, C. K., Blumenschein, G. R., and Gutterman, J. U. (1976): Comparison of adriamycin combination drug program with BCG immunotherapy versus MER immunotherapy for metastatic breast cancer. *Am. Soc. Clin. Oncol.,* 17:288 #C-207.

31. Thulin, H., Thestrup-Pedersen, K., and Ellegaard, J. (1975): In vitro parameters of cell-mediated immune reactions in healthy individuals following immune-stimulation attempts with levamisole. *Acta Allergol. (Kbh.),* 30:9–18.

32. Tripodi, D., Parks, L. C., and Brugmans, J. (1973): Drug-induced restoration of cutaneous delayed hypersensitivity in anergic patients with cancer. *N. Engl. J. Med.,* 289:354–357.

33. Van Eygen, M., Znamensky, P. Y., Heck, E., and Raymalkers, I. (1976): Levamisole in prevention of recurrent upper-respiratory-tract infections in children. *Lancet,* 1:382–385.

34. Verhaegen, H., DeCree, J., DeCock, W., and Verbruggen, F. (1973): Levamisole and the immune response. *N. Engl. J. Med.,* 289:1148–1149.

35. Verhaegen, H., DeCree, J., Verbruggen, F., Hoebeke, J., DeBrabander, N., and Brugmans, J. (1973): Immune responses in elderly cuti-negative subjects and the effect of levamisole. *Verh. Dtsch. Ges. Inn. Med.,* 79:823–828.

36. Wanebo, H. J., Rosen, P. P., Thaler, T., Urban, J. A., and Oettgen, H. F. (1976): Immunobiology of operable breast cancer: An assessment of biologic risks by immuno-parameters. *Ann. Surg.,* 184:258–266.

37. Whitehead, R. H., Bolten, P. N., Newcomb, R. G., James, S. L., and Hughes, L. E. (1975): Lymphocyte response to PHA in breast cancer: Correlation of predicted prognosis to response to different PHA concentrations. *Clin. Oncol.,* 1:191–200.

Immune Modulation and Control of Neoplasia by Adjuvant Therapy, edited by M. A. Chirigos. Raven Press, New York, 1978.

Unblocking Effect of Levamisole on a Subpopulation of T Lymphocytes in Hodgkin's Disease Patients

Bracha Ramot, Miriam Biniaminov, and Esther Rosenthal

Chaim Sheba Medical Center, Tel-Aviv University, Sackler School of Medicine, Tel-Hashomer, Israel

The immunomodulating effect of levamisole in experimental tumors has been clearly demonstrated. However, the mechanism of its action is as yet unclear. We have chosen Hodgkin's disease (HD) lymphocytes as an experimental model for the study of the *in vivo* and *in vitro* effect of levamisole since a cellular immune defect exists in this disease as evidenced by a decrease in the number of E-rosette-forming cells (ERFC), decreased cutaneous response to antigens, and poor lymphocyte response to low doses of phytohemagglutinin. In previous studies we were able to show that *in vivo* administration of levamisole, 150 mg $\times$ 3, raised the ERFC of HD patients with low ERFC numbers to normal levels (2). This effect persisted for at least 2 months (4). Incubation of peripheral blood lymphocytes of HD patients *in vitro* with 40 μg/ml levamisole raised their ERFC number to normal levels (1). There was no such *in vitro* effect after *in vivo* levamisole administration (4).

The questions we posed were as follows: (a) Is there a substance blocking the ERFC that is removed from cell surface by levamisole? (b) Is there a subpopulation of lymphocytes that is blocked and is affected by the drug? (c) Is the lymphocyte blocking and unblocking by levamisole related to extent of disease, histologic pattern, or therapy? and finally, (d) Does ERFC blocking occur also in spleen or lymph node lymphocytes, or both?

The nature of the blocking substance on peripheral blood lymphocytes of HD patients was studied in collaboration with Moroz (3).

It was found that a blocking substance removed from lymphocyte surface by levamisole is apoferritin. Twenty to sixty percent of the radioactive peak separated on acrylamide SDS isolated from the ^{125}I-iodinated surface proteins precipitated with antispleen ferritin. Reduction and alkylation of this protein peak dissociated it into a single monomeric unit of a molecular weight of about 18,000. The profile of HD lymphocytes after levamisole treatment was normal.

These results raised the next questions—Which are the cells that have the apoferritin on their surface? Is it a random adsorption of serum ferritin on peripheral blood lymphocytes or is ferritin bound to a specific subpopulation of cells? To answer these questions, Ficoll-hypaque-isolated lymphocytes were passed through a nylon column. The adherent cells were removed mechanically and compared to the cells in the void volume and in the total lymphocyte population. As can be seen from Fig. 1, the cells that are affected by levamisole are those that adhere to nylon. Furthermore, these cells can be eluted from the nylon by levamisole *(unpublished observations)*. These results indicate that we are dealing with a subpopulation of lymphocytes that adheres to nylon and has apoferritin on its surface. Reconstitution experiments were performed in the following way; HD and normal lymphocytes were incubated with 40 µg/

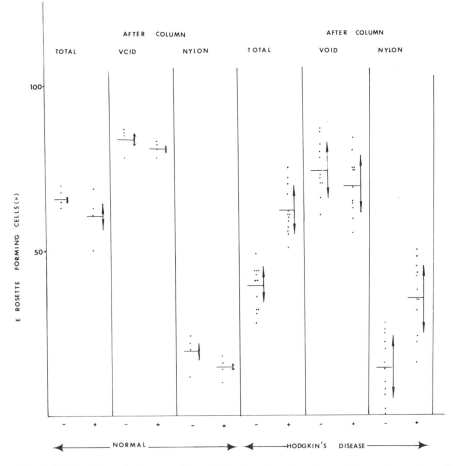

FIG. 1. Effect of levamisole on peripheral blood lymphocyte subpopulations of normals and Hodgkin's disease patients. E, E rosettes in total cell population; T, T cells which appear in the void volume; B, B cells—adherent to nylon; +, after *in vitro* incubation with levamisole; −, without incubation with levamisole. *Vertical arrows,* mean ± SD.

TABLE 1. In vitro *E-rosette-blocking effect of ferritin on Hodgkin's disease lymphocytes after levamisole treatment*

Patients	Cell treatment (%)					
	Lev *in vitro*	Lev	Lev + ferr	Lev + ferr + lev	Ferr	Ferr + lev
Normal no. 1	65	67	68	58	64	59
Normal no. 2	64	65	64	56	66	60
HD no. 1	28	51	30	56	27	49
HD no. 2	42	67	34	60	44	55

Lev, levamisole; ferr, ferritin.

ml levamisole, washed, and incubated with 150 µg of human spleen ferritin for an hour. The cells were again incubated with levamisole. The ERFC were counted after each incubation. As can be seen (Table 1), ferritin blocked E-rosettes, and levamisole reversed the reaction. Ferritin had no effect on lymphocytes isolated from normal individuals.

The next question to be answered was, Is this effect specific for ferritin or will any glycoprotein or protein do it? Our preliminary data using fetuin, α acid glycoprotein, and albumin show that only ferritin, and not the others, blocks ERFC and is removed by levamisole.

Although these are interesting laboratory findings, the basic questions remain, namely, Is the ferritin on the surface of a subpopulation of lymphocytes causally related to the disease? Is its amount an indication of the clinical state of the patient?

Since the ERFC number is not always low in HD, we have during the last year studied patients untreated as well as treated by radiotherapy and chemotherapy. No correlation could be found between low E-rosettes, histologic type, or clinical stage. Unexpectedly, we found that chemotherapy raised the ERFC number close to normal levels, whereas radiotherapy caused a long persistent decrease in ERFC number. In both groups of patients, however, there was still a population of lymphocytes affected by levamisole (Fig. 2).

As to the question whether ferritin is present on the surface of a subpopulation of spleen or lymph node lymphocytes, or both, in HD patients, our data are very preliminary. Levamisole has no effect on these tissues. However, reconstitution experiments with ferritin after incubation with levamisole have to be performed.

In summary, it would appear that apoferritin is a blocking substance on HD peripheral blood lymphocytes (3). This substance can be removed by incubation of the cells with levamisole *in vitro* or by administration of the drug *in vivo,* or both. It is present on a subpopulation of T lymphocytes but not on all T cells, which causes them to adhere to nylon, persists after radiotherapy, but is much less evident after combined chemotherapy. *In vitro* experiments

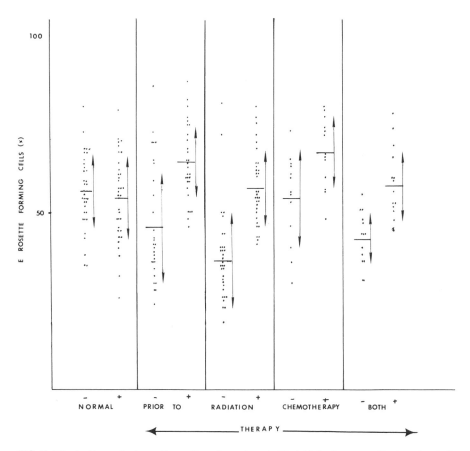

FIG. 2. Effect of levamisole on E-rosette cell numbers in Hodgkin's disease patients untreated and treated with radiotherapy and combined chemotherapy. +, after *in vitro* incubation with levamisole; —, without incubation with levamisole. *Vertical arrows,* mean ± SD.

indicate that the blocking can be reproduced *in vitro* by ferritin only on HD lymphocytes. Other glycoproteins studied did not show a similar effect. Although a relationship between ferritin blocking and E-rosette number *in vitro* and *in vivo* seems to exist, it remains to be determined if it has a real pathogenetic significance.

ACKNOWLEDGMENTS

These studies were supported by Janssen Pharmaceutica, the Freddy Marke-vitz Cancer Research Fund, and the Tali Carasso Leukemia Research Fund.

REFERENCES

1. Biniaminov, M., and Ramot, B. (1975): *In vitro* restoration by levamisole of thymus derived lymphocyte function in Hodgkin's disease. Letter to the Editor. *Lancet,* 1:464.

2. Levo, Y., Ramot, B., and Rotter, V. (1975): Restoration of cellular immune response by levamisole in patients with Hodgkin's disease. *Biomedicine,* 23:198.
3. Moroz, Ch., Lahat, N., Biniaminov, M., and Ramot, B. (1977): Ferritin on the surface of lymphocytes of Hodgkin's disease patients—a possible blocking substance removed by levamisole. *Clin. Exp. Immunol.,* 28: *(in press).*
4. Ramot, B., Biniaminov, M., and Shoham, Ch. (1976): Effect of levamisole on E-rosette forming cells *in vivo* and *in vitro* in Hodgkin's disease. *N. Engl. J. Med.,* 294:809.

Immune Modulation and Control of Neoplasia by Adjuvant Therapy, edited by M. A. Chirigos. Raven Press, New York, 1978.

Combination Immunotherapy with Levamisole, BCG, and Tumor Vaccines: Toward a Rationale

*,**L. M. Jerry, *,***M. G. Lewis, †H. R. Shibata, **,† P. W. A. Mansell, *A. Capek, and **G. Marquis

*McGill Cancer Research Unit, and Departments of **Medicine, ***Pathology, and †Surgery, McGill University and Royal Victoria Hospital, Montreal, Canada

In human cancer, immunotherapy has been applied empirically in clinical trials, often with only long-term statistical survival data to attest to its efficacy. The incomplete state of knowledge in tumor immunology and the unavailability of adequate monitoring systems have necessitated this approach, but it is leading to confusion (24). In fact, evidence to show that putative immunotherapeutic agents even act through the stimulation of antitumor immunity is often lacking.

In human melanoma, specific antitumor humoral and cell-mediated immune responses can be measured. Certain of these parameters, in particular antimembrane antibody, may have prognostic significance in terms of the development of metastasis (2,14). Moreover, the clinical triad of anergy, antiantibodies, and immune complex disease in melanoma have led to the suggestion that the progressive failure of specific antitumor immunity with advancing disease results from deranged immune regulation subsequent to chronic antigenic stimulation by cytoplasmic tumor antigens (8,9,12).

In this study, the effects of specific (autologous tumor cells) and nonspecific [oral Bacillus Calmette-Guérin (BCG) and levamisole] immunotherapy on serial measurements of antitumor immunity in melanoma are described. The results suggest an advantage, and provide a rationale for the use of combinations of agents with differing mechanisms of action, and indicate that it may be possible to assess their efficacy by serial monitoring of immune parameters in individual patients.

THE SYNDROME OF DERANGED IMMUNE REGULATION IN MELANOMA

Antitumor Immunity in Human Melanoma

Circulating serum antibodies are directed against surface membrane antigens on living autologous tumor cells. These IgG antibodies show strong individual or private specificity for a patient's own tumor (2,15,21), but weak cross-reactivity

147

seen against allogeneic cell surface membranes indicates that there are minor cross-reactive or public membrane antibodies as well (15,21). Antimembrane antibodies are cytotoxic to membrane tumor cells in the presence of complement *in vitro* (2) and can prevent adherence of tumor cells to surfaces and to endothelium. They have been measured by a number of methods including complement dependent cytotoxicity (2) and immune adherence (21), and, for the studies to be described here, by indirect immunofluorescence on suspensions of live autologous tumor cells (15). These antibodies are most common in early localized disease, becoming undetectable prior to the appearance of widespread dissemination of tumor (2,13,14). This stage relationship of antimembrane antibodies may have prognostic value, since serial monitoring of individual patients indicates that these antibodies invariably become undetectable within weeks or months before the clinical appearance of deep organ metastases.

Anticytoplasmic antibodies are detected by indirect immunofluorescence using snap-frozen tumor cell smears on glass slides (18). In contrast to the antimembrane system, anticytoplasmic antibodies show wide, but tumor-specific, cross-reactivity with allogeneic melanoma tumor cells (8,11). They are directed against internal components of the tumor cells and presumably represent an immune response against contents of tumor cells released through necrosis. Anticytoplasmic antibodies show a less clear stage relationship. They are seen throughout the growth of the tumor and are often present in largest amounts in patients with advanced disease (8,11).

The measurement of antitumor cellular immunity in melanoma is controversial. There is no universal agreement on whether the various assays that have been employed are capable of demonstrating tumor specificity or correlation with clinical stage. The microcytotoxicity assay of Takasugi and Klein (23) has been used in the studies to be reported here.

Lymphocyte cytotoxicity in melanoma patients shows a stage relationship, being elevated when the tumor is localized and falling progressively with advancing disease (8). The 40% of cytotoxicity distinguishes best between normal and abnormal ranges. Although cytotoxicity disappears in advanced disease, it can be readily revived by specific (immunization with irradiated tumor cells) or nonspecific (oral BCG or levamisole) immunotherapy. It has considerable value in sequential monitoring of the response of individual patients with malignancy to immunotherapy (20).

Deranged Immune Regulation in Melanoma

The discovery of antiantibodies and immune complexes in melanoma (1,8, 9,12), in addition to anergy, has led to the suggestion that immune failure in cancer can be thought to be a consequence of disordered immune regulation and control resulting from persistent antigenic stimulation, and manifesting clinically as the triad of anergy, antiantibodies, and immune complex disease (8,9,12).

Several antiantibody systems have been described in human melanoma. IgG anti-γ-globulins of the antiidiotypic variety are directed against determinants in the variable region, including the antigen-binding site, of antimembrane tumor antibody (8,12,16). Evidence suggests that these anti-γ-globulins mediate the disappearance of antimembrane tumor antibodies from the circulation in advancing melanoma (9,16). The formation of immune complexes between tumor antibody and antiidiotypic antibody results in immune elimination of the former from the circulation just prior to the appearance of deep metastases (9). Anti-γ-globulins of the serum (or pepsin) agglutinator (or anti-F(ab')$_2$) type have also been described (5). These are directed against determinants in the hinge region of the anticytoplasmic tumor antibodies, with which they show a reciprocal relationship in serum (4). More recently antiantibodies with rheumatoid factor-like activity have been described in the sera of melanoma patients as well (8).

There are some clues to the significance of antiantibody systems in melanoma. Antiidiotypic antibodies can be specifically immunosuppressive in experimental situations, and an idiotypic immune response against lymphoid cell immunoglobulin receptors has been proposed as one mechanism for regulating and limiting the extent of a normal antibody response (7,10). Serum agglutinators have been described in many conditions, including the rheumatic diseases (17) and chronic gram-positive infections (25). It has been suggested that they represent an attempt by the immune system to respond to a persistent antigenic stimulation (25). The production of F(ab')$_2$ fragments necessary for their elicitation could result from proteolysis of anticytoplasmic antibodies by host-cell infiltrates in the tumor (12). The origin and significance of rheumatoid factor-like anti-γ-globulins in malignancy are less clear. They may represent a response to circulating immune complexes in these patients.

There is growing evidence for immune complex-mediated phenomena in a variety of human and animal tumors, including melanoma (8,9). Although frank nephrotic syndrome due to immune complex nephritis occurs rarely in cancer patients, subclinical varieties may be common. Assays employing human Cl$_q$ or polyclonal rheumatoid factors (9) have been used to detect and quantitate circulating immune complexes in melanoma (9). Moderate levels of complexes of intermediate and large types circulate in increasing frequency with advancing disease. Such complexes may contain tumor antigen and tumor antibody, or antiantibody and tumor antibody. In addition to circadian fluctuations, the levels of complexes are altered by surgery, chemotherapy, and immunotherapy.

In addition to cancer, one or more of these three phenomena of anergy, antiantibodies, and immune complexes have been found in a number of disorders including chronic infections (bacterial endocarditis, tuberculosis, gram-positive infections), chronic parasitic disease (malaria, trypanosomiasis), and the rheumatic disorders (rheumatoid arthritis, lupus erythematosus). Many of these disorders share in common a persistent antigenic stimulus to the immune system (25), a system designed ordinarily to eliminate its antigenic stimulus and then shut itself off by negative feedback. This phasic regulatory action and reaction within the immune system would be expected to be disturbed by persistent antigenic stimulation. It is postulated that the ensuing deranged regulation is signalled by the syndrome of anergy, antiantibodies, and immune complex disease in varying proportions, followed later by failure of the antitumor immune response itself (8,9,12). The locus of the lesion presumably involves the cooperative cell-cell interactions among T cells, B cells, and macrophages that are necessary for a coordinated immune response. Defective regulator cell activity may be involved.

This model has several important clinical implications (Fig. 1). It can, for example, predict different mechanisms of action for certain immunotherapeutic agents and can provide a rationale for their combined use. The antianergic drug levamisole is active in several disorders that share defective immune regulation. These include recurrent and chronic infections of skin, mucous membranes, and the eye as well as respiratory and systemic infections caused by viruses, bacteria, or fungi: postviral anergy following influenza and measles; rheumatic disorders such as rheumatoid arthritis, systemic lupus erythematosus, and Reiter's syndrome; and cancer, where the drug stabilizes remission (22). Thus levamisole is immunoregulatory in action in contrast to an immunostimulant such as BCG. In addition to restoring defective function to many cell types involved in the immune response, perhaps through favorably influencing the intracellular balance of cyclic GMP and cyclic AMP (3), it also enhances suppressor cell activity in man (19).

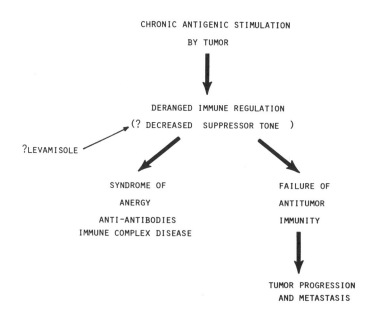

FIG. 1. Hypothesis—production of deranged immune regulation with subsequent failure of antitumor immunity in melanoma.

The object of immunotherapy in cancer then should be to restore immune regulation rather than to hyperstimulate a patient's immune response blindly. To achieve this end, however, it is necessary to monitor the effectiveness of immunotherapy by measurements of specific antitumor immunity.

COMBINATION IMMUNOTHERAPY WITH TUMOR VACCINES, LEVAMISOLE, AND BCG

Studies were carried out in 88 patients with stages I to IV malignant melanoma on the effects of various specific and nonspecific immunotherapy regimens on specific antitumor immunity (20). Fifty-one patients received levamisole and 37 were given oral BCG. Thirty-seven patients received levamisole alone, and 17 patients were given oral BCG alone, whereas 6 patients received oral BCG followed by levamisole and 11 patients received levamisole followed by oral BCG. Twelve patients were autoimmunized; five then received levamisole and seven had oral BCG. Because of a lack of tumor cells five patients were alloimmunized; three subsequently received levamisole and two had oral BCG.

In initial studies patients were given 8-week courses of either lyophilized reconstituted oral BCG (Institut Armand Frappier, Montreal, Canada; derived from Pasteur strain), 120 mg weekly, or levamisole, 150 mg for 3 days weekly. Measures of specific antitumor immunity were carried out before, at weekly intervals during, and at the end of each treatment course. Results are summarized in Table 1. Only 2 of 17 patients showed large elevations of antitumor antibody, but half of the patients had marked elevations in lymphocyte cytotoxicity in response to an 8-week course of oral BCG. Similar results were obtained with oral levamisole given alone for 8 weeks. Seven of 39 patients showed large rises in levels of antitumor antibodies and 11 of 28 had striking increases in lymphocyte cytotoxicity. These agents used alone seem about equally effective in stimulating antitumor immunity in melanoma patients and show a greater

TABLE 1. *Effect of immunotherapy on antitumor immunity in human melanoma*

	Increase in antimembrane antibody	Increase in anticytoplasmic antibody	Increase in lymphocyte cytotoxicity
BCG	0/1[a]	2/17[a]	5/10[a]
Levamisole	0/2	7/37	11/28
BCG → levamisole	ND	4/6	3/5
Levamisole → BCG	ND	2/11	3/7
Tumor vaccine + BCG	3/8[b]	0/9[b]	2/6[b]
Tumor vaccine + levamisole	2/5	1/8	2/5

ND, not done: Autologous cells unavailable.

[a]Number of patients showing large increase (> 30%) per number studied.

[b]Number of patients showing prolongation of response initiated by tumor vaccine per number studied.

effect on cellular immunity. Nearly all patients showed some response to the drugs, but because of the relative insensitivity of the assays for antitumor immunity only large changes (> 30%) are recorded in the table.

When six patients who had received three, 8-week courses of oral BCG with no antitumor response were subsequently given 8 weeks of levamisole, an unexpected result was obtained (Table 1). Four of six patients now showed striking antitumor antibody responses and three of five patients had marked increases in lymphocyte cytotoxicity. One of the two patients in stage I, both in stage II, and one of two patients with stage IV disease showed responses. The levamisole response tended to occur after 4 weeks of treatment and was often prolonged for two or three subsequent courses. No unusual toxicity was noted with the combined use of these two agents. Because of a lack of autologous tumor cells, only allogeneic anticytoplasmic melanoma antibodies were determined in these patients. However, the reverse sequence in which patients were given 8 weeks of levamisole followed by 8 weeks of oral BCG was about as effective as either drug used alone.

These early observations indicate differences in the mechanisms of action of these two agents and suggest using immunotherapeutic agents in combination. Until now we have relied on tumor cell vaccines to elicit immunity in melanoma patients (2,6,13,14). The proper combined use of levamisole and BCG now allows good responses to be obtained in over half of the patients in situations where tumor cells are unavailable for vaccination. An example of the combined sequential use of oral BCG and levamisole over a period of 22 months is shown in Fig. 2 in a stage II melanoma patient after complete surgical resection of tumor. Stimulation of both anticytoplasmic antibodies and lymphocyte cytotoxicity is achieved with oral BCG. Following initial stimulation, the immunoregula-

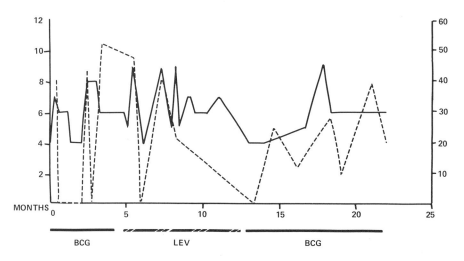

FIG. 2. Combined sequential oral BCG and levamisole immunotherapy in a stage II melanoma patient. ———, Anticytoplasmic antibody; ------, lymphocyte cytotoxicity.

tory action of the levamisole is then evident with subsiding levels of antitumor immunity. Restimulation with oral BCG then follows.

Since antimembrane antibodies in melanoma are present in localized or regional disease and appear to be related to control of blood-borne metastasis (2,14), it would seem reasonable that efforts to induce and maintain their levels in the circulation should be beneficial to individual patients (20). Immunization with irradiated autologous tumor cells regularly produces such responses, but the effects are transient, lasting 14 to 21 days (6). Although repeated immunizations are effective, the shortage of autologous tumor cells in most instances prevents this procedure from being a clinically practical way to maintain the response. Attempts were made, therefore, to prolong a vaccine-induced response by adding oral BCG or levamisole to the regimen (Table 1) (20). Immunizations used 100 to 200 million irradiated (12,000 rads) tumor cells injected in Hank's culture medium into multiple intradermal sites to stimulate as many regional lymph node areas as possible (6,13,16,20). Antitumor immunity was measured before and thrice weekly for the ensuing 14 days so that the response was not missed. On day 15 patients began successive 8-week courses of either oral BCG (120 mg weekly) or levamisole (150 mg for 3 days weekly), and antitumor immunity was monitored weekly. The responses in Table 1 (bottom) signify prolongation of the antitumor immunity initiated with the vaccine. Nine melanoma patients received tumor cells followed by oral BCG. Seven had autologous immunizations, and in two patients allogeneic melanoma cells were used. The antitumor antibody response obtained by immunization could be prolonged for 2 to 6 months by the addition of oral BCG in three of the nine patients, and prolongations of lymphocyte cytotoxicity were seen in two of six patients. The response lasted up to 6 months in some patients, but eventually further immunizations were required (20).

A similar effect was achieved with levamisole in eight patients, five of whom received autologous and three allogeneic tumor cells. Three of the eight patients showed prolongation of the antitumor antibody response initiated by immunization, and two of five patients showed effects on lymphocyte cytotoxicity. Thus in some patients oral BCG and levamisole showed similar effectiveness in prolonging immunization-induced antitumor immune responses for clinically practical periods of time measured in months. Similar results have been achieved also in patients with other tumors (four osteogenic sarcomas, one fibrosarcoma, one chondrosarcoma, two teratomas, and two colorectal cancers). In addition, levamisole showed an adjuvant effect when given just prior to immunization (20). Ordinarily effective doses of 10^8 irradiated tumor cells could be reduced to 3×10^6 and 11×10^6 in two patients with good antitumor responses.

An example of prolongation of vaccine-induced antitumor immunity by combined oral BCG and levamisole is illustrated in Fig. 3 for a stage II melanoma patient after complete surgical resection of tumor. The initial response in membrane antibody and lymphocyte cytotoxicity was short-lived. However, the sequential use of BCG and levamisole prolonged the response for nearly 7 months,

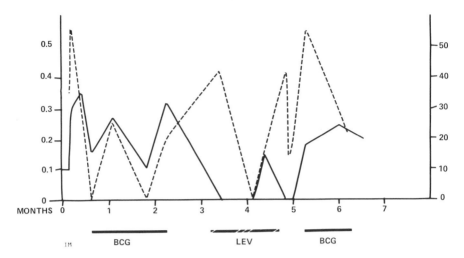

FIG. 3. Combination immunotherapy in a stage II melanoma patient using tumor vaccine followed by sequential oral BCG and levamisole. ———, Antimembrane antibody; -----, lymphocyte cytotoxicity. IM, immunization.

until the appearance of brain metastases. Indeed the first appearance of tumor in the brain, to the exclusion of other metastatic sites, in some of our patients may point to a potential limitation in dealing with immunologically privileged sites such as the central nervous system.

PROSPECTUS

Immunotherapy in man is in its infancy, and of necessity the approach has been empiric. The modest gains obtained thus far have been derived often from extrapolations from artificial animal models of uncertain significance to human cancer, and from empirically designed clinical trials. Unfortunately, in the case of clinical trials, the reasons for success, or more importantly failure, are not known, since in most instances reliable parameters other than long-term survival statistics are not available to guide the choice of therapy. If immunotherapeutic agents are effective in cancer because of their action on the immune response, then effects on specific antitumor immunity should be measurable and presumably could be used ultimately to design optimal regimens for use in clinical trials and to monitor the ongoing effectiveness of immunotherapy in individual patients. The studies reported here are early attempts to monitor immunotherapy of cancer patients by measurements of specific antitumor immunity, and show the feasibility of such an approach. These studies point out differences in the mechanism of action of immunotherapeutic agents. They allow the design of regimens using combinations of agents for optimum antitumor immune stimulation in individual patients that could then be tested in clinical trials. The concept of immune failure in cancer as a reflection of deranged immune regulation suggests the potential folly of blind hyperstimulation of the cancer patient's immune response (8). Effective therapy may require, at least in part, restoration of the disordered cooperation between the B and T arms of the immune response. To do this effectively will require monitored, and perhaps individually designed, regimens.

ACKNOWLEDGMENTS

The authors express their thanks to Chitra Roy, Helen Lyons, and Narcisso Mejia for expert technical assistance and to Mrs. Joan Bierd for preparation of the manuscript. The work reported in this chapter has been supported by the National Cancer Institute of Canada and by Ortho Pharmaceutical (Canada), Ltd.

L.M.J. is Scholar of the Medical Research Council of Canada and M.G.L. is Director of NCI, Canada Research Unit.

REFERENCES

1. Baldwin, R. W., and Robins, R. A. (1976): Factors interfering with immunological rejection of tumors. *Br. Med. Bull.,* 32:118.
2. Bodurtha, A. J., Chee, D. O., Laucius, J. F., Mastrangelo, J. J., and Prehn, R. T. (1975): Clinical and immunological significance of human melanoma cytotoxic antibody. *Cancer Res.,* 35:189.
3. Hadden, J. W., Coffey, R. G., Hadden, E. M., Lapezcar, E., and Sunshine, G. H. (1975): Effects of levamisole and imidazole on lymphocyte proliferation and cyclic nucleotide levels. *Cell. Immunol.,* 20:98.
4. Hartmann, D. (1976): *Anti-Immunologloblulins in Human Malignancy.* Thesis. McGill University, Montreal.
5. Hartmann, D., Lewis, M. G., Proctor, J. W., and Lyons, H. (1974): *In vitro* interactions between antitumor antibodies and antiantibodies in malignancy. *Lancet,* 2:1481.
6. Ikonopisov, R. L., Lewis, M. G., Hunter-Craig, I. D., Bodenham, D. C., Phillips, T. M., Cooling, C. I., Proctor, J., Hamilton Fairley, G., and Alexander, P. (1970): Auto-immunization with irradiated tumor cells in malignant melanomas. *Br. Med. J.,* 2:752.
7. Jerne, N. K. (1973): The immune system. *Sci. Am.,* 229:52.
8. Jerry, L. M., Lewis, M. G., and Cano, P. O. (1976): Anergy, anti-antibodies and immune complex disease: A syndrome of disordered immune regulation in human cancer. In: *Immunocancerology in Solid Tumors,* edited by M. Martin and L. Dionne, p. 63. Symposia Specialists, Miami.
9. Jerry, L. M., Rowden, G., Cano, P. O., Phillips, T. M., Deutsch, G. F., Capek, A., Hartmann, D., and Lewis, M. G. (1976): Immune complexes in human melanoma: A consequence of deranged regulation of humoral immunity. *Scand. J. Immunol.,* 5:845.
10. Kohler, H. (1975): The response to phosphorylcholine: Dissecting and immune response. *Transplant Rev.,* 27:24.
11. Lewis, M. G. (1974): Immunology and the melanomas. *Curr. Top. Microbiol. Immunol.,* 63:49.
12. Lewis, M. G., Hartmann, D. P., and Jerry, L. M. (1976): Antibodies and anti-antibodies in human malignancy. An expression of deranged immune regulation. *Ann. N.Y. Acad. Sci.,* 276:316.
13. Lewis, M. G., Ikonopisov, R. N., Nairn, R. C., Phillips, T. M., Hamilton Fairley, G., Bodenham, D. C., and Alexander, P. (1969): Tumor specific antibodies in human malignant melanomas and their relationship to the extent of the disease. *Br. Med. J.,* 3:547.
14. Lewis, M. G., McCloy, E., and Blake, J. (1973): The significance of humoral antibodies in the localization of human malignant melanoma. *Br. J. Surg.,* 60:443.
15. Lewis, M. G., and Phillips, T. M. (1972): The specificity of surface membrane immunofluorescence in human malignant melanoma. *Int. J. Cancer,* 10:105.

16. Lewis, M. G., Phillips, T. M., Cook, K. B., and Blake, J. (1971): Possible explanation for loss of detectable antibody in patients with disseminated malignant melanoma. *Nature,* 232:52.
17. Osterland, C. K., Harbo, M., and Kunkel, H. G. (1963): Anti-γ-globulin factors in human sera revealed in enzymatic splitting of anti-Rh antibodies. *Vox. Surg.,* 8:133.
18. Phillips, T. M., and Lewis, M. G. (1970): A system of immunofluorescence in the study of tumor cells. *Rev. Eur. Etudes Clin. Biol.,* 15:1016.
19. Sampson, D., and Lui, A. (1976): The effect of Levamisole on cell-mediated immunity and suppressor cell function. *Cancer Res.,* 36:952.
20. Shibata, H. R., Jerry, L. M., Lewis, M. G., Mansell, P. W. A., Capek, A., and Marquis, G. (1976): Immunotherapy of human malignant melanoma with irradiated tumor cells, oral Bacillus Calmette-Guérin, and levamisole. *Ann. N.Y. Acad. Sci.,* 277:355.
21. Shiku, H., Takahashi, T., Oettgen, H. F., and Old, L. J. (1976): Cell surface antigens of human malignant melanoma. II. Serological typing with immune adherence assays and definition of two new surface antigens. *J. Exp. Med.,* 144:873.
22. Symoens, J. (1977): Levamisole: An anti-anergic chemotherapeutic agent. In: *Control of Neoplasia by Modulation of the Immune System (Progress in Cancer Research and Therapy, Vol. 2),* edited by M. A. Chirigis, p. 1. Raven Press, New York.
23. Takasugi, M., and Klein, E. (1970): A microassay for cell-mediated immunity. *Transplantation,* 9:219.
24. Terry, W. D., and Windhorst, D. (Eds.) (1977): *Immunotherapy of Cancer: Present Status of Trials in Man (Progress in Cancer Research and Therapy, Vol. 6).* Raven Press, New York.
25. Waller, M., Curry, S., and Richard, A. (1968): Serological specificity of IgG and IgM antiglobulin antibodies in anti-Gm(a) antisera. *Clin. Exp. Immunol.,* 3:631.

Immune Modulation and Control of Neoplasia by Adjuvant Therapy, edited by M. A. Chirigos. Raven Press, New York, 1978.

Interpretation of Management of Levamisole-Associated Side Effects

R. Douglas Thornes

Department of Experimental Medicine, Royal College of Surgeons in Ireland, St. Laurence's Hospital, Dublin, Ireland

It is now 4 years since we first succeeded in restoring activity to the cellular immune mechanism in patients with cancer (5). First we used proteolytic enzymes such as streptokinase or Brinase, which are still the most effective (3), but the possible hemorrhagic side effects and difficulty of repeated intravenous injections made us welcome the discovery of the effect of orally administered levamisole on the immune mechanism (6).

A total of 301 patients have been treated with levamisole, and side effects have been observed in 128 patients, or 43%. These patients can be divided into those in the double-blind trial of levamisole to prevent recurrence of cancer and those in an open trial to correct anergy associated with cancer, brucellosis, or virus infections. The dosage used in the double-blind trial was 150 mg for 2 consecutive days each week, whereas the dosage in the open trial in most cases was 150 mg daily for 1 month and thereafter on 2 consecutive days each week. Results are in Table 1 and Fig. 1.

It is important to appreciate that most symptoms of disease are due to the patient's reactivity against invading organisms or noxious stimuli. It became clear from observing the above patients that the intensity of symptoms was related to the activity of the cellular immune system. It further became obvious that a totally anergic individual was tolerant of infections and antigens. Restoration of the allergic state resulted in the appearance of symptoms of disease. This was exemplified where restoration of the cellular immune mechanism produced an acute exacerbation of symptoms in chronic brucellosis. (4). The converse is also true, for inhibition of the cellular immune mechanism by steroids and cytotoxic agents suppresses symptoms of disease.

These observations were carried a stage further when inadequate or partial restoration of the allergic state resulted in prolonged mild symptoms with extreme tiredness. The tiredness is enhanced by repeated efforts to restore function to the cellular immune mechanism resistant to treatment. Thus partial restoration of the activity of the cellular immune system can produce side effects. These side effects differ depending on the underlying disease and whether or not the patient in the anergic state is carrying infection (See Fig. 2).

157

TABLE 1. *Side effects observed following levamisole therapy*

Trial	No. of patients	Side effects	Percentage
Double-blind	167	17	10
Open	134	111	82
Total	301	128	43

Patients with symptoms and a depressed T-lymphocyte function, as measured by E-rosetting, become symptom free when T-lymphocyte function is restored.

Thus, if the above observations are accurate, agents that influence the cellular immune system will produce side effects, and these must then be appraised in the context of the diseased state of the patient.

We define the cellular immune mechanism as involving all the white blood cells and their interactions. The difficulty has been in finding appropriate tests for function and inhibition. Anergy at present is defined as any one of the following:

1. An absolute lymphocyte count below $1,500/mm^3$

2. Lymphocyte phytohemagglutinin response less than 50% (visual method) (1)

3. Lymphocyte E-rosetting less than 50% (2)

4. Negative skin tests for delayed hypersensitivity after attempts to sensitize the patients to the antigen.

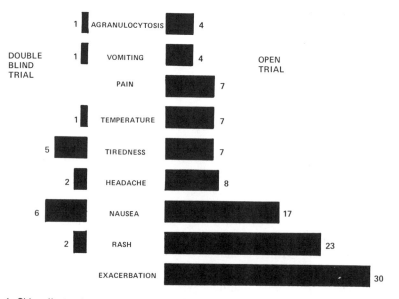

FIG. 1. Side effects observed following levamisole therapy. Double-blind trial, 167 patients; open trial, 134 patients.

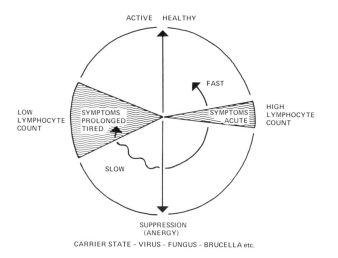

FIG. 2. Diagrammatic representation of production of symptoms following fast and slow stimulation of the cellular immune mechanism.

Patients with low absolute lymphocyte counts tend to have prolonging symptoms, and attempts at restoration often fail. The patients with a high lymphocyte count but low T-cell counts respond with acute symptoms if restoration is successful with levamisole or other antianergic agents (see Fig. 2).

SIDE EFFECTS

It was necessary to suspend treatment with levamisole because of the following side effects.

Nausea and Vomiting

Fifteen patients developed severe nausea and vomiting within the first month of treatment. Repeated attempts to restart therapy in all these patients failed even after an interval of months and the use of antiacids or antiemetics. Patients with mild nausea were helped by combining tablets with food and sometimes by taking all three tablets together instead of one three times a day, as was initially prescribed. Severe nausea is not associated with a good prognosis for the underlying disease.

Rash

Widespread erythematous rashes that were intensely itchy and uncomfortable developed in 25 patients. These rashes appeared between 2 weeks and 3 months after the start of therapy. Provided therapy was stopped immediately the rashes lasted about 48 hr. Continuation of levamisole for several days in the presence of a rash resulted in a miserable state in two patients who required heavy sedation combined with steroids and antihistamines for a week or more. Another patient had the rash for 3 weeks; the pruritis was controlled by antihistamines except at night when sedation was required. Despite the discomfort we associate rash formation with a good prognosis for the underlying disease.

Exacerbation of Symptoms

Severe exacerbation of underlying infections sufficient to suspend levamisole occurred in 30 patients within 28 days of the start of therapy. These patients were on continuous levamisole, 150 mg daily; 20 were anergic with brucellosis or other infection, and 10 had cancer. The symptoms and signs were those of inflammation or infection with coryza, joint pains, sweats, and fever in excess of 39°C lasting 48 hr. In three patients, two with brucellosis and one with cancer, psoriatic lesions reappeared after having been dormant for several years. Two patients both with brucellosis had rigors with fever of 41°C within 1 week of starting levamisole therapy. Reintroduction of levamisole after 7 days interval resulted in further milder symptoms in 21 patients, and treatment was continued intermittently. The two cases with psoriasis got worse, and levamisole was finally withdrawn. One patient on the monoamine oxidase inhibitor tranylcypromine sulphate had a severe reaction 11 days after start of levamisole and was in coma for 2 days. He recovered.

Exacerbation of tumor growth was not seen except possibly in one patient with stage IVb Hodgkin's disease who had responded to MOPP chemotherapy. Introduction of levamisole after the second course of chemotherapy was followed within 1 week by painful glandular enlargement to prefirst-treatment levels. A repeat course of MOPP[1] again reduced glandular enlargement. Levamisole was again given, and rapid glandular enlargement followed within 1 week. This patient later responded favorably to further chemotherapy without levamisole.

Agranulocytosis

There were five cases of agranulocytosis. One occurred in a case of lymphoma in the double-blind trial after 2 months; the absolute lymphocyte count fell by 50% 2 weeks before the peripheral granulocyte count fell by 80%. Dexamethasone was given, and recovery took 7 days.

In the case of multiple sclerosis, treated for 18 months with levamisole, 150 mg, for 3 days every fortnight, the granulocytes fell from 1,500 to 200/mm³. Recovery took 7 days. The patient with squamous cell carcinoma of the lung was treated with levamisole on 2 consecutive days each week for 4 months. Following radiation therapy there was was a sudden unexpected fall in granulo-

---

MOPP = mustine, oncovin, prednisone, and procarbazine.

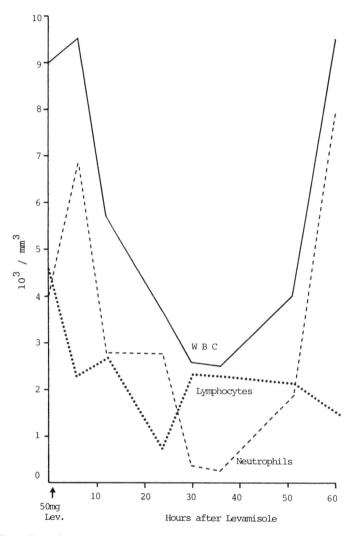

FIG. 3. The effect of a test oral dose of 50 mg levamisole in a sensitized patient. WBC, white blood count.

cytes to almost zero. Recovery took 1 week. Reintroduction of levamisole resulted again in a fall in granulocytes to zero.

The two cases of adenocarcinoma of the breast were both on levamisole, 150 mg daily, for two consecutive days each week combined with monthly cytotoxic therapy. Agranulocytosis occurred after 4 months. No antibodies to leukocytes or agglutination of leukocyte/levamisole mixtures was observed *in vitro*. Recovery took 5 days in one patient and 21 days in the other. Bone marrow examination showed myeloid series reduced to 6%, but eosinophils,

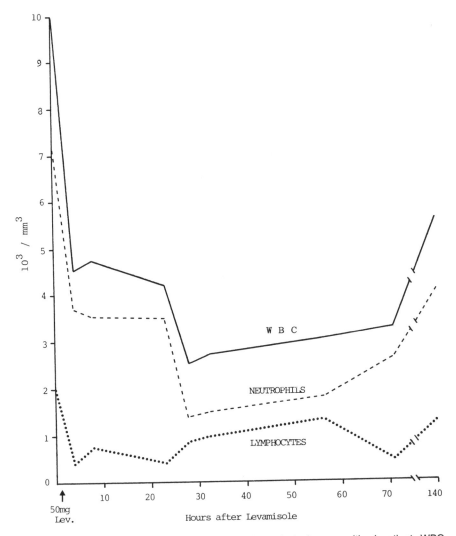

FIG. 4. The effect of a test oral dose of 50 mg levamisole in a sensitized patient. WBC, white blood count.

megakaryocytes, and erythroid series normoblastic. After recovery test doses of levamisole, 50 mg orally to each patient, produced leukopenia (see Figs. 3 and 4).

LEVAMISOLE IN BREAST CANCER

In a randomized ongoing clinical trial 44 cases of stage IV (International) carcinoma of the breast are being treated with monthly combination chemother-

TABLE 2. *Matching qualities of 44 patients with breast cancer*

	Group A. Adjuvant immunotherapy chemotherapy		Group B. Chemotherapy only	
Average age (yr)				
(range)	52.5	(33–76)	55.4	(37–70)
Premenopausal (%)	7	(31.8)	4	(18.1)
Postmenopausal (%)	15	(68.2)	18	(81.9)
Metastasis site				
Bone (%)	17	(77.3)	15	(68.2)
Liver (%)	13	(59.1)	15	(68.2)
Lung (%)	3	(13.6)	6	(27.3)
Brain (%)	2	(9.1)	2	(9.1)

apy. Half of these cases (group A) are receiving adjuvant immunotherapy with levamisole, 150 mg, on 2 consecutive days each week, Bacillus Calmette Guérin (BCG) (Glaxo percutaneous) monthly 15 days after chemotherapy, and anticoagulant therapy with sodium warfarin. For matching see Table 2.

All patients will be followed for at least 2 years. To date patients have been followed for 15 months (see survival curve in Fig. 5). There were two deaths in group A compared to 9 deaths in group B. The quality of life has been much better with adjuvant therapy, and the toxicity of chemotherapy has been diminished.

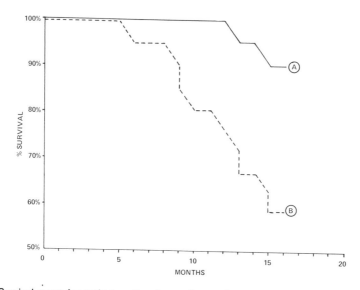

FIG. 5. Survival curve for patients with advanced stage IV breast cancer in randomized trial of monthly chemotherapy (FACOM) and chemotherapy plus immunotherapy with levamisole, warfarin, and BCG. A, FACOM + warfarin + BCG + levamisole (total 22, dead 2); B, FACOM (total 22, dead 9); FACOM, 5-fluorouracil, adriamycin, cytoxan, oncovin, and methotrexate.

It is our belief that for successful immunotherapy the function of the cellular immune mechanism must first be restored and then maintained so that stimulation can then be effective, hence the choice of levamisole for restoration, combined with warfarin for maintenance, and BCG for stimulation.

REFERENCES

1. Braeman, J. and Deeley T. J. (1973): Radiotherapy and the immune response in cancer of the lung. *Br. J. Radiol.,* 46:446–449.
2. Holland, P. D. J., Browne, O., and Thornes, R. D. (1975): The enhancing influence of proteolysis on E-rosette forming lymphocytes (T-cells) *in vivo* and *in vitro. Br. J. Cancer,* 31:164–169.
3. Thornes, R. D. (1974): Unblocking or activation of the cellular immune mechanism by induced proteolysis in patients with cancer. *Lancet,* II:382–384.
4. Thornes, R. D. (1977): Treatment of human brucellosis by antianergic therapy with levamisole. *Vet. Rec. (in press).*
5. Thornes, R. D., Smyth, H., Browne, O., and Holland, P. D. J. (1973): B.C.G. plus protease I in malignant melanoma. *Lancet,* I:1386.
6. Tripodi, D., Parks, L. C., and Brugmans, J. (1973): Drug-induced restoration of cutaneous delayed hypersensitivity in anergic patients with cancer. *N. Engl. J. Med.,* 289:354.

Immune Modulation and Control of Neo-plasia by Adjuvant Therapy, edited by M. A. Chirigos. Raven Press, New York, 1978.

Levamisole Therapy in Congenital Immunodeficiencies

C. Griscelli, A. M. Prieur, and F. DaGuillard

Groupe de Recherches d'Immunologie et de Rhumatologie Pédiatriques, Inserm U 132, Pr. Mozziconacci, Hôpital des Enfants Malades, 75015 Paris, France

Although levamisole seems to have no consistent effect on humoral immunity, several studies have established that this drug can restore cell-mediated functions when they are deficient or depressed (2,11). The present work was aimed at studying the effect of levamisole in various congenital immunodeficiency syndromes. Our results indicate that levamisole had no effect on patients with a selective humoral defect but can exert a positive influence on the clinical condition of various patients with an apparent T-cell defect, often improving both the *in vitro* and *in vivo* parameters of cell-mediated immunity.

MATERIAL AND METHODS

Patients

Twenty-three children with congenital immunodeficiency syndromes according to the World Health Organization classification (3) were studied: 12 ataxia telangiectasia (AT), two Wiskott-Aldrich, four common variable hypogamma-globulinemia, four Bruton disease, and one severe combined immunodeficiency (SCID). All patients showed evidence of chronic infections mainly of the upper respiratory tract.

Levamisole

Levamisole was administered orally at a dose of 3 to 5 mg/kg daily, 3 days a week for 5 weeks to 14 months.

Clinical Assessment

Medical examinations were performed monthly to assess the rate and severity of infectious episodes as well as the drug tolerance. At the same time cutaneous delayed hypersensitivity was tested with phytohemagglutinin (PHA) antigen or 2,4-dinitrochlorobenzene (DNCB), or both.

TABLE 1. *Modifications observed in Wiskott-Aldrich syndrome and variable hypogammaglobulinemia after levamisole therapy*

	Age	Infections	Cellular defect[a]	Humoral immunity	Skin Tests Positivation	Skin Tests Increased	Proliferative responses Positivation	Proliferative responses Increased	Clinical improvement
WA no. 1	8	+++	+++	IgM ≤ 10 mg/ml	PHA, CD		PWM	Con A	No
WA no. 2	7	±	+	IgM < 10		CD, PHA		PWM, CD	?
VHG no. 1	10	++	+	IgM < 10 Low IgG					+
VHG no. 2	4	++	+++	A G	PHA, Con A	PWM		PPD, CD	+
VHG no. 3	19	++	+	Hypo G					No
VHG no. 4	7	+++	++	Hypo G	PHA, SKSD, CD, DNCB				+
						4/6[b]		3/6[b]	3/6[b]

Con A, Concanavalin A; PPD, purified protein derivative; PWM, pokeweed mitogen; SKSD, streptokinase-streptodornase; VHG, variable hypogammaglobulinemia; WA, Wiskott-Aldrich.

[a] The intensity of cellular defect was appreciated on skin reactions to various antigens, percentage of E-rosette-forming cells and proliferative responses *in vitro* to mitogens (CONA, PHA, and PKW). + to +++ indicated various degrees of cellular defect. +, mild; +++, profound.

[b] Total number of patients who presented a modification of skin test and proliferative responses or a clinical improvement under levamisole therapy.

TABLE 2. Modifications observed in AT after levamisole therapy

AT no.	Age (years)	Infections	Cellular defect[a]	IgA mg%	Skin tests Positivation	Skin tests Increased	Proliferative responses Positivation	Proliferative responses Increased	Clinical improvement
AT 1	14	+++	+++	≤10	PPD, CD, DNCB		CD		No
2	9	+++	+++	150	CD, SKSD, PPD	PHA	PWM[b]	PHA	No
3	7	++	+++	≤10		PHA			No
4	7	++	+++	200	PHA, PPD, CD		PHA, Con A	PPD	+
5	5	++	+++	≤10	PPD, CD	PHA	PHA, Con A	PWM	+
6	6	+	++	160					+
7	3	++	++	20	CD	PPD			No
8	7	++	++	<10	PHA				+
9	13	+++	+	12					+
10	12	+	+	≤10	CD	SKSD		PHA, Con A, CD	?
11	3	+	+	90	DNCB	CD		CD	?
12	7	+	+	≤10					
					8/12[c]		7/12[c]		6/12[c]

Con A, Concanavalin A; PPD, purified protein derivative; PWM, pokeweed mitogen; SKSD, streptokinase-streptodornase; VHG, variable hypogamma-globulinemia; WA, Wiskott-Aldrich.

[a] The intensity of cellular defect was appreciated on skin reactions to various antigens, percentage of E-rosette-forming cells and proliferative responses in vitro to mitogens (CONA, PHA, and PKW). + to +++ indicated various degrees of cellular defect. +, mild. +++, profound.

[b] Con A not tested.

[c] Total number of patients who presented a modification of skin test and proliferative responses or a clinical improvement under levamisole therapy.

Biological Assessment

In each peripheral blood cell counts and levels of blood urea nitrogen were obtained.

Immunological Studies

Rosettes with sheep erythrocytes (E and EAC), membrane fluorescence for Ig and Fc receptors, lymphocyte proliferative response in the presence of mitogens and antigens, and serum levels of immunoglobulins and antibodies were performed as described (1,4,5,9).

RESULTS

No effect of levamisole on the clinical condition of patients with SCID and Bruton disease was observed. One out of two patients with Wiskott-Aldrich improved his clinical condition but died later from herpes virus encephalitis. In three out of four patients with common variable hypogammaglobulinemia, a decrease in the rate and severity of infections was observed (Table 1). The same was true for six out of 12 patients with AT (Table 2). No changes in blood cell counts or kidney functions were observed.

Humoral immunity was not modified. Cellular immune functions were improved, however, in several cases, although there was not always a good correlation with the clinical condition. For instance the patient with Wiskott-Aldrich who did not show any clinical improvement acquired positive skin tests and became responsive or improved his response to polyclonal mitogens. Similar biological improvements were observed in three out of four patients with AT who did not have any clinical improvement.

DISCUSSION

As expected levamisole had no effect on patients with a sole humoral defect, namely Bruton-type disease. No improvement was also observed in a SCID patient where one might have expected an amelioration of T-cell functions. However this patient died quickly of Pneumocystis carinii pneumonia, and no conclusion can be drawn from a single observation.

Our study confirms previous work indicating that levamisole can influence cell-mediated functions (2,8,11,12). It shows also that there is no correlation between the amelioration of various biological data and the clinical condition as assessed by our parameters. The clinical condition of several patients however seems to have benefited from this therapy. One must yet be cautious before drawing definite conclusions on these clinical results since these children were also receiving more conventional types of therapy and since frequent fluctuations can be seen in the course of these diseases.

Our study shows clearly that levamisole has a favorable action on both *in vivo* and *in vitro* immune functions. Particularly striking was the increase in the proliferative response to various mitogens, which in several cases increased by a factor of more than 30. The skin test also became positive in some patients. It is always difficult to show an immunostimulatory effect of a drug on normal cell populations. In the case of some of our children who often had strongly depressed or no cell-mediated functions, the effect of levamisole could be fully appreciated. A previous study in our laboratory had similarly established the immunostimulant action of transfer factor (6,7). It is very important to note that some patients who received successively both types of therapy were able to respond equally well to either one. Like transfer factor, levamisole had a positive effect on *in vitro* response to antigens and delayed skin reactions. It seems therefore, as we had suggested for transfer factor, that both immunostimulants act by inducing nonspecifically the expression of a previously acquired cellular hypersensitivity.

In contrast to the neutropenia reported in rheumatoid arthritis treated with levamisole (10), no adverse reaction was observed in our series. This encourages us to advocate the use of levamisole in congenital immunodeficiencies where the improvement of various biological parameters can be taken as objective criteria of its action.

ACKNOWLEDGMENT

We thank Laboratoire Lebrun for kindly supplying the levamisole used in this study. We wish also to acknowledge the technical help of Monique Agrapart and Lucienne Vaillant. This work was supported by INSERM grants ATP 7–74–28 and 8–74–29 and by Laboratoire Lebrun (Paris).

REFERENCES

1. Bianco, C., Patrick, R., and Nussensweig, V. (1971): A population of lymphocytes bearing a membrane receptor for antigen-antibody complement complexes. *J. Exp. Med.,* 132:702–710.
2. Churchill, W. H., and David, J. R. (1973): Editorial: Levamisole and cell-mediated immunity. *N. Engl. J. Med.,* 289:375–376.
3. Cooper, M. D., Faulk, W. P., Fudenberg, H. H., Good, R. A., Hitzig, W., Kunkel, H., Rosen, F. S., Seligmann, M., Soothill, Y., and Wedgwood, R. J. (1973): Classification of primary immunodeficiencies. *N. Engl. J. Med.,* 288:966–967.
4. Dickler, H. B., and Kunkel, H. G. (1972): Interaction of aggregated globulin with B lymphocytes. *J. Exp. Med.,* 136:191–196.
5. Froland, S., Natvig, J. B., and Berdal, P. (1971): Surface bound immunoglobulin as a marker of B lymphocyte in man. *Nature,* 234:251–252.
6. Griscelli, C., Revillard, J. P., Betuel, H., Herzog, C., and Touraine, J. L. (1973): Transfer factor therapy in immunodeficiencies. *Biomedicine,* 18:220–227.
7. Griscelli, C. (1974): Transfer factor in immunodeficiencies. In: *Clinical Immunobiology,* Vol. 2, edited by F. H. Bach and R. A. Good, Academic Press, New York.
8. Hirshaut, Y., Pinsky, C., Marquardt, H., and Oettgen, H. F. (1973): Effects of Levamisole on delayed hypersensitivity reactions in cancer patients. *Proc. Am. Assoc. Cancer Res.,* 14:109.
9. Jondal, M., Holm, G., and Wigzell, H. (1972): Surfaces markers on T and B lymphocytes. I. A large population of lymphocytes forming nonimmune rosettes with sheep red blood cells. *J. Exp. Med.,* 136:207–215.

10. Ruuskanen, O., Remes, M., Mäkela, A. L., Isomaki, H., and Toivanen, A. (1976): Levamisole and agranulocytosis. *Lancet,* ii:958–959.
11. Tripodi, D., Parks, L. C., and Brugmans, J. (1973): Drug-induced restoration of cutaneous delayed hypersensitivity in anergic patients with cancer. *N. Engl. J. Med.,* 289:354–357.
12. Verhaegen, H., De Gree, J., De Cock, W., and Verbruggen, F. (1973): Levamisole and the immune response. *N. Engl. J. Med.,* 229:1148–1149.

Immune Modulation and Control of Neoplasia by Adjuvant Therapy, edited by M. A. Chirigos. Raven Press, New York, 1978.

Enhancement of the Inhibitory Effect of Cyclophosphamide on Experimental Acute Myelogenous Leukemia by Glucan Immunopotentiation and Response of Serum Lysozyme

N. R. Di Luzio, J. A. Cook, C. Cohen, J. Rodrigue, P. Kokoshis, and R. B. McNamee

Department of Physiology, Tulane University School of Medicine, New Orleans, Louisiana 70112

Glucan, a unique β-1,3-polyglucose fraction isolated from *Saccharomyces cerevisiae,* has been demonstrated to be a profound reticuloendothelial (RE)-stimulating agent (1,12–14,24,26,30,32). The administration of glucan to mice or rats is associated with the induction of a hyperphagocytic state and the hypertrophy of major RE organs due to an increase in both size and number of macrophages (1,12–14,24,26,30,32). In association with the enhanced state of macrophage activation, glucan profoundly enhanced both the primary and secondary hemolysin response of mice to sheep red cells (30), as well as the intravascular clearance of the foreign red cell (12,24). Cell-mediated immunity appears also to be potentiated by glucan, since glucan administration modified the acceptance of allogeneic bone marrow in X-irradiated mice but had no effect on acceptance of syngeneic bone marrow (29,31). Similarly, the administration of glucan to radiation chimeras was associated with rejection of allogeneic and xenogeneic transplants, but was without effect in the syngeneic model (29). These composite studies denote that glucan is an immunopotentiator that has the ability to enhance the selective rejection of normal, nonmalignant cells if these cells are allogeneic or xenogeneic. Additionally, graft-versus-host reactions in F_1-hybrid mice were significantly enhanced in mice that received spleen cells derived from glucan-treated mice (6), denoting enhanced immunological capabilities of the transferred spleen cells.

In view of the unique enhancement in host defense mechanisms initiated by glucan, experimental studies were conducted to define the influence of glucan-induced macrophage activation on tumor growth (7,9,11). It was observed that the simultaneous subcutaneous administration of glucan with Shay acute myelogenous leukemia cells significantly inhibited growth of the primary tumor

(7,9) and reduced metastases. The intravenous administration of glucan prior to tumor cell transplantation also resulted in significant modification of tumor growth and prolongation in survival (7,9,11). Indeed, it was also found possible in the acute myelogenous leukemia model to modify significantly tumor growth when the primary tumor approximated 2 to 3% body weight and metastases to internal organs had developed (9).

In essential agreement with observations employing the allogeneic Shay myelogenous leukemia model, glucan-treated mice showed a significant inhibition of growth of a syngeneic adenocarcinoma (BW10232) and a melanoma B16 tumor (9). In preliminary clinical studies involving three types of metastatic lesions, the intralesional administration of glucan produced, in all cases studied, a prompt and striking reduction in the size of the lesion (23). Regression of the glucan-injected tumor was associated with a pronounced monocytic infiltrate and necrosis of the malignant cells. The degree of regression was dependent on the amount of glucan injected into the lesion which, in turn, because of its chemotactic nature, appeared to influence the mobilization of macrophages. To date, there has been no reported recurrence of the tumor at the injection site (22). The initial findings of regression of human tumors have been extended by additional studies that identify glucan-containing macrophages in close association with malignant cells (22).

Since glucan appeared to offer certain advantages over other currently employed forms of immunotherapy (8,10,23), studies were undertaken to ascertain whether glucan could be effectively employed in the presence of a chemotherapeutic agent.

It is overtly apparent that clinically employed immunostimulants must be effective in the presence of routinely employed chemotherapeutic agents. In the present study the influence of conjoint glucan and cyclophosphamide (CY) administration on tumor growth and survival of rats transplanted with acute myelogenous leukemia tumor cells was ascertained. Additionally, the influence of CY on macrophage function of control and glucan-treated rats was also evaluated.

Since Cappuccino et al. (4) have demonstrated that RE-stimulating agents such as Bacillus Calmette-Guérin (BCG) and zymosan induced an elevation in tissue lysozyme concentration that was related to RES stimulation, serum lysozyme levels were measured in control and glucan-treated rats, in both the presence and the absence of CY administration, to ascertain the possible employment of serum lysozyme as an index of the functional state of the RES.

MATERIALS AND METHODS

Male Long Evans rats weighing approximately 200 g were injected subcutaneously with Shay acute myelogenous leukemia cells in the dose of 15×10^6 viable cells. Following the administration of tumor cells, glucose (10 mg/kg) was administered intravenously to control rats, whereas glucan in the amount of 10 mg/

kg was injected intravenously on days 3 and 6. CY (40 mg/kg) or saline was administered intraperitoneally at the same time periods. The rats were killed on day 10 for determination of tumor weight and histology of liver, lung, and spleen.

Phagocytic function was measured by determining the intravascular clearance rate of gelatinized ^{131}I-triolein-labeled RE test lipid emulsion as previously described (27) in glucose, glucan, CY, or glucan + CY-treated rats. The dosage and times of injection were as described above. The RE test lipid emulsion was injected intravenously at a dose of 50 mg/100 g body weight. Following the injection, serial 0.1-ml aliquots of blood were obtained from the tail vein at approximate 2-min intervals for a 10-min period and evaluated for radioactivity. Blood radioactivity, expressed as the percentage of the injected dose/ml, was plotted semilogarithmically against time in minutes, and half-times (t/2) were determined. Liver, lung, and spleen were removed at the 10-min period and the distribution of the labeled emulsion determined. Tumors were also removed and weighed and radioactivity ascertained. Tissue uptake of the RE test lipid emulsion is expressed as the percentage of the injected dose per total organ (%ID/TO) and as the percentage of the injected dose per g of tissue (%ID/g).

To further define the interaction of glucan and CY, studies on the survival of rats that received 1×10^7 leukemic cells intravenously were undertaken. In these studies, glucan and CY were administered alone or conjointly. Glucan was administered intravenously in two different doses—5 mg/kg or 10 mg/ kg. CY was given intraperitoneally in the dose of 20 mg/kg. All injections were given on days 3 and 5 in order to ascertain possible additive or synergistic influences of CY and glucan.

Serum lysozyme concentrations of glucose- or glucan-treated Long Evans rats were measured by ascertaining the rate of lysis of a suspension of *Micrococcus lysodeikticus* cells (25). Glucan, in the amount of 1 mg/100 g, was injected intravenously on days 0, 2, and 4, with serum lysozyme concentration measured 24 hr later. Additional studies of a chronic nature were conducted employing glucan, CY, or glucan + CY-treated rats. One group of rats received glucan intravenously on days 0, 3, 6, 8, and 11. CY (20 mg/kg) was injected intraperitoneally in another group of rats at the same time intervals, while the third group received injections of both glucan plus CY. In this study, serum lysozyme concentrations were measured on day 14.

RESULTS

The administration of CY on days 3 and 6 significantly reduced ($p < 0.001$) primary tumor growth 90% by day 10 (Table 1). On a comparative basis, glucan administration was not as effective as CY since the reduction in mean tumor weight was approximately 62% ($p < 0.001$). The combination of CY + glucan was, however, most effective as mean tumor weight decreased by 97.4%. This

TABLE 1. *Influence of CY and glucan on growth of Shay acute myelogenous leukemia cells*

Group	N	Tumor weight (g)
Glucose	19	15.2 ± 1.43
Glucan	21	5.8 ± 0.59
CY	20	1.37 ± 0.22
Glucan + CY	20	0.40± 0.07

Tumor weights, expressed as means ± standard error, were ascertained on day 10 following subcutaneous administration of 15 X 10[6] viable leukemia cells.

degree of tumor inhibition was significantly different from the glucose, glucan, or CY groups ($p < 0.001$).

The influence of glucan and CY administered alone or conjointly on organ weight and phagocytic activity is presented in Tables 2 through 4. Glucan administration increased lung and spleen weight. CY significantly reduced liver and spleen weight ($p < 0.01$) and body weight ($p < 0.01$). The glucan-induced enhancement in lung and spleen weight was effectively inhibited by CY. Liver weight and body weight were also significantly decreased.

The intravenous administration of glucan to rats following the subcutaneous injection of leukemic cells significantly enhanced ($p < 0.001$) the intravascular clearance of the gelatinized RE test lipid emulsion by 47% (Table 3). CY alone did not significantly modify the clearance of the lipid emulsion. CY did, however, prevent the glucan-induced enhancement in vascular clearance (Table 3). The enhanced removal of the lipid emulsion in the glucan-treated group was not associated with an increased uptake by liver on a total organ basis (Table 4). CY did not modify the uptake by liver when administered alone or in conjunction with glucan.

Although the localization of the lipid emulsion by lung was not overtly influ-

TABLE 2. *Influence of CY and glucan on body and organ weights of rats injected subcutaneously with Shay acute myelogenous leukemia cells*

Group	N	Weight (g)			
		Body	Liver	Lung	Spleen
Saline	19	218 ± 7.9	12.7 ± 0.76	1.33 ± 0.07	1.57 ± 0.15
Glucan	20	206 ± 6.4	12.9 ± 0.59	1.96 ± 0.10	1.87 ± 0.22
CY	20	190 ± 6.9	9.3 ± 0.33	1.19 ± 0.07	1.00 ± 0.09
Glucan + CY	10	185 ± 6.8	9.4 ± 0.34	1.24 ± 0.08	0.69 ± 0.04

Body and organ weights were ascertained on day 10 following the administration of 15 X 10[6] viable leukemia cells. Glucan (10 mg/kg) was administered intravenously whereas CY (40 mg/kg) was administered intraperitoneally on days 3 and 6 following leukemic cell administration.

TABLE 3. *Influence of glucan and CY alone or conjointly on vascular clearance of the RE test lipid emulsion*

Group	N	Clearance (t/2, min)
Glucose	10	8.1 ± 0.38
Glucan	10	3.9 ± 0.49
CY	9	6.3 ± 0.80
Glucan + CY	10	7.9 ± 0.75

Intravascular clearance rate ascertained on day 10 following the subcutaneous injection of 15×10^6 cells. Glucan and/or CY was administered on days 3 and 6.

enced by either CY or glucan, insofar as total organ uptake, the uptake of the lipid emulsion by lung on a per g basis was significantly reduced in the glucan group due to the induced hyperplasia. Likewise, uptake of the lipid emulsion by spleen on an organ basis was not significantly altered. On a unit-weight basis, however, splenic uptake was significantly reduced in the glucan-treated group—by 43%. The CY and CY-glucan-treated group showed a 178 and 229% increase in spleen uptake of the gelatinized RE test lipid emulsion on a per g basis. These changes are due to alteration in organ weight due to lymphoid atrophy.

The uptake of the labeled lipid emulsion by the tumor was essentially constant on a per g basis ranging from 0.03 to 0.07% per g. On a tumor basis approximately 0.5% of the injected dose was localized in the tumor of the control group that had the largest tumor mass. The reduction in tumor weight in the glucan and CY-treated group was associated with a decrease in localization of the lipid emulsion (Table 4).

The influence of glucan and CY administration, alone or conjointly, on survival of rats following intravenous administration of leukemic cells is presented in Fig. 1 and 2. The administration of low-dose glucan (5 mg/kg) did not significantly modify mortality when compared to the glucose control group. In contrast, a significant enhancement in survival was observed in the group treated with a high dose (10 mg/kg) of glucan. Although CY significantly prolonged the time of survival, all CY-treated rats succumbed by day 17 (Fig. 1). When glucan and CY were administered together, a significant enhancement was observed in survival in the group that received the intravenous challenge of tumor cells. In contrast to zero survival in the CY group and 20% survival in the glucan group, the administration of CY + glucan was associated with 80% survival (Fig. 2).

The administration of glucan to normal rats produced a 6.4-fold elevation in serum lysozyme concentration by day 5 (Table 5). The prolonged administration of glucan produced a further elevation in serum lysozyme (Table 6) that was not significantly modified by the simultaneous administration of CY.

TABLE 4. *Influence of glucan and CY on tissue uptake of the RE test lipid emulsion*

Group	Liver		Lung		Spleen		Tumor	
	%ID/g	%ID/TO	%ID/g	%ID/TO	%ID/g	%ID/TO	%ID/g	%ID/TO
Glucose	4.4 ±0.74	59.6 ±6.0	0.41 ±0.11	0.55 ±0.13	0.79 ±0.08	1.20 ±0.10	0.04 ±0.004	0.47 ±0.06
Glucan	4.3 ±0.29	63.8 ±4.8	0.16 ±0.01	0.43 ±0.05	0.45 ±0.06	1.15 ±0.14	0.03 ±0.004	0.17 ±0.04
CY	5.8 ±0.48	59.2 ±4.2	0.40 ±0.07	0.45 ±0.08	2.21 ±0.29	1.51 ±0.11	0.06 ±0.011	0.030 ±0.008
Glucan + CY	5.6 ±0.45	51.5 ±4.1	0.43 ±0.08	0.54 ±0.10	2.58 ±0.48	1.82 ±0.31	0.07 ±0.028	0.027 ±0.008

Values are expressed as mean ± standard error and are derived from nine to 10 rats per group.

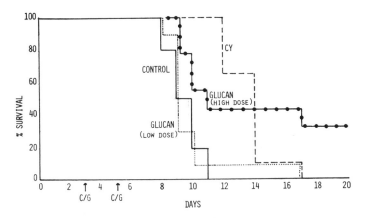

FIG. 1. The comparative influence of glucan at differential intravenous doses of 5 mg/kg (---), and 10 mg/kg (-●-●-), and CY (Cytoxan®) administered intraperitoneally at a dose of 20 mg/kg (--) on survival of Long Evans rats administered intravenously 1×10^7 acute myelogenous leukemia cells. The control group received glucose. All injections were made on days 3 and 5 following tumor cell administration. Each group was composed of 10 rats.

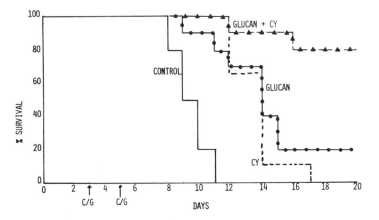

FIG. 2. The synergistic influence of combined glucan and CY (Cytoxan ®) therapy on survival of Long Evans rats intravenously administered 1×10^7 acute myelogenous leukemia cells. Treatment procedures: glucose, 10 mg/kg (-); glucan, 10 mg/kg (-●-●-); CY, 20 mg/kg i.p. (---), and glucan + CY (-▲-▲-). All injections were made on days 3 and 5 following tumor cell administration. Each group consisted of 10 animals.

TABLE 5. *Elevation in serum lysozyme concentration by the administration of glucan*

Group	Serum lysozyme (μg/ml)
Saline	2.06 ± 0.16
Glucan	13.37 ± 2.67

Saline or glucan (1 mg/100 g) was administered to male Long Evans rats on days 0, 2, and 4. Serum lysozyme concentrations were measured on day 5. Values are expressed as mean ± standard error of six rats per group.

TABLE 6. *Influence of glucan and CY administered alone or conjointly on serum lysozyme concentrations of normal Long Evans rats*[a]

Treatment	Serum lysozyme (μg/ml)
Glucan	29.6 ± 1.46
CY	9.8 ± 1.00
Glucan + CY	23.2 ± 1.16

[a]Values are expressed as means ± standard error and are compiled from seven rats per group. Glucan (1 mg/100 g) was administered intravenously on days 0, 3, 6, 8, and 11. CY was administered intraperitoneally at a dose of 2 mg/100 g on day 0 and at a dose of 0.5 mg/100 g on days 3, 6, 8, and 11. Serum lysozyme activity was measured on day 14.

DISCUSSION

The present studies confirm previous observations about the inhibitory activity of glucan on the growth of Shay acute myelogenous leukemia tumor cells when implanted subcutaneously (7,9,11). Additionally, the increased survival of glucan-treated rats following the intravenous administration of leukemic cells was also confirmed (9). However, when the administration of glucan was delayed to 3 days following the intravenous administration of leukemic cells, the protective influence of glucan on survival was significantly reduced from that observed when it was administered prior to or simultaneously with the intravenous injection of tumor cells (9). This reduction in the protective influence of glucan on survival was, however, purposefully employed to ascertain the conjoint use of glucan and CY. Indeed, if the glucan dose and time schedule employed were 100% effective in promoting survival, it would have been impossible to ascertain any additive influence of CY. Likewise, in order to determine the possible additive influence of glucan, CY dose was also reduced to a level where, although survival time was prolonged, a 100% mortality occurred. The most effective therapeutic procedure employed was when both CY and glucan were administered simultaneously. Depending on the experimental design, this combined drug approach resulted in enhancement in survival and decreased tumor growth. Since CY effectively blocked glucan-induced phagocytic enhancement, as denoted by changes in intravascular clearance rates, it is obvious that the macrophage-mediated antitumor action of glucan cannot be by a phagocytic mechanism.

CY has been demonstrated to be a potent immunosuppressant compound that possesses the ability to inhibit expression of both T- and B-lymphocyte function (3,16,20). Fisher et al. (16) studied the combined use of such macrophage stimulants as *Corynebacterium parvum* and BCG, in conjunction with CY in mice employing a syngeneic mammary carcinoma tumor model. The dosage sequence employed was that either *C. parvum* or BCG was administered 4 days following the administration of CY. Fisher et al. observed that the conjoint use of *C. parvum* and CY induced a degree of inhibition of tumor growth not achieved by either agent alone. The combination of *C. parvum* and CY also resulted in a survival period that was more prolonged than that induced by either agent alone. The present studies with glucan administered simultaneously with CY essentially are in accord with the observations of Fisher et al. (16,17).

The initial study of the conjoint influence of an oncolytic drug and a macrophage-stimulating agent on tumor growth and drug toxicity was undertaken by Sokoloff et al. (28). Mitomycin C toxicity could be significantly reduced by the administration of zymosan, an effective RES-stimulating agent (2,26) from which glucan was originally isolated (26). The reduction in phagocytosis of colloidal carbon induced by mitomycin C was prevented to a significant degree by the prior administration of zymosan. Additionally, it was observed that the greatest degree of inhibition of Sarcoma 180 tumor growth was when zymosan was administered first, followed by mitomycin C. Sokoloff et al. (28) concluded that by activating RES and enhancing host defense mechanisms the oncolytic effect of mitomycin C could be enhanced. In a similar fashion, the present studies indicate that glucan can be employed with a cytostatic agent to produce an additive effect relative to tumor inhibition. More importantly, not only was the tumor inhibitory effect additive, but histologically the combination of CY + glucan resulted in a significant modification of the classic glucan-induced pulmonary and hepatic granuloma. These studies indicate that it may be advantageous to combine glucan with agents such as CY to minimize glucan-induced cellular changes while maximizing the therapeutic effectiveness of both agents.

The present study on enhanced survival of the glucan + CY-treated rats suggests that glucan prolongs the chemotherapeutic-induced remission in acute leukemia. Since glucan has a prolonged state of retention in macrophages (18), the maintenance of an activated RES state following the cessation of chemotherapy may be the basis of the enhanced survival.

In addition to the enhancement of the antitumor effect of CY, the employment of glucan may have another beneficial effect on host survival. Infectious complications are of major concern in oncology patients, particularly those with acute leukemia (15). Enhanced susceptibility of Long Evans rats to *Escherichia coli* at early stages of the leukemia state has been demonstrated (9). It remains to be established if by increasing host immune response with glucan one can modify the predisposition of this patient population to opportunistic infections. The elevation in plasma lysozyme levels by glucan and the maintenance of such an elevation in the presence of repeated CY administration are suggestive that increased resistance to certain infectious agents appears feasible since lysozyme hydrolyzes β 1,4 glucosidic linkages in cell walls of a variety of microorganisms. An enhanced host resistance to infectious agents due to an elevation in lysozyme levels may also be mediated by lysozyme stimulation of phagocytosis (21).

Currie and Eccles (5) have recently reported that the serum lysozyme concentrations may reflect macrophage content of tumors and may "under well defined conditions" be employed as an index of macrophage-mediated host response to tumors. Since the synthesis and secretion of lysozyme have been demonstrated to be a function of macrophages (19) and production a measure of macrophage cell number (5), it appears that a useful index of glucan-induced macrophage activation in both normal and tumor-bearing rats is the serum lysozyme levels. Since the lysozyme levels induced by glucan were not appreciably altered by simultaneous CY administration, which markedly reduced glucan granuloma, the elevation in serum lysozyme level may well reflect glucan-induced stimulation of macrophage function. Based on the present observations, it appears that the employment of serum lysozyme concentration merits further evaluation as a practical clinical test to determine the therapeutic effectiveness of macrophage stimulating agents such as glucan, BCG, *C. parvum,* and MER.

Although additional studies are obviously essential, our preliminary studies denote that glucan may be effectively employed in combined drug therapy procedures involving chemo- and immunotherapy. The ideal therapeutic procedure, about the synchronous or asynchronous administration of glucan and CY, is yet to be established as is the extension of these studies to other spontaneous and syngeneic tumor models. It also appears highly desirable in the continued investigation of the immunopotentiation by glucan to interface glucan with other currently employed chemotherapeutic agents. It is important not only to ascertain possible additive or synergistic effects on the inhibition of tumor growth and metastases, but also to evaluate whether the toxicity and immunosuppressive activity of certain chemotherapeutic agents are modified in the presence of glucan, leading to an increase of host resistance to opportunistic infections or a reduction in drug toxicity, or both.

SUMMARY

The present experiments were undertaken to evaluate whether the antineoplastic activity of CY could be potentiated by conjoint therapy with the immunostimulant glucan. Long Evans rats were injected subcutaneously with Shay myelogenous leukemia cells (15×10^6 cells/rat). The rats were subsequently administered glucan (1 mg/100 g) intravenously or CY (4 mg/100 g) intraperitoneally, or both, on days 3 and 6 after injection of tumor cells and sacrificed on day 10. Tumor growth was significantly reduced in rats receiving either CY or glucan alone compared to control rats. The most effective antineoplastic action, however, was evident with concurrent glucan and CY therapy as denoted by a mean 97% decrease in tumor weight compared to control rats. Phagocytic activity of the RES was subsequently evaluated following singular or combined administration of glucan and CY. CY abrogated the glucan-induced hyperphagocytic state even though interaction of these two agents was extremely effective in inducing tumor regression. Increased survival to intravenously administered acute myelogenous leukemic cells was also observed in the glucan- and CY-treated group. CY significantly inhibited the glucan-induced hepatic and pulmonary granuloma.

Glucan profoundly elevated serum lysozyme concentrations in both the presence and absence of CY. The use of serum lysozyme concentrations to evaluate the therapeutic effectiveness of certain immunotherapeutic agents merits further investigation. These composite studies denote that glucan may be a valuable adjunct to conventional cancer chemotherapy.

ACKNOWLEDGMENT

These studies were supported, in part, by the Cancer Research Institute, Inc. and National Institutes of Health grant no. CA 13746.

REFERENCES

1. Ashworth, C. T., Di Luzio, N. R., and Riggi, S. J. (1963): A morphologic study of the effect of reticuloendothelial stimulation upon hepatic removal of minute particles from the blood of rats. *J. Exp. Mol. Pathol.,* 2(Suppl 1):83–103.

3. Benacerraf, B., and Sebestyen, M. M. (1957): Effect of bacterial endotoxins on the reticuloendothelial system. *Fed. Proc.,* 16:860–867.

3. Bodey, G. P., Hersh, E. M., Valdivieso, M., Feld, R., and Rodriguez, V. (1975): Effects of cytotoxic and immunosuppressive agents on the immune system. *Postgrad. Med.,* 68(7):67–74.

4. Cappuccino, J. G., Winston, S., and Perri, G. C. (1964): Muramidase activity of kidney and spleen in Swiss mice challenged with BCG, zymosan and bacterial endotoxins. *Proc. Soc. Exp. Biol. Med.,* 116:869–872.

5. Currie, G. A., and Eccles, S. A. (1976): Serum lysozyme as a marker of host resistance. I. Production by macrophages resident in rat sarcomata. *Br. J. Cancer,* 33:51–59.

6. Di Luzio, N. R. (1967): Evaluation by the graft-versus-host reaction of the immune competence of lymphoid cells of mice with altered reticuloendothelial function. *J. Reticuloendothel. Soc.,* 4:439–475.

7. Di Luzio, N. R. (1975): Macrophages, recognition factors and neoplasia. In: *The Reticuloendothelial System: IAP Monograph No. 16,* Chapter 5, edited by J. W. Rebuck, C. W. Berard, and M. R. Abell, pp. 49–64. Williams & Wilkins, New York.

8. Di Luzio, N. R. (1976): Pharmacology of the reticuloendothelial system—Accent on glucan. In: *The Reticuloendothelial System in Health and Disease: Functions and Characteristics (Advances in Experimental Medicine and Biology),* edited by S. M. Reichard, M. R. Escobar, and H. Friedman, pp. 412–421. Plenum Press, New York.

9. Di Luzio, N. R., Hoffmann, E. O., Cook, J. A., Browder, W., and Mansell, P. W. A. (1976): Glucan-induced enhancement in host resistance to experimental tumors. In: *Control of Neoplasia by the Modulation of the Immune System,* edited by M. A. Chirigos, pp. 475–499. Raven Press, New York.

10. Di Luzio, N. R., McNamee, R., Jones, E., Cook, J. A., and Hoffmann, E. O. (1976): The employment of glucan and glucan activated macrophages in the enhancement of host resistance to malignancies in experimental animals. In: *The Macrophage in Neoplasia,* edited by M. Fink, pp. 181–198. Academic Press, New York.

11. Di Luzio, N. R., McNamee, R., Jones, E., Lassoff, S., Sear, W., and Hoffmann, E. O. (1976): Inhibition of growth and dissemination of Shay myelogenous leukemic tumor in rats by glucan and glucan activated macrophages. In: *The Reticuloendothelial System in Health and Disease: Immunologic and Pathologic Aspects (Advances in Experimental Medicine and Biology),* edited by E. M. Reichard, M. R. Escobar, and H. Friedman, pp. 397–413. Plenum Press, New York.

12. Di Luzio, N. R., and Riggi, S. J. (1964): The development of a lipid emulsion for the measurement of reticuloendothelial function. *J. Reticuloendothel. Soc.,* 1:136–149.

13. Di Luzio, N. R., and Riggi, S. J. (1970): The effects of laminarin, sulfated glucan and oligosaccharide of glucan on RE activity. *J. Reticuloendothel. Soc.,* 8:464–473.

14. Di Luzio, N. R., Wooles, W. R., and Morrow, S. H. (1964): The effect of splenectomy and x-irradiation on antibody formation in RE hyperfunctional mice. *J. Reticuloendothel. Soc.,* 1:429–441.
15. Donaldson, S. S., Moore, M. R., Rosenberg, S. A., and Vosti, K. L. (1972): Characterization of post-splenectomy bacteremia among patients with and without lymphoma. *N. Engl. J. Med.,* 287:69–71.
16. Fisher, B., Rubin, H., and Wolmark, N. (1976): Further observations on the inhibition of tumor growth by Corynebacterium parvum with cyclophosphamide. IV. Effect of Rifampin on tumor growth inhibition, bone marrow macrophages precursor stimulation and macrophage cytotoxicity. *J. Natl. Cancer Inst.,* 57:317–322.
17. Fisher, B., Wolmark, N., and Fisher, E. R. (1975): Results of investigations with Corynebacterium parvum in an experimental animal system. In: *Corynebacterium parvum,* edited by B. Halpern, pp. 218–243. Plenum Press, New York.
18. Gilbert, K., Chu, F., and Di Luzio, N. R. (1977): Fate of ^{14}C-labeled glucan in normal and tumor bearing rats. *J. Reticuloendothel. Soc. (in press).*
19. Gordon, S., Todd, J., and Cohn, Z. A. (1974): *In vitro* synthesis and secretion of lysozyme by mononuclear phagocytes. *J. Exp. Med.,* 139:1228–1248.
20. Hersh, E. M., and Freireich, E. J. (1968): Host defense mechanisms and their modification by cancer chemotherapy. *Methods Cancer Res.,* 4:355–451.
21. Klockars, M., and Roberts, P. (1976): Stimulation of phagocytosis by human lysozyme. *Acta Haematol.,* 55:289–295.
22. Mansell, P. W. A., Di Luzio, N. R., McNamee, R., Rowden, G., and Proctor, J. W. (1976): Recognition factors and non-specific macrophage activation in the treatment of neoplastic disease. In: *Immunotherapy of Cancer,* edited by H. Friedman and C. M. Southam. *Ann. NY Acad. Sci.,* 277:20–44.
23. Mansell, P. W. A., Ichinose, H., Reed, R. J., Krementz, E. T., McNamee, R., and Di Luzio, N. R. (1975): Macrophage mediated destruction of human malignant cells *in vivo. J. Natl. Cancer Inst.,* 54:571–580.
24. Morrow, S. H., and Di Luzio, N. R. (1965): The fate of foreign red cells in mice with altered reticuloendothelial function. *Proc. Soc. Exp. Biol. Med.,* 119:647–652.
25. Parry, R. M., Jr., Chandan, R. C., and Shahani, K. M. (1965): A rapid and sensitive assay of muramidase. *Proc. Soc. Exp. Biol. Med.,* 119:384–386.
26. Riggi, S. J., and Di Luzio, N. R. (1961): Identification of a reticuloendothelial stimulating agent in zymosan. *Am. J. Physiol.,* 200:297–300.
27. Saba, T. M., and Di Luzio, N. R. (1968): Involvement of the opsonic system in starvation induced depression of the reticuloendothelial system. *Proc. Soc. Exp. Biol. Med.,* 128:869–875.
28. Sokoloff, B., Toda, Y., Fujisawa, M., Enomoto, K., Saelhof, C. C., Bird, L., and Miller, C. (1961): Experimental studies on mitomycin C. 4. Zymosan and the RES. *Growth,* 25:249–263.
29. Wooles, W. R., and Di Luzio, N. R. (1962): Influence of reticuloendothelial hyperfunction on bone marrow transplantation. *Am. J. Physiol.,* 203:404–408.
30. Wooles, W. R., and Di Luzio, N. R. (1963): Reticuloendothelial function and immune response. *Science,* 142:1078–1080.
31. Wooles, W. R., and Di Luzio, N. R. (1964): Inhibition of homograft acceptance and homo- and hetero-graft rejection in chimeras by reticuloendothelial system stimulation. *Proc. Soc. Exp. Biol. Med.,* 115:756–759.
32. Wooles, W. R., and Di Luzio, N. R. (1964): The phagocytic and proliferative response of the RES following glucan administration. *J. Reticuloendothel. Soc.,* 1:160–169.

Immune Modulation and Control of Neo-plasia by Adjuvant Therapy, edited by M. A. Chirigos. Raven Press, New York, 1978.

Comparative Evaluation of the Role of Macrophages and Lymphocytes in Mediating the Antitumor Action of Glucan

J. A. Cook, D. Taylor, C. Cohen, J. Rodrigue, V. Malshet, and N. R. Di Luzio

Department of Physiology, Tulane University School of Medicine, New Orleans, Louisiana 70112

The purpose of this chapter is to review evidence delineating the role of macrophages and lymphocytes in mediating the antineoplastic activity of the β 1–3 polyglucose, glucan. Previous studies conducted in our laboratory have shown glucan, an insoluble polysaccharide component of the inner cell wall of *Saccharomyces cerevisiae,* to be a potent stimulant of the reticuloendothelial system (RES) (20). Administration of glucan was also demonstrated to markedly retard the growth of Shay acute myelogenous leukemia in the rat as well as the adenocarcinoma and melanoma B16 tumors in mice (3). In subsequent clinical studies involving three types of metastatic lesions in man, the intralesional administration of glucan produced a prompt and striking reduction in the size of the lesion (16). Regression of the glucan-injected tumor was associated with necrosis of the malignant cells and a pronounced monocytic infiltrate.

The mechanism by which glucan induces tumor regression remains to be delineated. Since glucan enhances reticuloendothelial function (20) and macrophages have been demonstrated to be cytotoxic toward tumor cells (5,12), the antitumor action of glucan may well be mediated by macrophages. However, the T lymphocyte has also been postulated to mediate cytotoxicity toward tumor cells (10,14,18). Furthermore, Maeda and Chihara (15) have reported that lentinan, a linear β 1,3 soluble glucan isolated from the mushroom *lentinus edodes,* exhibits an antitumor response in normal, but not in neonatally thymectomized, mice. Glucan, like lentinan, therefore, may mediate part of its antitumor effects through activation of thymus-dependent lymphocytes. In an effort to evaluate this possibility, the influence of glucan on lymphocyte blastogenesis was evaluated. To further assess the role of the T lymphocyte in glucan-induced tumor regression, studies on the antitumor action of glucan were undertaken employing congenital nude athymic mice (C57B1/10 nu/nu). Additionally, phagocytic activity of the RES of athymic mice following glucan administration was ascertained by employing the ^{131}I RE test lipid emulsion.

In view of the evidence for macrophage-induced tumoricidal activity following administration of certain immunological adjuvants (22), we also evaluated the effect of glucan on *in vitro* macrophage-mediated cytotoxicity toward malignant cells.

MATERIALS AND METHODS

Animals

Male C57B1/6J inbred mice were employed as recipients for the syngeneic melanoma B16 tumors (Jackson Laboratory, Bar Harbor, Maine). The mice were maintained on Purina laboratory chow and tap water *ad libitum*. C3H/HeJ and A/J inbred strains of mice were used as host animals for the anaplastic mammary carcinoma 15091A. C57B1/10 nu/nu athymic mice were employed as T-lymphocyte-deficient mice. The athymic mice were maintained under asceptic conditions in standard laboratory cages that were cleaned, autoclaved, and covered with germ-free filtered lids (Negus Container Co., Madison, Wisconsin). Both food (Purina lab chow) and water source were sterilized by autoclaving. The nude mice were transferred under sterile conditions to a sterile plastic container during cage cleaning and always returned to their original cages.

Tumor Cells

Tumor cells (melanoma B16 or anaplastic carcinoma) were dispersed under sterile conditions by means of a glass tissue grinder. The cells were suspended in 0.9% saline, and the number of viable cells were determined employing trypan blue exclusion. Established dilutions of the tumor cells were then injected subcutaneously utilizing the appropriate host mouse strain.

Anaplastic mammary carcinoma (15091A) were also maintained as suspension cultures in RPMI 1640 medium supplemented with 10% fetal calf serum, streptomycin (100 μg/ml), and penicillin (100 U/ml). The cells were maintained in sterile plastic culture flasks (Falcon Plastics) at 37°C and 5% CO_2. Viability of the cells, as determined by trypan blue exclusion, for all experiments was greater than 95%.

Glucan Preparation

Yeast glucan, the source of glucan employed in these studies, was prepared from baker's yeast (Fleischmanns) by a modification of the acidic and alkaline hydrolysis method of Hassid et al. (9). As determined by scanning electron microscopy, glucan has a particle diameter of approximately 1 μm.

T- and B-Lymphocyte Stimulation

Splenic lymphocytes were tested for their reactivity in culture to class-specific mitogens (8). Spleen cells were isolated under sterile conditions from glucan-

(0.3 mg/animal intravenously) or saline-treated (control) C57B1/6J mice. One group of mice, designated group 1, was injected on days 0 and 2 and sacrificed on day 5. Another group, designated group 2, was given more prolonged treatment of glucan or saline (days 1, 3, 7, 11, 14, and 17 prior to sacrifice). The spleen cell isolation and culture procedures were modifications of the method of Gery et al. (6). Spleen cells were isolated and cultured in RPMI 1640 medium containing 10% fetal calf serum, streptomycin (100 μg/ml), and penicillin (100 U/ml). The cell cultures of splenocytes (1 $\times$ 10^6/ml) had an initial viability of greater than 95% as denoted by trypan blue exclusion. The mitogens concanavalin A (Sigma) (2 μg) or *Escherichia coli* 0.26:B6 endotoxin (Difco) (50 μg) were added in 0.1-ml volumes. Cells were cultured at 37°C under 5% CO_2 in air for a 48-hr period at which time 1 μCi (0.1 ml) of methyl ^{3}H-thymidine was added. Cells were harvested 24 hr later by an initial centrifugation of 750 $\times$ g for 15 min. The pellet was precipitated and washed three times with cold 5% trichloracetic acid. The precipitate was dissolved in NCS tissue solubilizer, suspended in Aquafluor (New England Nuclear), and counted by means of a liquid scintillation spectrophotometer.

Phagocytic Activity

Phagocytic activity of the RES was evaluated with gelatinized ^{131}I-labeled RE test lipid emulsion (4). The lipid base was used to make a 10% emulsion in aqueous solution of 5% dextrose and 0.3% gelatin. Mice were injected intravenously with the gelatinized ^{131}I-labeled RE test lipid emulsion at a dose of 100 mg/100 g. Tail blood samples, 0.01-ml aliquots, were obtained at timed intervals and radioactivity measured and expressed as per cent injected dose/ml. The values were plotted semilogarithmically against time, and half-time (t/2) values for the clearance of the test lipid emulsion were plotted. Ten minutes after injection, the animals were sacrificed and tissue distribution of the emulsion was evaluated.

Test for Macrophage-Mediated Cytotoxicity

Either C3H/HeJ or A/J mice were administered intraperitoneal injections of saline (1 ml) or glucan (1 mg/mouse). On day 3 after treatment, peritoneal exudate cells were harvested by injecting 6 ml of culture media (RPMI) into the peritoneal cavity. Exudates from 10 mice per group were employed for each experiment. The peritoneal exudate cells were placed in 15-cm sterile glass Petri dishes. The cells were then incubated for 2 hr at 37°C under 5% CO_2. Nonadherent cells were then washed off the Petri dish, and the adherent macrophage cell population was gently removed. The cells were kept in sterile silicone-coated vacutainers (Becton Dickinson) in an ice bath before counting and appropriate dilutions were computed. Initial viability was measured by trypan blue exclusion.

An aliquot of the adherent cell population (5 $\times$ 10^5 cells) was added to 1 ml of 5×10^4 or 1×10^4 anaplastic carcinoma cells in RMPI 1640 medium with 10% fetal calf serum. Tumor cells and macrophages were then allowed to incubate for 16 hr at 37°C at 5% CO_2 in sterile 13×10 mm culture tubes. The cultures were subsequently labeled with 4 μCi of methyl ^{3}H-thymidine (0.2 ml) for 4 hr. Cells were then harvested by centrifugation at $750 \times g$ for 15 min. The pellet was precipitated, washed, and solubilized and radioactivity ascertained. Results are expressed as percent inhibition of tumor cell proliferation at effector:target cell ratios of 10:1 and 50:1.

$$\% \text{ inhibition} = \frac{CPM_M - CPM_E \times 100}{CPM_M}$$

where CPM_M = maximum uptake of ^{3}H-thymidine by tumor cells alone + macrophages alone

and CPM_E = uptake of ^{3}H-thymidine by tumor cells in combination with macrophages.

Statistics

Data were analyzed by employing the Student's t-test. All data were compared for statistical significance employing a confidence level of 95%.

RESULTS

Effect of Glucan Administration on the Response of Spleen Cells to Mitogens

The mitotic response of splenocytes from glucan- or saline-treated mice to various mitogens was enhanced ($p < 0.01$) relative to the unstimulated spleen cell controls (Table 1). Uptake of the ^{3}H-thymidine did not, however, vary significantly between unstimulated control spleens and unstimulated spleen cells from glucan-treated mice. The direct *in vitro* addition of glucan (Table 2) at a concentration of 100 μg per 1×10^6 spleen cells also failed to significantly modify thymidine incorporation.

Spleen cells of mice in group 1 were tested for reactivity to the added mitogens on day 5 after administration of glucan (0.3 mg/mouse) or saline on days 0 and 2. The splenocytes from these glucan-treated mice manifested a significantly ($p < 0.05$) greater incorporation of the ^{3}H-thymidine in response to *E. coli* lipopolysaccharide than did spleen cells from control mice (Table 1). There was a 49% greater increase in labeling of spleen cells from glucan-treated mice in the presence of endotoxin relative to the respective endotoxin control group. An enhanced responsiveness ($p < 0.05$) to concanavalin A was also observed in spleen cells from glucan-treated mice compared to the control. Spleen cells from glucan-treated mice demonstrated an approximate 42% greater increase

TABLE 1. *Biphasic response of splenocytes from acute and chronic glucan-treated C57B1/ 6J mice to T- and B-Lymphocyte mitogens*

| Group | ^{3}H-thymidine (cpm) | |
	Control	Glucan
1 [a]		
(Day 5)		
Buffer	604 ± 65	718 ± 59
Endotoxin	4,253 ± 434	8,298 ± 1,147 [b]
Con A	12,754 ± 2,054	22,101 ± 3,324 [b]
2 [c]		
(Day 18)		
Buffer	422 ± 69	336 ± 33
Endotoxin	1,622 ± 187	719 ± 114 [b]
Con A	13,940 ± 2,027	3,513 ± 753 [b]

[a] Glucan (0.3 mg/mouse) or saline was administered on days 0 and 2 before sacrifice on day 5. Data represent the mean standard error of nine separate experiments. In each experiment spleen cells were harvested and pooled from four mice.
[b] $p < 0.05$.
[c] Glucan (0.3 mg/mouse) or saline was administered on days 1, 3, 7, 11, 14, and 17 prior to sacrifice. In each group spleen cells were harvested from six to nine mice.

in thymidine incorporation in response to concanavalin A than did those of concanavalin A-treated controls.

In marked contrast to the enhanced reactivity of splenocytes to T- and B-cell mitogens after two injections of glucan, a suppression of blastogenic responses occurred after more prolonged administration of glucan (group 2) (Table 1). The spleen cell response of chronic glucan-treated mice to *E. coli* endotoxin was depressed 56.7% ($p < 0.001$) relative to the respective saline control group. In a similar fashion, spleen cell response to concanavalin A was significantly reduced 75% when compared to the response by splenocytes of the control group.

TABLE 2. *Effect of in vitro glucan addition on ^{3}H-thymidine incorporation of spleen and tumor cells*

Cells	In vitro addition	Counts per minute of ^{3}H-thymidine
Spleen	—	912 ± 127
Spleen	Glucan	598 ± 149
Tumor	—	169,112 ± 11,550
Tumor	Glucan	166,264 ± 12,504

Glucan was added *in vitro*, 100 μg to 1×10^6/ml spleen cells (C57B1/ 6J mice) and 50 μg to 5×10^5/ml anaplastic carcinoma cells. Spleen cells were incubated with glucan for 72 hr. Tumor cells were incubated for 20 hr in the presence of glucan. $N = 8$ to 10.

TABLE 3. *Inhibitory effect of glucan on growth of melanoma B16 in syngeneic C57B1/6J mice*

Group	N	Body weight (g)	Tumor weight (mg)
Control	9	21.6 ± 1.2	1,743 ± 348
Glucan	6	18.3 ± 0.8	610 ± 55 [a]

C57 mice were injected s.c. with 5×10^6 melanoma B16 cells on day 0. Mice were given glucan (0.3 mg/mouse) or saline on days 1, 4, 8, 12, and 15. Mice were sacrificed on day 18.

[a] Significant $p < 0.05$.

Antitumor Effect of Glucan in Athymic and Normal Mice

To evaluate the role of the T lymphocyte as an effector cell mediating the antitumor effects of glucan, studies were conducted employing congenitally athymic mice (C57B1/10 nu/nu) and normal C57B1/6J syngeneic recipients of the melanoma B16 tumors. C57B1/6J mice were administered 5×10^6 melanoma B16 cells subcutaneously (day 0) followed by intravenous glucan (0.3 mg/mouse) or saline on days 1, 4, 8, 12, and 15. The mice were subsequently sacrificed on day 18, and the tumors excised and weighed (Table 3). Tumor weights from the glucan-treated mice were approximately 65% less than the saline-treated control group ($p < 0.05$).

The antitumor action of glucan was also evaluated in athymic mice following the injection of 5×10^6 melanoma cells subcutaneously (Table 4). Glucan was subsequently injected intravenously (0.3 mg/mouse) on days 1, 4, 8, and 12 after tumor inoculation. As with normal mice, an approximate 67% reduction in tumor weight was observed in athymic mice treated with glucan, as compared to the control group. Glucan, therefore, significantly inhibited growth of melanoma cells in T-lymphocyte-deficient mice as well as in normal mice.

One noticeable feature of these experiments is the apparent slower growth of tumors in athymic mice as opposed to control mice even though the initial tumor cell burden was identical (Tables 3 and 4). Primary tumor weights of normal mice treated with either saline or glucan were substantially greater than the tumor weights of respective groups in the athymic mice.

TABLE 4. *Inhibitory effect of glucan on growth of melanoma B16 in C57B1/10 nu/nu mice*

Group	N	Body weight (g)	Tumor weight (mg)
Saline	8	20.2 ± 1.0	298.6 ± 75.3
Glucan	5	18.0 ± 1.3	98.3 ± 44.9 [a]

Melanoma cells were injected s.c. 5×10^6 on day 0. Mice were given saline or glucan (0.3 mg/mouse) on days 1, 4, 8, and 12 and sacrificed on day 18.

[a] Significant $p < 0.05$.

TABLE 5. *Clearance and tissue distribution of* ^{131}I-*triolein-labeled RE test lipid emulsion in control and glucan-treated nude athymic mice*

Group	T/2 (min)	Organ distribution (%ID/TO)		
		Liver	Lung	Spleen
Control	6.2 ± 0.40	47.8 ± 3.4	2.18 ± 0.64	1.72 ± 0.29
Glucan	4.6 ± 0.61	66.0 ± 7.4 [a]	1.56 ± 0.18	2.17 ± 0.30

Mice were administered glucan (0.3 mg/mouse) or isovolumetric saline on days 0, 3, and 7. The ^{131}I-labeled RE test lipid clearance and tissue distribution was ascertained on day 9. Lipid was given intravenously 100 mg/100 g. Values are expressed as mean ± standard error and are derived from seven to eight mice per group.

[a] Significant $p < 0.05$.

Effect of Glucan on Phagocytic Activity of the RES of Athymic Mice

C57B1/10 nu/nu mice were administered glucan (0.3 mg/mouse) or saline intravenously on days 0, 3, and 7. On day 9, the animals were injected with the ^{131}I-triolein-labeled RE test lipid emulsion at which time clearance and tissue distribution of the lipid emulsion were ascertained (Table 5). In regard to tissue distribution of the lipid emulsion, glucan treatment significantly enhanced hepatic phagocytosis of the labeled emulsion ($p < 0.05$) relative to the saline-treated control athymic mice. This increase in hepatic phagocytosis is denoted by 28% increase in localization of the emulsion in the glucan group compared to the control group. Glucan did not significantly modify lung or spleen localization of the emulsion. The vascular clearance rate of the lipid emulsion was 25% faster in glucan-treated athymic mice than in control, although the values were of border-line significance ($0.05 < p < 0.1$).

Cytostasis of Anaplastic Carcinoma Cells by Adherent Peritoneal Cells

To ascertain the role of the macrophage as an effector cell mediating the antitumor effect of glucan, the *in vitro* cytostasis of control and glucan-activated adherent peritoneal cell populations against mammary carcinoma cells was measured. Tumoricidal activity, as reflected by inhibition of ^3H-thymidine incorporation by cultured anaplastic carcinoma cells, was evaluated in the presence of adherent peritoneal exudate cells from either A/J or C3H/HeJ mice. A significant ($p < 0.001$) cytostasis of tumor cell proliferation was evident in the presence of noninduced or glucan-activated adherent cells from both species of mice after 20 hr in culture at effector : target cell ratios of 50 : 1 or 10 : 1 (Table 6). However, a more pronounced inhibition of thymidine uptake (approximately double) was evident when tumor cells were incubated with glucan-activated adherent cells from A/J or C3H/HeJ mice, respectively, compared to nonstimulated adherent cells ($p < 0.001$). This enhanced cytostasis with adherent peritoneal cells from glucan-treated mice does not appear to reflect any direct tumoricidal effect of particulate glucan because the addition of 50 μg of glucan to 5×10^5

TABLE 6. *Cytostasis of anaplastic carcinoma cells* in vitro—*control vs. glucan-stimulated macrophages*

| Group | Mice | % Inhibition with effector target cell ratios [a] | |
		10 : 1	50 : 1
Control	A/J	21.8 ± 4.8	26.4 ± 4.3
Glucan	A/J	41.1 ± 5.2 [b]	49.2 ± 3.2 [b]
Control	C3H	24.7 ± 3.3	2.9 ± 1.9
Glucan	C3H	45.7 ± 3.4 [b]	40.4 ± 5.1 [b]

AJ or C3H/HeJ mice were administered saline or glucan (1 mg) i.p. on day 0, and on day 3 adherent peritoneal exudate cells were harvested.
[a] Percent inhibition of thymidine incorporation elicited by control or glucan-stimulated adherent cells. $N = 10$ to 18.
[b] Significant $p < 0.001$.

tumor cells did not induce an inhibitory effect on thymidine incorporation by tumor cell cultures (Table 2).

To further corroborate our *in vitro* studies, we also ascertained the effectiveness of glucan in inhibiting growth of the anaplastic carcinoma cells *in vivo.* Tumor cells were administered subcutaneously (10×10^6) on day 0 in A/J mice and followed by intravenous glucan injections (0.3 mg/mouse) on days 0, 2, 4, 6, and 8. The tumors were removed and weighed on day 11. Glucan significantly ($p < 0.001$) retarded growth of the anaplastic carcinoma by approximately 48% relative to control mice (Table 7). Associated with the marked reduction of tumor weight was significant glucan-induced hepatomegaly and splenomegaly ($p < 0.01$).

DISCUSSION

Glucan, an insoluble polyglucose derived from the inner cell wall of *Saccharomyces cerevisiae,* has been shown a potent modulator of immunological responsiveness with respect to both humoral and cellular types. Previous studies have demonstrated that administration of glucan to mice evokes a marked increase in the primary and secondary immune response to sheep red blood cells

TABLE 7. *Inhibitory effect of glucan on growth of anaplastic carcinoma in A/J mice*

Group	Liver (g)	Spleen (g)	Tumor (mg)
Control	1.04 ± 0.03	0.12 ± 0.01	1,369 ± 56
Glucan	1.24 ± 0.05	0.20 ± 0.01	717 ± 25

Glucan was administered i.v. 0.3 mg on days 0, 2, 4, 6, and 8 following subcutaneous administration of 10×10^6 anaplastic carcinoma cells. Tumors were excised on day 11 after injection. $N = 17$ to 19.

(26). Glucan treatment prior to whole body radiation exposure selectively abolished the acceptance of genetically foreign bone marrow, thus denoting an enhanced cellular immune response (25). The administration of glucan to radiation chimeras resulted in a 100% mortality when the animals were bearing allogeneic or xenogeneic grafts, but did not modify survival of mice with syngeneic bone marrow grafts (25). Administration of glucan has also been demonstrated to enhance the graft-versus-host reaction induced in F_1 hybrid mice by the injection of immunologically competent spleen cells from a parent strain (1).

The enhanced *in vitro* reactivity of splenocytes from mice given glucan injections on days 3 and 5 prior to sacrifice in the presence of concanavalin A and endotoxin, as opposed to the decreased responsiveness following more prolonged glucan treatment, may be a more accurate reflection of the *in vivo* immunocompetence of glucan-treated animals. The apparent suppression in reactivity to the mitogenic agents following repeated injections of glucan may well be due to the increased numbers of activated macrophages within the spleen cell population. Indeed, Keller (13) has demonstrated either enhancement or suppression of lymphocyte proliferation induced by concanavalin A or endotoxin depending on the ratio of activated macrophages to lymphocytes in culture. When the number of activated macrophages equals or exceeds the number of lymphocytes in culture, a significant inhibition of thymidine incorporation is observed, whereas fewer numbers of activated macrophages in the presence of lymphocytes often markedly enhances proliferation in response to the mitogens (13).

T lymphocytes have been implicated as effector or killer cells in cell-mediated immunity controlling the growth of tumors (10,14,18). Our results denote that glucan effectively retarded growth of the melanoma B16 tumors in mice congenitally depleted of thymus-derived cells as well as in normal mice. The mechanism, therefore, by which glucan exerts its antitumor effect appears to be a thymic-independent process. Associated with the tumor inhibitory action of glucan in athymic mice was an increase in functional activity of the RES. Hepatic phagocytosis of the ^{131}I RE test lipid emulsion was significantly enhanced relative to control athymic mice, thus denoting that glucan can activate macrophages in T-lymphocyte-deficient mice. These observations with yeast glucan differ from the tumor inhibitory effect of lentinan, a water soluble linear β 1,3 glucan, where the antitumor action is absent in thymectomized mice (15). Tumoricidal activity of lentinan appears to differ from yeast glucan since neither macrophage stimulation nor enhancement in cell or humoral immunity has been observed (15).

The tumor inhibitory action of yeast glucan in athymic mice, we have observed, appears to be similar to that of certain RE stimulants possessing significant antitumor activity. For example, *Corynebacterium parvum* was demonstrated to have antitumor action in neonatally thymectomized mice implanted with fibrosarcoma (24). Indeed, in subsequent investigations, peritoneal macrophages from normal as well as athymic mice stimulated with *C. parvum* were shown to be markedly cytotoxic to tumor cells *in vitro* (7). The antitumor effect of pyran copolymer has also been shown to be mediated through a thymus-independent process (21). In a similar fashion, Bacillus Calmette-Guérin (BCG) has been shown to prevent growth of tumor cells in athymic mice (19). The importance of macrophages in the mediation of the antitumor action of BCG and methanol extraction residue (MER) is also denoted by the observation that macrophage depletion by silica administration inhibited the antitumor effect of BCG and its methanol extraction residue (11).

Our results have also demonstrated that melanoma B16 cells apparently grow at a slower rate in nude athymic mice than in normal mice. The reason for slower growth of tumors in T-lymphocyte-deficient mice remains to be elucidated, but it is consistent with the findings of other investigators. Woodruff et al. (24) observed a decreased growth of fibrosarcoma isotransplants in neonatally thymectomized mice relative to normal mice although rejection of skin allotransplants was grossly impaired. Skov et al. (23) observed a marked reduction of lung metastases in athymic mice relative to normal littermate mice after injection of transplantable syngeneic tumor cells. Decreased tumor growth was evident in the athymic mice when challenged with five different syngeneic tumor types, including the melanoma B16. Additionally, malignant hamster tumor cells transplanted to nude mice grow at a slower rate than in normal hamsters and with a higher incidence of spontaneous regression (17).

In an effort to further elucidate effector mechanisms by which glucan initiates tumoricidal activity, *in vitro* cytotoxicity of glucan-stimulated peritoneal macrophages against anaplastic carcinoma cells was assessed. Our findings revealed that glucan-stimulated macrophages, as opposed to unstimulated control macrophages, elicit a markedly enhanced cytostasis of malignant cells indicated by reduced thymidine incorporation. The enhanced capacity of glucan-stimulated macrophages to inhibit proliferation of tumor cells was evident with adherent peritoneal exudate cells from both A/J and C3H/HeJ mice. Since the addition of glucan directly to cultures of the malignant cells did not interfere with thymidine uptake, our findings cannot be attributed to a direct cytocidal effect of glucan. Glucan administration also inhibited growth of the anaplastic carcinoma cells when transplanted to A/J mice—an *in vivo* counterpart of our *in vitro* observation. Furthermore, it has been previously demonstrated that injection of glucan-activated peritoneal macrophages conjointly with Shay myelogenous tumor cells in the rat significantly inhibits primary tumor growth as well as metastasis (3).

There is increasing evidence that macrophages activated specifically or nonspecifically may be primary cells in the control of tumor growth and metastasis (5,7,12,21,22). Although a lymphocytic involvement certainly cannot be negated, our composite observations are consistent with the hypothesis that glucan mediates its antitumor effects by activating macrophages. Conjoint activation of macrophages with tumor antigen and certain immunological adjuvants has been recently demonstrated by Schultz et al. (22) to act synergistically in potentiating specific macrophage tumoricidal activity. Such a mechanism, therefore, may explain the *in vivo* observation from our laboratory (2) that concurrent immuno-stimulation with attenuated tumor cells and glucan is markedly more effective in inhibiting metastasis and promoting survival in leukemic rats than either treatment alone.

SUMMARY

Depending on the duration of administration, glucan either enhanced or depressed the *in vitro* response of isolated splenocytes to the T-cell mitogen concanavalin A and the B-cell mitogen *E. coli* endotoxin. Spleen cells from mice given glucan (0.3 mg) 5 and 3 days prior to sacrifice manifested an enhanced response to the mitogens, whereas those from mice given more prolonged administration, i.e., injections over an 18-day period, showed a suppressed blastogenic response. To evaluate the possible relationship between the T-lymphocytic effects of glucan and its antitumor action, studies were conducted in congenitally athymic mice. Administration of glucan significantly inhibited the growth of melanoma B16 cells in nude athymic as well as in normal syngeneic mice. Glucan, therefore, may promote antitumor activity through a thymus-independent mechanism. Associated with the antitumor action of glucan in athymic mice was an enhanced phagocytic activity. Glucan-activated peritoneal macrophages, as opposed to unstimulated macrophages from C3H/HeJ and AJ host mice, were markedly more effective in inhibiting *in vitro* proliferation of anaplastic mammary carcinoma cells. Although lymphocytic involvement certainly cannot be negated, these composite observations suggest that activated macrophages play a significant role in mediating the antitumor action of glucan.

ACKNOWLEDGMENT

These studies were supported, in part, by the Cancer Research Institute, Inc. and National Institutes of Health grant CA 13746.

REFERENCES

1. Di Luzio, N. R. (1967): Evaluation by the graft-versus-host reaction of the immune competence of lymphoid cells of mice with altered reticuloendothelial function. *J. Reticuloendothel. Soc.,* 4:459–475.
2. Di Luzio, N. R., Browder, W., McNamee, R., and Cook, J. A. (1976): Induction of tumor immunity by conjoint use of attenuated tumor cells and glucan. *Fed. Proc. (in press).*
3. Di Luzio, N. R., Hoffmann, E. O., Cook, J. A., Browder, W., and Mansell, P. (1976): Glucan-induced enhancement in host resistance to experimental tumors. *Natl. Cancer Inst. Monogr. (in press).*
4. Di Luzio, N. R., and Riggi, S. J. (1964): The development of a lipid emulsion for the measurement of reticuloendothelial function. *J. Reticuloendothel. Soc.,* 1:136–149.
5. Evans, R. (1973): Macrophages and the tumor bearing host. *Br. J. Cancer,* 28 (Suppl.1):19–25.

6. Gery, I., Baer, A., Stupp, Y., and Weiss, D. (1974): Further studies on the effects of the methanol extraction residue fraction on tubercle bacilli on lymphoid cells and macrophages. *Isr. J. Med. Sci.,* 10:170–177.

7. Ghaffer, A., Cullen, R. T., and Woodruff, M. F. (1975): Further analysis of the anti-tumor effect *in vitro* of peritoneal exudate cells from mice treated with *Corynebacterium parvum. Br. J. Cancer,* 31:15–24.

8. Greaves, M., and Janossy, G. (1972): Elucidation of selective T and B lymphocyte responses by cell surface binding. *Transplant. Rev.,* 11:87.

9. Hassid, W. Z., Joslyn, M. A., and McCready, R. M. (1941): The molecular constitution of an insoluble polysaccharide from yeast, *Saccharomyces cerevisiae. J. Am. Chem. Soc.,* 63:295–298.

10. Hellstrom, K. E., and Hellstrom, I. (1974): The role of cell mediated immunity in control and growth of tumors. *Clin. Immunobiol.,* 2:233–264.

11. Hopper, D. G., Pimm, M. V., and Baldwin, R. W. (1976): Silica abrogation of mycobacterial adjuvant contact suppression of tumor growth in athymic mice. *Cancer Immunol. Immunother.,* 1:143–144.

12. Keller, R. (1973): Cytostatic elimination of syngeneic rat tumor cells *in vitro* by nonspecifically activated macrophages. *J. Exp. Med.,* 138:625–644.

13. Keller, R. (1975): Major changes in lymphocyte proliferation evoked by activated macrophages. *Cell. Immunol.,* 17:542–551.

14. Kumar, S., and Taylor, G. (1973): Specific lymphocytotoxicity and blocking factors in tumors of the central nervous system. *Br. J. Cancer,* (Suppl. 1) 28:135.

15. Maeda, Y. Y., and Chihara, G. (1973): The effects of neonatal thymectomy on the antitumor activity of lentinan carboxymethyl pachymaran and zymosan and their effect on various immune responses. *Int. J. Cancer,* 11:153–161.

16. Mansell, P. W. A., Ichinose, H., Reed, R. J., Krementz, E. T., McNamee, R., and Di Luzio, N. R. (1975): Macrophage mediated destruction of human malignant cells *in vivo. J. Natl. Cancer Inst.,* 54:571–580.

17. Maguire, H. (1976): Invasion and metastasis of xenogenic tumors in nude mice. *J. Natl. Cancer Inst.,* 57:439–442.

18. Perlmann, P., and Holm, G. (1969): Cytotoxic effects of lymphoid cells *in vitro. Adv. Immunol.,* 11:117–193.

19. Pimm, M. V., and Baldwin, R. W. (1975): BCG immunotherapy of rat tumors in nude athymic mice. *Nature,* 254:77–78.

20. Riggi, S. J., and Di Luzio, N. R. (1961): Identification of a reticuloendothelial stimulating agent in zymosan. *Am. J. Physiol.,* 200:297–300.

21. Schultz, R. M., Woods, W. A., Mohr, S. J., and Chirigos, M. A. (1976): Immune response of Balb/C X DBA/2F$_1$ mice to a tumor allograft during pyran copolymer induced tumor enhancement. *Cancer Res.,* 36:1641–1646.

22. Schultz, R., Papamatheakis, J. D., Stylos, W. A., and Chirigos, M. A. (1976): Augmentation of specific macrophage mediated cytotoxicity: Correlation with agents which enhance antitumor resistance. *Cell. Immunol.,* 25:309–316.

23. Skov, C. B., Holland, J. M., and Perkins, E. H. (1976): Development of fewer tumor colonies in lungs of athymic mice after intravenous injection of tumor cells. *J. Natl. Cancer Inst.,* 56:193–195.

24. Woodruff, M. F. A., Dunbar, N., and Ghaffar, A. (1973): The growth of tumors in T cell deprived mice and their response to treatment with *Corynebacterium parvum. Proc. R. Soc. Lond. [Biol.],* 184:97–102.

25. Wooles, W. R., and Di Luzio, N. R. (1962): Influence of reticuloendothelial hyperfunction on bone marrow transplantation. *Am. J. Physiol.,* 203:404–408.

26. Wooles, W. R., and Di Luzio, N. R. (1963): Reticuloendothelial function and the immune response. *Science,* 142:1078–1080.

Immune Modulation and Control of Neoplasia by Adjuvant Therapy, edited by M. A. Chirigos. Raven Press, New York, 1978.

Increased Granulopoiesis and Macrophage Production in Glucan-Treated Mice

Carmen Burgaleta and David W. Golde

Division of Hematology-Oncology, Department of Medicine, UCLA School of Medicine, Los Angeles, California 90024

Macrophage activation can occur in response to a wide variety of biological agents. There is now considerable experimental data indicating that nonspecifically activated macrophages have the capacity for syngeneic tumor cell cytotoxicity *in vitro* and that they probably play an important role in the prevention and limitation of tumor cell growth *in vivo* (1,4,9,11,17). The number of macrophages present at the tumor site also appears to be an important variable (7).

Glucan is a partially purified derivative of zymosan obtainable from the cell wall of *Saccharomyces cerevisiae*. Glucan has a molecular weight of 6,500 daltons and represents most of the polysaccharide content of zymosan (5,15). The administration of glucan results in marked stimulation of the reticuloendothelial system, and it appears to have most of the biological properties of zymosan (22). There is evidence for the immunotherapeutic utility of glucan in several experimental tumor systems (6) and very limited experience in man (19).

We performed a series of experiments to determine the effect of glucan on granulopoiesis and macrophage production in the mouse.

MATERIALS AND METHODS

Glucan was provided by N. Di Luzio and was prepared in his laboratory by previously described methods (15). Female DBA-2 mice, 8 to 10 weeks old, were used in all experiments. The mice were injected intraperitoneally on day 0 and 1 with 2 mg of glucan, and control mice received equal volumes of 5% dextrose. The mice were sacrificed 6 and 20 days after injection by cervical dislocation. The femoral bone marrow and spleen were removed and single-cell suspensions prepared in α medium with 15% fetal calf serum and antibiotics. Peritoneal cells were obtained by washing the peritoneal cavity with Hanks' balanced salt solution containing 10 U/ml of preservative-free heparin and antibiotics. The cells were washed twice and resuspended in complete medium. The total number of nucleated cells was determined in all samples. The liver was also removed and minced in Hanks' solution with 0.125% trypsin. The hepatic cells were washed twice and resuspended in complete α medium.

In vitro colony-forming capacity was determined in cell suspensions from these tissues. Granulocyte-monocyte progenitors (CFU-C) were assayed with a single-layer agar technique using methods previously described (12,14). Fifty microliters of pregnant mouse uterus extract was added to each culture as the source of colony-stimulating activity (CSA) (2). Cultures were incubated in a humidified atmosphere of 7.5% CO_2 in air at 37° for 7 to 10 days and colonies of 50 or more cells enumerated with an inverted microscope. Colonies from peritoneal cells are all of the macrophage type and were counted at 15 to 20 days. Selected colonies were picked with a finely drawn pipette and deposited on glass slides for morphological examination after Giemsa staining.

To determine the cloning capacity of spleen cells without added CSA (auto-stimulation), high-cell concentrations (1 to 4×10^6) were plated, and the number of colonies and clusters (8 to 50 cells) were counted after 7 days in culture. To test for macrophage CSA production, 2×10^5 normal mouse bone marrow cells were cultured in the upper layer of the double-layer agar system (12), using control and glucan-stimulated macrophages (1 to 2×10^5 per plate) as feeder layers.

The number of macrophages in bone marrow, spleen, and peritoneal cavity was determined by α-naphthyl butyrase stain of cytocentrifuge preparations from these tissues (24). Blood was obtained by heart puncture from etherized mice, and white blood cell counts and differentials were performed.

RESULTS

Glucan administration did not have a statistically significant effect on total spleen or bone marrow cellularity, although viable cell counts were higher in the treated animals (Table 1). There was a 10-fold increase in splenic CFU-C and a 75% increase in bone marrow CFU-C 1 week after glucan injection (Tables 1 and 2). Twenty days after treatment, a further two- and fourfold increase occurred, respectively, in bone marrow and spleen CFU-C. The cloning efficiency of liver cell preparations from glucan-treated mice was four times greater than that observed in control animals (Table 3). Almost all of the liver-derived colonies were composed of macrophages. Colonies grown from bone marrow and spleen were usually of pure macrophage or mixed granulocyte-

TABLE 1. *Effect of glucan on bone marrow cellularity and CFU-C*

Days after treatment	Total viable cells $\times 10^7$			Total CFU-C per femur $\times 10^3$		
	Glucan		Control	Glucan		Control
6	1.6 ± 2	$(p = 0.5)$	1.4 ± 1	9.3 ± 1	$(p = 0.05)$	5.6 ± 1
20	4.1 ± 0.3	$(p \leq 0.1)$	2.6 ± 2	20 ± 0.6	$(p = 0.05)$	11 ± 0.4

Mean ± SE of seven experiments.

TABLE 2. *Effect of glucan on spleen cellularity and CFU-C*

Days after treatment	Total number of cells $\times 10^8$			Total CFU-C $\times 10^3$		
	Glucan		Control	Glucan		Control
6	1.3 ± 1	$(p \le 0.5)$	1 ± 2	9.3 ± 2	$(p \le 0.01)$	0.9 ± 0.3
20	2.1 ± 0.3	$(p \le 0.1)$	1.4 ± 1	42 ± 2	$(p \le 0.01)$	1.1 ± 0.3

Mean $\pm$ SE of seven experiments.

TABLE 3. *Effect of glucan on liver CFU-C*

	Colonies	
	2×10^5	1×10^6
Glucan	7	25
Control	1	6

TABLE 4. *Effect of glucan on peritoneal macrophages*

	Total viable peritoneal cells $\times 10^6$	Total macrophage colonies $\times 10^2$	Macrophages (%)	Total macrophages $\times 10^6$
Glucan	7.3 ± 0.7	2 ± 0.2	60 ± 2.5	4.4 ± 0.4
	$(p \le 0.01)$	$(p \le 0.01)$		$(p \le 0.01)$
Control	2.4 ± 0.3	1 ± 0.2	74 ± 3.6	1.8 ± 0.2

Mean $\pm$ SE of seven experiments.

TABLE 5. *Effect of glucan on CSA elaboration*

	CFU-C generation without added CSA		CFU-C generation with macrophage feeder layers		
	Spleen cells	Colonies	Bone marrow cells	Macrophages	Clusters
Glucan	1×10^6	2	2×10^5	2×10^5	50
	2×10^6	9			
	4×10^6	20			
Control	1×10^6	0	2×10^5	2×10^5	11
	2×10^6	3			
	4×10^6	4			

macrophage type in glucan-treated animals, whereas granulocytic colonies predominated in control mice.

There was a significantly greater total number of cells in the peritoneal cavity of treated mice with approximately a twofold increase in total macrophages and macrophage colony-forming cells (Table 4). Spleen cells from glucan-treated mice exhibited prominent colony formation at high plating densities without added CSA (Table 5). This phenomenon of autostimulation is ascribed to augmented CSA elaboration in the culture dish (14). Peritoneal macrophages from glucan-injected animals also elaborated greater amounts of CSA *in vitro* than an equal number of control cells (Table 5). Total macrophage counts in bone marrow and spleen were increased in glucan-treated mice. Also, there was a consistent twofold higher total peripheral white blood cell count in the glucan-injected mice, although there was no change in the differential count.

DISCUSSION

Activated macrophages manifest a general increase in functional capacity and exhibit measurable antitumor activity in several experimental systems (1, 4,8,9,17). Generally, a high ratio of macrophages to target cells is necessary to demonstrate syngeneic cytotoxicity *in vitro* (21). *In vivo* studies suggest that the number of macrophages present in tumor tissue relates importantly to tumor growth and dissemination (7). Bacillus Calmette-Guérin and *Corynebacterium parvum* are nonspecific immunotherapeutic agents that activate macrophages and have been shown to increase macrophage production in experimental animals (10,25). Because of glucan's potential utility in immunotherapy, we undertook studies designed to define the effect of glucan on granulopoiesis and macrophage genesis.

Glucan administration in mice resulted in a prominent increase in precursor cells capable of colony formation *in vitro* (CFU-C) in various tissues. Total splenic CFU-C increased by tenfold 1 week after treatment, whereas bone marrow CFU-C increased to a smaller but significant degree compared to control. Twenty days after glucan injection there was a further increase in total splenic and femoral CFU-C. The colonies from glucan-treated animals were often of the pure macrophage type (approximately 50%), whereas granulocytic colonies predominated in control animals. CFU-C in the liver were also markedly increased in treated animals. Usually few of these progenitor cells are found in normal murine liver (16). Cells in the peritoneal cavity are capable of pure macrophage-colony formation in soft-gel culture (18). Glucan-treated mice had a twofold increase in these cells compared to controls.

Total numbers of macrophages were increased in the peritoneal cavity, spleen, and bone marrow of treated mice, suggesting that the expansion of the progenitor cell compartment related to augmented macrophage production *in vivo*. The elevated peripheral white counts also provide evidence that the enhanced leukopoiesis demonstrated *in vitro* was also reflected *in vivo*.

Macrophages play an important role in the feedback regulation of granulopoiesis and monocytopoiesis because they are a major source of CSA production (13,20). Macrophages activated by endotoxin elaborate increased quantities of CSA (3,23), and the enhanced leukopoiesis associated with macrophage activation *in vivo* may also be mediated by CSA. We performed studies of CSA production in glucan-treated mice and were able to demonstrate increased CSA elaboration by macrophages from treated animals.

These studies indicate that glucan administration results in increased granulopoiesis and macrophage production in mice. The increased white cell production is probably related to augmented macrophage CSA production. In terms of immunotherapy, the important implication of these experiments is that glucan administration can result in increased availability of effector cells.

ACKNOWLEDGMENTS

Supported by USPHS grants CA 15619 and CA 15688. The authors gratefully acknowledge Dr. N. Di Luzio's help with these studies.

REFERENCES

1. Alexander, P., and Evans, R. (1971): Endotoxin and double stranded RNA render macrophages cytotoxic. *Nature (New Biol.),* 232:76–78.
2. Bradley, T. R., Stanley, E. R., and Sumner, M. A. (1971): Factors from mouse tissues stimulating colony growth of mouse bone marrow cells *in vitro. Aust. J. Exp. Biol. Med. Sci.,* 49:595–603.
3. Cline, M. J., Rothman, B., and Golde, D. W. (1974): Effect of endotoxin on the production of colony-stimulating factor by human monocytes and macrophages. *J. Cell. Physiol.,* 84:193–196.
4. David, J. R. (1975): Macrophage activation by lymphocyte mediators. *Fed. Proc.,* 34:1730–1736.
5. Di Carlo, F. J., and Fiore, J. V. (1958): On the composition of zymosan. *Science,* 127:756–757.
6. Di Luzio, N. R., McNamee, R., Jones, E., Cook, J. A., and Hoffman, E. O. (1976): The employment of glucan and glucan activated macrophages in the enhancement of host resistance to malignancies in experimental animals. In: *The Macrophage in Neoplasia,* edited by M. Fink. Academic Press, New York.
7. Evans, R. (1973): Macrophages and the tumour bearing host. *Br. J. Cancer,* 28 (Suppl. I): 19–25.
8. Fidler, I. J., Darnell, J. H., and Budmen, M. B. (1976): Tumoricidal properties of mouse macrophages activated with mediators from rat lymphocytes stimulated with concanavalin A. *Cancer Res.,* 36:3608–3615.
9. Fink, M. A. (editor) (1976): *The Macrophage in Neoplasia.* Academic Press, New York.
10. Fisher, B., Taylor, S., Levine, M., Saffer, E., and Fisher, E. R. (1974): Effect of *Mycobacterium bovis* (Strain *Bacillus Calmette-Guérin*) on macrophage production by the bone marrow of tumor-bearing mice. *Cancer Res.,* 34:1668–1670.
11. Ghaffar, A., Cullen, R. T., and Woodruff, M. F. A. (1975): Further analysis of the anti-tumour effect *in vitro* of peritoneal exudate cells from mice treated with *Corynebacterium parvum. Br. J. Cancer,* 31:15–24.
12. Golde, D. W., and Cline, M. J. (1972): Identification of the colony-stimulating cell in human peripheral blood. *J. Clin. Invest.,* 51: 2981–2983.
13. Golde, D. W., and Cline, M. J. (1974): Regulation of granulopoiesis. *N. Engl. J. Med.,* 291:1388–1395.

14. Golde, D. W., Faille, A., Sullivan, A., and Friend, C. (1976): Granulocytic stem cells in Friend leukemia. *Cancer Res.,* 36:115–119.
15. Hassid, W. Z., Joslyn, M. A., and McCready, R. M. (1941): The molecular constitution of an insoluble polysaccharide from yeast *Saccharomyces cerevisiae. J. Am. Chem. Soc.,* 63:295–298.
16. Hays, E. F., Firkin, F. C., Koga, Y., and Hays, D. M. (1975): Hemopoietic colony forming cells in regenerating mouse liver. *J. Cell. Physiol.,* 86:213–220.
17. Hibbs, J. B., Jr., Lambert, L. H., Jr., and Remington, J. S. (1972): Control of carcinogenesis: A possible role for the activated macrophage. *Science,* 177:998–1000.
18. Lin, H.-S., and Stewart, C. C. (1973): Colony formation by mouse peritoneal exudate cells *in vitro. Nature (New Biol.),* 243:176–177.
19. Mansell, P. W. A., Ichinose, H., Reed, R. J., Krementz, E. T., McNamee, R., and Di Luzio, N. R. (1975): Macrophage-mediated destruction of human malignant cells *in vivo. J. Natl. Cancer Inst.,* 54:571–580.
20. Moore, M. A. S. (1976): Regulatory role of macrophages in hemopoiesis. *J. Reticuloendothel. Soc.,* 20:89–91.
21. Norbury, K. C., and Fidler, I. J. (1975): *In vitro* tumor cell destruction by syngeneic mouse macrophages: Methods for assaying cytotoxicity. *J. Immunol. Methods,* 7:109–122.
22. Riggi, S. J., and Di Luzio, N. R. (1961): Identification of a reticuloendothelial stimulatory agent in zymosan. *Am. J. Physiol.,* 200:297–300.
23. Ruscetti, F. W., and Chervenick, P. A. (1974): Release of colony-stimulating factor from monocytes by endotoxin and polyinosinic-polycytidylic acid. *J. Lab. Clin. Med.,* 83:64–72.
24. Willcox, M. B., Golde, D. W., and Cline, M. J. (1976): Cytochemical reactions of human hematopoietic cells in liquid culture. *J. Histochem. Cytochem.,* 24:979–983.
25. Wolmark, N., Levine, M., and Fisher, B. (1974): The effect of a single and repeated administration of *Corynebacterium parvum* on bone marrow macrophage colony production in normal mice. *J. Reticuloendothel. Soc.,* 16:252–256.

Immune Modulation and Control of Neoplasia by Adjuvant Therapy, edited by M. A. Chirigos. Raven Press, New York, 1978.

Glucan-Activated Macrophages: Functional Properties and Cytotoxicity Against Syngeneic Leukemia Cells

David W. Golde and Carmen Burgaleta

Division of Hematology-Oncology, Department of Medicine, UCLA School of Medicine, Los Angeles, California 90024

Nonspecifically activated macrophages exhibit morphological alterations and increased cellular functional capacity (2). These activated cells are usually larger, show increased adherence and spreading on glass, have greater chemotactic and microbicidal activity, and are capable of syngeneic tumor cell cytotoxicity (1,2,8,9). A number of biological products referred to as reticuloendothelial stimulants are macrophage activators. These activators are presently under intensive study because of their potential role in the nonspecific immunotherapy of cancer (4,10,12).

Glucan, a polysaccharide derived from zymosan, is composed of glucopyranose units joined by 1-β glucoside linkages. This partially purified derivative has most of the biological properties of zymosan (13). Glucan is a potent reticuloendothelial stimulant and is reported to cause tumor regression *in vivo* in syngeneic tumor models (3). We performed a series of *in vitro* studies on glucan-activated mouse macrophages to assess their functional and cytotoxic characteristics.

MATERIALS AND METHODS

Glucan was prepared in the laboratory of N. Di Luzio by techniques previously described (7). Solutions of 4 mg/ml were made by dilution in 5% glucose from a 36 mg/ml stock vial.

Female DBA-2 mice (8 to 10 weeks old) were used in all studies. They received an intraperitoneal injection of 4 mg of glucan on days 0 and 1 and were sacrificed by cervical dislocation on day 7. Control mice were injected with equal volumes of 5% glucose in water. Macrophages were obtained by washing the peritoneal cavity with Hanks' balanced salt solution containing 10 units of preservative-free heparin per ml and antibiotics. Cells were washed twice and resuspended in α medium with 15% fetal calf serum and antibiotics. Viable and differential cell counts were performed and the cell suspensions adjusted to 1×10^6 macrophages per ml.

To quantitate macrophage adherence to glass, 5×10^5 macrophages were added to small Leighton tubes and allowed to attach to coverslips during a 1-hr incubation at 37°C. The cover glasses were then washed three times with warm phosphate-buffered saline to remove nonadherent cells. Total and differential counts were performed on the nonadherent cells. The percent macrophage adherence was calculated according to the following formula:

$$\frac{\text{\% macrophage}}{\text{adherence}} = \frac{\text{total macrophages added} - \text{nonadherent macrophages}}{\text{total macrophages added}} \times 100$$

For scanning electron microscopic examination, 5×10^5 macrophages were allowed to settle on glass coverslips for 1 hr. The coverslips were fixed in 3% glutaraldehyde for 30 min, washed with cacodylate buffer, and dehydrated with ethanol and freon. Cells were dried using the critical point method with a Bomar SPC 900/EX dryer. The coverslips were then vacuum coated with gold or carbon and gold and examined with an ETEC autoscan at 10 kV. Mean cell diameter was also measured in these samples.

Friend erythroleukemia cells (GM-86, clone 745) were obtained (Institute for Medical Research, Camden, N.J.) and kept in continuous culture with Eagle's medium (5). This cell line is derived from the DBA-2 mouse. Cytotoxicity of glucan macrophages against the syngeneic Friend leukemia cells was assayed by a ^{3}H-thymidine uptake inhibition method. Macrophages (2×10^5) were added to multiwells (Falcon Plastics, Los Angeles, Cal.) and incubated overnight in a CO_2 incubator. The nonadherent cells were removed by washing three times with Hanks' balanced salt solution containing 15% fetal calf serum. Friend leukemia cells were added to the macrophage monolayers. A ratio of effector to target cells of 10:1 and 100:1 was used, and correction was made for differences in macrophage adherence. Macrophages were cultured in contact with leukemic cells for 1 and 3 days and pulsed with 1 μCi/ml of ^{3}H-thymidine (SA: 6.7 Ci/mM) for 4 hr. The ^{3}H-thymidine uptake was measured by well scintillation counting and the percent inhibition calculated (9,11).

Macrophage cytotoxicity was also measured by a cloning inhibition assay. Macrophages were adhered to 35-mm Lux Petri dishes, and nonadherent cells were removed by washing after 1 hr incubation. One thousand Friend cells were plated in 0.8% methylcellulose in α medium (6) over the macrophage monolayers and the culture incubated at 37° in a CO_2 incubator. Adjustment was made for differences in macrophage adherence, so that 2×10^5 were present on each plate. Friend leukemic cell colonies of six or more cells were counted after 72 hr incubation with an inverted microscope.

RESULTS

Glucan-activated macrophages were 20% more adherent to glass than control cells after 60 min incubation (Table 1). Measurement of the longest cell diameter by optical microscopy and scanning electron microscopy showed that macro-

TABLE 1. *Macrophage adherence (60 min)*

	Mean (%)		SE
Glucan	93	±	1.3
Control	72	±	3

Six experiments.

TABLE 2. *Effect of glucan on macrophage cell length (60-min adherence)*

	Optical microscopy		Scanning electron microscopy	
	Mean (μm)	Range	Mean (μm)	Range
Glucan	17.2 ± 2	14–21	32.8	21–67
Control	12.2 ± 1.6	12–19	14.8	10–14

Mean ± SE of five experiments.

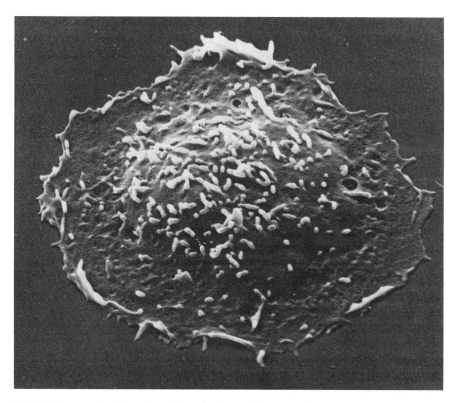

FIG. 1. Glucan-activated peritoneal macrophage adhered to glass for 1 hr. The cell is flat and spread with few blebs and microvilli on the surface. There is ruffling at the marginal edge.

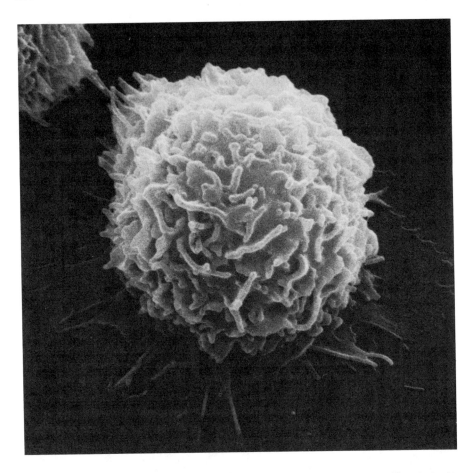

FIG. 2. Normal peritoneal macrophage adhered to glass for 1 hr. The cell is spherical with extensive ruffled membrane. Attachment is by smooth lamellipodia and filopodia and is not extensive.

phages from glucan-treated animals were 30 to 50% longer than control macrophages (Table 2). The surface morphology of the glucan-activated macrophages was also clearly different from control. Scanning electron microscopy showed the activated macrophages to be spread and flattened on the glass with extensive adherent lamellipodia (Fig. 1). There also were blebs and microvilli on the surface. After 60 min adherence, a number of cells developed a polar morphology with markedly elongated asymmetric lamellipodia. In contrast, control macrophages were spherical, showed little spreading, and had small, smooth lamellipodia and filopodia attachments (Fig. 2). There were no elongated cells.

Studies of syngeneic leukemia cell cytotoxicity *in vitro* using ^{3}H-thymidine incorporation showed modest inhibition (9 to 13%) after 1 day's exposure to

TABLE 3. *Cytotoxicity by ³H-thymidine uptake inhibition (3 days, 100 : 1 effector-target ratio)*

Glucan	Control	% Inhibition
20,822	28,142	26
4,370	6,006	27
12,443	18,104	32
17,118	29,070	41

TABLE 4. *Macrophage cytotoxicity (clonogenic assay)*

Effector cells	Colonies per 10³ 745 cells
Glucan	53
Control	136
None	146

macrophages at a 100:1 ratio of effector-target cells. No activity was seen with a 10:1 ratio. With 3 days' exposure at 100:1 ratio, ^{3}H-thymidine uptake inhibition was prominent (26 to 41%) (Table 3). The results of the clonogenic assays for cytotoxicity paralleled the ^{3}H-thymidine uptake data. Inhibition of cloning ranged from 30 to 60% (Table 4).

DISCUSSION

Glucan is a potent reticuloendothelial stimulant, and there is evidence that it may have use as an immunotherapeutic agent. We performed *in vitro* studies to evaluate the effect of glucan on macrophage morphology and function. The glucan-activated macrophages showed greater glass adherence than control cells. The increased adherence was reflected in their surface morphology. Activated macrophages were flattened and had extensive lamellipodia attachments. There was evidence from surface morphology and direct measurement of increased cell spreading. Increased cell movement was suggested by the frequent appearance of elongated cells with pseudopodia.

Tests of syngeneic cytoxocity were performed with the 745 Friend leukemia cell line. Using ^{3}H-thymidine incorporation and a direct clonogenic assay, we were able to demonstrate syngeneic cytotoxicity by both techniques at an effector-target ratio of 100:1 and 200:1, respectively. These preliminary cytotoxicity data, however, must be interpreted with caution. For example, it may be that the activated cells liberate some products that are toxic to the 745 cells.

These studies require considerable expansion and application of other assay techniques, as well as *in vivo* testing. The present information, however, suggests that glucan-activated macrophages exhibit many of the properties of macrophages activated by other nonspecific agents.

ACKNOWLEDGMENTS

Supported by USPHS grants CA 15688 and CA 15619. The authors thank N. Di Luzio for help with this work.

REFERENCES

1. Alexander, P., and Evans, R. (1971): Endotoxin and double stranded RNA render macrophages cytotoxic. *Nature (New Biol.)*, 232:76–78.
2. David, J. R. (1975): Macrophage activation by lymphocyte mediators. *Fed. Proc.*, 34:1730–1736.
3. Di Luzio, N. R., McNamee, R., Jones, E., Cook, J. A., and Hoffmann, E. O. (1976): The employment of glucan and glucan activated macrophages in the enhancement of host resistance to malignancies in experimental animals. In: *The Macrophage in Neoplasia*, edited by M. A. Fink, pp. 181–198. Academic Press, New York.
4. Fink, M. A. (editor) (1976): *The Macrophage in Neoplasia*. Academic Press, New York.
5. Friend, C., Scher, W., Holland, J. G., and Sato, T. (1971): Hemoglobin synthesis in murine virus-induced leukemic cells *in vitro:* Stimulation of erythroid differentiation by dimethyl sulfoxide. *Proc. Natl. Acad. Sci. USA*, 68:378–382.
6. Golde, D. W., Bersch, N., and Cline, M. J. (1976): Potentiation of erythropoiesis *in vitro* by dexamethasone. *J. Clin. Invest.*, 57:57–62.
7. Hassid, W. Z., Joslyn, M. A., and McCready, R. M. (1941): The molecular constitution of an insoluble polysaccharide from yeast *Saccharomyces cerevisiae*. *J. Am. Chem. Soc.*, 63:295–298.
8. Hibbs, J. B., Jr., Lambert, L. H., Jr., and Remington, J. S. (1972): Control of carcinogenesis: A possible role for the activated macrophage. *Science*, 177:998–1000.
9. Krahenbuhl, J. L., and Remington, J. S. (1974): The role of activated macrophages in specific and nonspecific cytostasis of tumor cells *J. Immunol.*, 113:507–516.
10. Mohr, S. J., Chirigos, M. A., Fuhrman, F. S., and Pryor, J. W. (1975): Pyran copolymer as an effective adjuvant to chemotherapy against a murine leukemia and solid tumor. *Cancer Res.*, 35:3750–3754.
11. Norbury, K. C., and Fidler, I. J. (1975): *In vitro* tumor cell destruction by syngeneic mouse macrophages: Methods for assaying cytotoxicity. *J. Immunol. Methods*, 7:109–122.
12. Olivotto, M., and Bomford, R. (1974): *In vitro* inhibition of tumour cell growth and DNA synthesis by peritoneal and lung macrophages from mice injected with *Corynebacterium parvum*. *Int. J. Cancer*, 13:478–488.
13. Riggi, S. J., and Di Luzio, N. R. (1961): Identification of a reticuloendothelial stimulatory agent in zymosan. *Am. J. Physiol.*, 200:297–300.

Immune Modulation and Control of Neoplasia by Adjuvant Therapy, edited by M. A. Chirigos. Raven Press, New York, 1978.

Suppression of Hepatic Metastases by Immunization with Glucan

*William Browder, Craig Cohen, Rose McNamee, **E. O. Hoffmann, and N. R. Di Luzio

*Departments of Physiology, and *Surgery, Tulane University School of Medicine; and ** Department of Pathology, Louisiana State University School of Medicine, New Orleans, Louisiana 70112*

Previous studies have demonstrated that a glucan fraction isolated from *Saccharomyces cerevisiae* is a profound reticuloendothelial-(RE) stimulating agent (2,13–15,25,26,32,33). The administration of glucan to mice or rats is associated with the induction of a hyperphagocytic state and the hypertrophy of major RE organs due to an increase in both size and number of macrophages (2,13–15,25,26,32,33). Since both the induced hyperfunction and hypertrophy of the reticuloendothelial system (RES) are rapidly reversible in nature (33), glucan is a unique agent for evaluating the role of macrophages in immunophysiology. In addition to utilizing glucan in the control of the RES function, it has been previously demonstrated that the administration of glucan profoundly enhances both the primary and secondary hemolysin response of mice to sheep red cells (32). Enhanced clearance of the foreign red cell was also observed in glucan-treated mice (25,32). In the area of transplantation, glucan-induced stimulation of the RES modified the acceptance of allogeneic bone marrow in X-irradiated mice but had no effect on acceptance of syngeneic bone marrow (31,34). Similarly, the administration of glucan to radiation chimeras was associated with rejection of allogeneic and xenogeneic transplants but was without effect in the syngeneic model (31). These composite studies denote that glucan is an excellent immunostimulant having the ability to enhance the selective rejection of normal, nonmalignant cells if these cells are allogeneic or xenogeneic. Additionally, graft-versus-host reactions in F_1 hybrid mice were significantly enhanced in mice that received spleen cells derived from glucan-treated mice (8), denoting enhanced immunological abilities for the transferred spleen cells.

In view of the unique alteration in host defense initiated by glucan, studies were conducted to define the influence of macrophage activation on tumor growth (9,11,12). It was observed that the simultaneous subcutaneous administration of glucan with Shay acute myelogenous leukemia cells significantly inhibited growth of the tumor (9,11). The intravenous administration of glucan prior to tumor cell transplantation resulted in significant modification of tumor growth and prolongation of survival (9,11). Indeed, it was also possible to significantly modify tumor growth when the primary tumor approximated 2 to 3% of body weight and metastases to internal organs had developed (9).

In essential agreement with observations employing the allogeneic Shay myelogenous leukemia model, glucan-treated mice showed a significant growth inhibition of a syngeneic adenocarcinoma (BW10232) and a melanoma (B16) tumor (4,11). In preliminary clinical studies involving three types of metastatic lesions in man, the intralesional administration of glucan produced, in all cases studied, a prompt and striking reduction in the size of the lesion (22). Regression of the glucan-injected tumor was associated with necrosis of the malignant cells and a pronounced monocytic infiltrate. The degree of regression was dependent on the amount of glucan injected into the lesion which in turn appeared to influence the mobilization of macrophages. The initial findings of regression of human tumors have been extended by additional studies (21).

Since glucan appeared to offer distinct advantages over most other currently employed forms of immunotherapy in which viable or nonviable microorganisms are employed (10,21), studies were undertaken to ascertain whether it could modify the development and progression of hepatic tumor induced by the intraportal administration of leukemia cells. These studies were undertaken to determine if glucan could be effective in modifying metastatic lesions. Additionally, when it was observed that the effectiveness of glucan could be overcome with the administration of an increased population of tumor cells, studies were undertaken to establish whether immunity to leukemia cells could be enhanced by the employment of glucan.

MATERIALS AND METHODS

Male Long Evans rats weighing approximately 200 g were anesthetized with ether and the portal vein exposed by means of midline abdominal incision. Leukemia cells in a dose of 1×10^6 or 1×10^7 viable cells were administered slowly in order to provide for maximum lodging of cells within the hepatic sinusoids. Following the administration of tumor cells and the closure of the incision, glucose was administered to controls while glucan in the amount of 20 mg/kg was injected intravenously. Subsequent intravenous injections were made on days 2, 6, 8, and 13 following tumor inoculation. Survival was followed for a 30-day period.

In the immunization studies, the acute myelogenous tumor cells were attenuated by treatment with glutaraldehyde as described by Sanderson and Frost (28). One hundred Long Evans male rats weighing approximately 150 g were divided into four groups; group 1 received 1×10^8 attenuated tumor cells i.p. and glucan 20 mg/kg i.v. on days -14 and -7, group 2 received only the attenuated cells on days -14 and -7, group 3 received glucan 20 mg/kg i.v., and control group 4 received 5% dextrose i.v., again on days -14 and -7. On day 0, the animals were operated on through a midline abdominal incision and 1×10^7 live leukemia cells were injected into the portal vein. Eight days later rats from each group were randomly selected for the assessment of liver function by determining the clearance of bromsulfophthalein (BSP) from plasma (18). BSP was administered in the amount of 50 mg/kg and blood samples obtained 30 min later for BSP determination. Liver sections were obtained from these control and experimental rats and fixed in buffered formalin, embedded in paraffin, and stained with hematoxylin and eosin.

Survival of the animals was established over a 30-day period. The Student's *t*-test and the Chi-square test were utilized to determine statistical significance.

RESULTS

Initial studies documented the ability of glucan to modify survival of animals that received intraportal injections of 1×10^6 leukemia cells. In contrast to the 13% survival in the saline-treated group, an 88% survival was manifested in the glucan group (Fig. 1). BSP retention studies reflected the beneficial effect of glucan in maintaining hepatic function compared to the control group (Table 1). In marked contrast to the protectiveness mediated when 1×10^6 cells were administered, when the tumor cell dose was increased to 10^7 cells, the protective effect of glucan was totally abolished (Fig. 2).

In the studies attempting to immunize rats against intraportal injection of leukemic cells, the prior administration of attenuated cells alone did not significantly modify survival (Fig. 3). However, when glucan and attenuated cells were simultaneously administered, survival was significantly enhanced; 68% of the rats survived the tumor challenge (Fig. 4).

Differences in survival between the various groups and the glucan-plus-attentu-

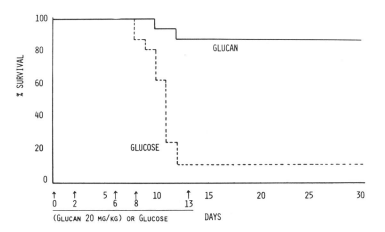

FIG. 1. Enhancement in survival of glucan-treated rats following the administration of 1×10^6 leukemic cells intraportally. The glucan-treated group (—) had an *N* of 16, and the glucose group (----) had an *N* of 15.

TABLE 1. *Plasma BSP concentration in rats following intraportal administration of leukemia cells as influenced by glucan*

Treatment	N	Plasma BSP concentration (mg%)
Normal	10	0.28 ± 0.02
Glucose	6	7.8 ± 1.8
Glucan	6	1.1 ± 0.76

Plasma BSP concentration determined 30 min following injection of BSP in the dose of 50 mg/kg. Studies were conducted on day 8 following the intraportal injection of 1×10^6 acute myelogenous leukemic cells.

ated-cells-immunized group were statistically significant by Chi-square analysis at the $p < 0.05$ level.

In essential agreement with the mortality pattern, liver function, as measured by plasma BSP retention evaluated on day 8 following tumor cell administration, revealed significant impairment in all tumor-injected animals compared to the normal group (Table 2). An approximate 10-fold enhancement in BSP retention occurred in the glucan, glucose, or attenuated cell group. A significant difference was observed in the glucan-attenuated-cell-treated group; an approximate 60% reduction in BSP retention was observed ($p < 0.02$) when comparisons were made with the control, glucan, or attenuated cell group. Hepatic function in the glucan-attenuated cell group was, however, not normalized as a mean 3.6-fold retention of BSP was noted.

In accordance with the BSP data, massive replacement of hepatic parenchyma by myeloblastic leukemia cells was observed in six of seven animals immunized with attenuated tumor cells (Fig. 5). Additionally, all seven animals in the attenuated cell-treated group had extensive tumor cells infiltrating the lung (Fig.

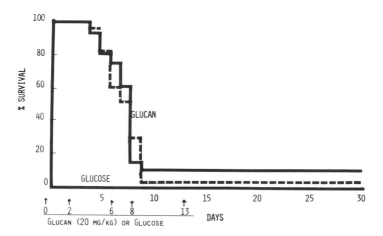

FIG. 2. Inability of glucan to modify the survival of rats that received 1×10^7 tumor cells intraportally. Glucan-treated group (—), $N = 36$; glucose (----), N = 40.

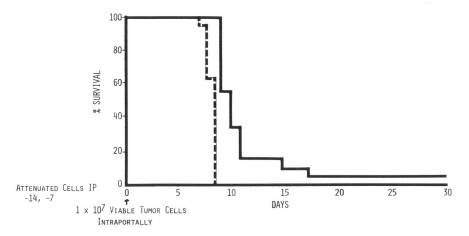

FIG. 3. Inability of glutaraldehyde-attenuated tumor cells to induce immunity to 1×10^7 leukemic cells injected intraportally. The survival of the 20 rats treated with attenuated cells (—) did not differ significantly from the 20 rats of the control group that received glucose (---).

6). Similar findings were present in the liver (Fig. 7) and lung of rats treated with glucan only. Eighty percent of the animals in the glucan group had pulmonary and hepatic lesions, whereas all the animals in dextrose control group had liver and lung metastases. In marked contrast, no animals in the attenuated cell and glucan group had tumor cells detectable in the lung (Fig. 8), whereas two of five animals had only microfoci of tumor in the liver (Fig. 9). The outstanding feature of the liver in this group was the presence of granuloma composed of reticuloendothelial cells.

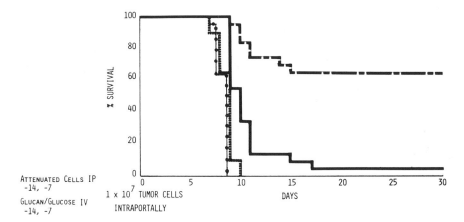

FIG. 4. Induction of tumor immunity to 1×10^7 leukemic cells injected into the portal vein by the conjoint use of glutaraldehyde-treated tumor cells and glucan. The mortality of rats treated with glucose alone (-●-●-), glucan alone (----), and attenuated cells alone (—) was comparable, whereas the increase in survival of the glucan-plus-attenuated-cell-treated group (-—-) is significantly enhanced. Each group had a population of 18 to 20 rats.

TABLE 2. *Plasma BSP concentration in rats that received an intraportal vein injection of leukemic cells as influenced by the presence and absence of immunotherapy*

Treatment	N	Plasma BSP concentration (mg%)
Normal	10	0.28 ± 0.02
Glucose	6	2.85 ± 0.47
Attenuated cells	6	2.42 ± 0.37
Glucan	6	2.69 ± 0.63
Glucan + attenuated cells	6	1.03 ± 0.27

Plasma BSP concentration determined 30 min following injection of BSP in the dose of 50 mg/kg. Studies were conducted on day 8 following the intraportal injection of 1×10^7 leukemic cells.

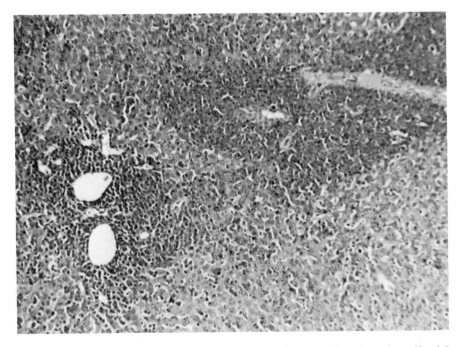

FIG. 5. Liver from rat treated with glutaraldehyde-treated tumor cells only and sacrificed 8 days following intraportal injection of 1×10^7 tumor cells. An extensive infiltration of tumor cells is present.

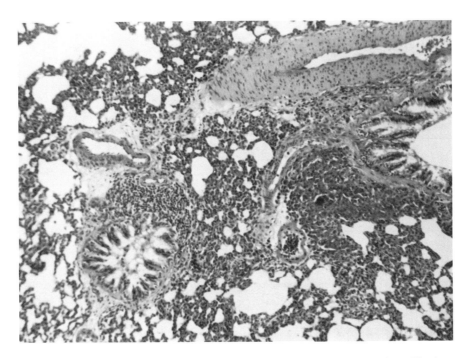

FIG. 6. Section of lung from rat treated with attenuated tumor cells only and sacrificed on day 8 following intraportal injection of 1×10^7 tumor cells denoting the extensive area of tumor cell involvement.

DISCUSSION

The present studies confirm our previous observations that the systemic administration of glucan following the administration of malignant cells results in a significant modification in the progression of tumor state (11,12,21,22). The effect of glucan has been demonstrated in both allogeneic and syngeneic tumor models (4,11,12).

Since direct contact between activated macrophages and tumor target cells is essential for the manifestation of cytotoxic action (3,20,23), the increased number and function of hepatic macrophages induced by glucan increases the opportunity for tumor cell destruction. Indeed, one of the most prominent histological findings in glucan-treated animals is the pronounced enhancement in macrophage cell populations of liver, lung, and spleen (2,26,33).

The present studies show that at increased tumor load the inhibitory effect of glucan on the proliferation and dissemination of leukemic cells is lost. The mechanism by which the protective effect of glucan is overcome when the number of tumor cells is increased 10-fold from 10^6 to 10^7 is not presently known.

In contrast to the observations of Sanderson and Frost (28) that tumor immunity in mice is induced with the use of glutaraldehyde-treated tumor cells, we

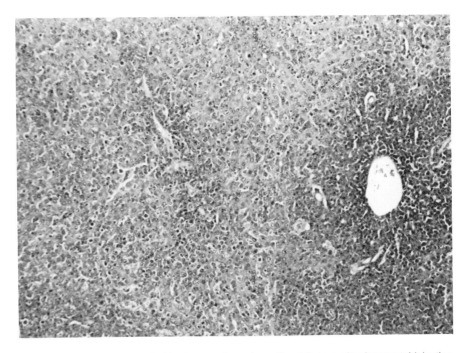

FIG. 7. Liver from rat treated with glucan only and sacrificed 8 days after intraportal injection of 1×10^7 tumor cells. Note massive tumor in periportal area as well as presence of tumor cells throughout the liver.

have not found it possible to use glutaraldehyde-treated leukemia cells to induce immunity to intraportally administered leukemia cells. The inability to induce immunity by the prior administration of glutaraldehyde-treated leukemia cells may well denote minimum antigenicity of the attenuated tumor cells that may be considerably enhanced in the presence of glucan. Indeed, it has been previously found that the administration of glucan to mice that received foreign red cells produced profound enhancement in both primary and secondary immune response (15,32). In agreement with the observations and conclusions of Sanderson and Frost, the glutaraldehyde-treated tumor cells were found to be nonviable and no growth occurred when the glutaraldehyde-treated cells were administered subcutaneously to normal animals. Since the glutaraldehyde-fixed cells can be stored for prolonged periods and intermixed with glucan, repeated immunization procedures are possible employing the identical tumor cell population. Since glucan has been administered intralesionally in man without any observable side effects (21,22), it remains to be established whether the combined use of glutaraldehyde-fixed tumor cells and glucan is advantageous for the mediation of tumor immunotherapy in man.

The present studies show the potentiation of tumor vaccine by glucan is essentially identical to the potentiation of L1210 vaccine employing pyran co-

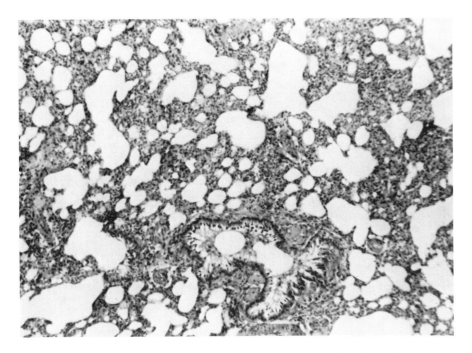

FIG. 8. Lung from animal treated with glucan plus attenuated cells and sacrificed 8 days after 1×10^7 tumor cell injection. Hypertrophy of macrophage elements is present, but no tumor is observed.

polymer (24). In the absence of pyran copolymer, which, like glucan, also enhances antibody production and macrophage activity, no potentiation of survival is seen. Thus, the use of X-irradiated tumor cells alone did not, in the absence of an immunostimulant, enhance survival of mice to subsequent challenges with viable tumor cells.

It has been observed that other macrophage-stimulating agents, such as Bacillus Calmette-Guérin (BCG) (19) and *Corynebacterium parvum* (30), have also induced immunity to malignant cells. A common feature of these agents, as well as glucan, is their ability to produce a significant enhancement in macrophage number and function (17). Additionally, Schultz et al. (29) have demonstrated the ability of nonspecific immunostimulants, such as BCG, *C. parvum,* and pyran copolymer, to act synergistically to enhance specific macrophage cytotoxicity toward the appropriate target cell. It may be that glucan acts as such an adjuvant when used in conjunction with the glutaraldehyde-fixed cells and that this synergistic enhancement of macrophage tumoricidal activity accounts for the increased survival when the regimen is utilized.

Sadler and Alexander (27) have reported leukemic cells administered intravenously were rapidly destroyed by the RES. Employing a lymphoid and myeloid leukemia system, Sadler and Alexander demonstrated rapid destruction of both

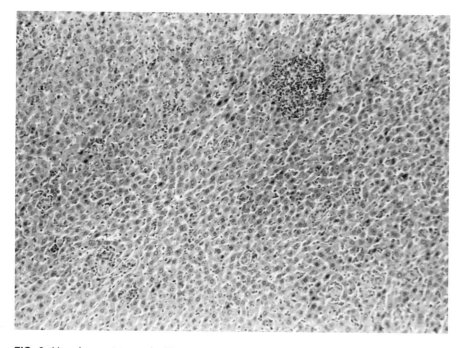

FIG. 9. Liver from rat treated with attenuated cells plus glucan and sacrificed 8 days after injection of 1×10^7 tumor cells intraportally. Multiple granulomas of varying sizes are seen, but no tumor is present. The striking differences in hepatic tumor state in the attenuated-cell-plus-glucan-treated group is readily apparent when the figure is compared to Figs. 5 and 7.

leukemia cell populations so that, by 24 hr, almost all of the injected cells were totally destroyed as denoted by the loss of radiolabel and histological observations. It remains to be established whether there is an increased destruction of leukemia cells by hepatic macrophages through either contact lysis (3, 20,23) or phagocytosis in the immunized state. The relative roles of cellular and humoral factors mediating enhanced survival of rats following the administration of attenuated tumor cells and in glucan remain to be established.

Frost et al. (16) have utilized glutaraldehyde-attenuated tumor cells to immunize a variety of syngeneic tumor models. Despite survival in the immunized group, no increase in serum antibody against the tumor cell could be detected. They hypothesized that glutaraldehyde fixation induces a cellular rather than humoral immune response. This concept is supported by the work of Dennert and Tucker (7) who showed that glutaraldehyde-treated sheep erythrocytes developed altered antigenicity that preferentially encouraged a cellular immune response.

The mechanism of inhibition of hepatic leukemia mediated by the administration of attenuated tumor cells and glucan is presently not known. It is entirely possible, in view of the role of macrophages in the phagocytosis and processing of antigen, that the activation of T- and B-lymphocytes to enhance both cellular and humoral immunity is an important facet. In support of this concept, it has recently been demonstrated that the administration of glucan increases splenic T- and B-lymphocyte response (6). It is, therefore, possible that tumor target cells are killed both by cell-mediated immunity initiated by the interaction of macrophages and lymphocytes, and by antibody-induced cytotoxicity.

The present studies demonstrate that glucan possesses the ability to mediate nonspecific immunotherapy as well as to induce active specific immunotherapy. In contrast to the significant number of variables involved in the use of BCG, as delineated by Carter (5), which not only involve viability, methods of preparation, and strain variation, the employment of glucan as a nonviable, highly purified molecular entity is worthy of further consideration in the induction of tumor immunity.

Because of the multiplicity of functions that macrophages exhibit, as noted in a recent review by Alexander (1), it is obviously impossible at the present to predict the mechanism by which enhanced survival to intraportal administration of leukemic cells develops in animals receiving attenuated cells plus glucan. Whether the manifestation of enhanced survival is due to cell-dependent antibody cytotoxicity or macrophage and/or lymphocyte cytotoxicity must be established.

ACKNOWLEDGMENT

These studies were supported, in part, by the Cancer Research Institute Inc. and National Institutes of Health grant no. CA13746.

REFERENCES

1. Alexander, P. (1976): The functions of the macrophage in malignant disease. *Annu. Rev. Med.,* 27:207–224.
2. Ashworth, C. T., Di Luzio, N. R., and Riggi, S. J. (1963): A morphologic study of the effect of reticuloendothelial stimulation upon hepatic removal of minute particles from the blood of rats. *Exp. Mol. Pathol.,* 2 (Suppl. 1):83–103.
3. Boyle, M. D. P., and Ormerod, M. G. (1975): The destruction of allogeneic tumour cells by peritoneal macrophages from immune mice: Purification of lytic effector cells. *Cell. Immunol.,* 17:247–258.
4. Browder, W., Jones, E., McNamee, R., and Di Luzio, N. R. (1976): Inhibition of tumor growth by glucan, a non-specific immunostimulant. *Surg. Forum,* 27:134–135.
5. Carter, S. K. (1976): Immunotherapy of cancer in man. *Am. Sci.,* 64:418–423.
6. Cook, J. A., Stege, T. E., and Di Luzio, N. R. (1976): Effect of glucan administration on *in vitro* response of splenic lymphocytes to T and B cell mitogens. *Physiologist (in press)* (Abst.).
7. Dennert, G., and Tucker, D. F. (1972): Selective priming of T cells by chemically altered cell antigens. *J. Exp. Med.,* 136:656–661.
8. Di Luzio, N. R. (1967): Evaluation by the graft-versus-host reaction of the immune competence of lymphoid cells of mice with altered reticuloendothelial function. *J. Reticuloendothel. Soc.,* 4:439–475.
9. Di Luzio, N. R. (1975): Macrophages, recognition factors and neoplasia. In: *The Reticuloendothelial System: IAP Monograph No. 16,* Chapter 5, pp. 49–64. Williams & Wilkins, Baltimore.
10. Di Luzio, N. R. (1976): Pharmacology of the reticuloendothelial system—Accent on glucan.

In: *The Reticuloendothelial System in Health and Disease: Functions and Characteristics,* edited by H. Friedman, M. Escobar, and S. Reichard, pp. 412–421. Plenum Press, New York.

11. Di Luzio, N. R., Hoffmann, E. O., Cook, J. A., Browder, W., and Mansell, P. W. A. (1976): Glucan-induced enhancement in host resistance to experimental tumors. In: *Control of Neoplasia by the Modulation of the Immune System,* edited by M. A. Chirigos, pp. 475–499. Raven Press, New York.

12. Di Luzio, N. R., McNamee, R., Jones, E., Lassoff, S., Sear, W., and Hoffmann, E. O. (1976): Inhibition of growth and dissemination of Shay myelogenous leukemic tumor in rats by glucan and glucan activated macrophages. In: *The Reticuloendothelial System in Health and Disease: Functions and Characteristics,* edited by H. Friedman, M. Escobar, and S. Reichard, pp. 397–413. Plenum Press, New York.

13. Di Luzio, N. R., and Riggi, S. J. (1964): The development of a lipid emulsion for the measurement of reticuloendothelial function. *J. Reticuloendothel. Soc.,* 1:136–149.

14. Di Luzio, N. R., and Riggi, S. J. (1970): The effects of laminarin, sulfated glucan and oligosaccharide of glucan on RE activity. *J. Reticuloendothel. Soc.,* 8:464–473.

15. Di Luzio, N. R., Wooles, W. R., and Morrow, S. H. (1964): The effect of splenectomy and x-irradiation on antibody formation in RE hyperfunctional mice. *J. Reticuloendothel. Soc.,* 1:429–441.

16. Frost, P., Edwards, A., and Sanderson, C. (1976): The use of glutaraldehyde fixation for the study of the immune response to syngeneic tumor antigen. *Ann. NY Acad. Sci.,* 276:91–96.

17. Halpern, B. N., Prevot, A. R., Biozzi, G., Stiffel, C., Mouton, D., Morard, J. C., Bouthillier, Y., and Decreuesefond, C. (1964): Stimulation de l'activite phagocytaire du systeme reticuloendothelial provoquee par *Corynebacterium parvum. J. Reticuloendothel. Soc.,* 1:77–96.

18. Hartman, A. D., Di Luzio, N. R., and Trumbull, M. L. (1968): Modification of chronic carbon tetrachloride hepatic injury by N,N'-diphenyl-p-phenylenediamine. *Exp. Mol. Pathol.,* 9:349–362.

19. Hawrylko, E. (1975): Immunopotentiation with BCG: Dimensions of a specific antitumor response. *J. Natl. Cancer Inst.,* 54:1189–1197.

20. Krahenbuhl, J., and Lambert, L. H., Jr. (1975): Cytokinetic studies of the effects of activated macrophages on tumor target cells. *J. Natl. Cancer Inst.,* 54:1433–1437.

21. Mansell, P. W. A., Di Luzio, N. R., McNamee, R., Rowden, G., and Proctor, J. W. (1976): Recognition factors and non-specific macrophage activation in the treatment of neoplastic disease. In: *Immunotherapy of Cancer,* edited by H. Friedman and C. M. Southam. New York Academy of Science *(in press).*

22. Mansell, P. W. A., Ichinose, H., Reed, R. J., Krementz, E. T., McNamee, R., and Di Luzio, N. R. (1975): Macrophage mediated destruction of human malignant cells *in vivo. J. Natl. Cancer Inst.,* 15:571–580.

23. Meltzer, M. S., Tucker, R. W., and Breuer, A. C. (1975): Interaction of BCG activated macrophages with neoplastic and non-neoplastic cell lines *in vitro.* Cinemicrographic analysis. *Cell. Immunol.,* 17:30–42.

24. Mohr, S. J., Chirigos, M. A., Smith, G. T., and Fuhrman, F. S. (1976): Specific potentiation of L1210 vaccine by pyran copolymer. *Cancer Res.,* 36:2035–2039.

25. Morrow, S. H., and Di Luzio, N. R. (1965): The fate of foreign red cells in mice with altered reticuloendothelial function. *Proc. Soc. Exp. Biol. Med.,* 119:647–652.

26. Riggi, S. J., and Di Luzio, N. R. (1961): Identification of a reticuloendothelial stimulating agent in zymosan. *Am. J. Physiol.,* 200:297–300.

27. Sadler, T. E., and Alexander, P. (1976): Trapping and destruction of blood-borne syngeneic leukemia cells in lung, liver and spleen of normal and leukemic cells. *Br. J. Cancer,* 33:512–520.

28. Sanderson, C. J., and Frost, P. (1974): The induction of tumour immunity in mice using glutaraldehyde-treated tumour cells. *Nature,* 248:690–691.

29. Schultz, R. M., Papamatheakis, J. D., Stylos, W. A., and Chirigos, M. A. (1976): Augmentation of specific macrophage-mediated cytotoxicity: Correlation with agents which enhance antitumor resistance. *Cell. Immunol.,* 25:309–316.

30. Scott, M. T. (1975): Potentiation of the tumor specific immune response by *Corynebacterium parvum. J. Natl. Cancer Inst.,* 55:65–72.

31. Wooles, W. R., and Di Luzio, N. R. (1962): Influence of reticuloendothelial hyperfunction on bone marrow transplantation. *Am. J. Physiol.,* 203:404–408.

32. Wooles, W. R., and Di Luzio, N. R. (1963): Reticuloendothelial function and the immune response. *Science,* 142:1078–1080.

33. Wooles, W. R., and Di Luzio, N. R. (1964): The phagocytic and proliferative response of the RES following glucan administration. *J. Reticuloendothel. Soc.,* 1:160–169.

34. Wooles, W. R., and Di Luzio, N. R. (1964): Inhibition of homograft acceptance and homo- and heterograft rejection in chimeras by reticuloendothelial system stimulation. *Proc. Soc. Exp. Biol. Med.,* 115:756–759.

Immune Modulation and Control of Neoplasia by Adjuvant Therapy, edited by M. A. Chirigos. Raven Press, New York, 1978.

Comparison of the Antitumor Effects of Glucan, BCG, and Levamisole

*,[1]J. W. Proctor, *B. G. Auclair, *L. Stokowski, and *†P. W. A. Mansell

*McGill University Cancer Research Unit; and †Division of Oncology, Royal Victoria Hospital, Montreal, P. Q., Canada

The recent upsurge in interest in immunotherapy has led to the large-scale use of immunomodulators, particularly the bacterial agents Bacillus Calmette-Guérin (BCG) and *Corynebacterium parvum.* Both have noticeable antitumor effects in experimental animal models (2,27), and some success has been claimed in a variety of human cancers (3,12). However, a number of side effects have been reported in man, including systemic infection and multiple granulomatosis with BCG (28,31) and transient but unpleasant sequelae following systemic injection of *C. parvum* (12). These side effects have been considered acceptable since widespread metastases are seldom amenable to more conventional modes of therapy. Nonetheless, there is every advantage in relatively nontoxic agents such as glucan and levamisole having the additional advantages of being nonimmunogenic and potentially safe for systemic use. A potent stimulator of the reticuloendothelial system (25), water insoluble forms of glucan from a yeast and other preparations known as lentinan from an Eastern mushroom have been demonstrated to exercise potent anti-tumor effects systemically in animal models (6,7,11,15) and following local intralesional injection in man (15). Levamisole has been reported to cure blood-borne metastases in animals (24) and to have useful effects in man (1).

The present study was designed to compare the effects of irradiated autologous tumor cells, BCG, and levamisole with glucan on blood-borne metastatic spread from the B16 mouse melanoma.

An attempt has been made also to assess whether it is possible to predict the effects of combining an immunomodulator with irradiated cells from knowledge of their separate effects when used alone.

---

[1] *Present address:* Division of Radiation Oncology, Clinical Radiation Therapy Research Center, Allegheny General Hospital, Pittsburgh, Pennsylvania 15212.

MATERIALS AND METHODS

Mice

Conventionally housed 8-week-old inbred male C57B1/6J mice were obtained from Jackson Laboratories and maintained on rat cake and tap water *ad libitum* in all experiments.

Tumor

The B16 melanoma, which arose spontaneously in the above strain and has been maintained by long-term transplantation, metastasizes reproducibly to the lung in 100% of animals when grown as a subcutaneous implant in the right hindlimb in this laboratory.

Tumor Vaccine

Areas of the leg tumor appearing most viable were selected and incubated at room temperature for 1 hr in 25 ml of minimum essential medium (MEM) containing 13 mg trypsin, 15 mg collagenase, and a trace of DNA'ase (all Sigma Type 1, England) with a magnetic stirrer. The resulting suspension was filtered through gauze to obtain a single-cell suspension of greater than 97% viability on phase microscopy. Following incubation overnight at 4°C in MEM medium (Grand Island Biological Co., USA) containing 10% syngeneic mouse serum the cells were irradiated on a conventional X-ray machine at 800 R/min to a level of 15,000 R and 2×10^6, 2×10^5, 2×10^4, or 2×10^3 cells injected in 0.05-ml volumes into each of five sites (i.p. and i.d. to four limbs) per mouse.

BCG

Doses of 2.5, 25, and 250 μg of lyophilized viable BCG (Institut Microbiologie et Hygiene strain, Montreal) in a 0.25-ml volume of saline were injected in divided doses of 0.05 ml, into each of five sites (i.p. and i.d. to four limbs) per mouse for groups of 11 mice on a single occasion.

Glucan

Doses of 2.5, 25, and 250 μg of glucan (obtained from N. R. Di Luzio, Tulane University, USA) were injected as for BCG.

Levamisole

Doses of 2.5, 25, and 250 μg of levamisole (McNeill Laboratories, Canada) were injected as for BCG and glucan.

Immunomodulators and Irradiated Cells

The doses of agents outlined above were injected into five sites as above in 0.05-ml volumes containing either 4×10^6 or 4×10^4 tumor cells per ml.

Experimental Design

Aliquots of 10^3 tumor cells were injected into the righthind limb of 726 mice divided into 62 experimental groups of 11 and a control group of 44 mice (see Table 1 for outline of experimental design). Half of the experimental groups were treated on day 8, and the remainder on day 19. The tumors were excised, by disarticulation of the femoral head of the tumor-bearing limb, from six mice of each group on day 18, and five on day 19, as the number of mice

TABLE 1. Experimental design

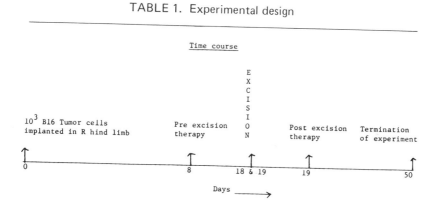

Immunomodulator	Dose (μgm/mouse)	Number of irradiated tumor cells/mouse				
		0	10^4	10^5	10^6	10^7
None	--	+	+	+	+	+
BCG	2.5	+	+	-	+	-
(L' I'nstitut Microbiologie et	25	+	+	-	+	-
Hygiene, Montreal)	250	+	+	-	+	-
Levamisole	2.5	+	+	-	+	-
(McNeill – Janssen)	25	+	+	-	+	-
	250	+	+	-	+	-
Glucan	2.5	+	+	-	+	-
(Dr. DiLuzio, New Orleans)	25	+	+	-	+	-
	250	+	+	-	+	-

in the experiment rendered it impossible to remove all the tumors on the same day. The tumor-bearing and contralateral hindlimbs were weighed to the nearest 0.01 g and the values for the latter subtracted from the former to give an approximate estimate of the tumor weight.

Analysis of Experiments

Thirty-one days after tumor excision the mice were exsanguinated under ether anesthesia, the lungs removed, and the metastases (mostly pigmented) counted macroscopically. There were no significant differences in the leg tumor weights or the number of metastases found within groups amputated on day 18 compared to those amputated on day 19, and the data are tabulated together.

The results were analyzed using the Mann Whitney nonparametric test, and values of $p < 0.05$ were considered significant. The predicted mean number of metastases following treatment with a combination of immunomodulator and autovaccine was compared retrospectively with the observed mean number of metastases in these groups on the basis of the formula below.

Let the mean number of metastases following autovaccine alone equals X and the mean number of metastases following treatment with an immunomodulator equals Y. The predicted number of metastases equals $(X + Y)/2$. Agreement within two metastases per mouse was taken arbitrarily to represent an accurate prediction and showed neither an antagonistic nor a synergistic effect. Antagonistic effects were considered to be values of greater than $(X + Y)/2$, whereas synergistic effects were considered to be values of less than $(X + Y)/2$. Significant antagonism was considered to have occurred when observed values reached $X + Y$, and synergism when values reached $(X + Y)/4$.

RESULTS

Groups of 11 mice were treated with irradiated cells or immunomodulators, or both, and the weight of the primary tumor (g wet weight) and the incidence and number of macroscopic lung metastases compared to those in the 44 controls.

No significant alterations in leg tumor weights were observed, the average for the control groups being 1.19 g whereas the range for experimental groups was 0.94 to 1.48 g.

At autopsy, a few mice (up to two in any one group) were observed to have tumor recurrence at the site of excision; these were excluded from the analysis. The incidence of metastases in the controls was 97%, and although in one experimental group it was as low as 50%, these differences were not considered significant.

The average number of macroscopic metastases per mouse in the control groups was 9.2, and a statistically significant degree of suppression or facilitation of metastatic spread occurred in a number of experimental groups (see below).

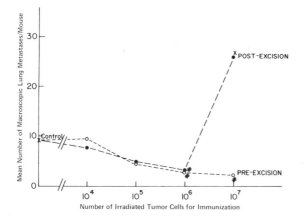

FIG. 1. Effect of immunization with irradiated tumor cells, comparison of preexcision with postexcision. Statistically significant ($p < 0.05$ level) suppression (#) and facilitation (X).

Effects of Irradiated Tumor Cells

When treated prior to tumor excision, a progressive reduction in metastatic spread occurred as the number of irradiated cells increased from 10^4 to 10^7 and the values for treatment with 10^6 and 10^7 cells were statistically significant (Fig. 1).

A similar reduction occurred when mice were treated following tumor excision, except in the group immunized with 10^7 cells in which there was a significant increase in metastatic spread compared to the controls.

Effect of Nonspecific Adjuvant Therapy

A significant reduction in metastatic spread resulted from treatment prior to tumor excision with either 2.5 μg of glucan, 25 μg, or 2.5 μg of levamisole,

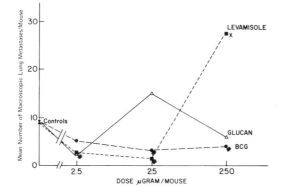

FIG. 2. Preexcision comparison of BCG, levamisole, and glucan. Statistically significant ($p < 0.05$ level) suppression (#) and facilitation (X).

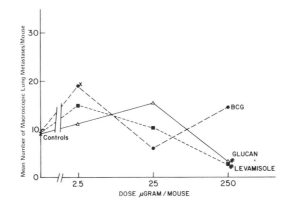

FIG. 3. Postexcision comparison of BCG, levamisole, and glucan. Statistically significant ($p < 0.05$ level) suppression ($\#$) and facilitation (X).

or 25 or 250 μg of BCG (Fig. 2). In contrast, treatment with 250 μg of levamisole produced a significant degree of facilitation, whereas other treatment schedules resulted in no detectable effects. Treatment with 250 μg of glucan or 250 μg of levamisole after surgical removal of the leg tumor resulted in a significant suppression of metastatic spread, whereas treatment with 2.5 μg of BCG produced a significant increase in the number of pulmonary metastases (Fig. 3). Other treatment schedules neither significantly facilitated nor suppressed metastatic spread.

Effect of Combining Immunomodulators with Irradiated Tumor Cells

A significant reduction in metastatic spread resulted from preoperative treatment with 10^6 irradiated tumor cells combined with either 25 or 2.5 μg of glucan and 250 μg of levamisole. Similar results followed an injection of 10^4 irradiated tumor cells combined with 2.5 μg of glucan and 250 and 2.5 μg of levamisole. A significant degree of facilitation resulted in only two groups—those treated with 25 μg of BCG and 10^4 irradiated tumor cells or 250 μg of glucan and 10^6 irradiated cells (Table 2).

Following postoperative treatment with a combination of 10^6 irradiated tumor cells and 250 μg of levamisole or BCG resulted in a decrease in the number of metastases, whereas a significant degree of facilitation occurred on combination with 2.5 μg of levamisole. In groups treated with 10^4 irradiated cells postoperatively, suppression of metastases resulted from combination with 25 and 2.5 μg of glucan and 25 μg of levamisole whereas an increased number of metastases occurred following combination with 25 and 2.5 μg of BCG (Table 1).

An attempt was made to assess the predictability of combining immunomodulators with irradiated cells from the results of treatment with the immunomodulator or the autograft alone.

TABLE 2. The number of spontaneous metastases following treatment with a combination of immunomodulators and irradiated B16 tumor cells

	Glucan (μg/mouse)			Levamisole (μg/mouse)			BCG (μg/mouse)		
	2.5	25	250	2.5	25	250	2.5	25	250
Number of irradiated tumor cells									
Preoperative									
10^6	2.7[b] (0–10)	1.8[c] (0–10)	18.5[d] (4–61)	2.9[b] (0–11)	6.2 (0–25)	3.3[a] (0–12)	4.8 (0–17)	9.3 (0–68)	4.6 (0–16)
10^4	3.9[a] (0–14)	9.0 (0–27)	6.3 (0–16)	2.7[b] (0–8)	9.2 (0–48)	0.9[c] (0–4)	10.2 (0–38)	31.8[d] (4–79)	6.6 (0–16)
Postoperative									
10^6	7.1 (0–19)	8.7 (0–23)	14.2 (6–19)	16.7[d] (5–48)	9.1 (3–17)	3.4[b] (0–12)	6.8 (1–16)	9.0 (0–16)	3.3[a] (0–11)
10^4	4.2[a] (0–24)	4.5[a] (0–34)	6.4 (0–24)	12.3 (0–39)	2.6[b] (0–8)	15.4 (3–71)	26.0[d] (0–72)	16.6[d] (2–49)	8.0 (0–33)

Average number of lung metastases per mouse (range in brackets). Statistical analyses (Mann Whitney).
[a] $p < 0.05$. Significant suppression.
[b] $p < 0.01$. Significant suppression.
[c] $p < 0.001$. Significant suppression.
[d] $p < 0.05$. Significant facilitation.

TABLE 3. Breakdown of analysis for percent of synergistic or antagonistic effects of immunomodulators and irradiated tumor cells

Effect	BCG	Levamisole	Glucan	10^6	10^4	Post-operative	Pre-operative
Synergism $< \dfrac{X+Y}{4}$	0 (0/12)	33 (4/12)	33 (4/12)	11 (2/18)	33 (6/18)	17 (3/18)	27 (5/18)
No effect $\simeq \dfrac{X+Y}{2}$	50 (6/12)	50 (6/12)	42 (5/12)	44 (6/18)	44 (8/18)	33 (6/18)	56 (10/18)
Antagonism $> X+Y$	50 (6/12)	17 (2/12)	25 (3/12)	44 (9/18)	22 (4/18)	50 (9/18)	17 (3/18)

The incidence (figures in brackets) and percentage of the groups exhibiting synergism or antagonism following combination of an immunomodulator and of irradiated cells are shown.
X represents mean number of metastases following treatment with irradiated cells alone.
Y represents mean number of metastases following treatment with an immunomodulator alone.

Thus the mean numbers of metastases observed from the combination of specific and nonspecific therapy were compared to the numbers that would have been predicted from the results of the relevant groups treated specifically or nonspecifically alone. A difference of less than two metastases per mouse between expected and observed values was considered arbitrarily to denote an accurate prediction of a negligible effect (e.g., neither antagonistic nor synergistic). Out of a total of 36 therapeutic attempts, a significant reduction in metastatic spread occurred in 12 groups and facilitation of metastatic spread in five groups. Accurate predictions (a difference of less than two metastases per mouse between expected and observed values) could have been made for two of 12 (16.7%) of the groups in which suppression was expected compared to none of five (0%) for those in which facilitation was expected and eight of 19 (47.3%) in which no effect was predicted. An overall accurate prediction could have been made for 10 of 36 (27.8%) of all groups.

On the basis of the arbitrary formulation (see Materials and Methods) antagonistic effects were seen in 12 of 36, synergistic effects in eight of 36, and no alteration in 16 of 36 groups undergoing combination therapy, indicating no obvious pattern overall (see Table 3). Nevertheless antagonistic effects occurred more readily following combination with BCG than with glucan and levamisole, and following combination with 10^6 than with 10^4 irradiated tumor cells. Furthermore such effects occurred more commonly following postoperative than preoperative treatment.

DISCUSSION

The results obtained with each of the agents depended on both the dose and whether they were administered before or after tumor excision.

These match previous observations on the effect in general of irradiated tumor cells (9,20,30), BCG (4,13,17,21), levamisole (16), and glucan (N. R. Di Luzio and Y. Yamamura, *personal communication,* 1976) in animal model systems. The route of administration of BCG (18,21) and glucan (N. R. Di Luzio and Y. Yamamura, *personal communication,* 1976) is also important. In light of such obvious dose dependence, little can be said of the relative merits of the immunomodulators, since only three doses of each agent were tested at only two time points, save only that glucan seemed at least comparable to the other two in its antitumor effect. Furthermore, this agent showed no evidence of tumor promotion when used by itself.

The reasons for facilitation of tumor spread are complex but may well involve excessive release of soluble antigen when large numbers of irradiated tumor cells are used. Such antigen alone or in complex form could block existing antitumor immune mechanisms (5). These blocking effects might outweigh the beneficial effects of maximally stimulating previously uncommitted lymph nodes distant from the tumor site. Certainly a large proportion of irradiated tumor cells die within the first 24 hr of injection into normal animals *(personal observa-*

tion) as do unattenuated tumor cells (22) concomitant with a transient rise in circulating soluble antigen (29). Such an increase of circulating antigen may well occur more readily in late stages of tumor growth, but since the levels are presumably already high, this further increase would not necessarily be harmful. However in situations of minimal residual disease, although perhaps more unlikely to reach harmful levels, the effects of an antigen overload on the progress of the disease could be expected to be far more sinister.

It is possible that the mechanisms accounting for tumor facilitation vary from one nonspecific agent to another. Thus immunostimulation possibly, as described by Prehn (19), or more possibly antigenic competition, as demonstrated by Liaocopoulos et al. (14), accounts for the bad results reported with BCG.

In the case of levamisole, the recent report by Sampson and Lui (26) may be relevant. They report increased stimulation of lymphocytes in PHA and MLC responses following incubation with certain doses of levamisole, but as the dose was increased the reactivity became depressed. It is conceivable that a nonspecific immune depression could have resulted with levamisole in our experiments leading to facilitation of metastatic spread.

Finally W. Lapp (personal communication, 1976) has suggested that macrophages exercise a modulating or "suppressor" effect on "helper" T cells involved in T- and B-lymphocyte effector functions. In the presence of a chronic persistent antigenic challenge such as during graft-versus-host disease, this control or suppressor mechanism is apparently extremely strong. A progressively growing tumor also constitutes a similar chronic antigenic challenge, and at certain stages in tumor growth, the provision of more macrophages after reticuloendothelial stimulation might increase the suppressor activity, rather than augment effector mechanisms. The dose dependence with levamisole observed by Sampson and Lui (26) was also associated with alterations in T-cell suppressor activity. Thus a single explanation can certainly be postulated for facilitation of tumor growth by all of the various agents.

One can only guess at the relevance to man of these findings in animal models. Nevertheless there seems to be no a priori reason why man should differ from mice in the importance of dose dependence and tumor burden in immunotherapy. Should dose dependence be important in man, for forms of cancer that do not present as a homogeneous population with respect to immunocompetence, immunogenicity of the tumor, and tumor burden, etc., it is unlikely that a dose of an immunomodulator which has a good effect in one patient will benefit many succeeding cases (23). However, patients with stage I to II melanoma are a heterogeneous population in many respects, and when considered in this light, the results reported (8,10) for man with BCG in the last few years are surprisingly good. However, considering the immense importance attached to a number of prognostic variables in this disease, these trials have not been properly controlled and the case, therefore, for a beneficial effect of BCG in such patients is far from proved.

In our study, the effects of combining the nonspecific agents and irradiated tumor cells were disappointing compared to a previous study with *C. parvum* on another tumor (20) and were more reminiscent of those reported more recently (32). There was very little obvious pattern, and synergistic and antagonistic effects were observed with comparable frequency.

In summary glucan appears to be as effective as other forms of specific or nonspecific therapy in this tumor model. With the added attractions of a lack of immunogenicity and a potential for systemic use without unwanted side effects, this substance appears currently to have a greater potential than bacterial immunomodulators in the immunotherapy of cancer. The importance of the dose and tumor burden, etc., however, should not be underestimated when considering the clinical use of glucan to treat systemic disease.

SUMMARY

Varying doses of BCG, levamisole, or glucan, alone or in combination with different numbers of irradiated tumor cells, were given at multiple sites on a single occasion before or after excision of the B16 melanoma growing in the hindlimbs of syngeneic C57B1/6J mice. Facilitation or suppression of spontaneous metastatic spread to the lung was observed with all of the agents studied and depended on the dose of the agent and the time point during tumor growth at which it was administered. No facilitation was observed, however, when glucan was used alone.

The result of combining irradiated cells with an immunomodulator could not be predicted from the effects of similar doses of these agents used alone.

ACKNOWLEDGMENT

We thank Drs. H. Shibata, M. Jerry, and M. G. Lewis for their helpful advice and Dru Ann Heath who prepared the manuscript.

The work reported here has been supported financially by the Quebec Cancer Research Society, Inc., The National Cancer Institute, and McNeill Laboratories, Canada.

REFERENCES

1. Amery, W. K. (1976): Double blind Levamisole trial in resectable lung cancer. *Ann. NY Acad. Sci.,* 277:260.
2. Bast, R. C., Zbar, B., Borsos, T., and Rapp, H. J. (1974): BCG and cancer. *N. Engl. J. Med.,* 290:1413.
3. Bast, R. C., Zbar, B., Borsos, T., and Rapp, H. J. (1974): BCG and cancer. *N. Engl. J. Med.,* 290:1458.
4. Chee, D. O., and Bodurtha, A. J. (1974): Facilitation and inhibition of B16 melanoma by BCG *in vivo* and by lymphoid cells from BCG treated mice *in vitro. Int. J. Cancer,* 14:137.
5. Currie, G. A., and Alexander, P. (1974): Spontaneous shedding of TSTA by viable sarcoma cells: Its possible role in facilitation of metastatic spread. *Br. J. Cancer,* 29:72.

6. Di Luzio, N. R., McNamee, R., Jones, E., Lassoff, S., Sear, W., and Hoffman, E. O. (1976): Inhibition of growth and dissemination of Shay myelogenous leukemic tumor in rats by Glucan and Glucan activated macrophages. In: *Proc. VII Int. Congr. Reticuloendothel. Soc.*, Plenum Publ., New York *(in press)*.

7. Di Luzio, N. R., McNamee, R., Jones, E., Cook, J. A., and Hoffman, E. O. (1976): Role of macrophages in neoplasia. *Proc. NCI Workshop (in press)*.

8. Eilber, F. R., Morton, D. L., Carmack Holmes, E., Sparks, F. C., and Ramming, K. P. (1976): Adjuvant immunotherapy with BCG in treatment of regional lymph node metastases from malignant melanomas. *N. Engl. J. Med.*, 294:237.

9. Godrick, E. A., Michaelson, J. S., Vanwijk, R. R., and Wilson, R. E. (1972): Immunotherapy combined with primary resection or murine fibrosarcoma. *Ann. Surg.*, 176: 544.

10. Gutterman, J. U., Mavligit, G. M., Reed, R. C., Gottlieb, J. A., Burgess, M. A., McBride, C. E., Einhorn, L., Freirich, E. J., and Hersh, E. M. (1975): Adjuvant BCG immunotherapy for minimal residual disease (M.R.D.). *N. Engl. J. Med.*, 291:592–597.

11. Ishimura, K., Maeda, Y. Y., and Chihara, G. (1975): A possibility of synergism between *Corynebacterium parvum* and Lentinan Serotonin, or Thyroid Hormone in potentiation of host resistance against cancer. In: *Corynebacterium parvum, Applications in Clinical Oncology*, edited by B. Halpern, pp. 298–313. Plenum Press, New York and London.

12. Israel, L. (1975): In: *Corynebacterium parvum, Applications in Clinical Oncology*, edited by B. Halpern, pp. 389. Plenum Press, New York and London.

13. Lemonde, P. (1974): Dual effects of BCG on tumor and tumor immunity. *Proc. Am. Assoc. Cancer Res.*, 15:41 (Abstr. 163).

14. Liacopoulos, P., Couderc, J., and Gille, M. F. (1971): Competition of antigens during induction of low zone tolerance. *Eur. J. Immunol.*, 1:359.

15. Mansell, P. W. A., Di Luzio, N. R., McNamee, R., Rowden, G., and Proctor, J. W. (1976): Recognition factors and nonspecific macrophage activation in the treatment of neoplastic disease. *Ann. NY Acad. Sci.*, 277:21.

16. Mantovani, A., and Spreafico, F. (1975): Allogenic tumor enhancement by Levamisole, a new immunostimulating compound: Studies on cell mediated immunity and humoral antibody response. *Eur. J. Cancer*, 11:537.

17. Piessens, W. F., Lachapelle, F. L., Legros, N., and Heuson, J. C. (1970): Facilitation of rat mammary tumor growth by BCG. *Nature*, 228:1210.

18. Pimm, M. V., and Baldwin, R. W. (1975): BCG therapy of pleural and peritoneal growth of transplanted rat tumors. *Int. J. Cancer*, 15:260.

19. Prehn, R. T. (1972): The immune reaction as a stimulation of tumor growth. *Science*, 176:179.

20. Proctor, J. W., Rudenstam, C. M., and Alexander, P. (1973): Increased incidence of lung metastases following treatment of rats bearing hepatomas with irradiated cells and the beneficial effect of *Corynebacterium parvum* in this system. *Biomedicine*, 19:248.

21. Proctor, J. W., Auclair, B. G., and Lewis, M. G. (1976): A comparison of the effects of BCG given by different routes on growth of B16 mouse melanoma at different anatomic locations. *Eur. J. Cancer*, 72:203.

22. Proctor, J. W., Auclair, B. G., Stokowski, L., and Rudenstam, C-M. (1976): The distribution and fate of bloodborne ^{125}IUdR-labelled tumor cells in immune syngeneic rats. *Int. J. Surg.*, 18:255.

23. Proctor, J. W., Lewis, M. G., and Mansell. P. W. A. (1976): Immunotherapy for cancer: An overview. *Can. J. Surg.*, 19:12.

24. Renoux, G., and Renoux, M. (1972): Levamisole inhibits and cures a solid malignant tumor and its pulmonary metastases. *Nature* [*New Biol.*], 240:217.

25. Riggi, S., and Di Luzio, N. R. (1961): Identification of a reticuloendothelial stimulating agent in zymosan. *Am. J. Physiol.*, 200:297.

26. Sampson, D., and Lui, A. (1976): The effect of Levamisole on cell mediated immunity and suppressor cell function. *Cancer Res.*, 36:952.

27. Scott, M. T. (1974): *Corynebacterium parvum* as an immunotherapeutic anti-cancer agent. *Semin. Oncol.*, 1:367.

28. Sparks, F. C., Silverstein, M. J., Hunt, J. S., Haskell, C. M., Pilch, Y. H., and Morton, D. L. (1973): Complications of BCG immunotherapy in patients with cancer. *N. Engl. J. Med.*, 289:827.

29. Thomson, D. M. P., Sellens, V., Eccles, S., and Alexander, P. (1973): Radioimmunoassay of

tumor specific transplantation antigen of a chemically induced rat sarcoma: Circulating soluble tumor antigen in tumor bearers. *Br. J. Cancer,* 28:377.

30. Vanwijk, R. R., Godrick, E. A., Smith, H. G., Goldweitz, J., and Wilson, R. E. (1971): Stimulation or suppression of metastases with graded doses of tumor cells. *Cancer Res.,* 13:1559.
31. Wilson, G. S. (1967): *Hazards of Immunization.* Oxford Univ. Press, London.
32. Woodruff, M. F. A., Ghaffar, A., Dunbar, N., and Whitehead, V. L. (1976): Effect of *C. parvum* on immunization with irradiated tumor cells. *Br. J. Cancer (in press).*

Immune Modulation and Control of Neoplasia by Adjuvant Therapy, edited by M. A. Chirigos. Raven Press, New York, 1978.

Comparative Evaluation of Tumor-Inhibitory Activity of Glucan and *Corynebacterium parvum* in a Mouse Fibrosarcoma Model

Herman D. Suit, Arthur Elman, Robert Sedlacek, and
*Vlatko Silobrcic

*Edwin L. Steele Laboratory of Radiation Biology, Department of Radiation Medicine, Massachusetts General Hospital, Boston, Massachusetts 02114; and *Institute of Immunology, Zagreb, Yugoslavia*

Potentiation of the immune rejection reaction against tumor has been convincingly demonstrated by several agents with a variety of laboratory animal tumor systems. Among the more thoroughly studied immunopotentiating agents are Freunds adjuvant, Bacillus Calmette-Guérin, *Corynebacterium parvum*, zymosan, and/or glucan and levamisole (5). Our own work has concentrated on *C. parvum* and has shown it to be effective in four of five animal tumor systems studied (2–4). Namely, *C. parvum* administered intravenously alone or combined with intralesional administration after tumor transplantation resulted in significant delay of growth, an occasional complete and permanent regression, and a reduction in radiation dose required to achieve tumor destruction. These effects have been observed for these four tumor systems—a methylcholanthrene-induced fibrosarcoma, two methylcholanthrene-induced squamous cell carcinomas, and a radiation-induced osteogenic sarcoma. Benefits of *C. parvum* treatment of mice bearing a nonimmunogenic mammary carcinoma were slight. These tumors have been studied as third to fifth generation isotransplants growing in the legs of mice. Although *C. parvum* is clearly effective in some animal tumor models, its administration to man is associated with significant toxicity. Because of reports of a high potency and low toxicity of glucan, a component of zymosan, we have compared the efficacy of glucan with that of *C. parvum* using our fibrosarcoma model, viz., the tumor system against which *C. parvum* has a high level of effectiveness (3).

MATERIALS AND METHODS

Animal Tumor System

The mice were C3H/f Sed; these were maintained in our own colony under defined flora-specific pathogen-free conditions (3). Mice of 10 to 12 weeks of age of both sexes were utilized in this investigation. The tumor was the same fibrosarcoma employed in our earlier work. This had been induced by methylcholanthrene injection in the subcutaneous tissue of a C3H mouse; it has been maintained in a liquid nitrogen refrigerator. Actual experiments were performed on fifth generation isotransplants. Tumor transplantation was performed using a suspension of tumor cells prepared by a nonenzymatic technique (3). For transplantation, 2.5×10^5 viable cells (trypan blue negative) were injected in a volume of 5 to 10 μl into the leg muscle. The tumor transplant take rate was essentially 100%. By 5 days after transplantation the tumor was $\simeq$ 5 mm in diameter.

C. Parvum

The formalin-killed bacteria suspended in thiomersalate was kindly provided by Burroughs Wellcome Company through John Whisnant. Material from several different batches has been used in these studies over the past 3 years. The bacterial preparation was diluted with sterile saline to a concentration of 350 μg in 0.4 ml. Administration was by the intravenous route. Glucan was generously provided by N. R. Di Luzio. The stock solution of glucan was diluted appropriately with saline immediately prior to experimental use. During this research project (11 months) three separate batches of glucan were received from Di Luzio.

Experimental Design

Normal mice or tumor-injected mice were assigned by random number scheme to one of the groups within an experiment. Treatment with *C. parvum* or glucan was given at a fixed time following transplantation or at a time that the mean tumor reached 5 mm in diameter as indicated by the individual experimental protocol. Mice have been followed for up to 120 days following the injection of either the glucan or the *C. parvum*. Weights of spleen or liver, or both, were measured by weighing the freshly excised and blotted organ on a standard laboratory balance.

Local Irradiation

Radiation was administered to the leg bearing the tumor through 3-cm diameter portals. A specially designed Cesium irradiator (137 Cs) was employed, the dose rate being approximately 950 rads/min to the center of the tumor-bearing tissues (1).

RESULTS

Acute Lethal Toxicity

Death due to glucan occurred within the first few hours (up to 14) after i.v. injection or did not occur at all. Proportions of mice dying after 0, 2,000,

3,000, or 4,000 µg were 0/10, 0/10, 4/16, and 8/10, respectively. From that experience, a single i.v. dose of 2,000 µg has been found to be entirely safe. There have been no grossly evident reactions and no deaths at that dose level. A single dose i.v. of 350 µg of *C. parvum* has caused no acute deaths in many hundreds of mice; a very occasional death has been observed at 750 µg i.v.

Splenomegaly

Spleen sizes were measured at 10 days following single intravenous injection of either *C. parvum* or glucan. Data are presented for the 10-day spleen weight in Table 1. The mean spleen weight following a single i.v. injection of 350 µg of *C. parvum* was 15.3 mg as compared with 3.5 mg for spleens from control mice. At this same dose level of 350 µg a significant increase in spleen weight was obtained using glucan batches 1 or 3. Batch 1 was slightly more effective than batch 3 in producing splenomegaly. Spleen weights at 10 days posttreatment were measured for glucan doses of 350, 1,000, and 2,000 µg. The data (Table 1) show that for batch 3, a dose of 2,000 µg of glucan produced a splenic weight increase equivalent to that for 350 µg of *C. parvum.*

Tumor Growth Delay

Delay in growth of fibrosarcoma was achieved by each of the three batches of glucan tested, although the dose level required to obtain a clear growth delay was variable. This tumor grows rapidly, and by $\simeq$ day 25 after transplantation some of the mice are dead of tumor. For this analysis the tumor volumes at 20 days after transplantation have been used. In Table 2, the ratios of tumor volume in the glucan-treated to tumor volume in control mice are listed for the various dose levels used for each of the three glucan batches. Delay of growth was greatest for glucan from batch 1. Namely, the tumor volume ratios for the 1,000 µg dose level were 0.43, 0.77, and 1.12 for batches 1, 2, and 3, respectively. In this work, 2,000 µg from batch 3 was of an effectiveness intermediate between that of 350 µg and 1,000 µg for batch 1.

TABLE 1. *Spleen weight at 10 days after i.v. injection of glucan or* C. parvum

Treatment	Spleen weight at 10 days (mg/10 g body weight) mg ± 1 SE
None	3.5 ± 0.2
350 µg *C. parvum*	15.3 ± 0.8
350 µg glucan	
Batch 1	6.4 ± 0.4
Batch 2	5.0 ± 0.4
1,000 µg glucan (batch 3)	11.2 ± 0.4
2,000 µg glucan (batch 3)	16.0 ± 0.7

TABLE 2. *Delay of growth of fibrosarcoma by glucan test of three batches of glucan*

Glucan dose (i.v. @ 5 days)	Tumor volume @ 20 days (glucan/control)		
	Batch nos.		
	1	2	3
350	0.80	0.93	
1,000	0.43	0.77	1.12
2.000		0.77	0.78

Complete and Permanent Regression of Fibrosarcoma by Glucan Injections

C. parvum administered 350 μg i.v. to mice with 5-mm isotransplants in the leg muscle achieved cure of 40 of 90 mice (44%). By giving three injections of 350 μg (injections at time the tumor was 5 mm and then at 5 and 10 days later), the yield was not increased, viz., seven cures of 15 treated mice (47%). Results obtained from the i.v. injections of glucan to mice bearing 5-day or ≃ 5-mm fibrosarcoma isotransplants are listed in Table 3 for batches 1, 2, and 3. Cure rates in the range of 10 to 33% were achieved using batch 1 glucan in doses of 200 to 350 μg × 3 up to 1,000 μg × 3. Thus at the highest dose level tested (1,000 μg × 3), the effectiveness was comparable to that obtained with *C. parvum*. Unfortunately these good response rates were not confirmed using glucan from batches 2 or 3, despite utilization of dose levels of 1,000 μg × 1 and 2,000 μg × 1 → 2,000 μg × 3.

Combination of i.v. Glucan and Local Irradiation

Mice were given 2,000 μg glucan i.v. when the fibrosarcoma isotransplants reached 5 mm, and local irradiation was performed ≃ 3 days later or when the tumor was 8 mm in diameter. Results are presented in Table 4. There is

TABLE 3. *Cure of mice bearing* ≃ 5-mm fibrosarcoma by glucan

Batch no.	Glucan dose (μg, i.v.)	No. cured/no. treated
1	350 × 1	0/15
	200–350 × 3	3/30
	1,000 × 1	3/15
	1,000 × 3	5/15
2	350 × 1	0/6
	1,000 × 1	0/10
	2,000 × 1	0/6
3	1,000 × 1	0/10
	2,000 × 1	0/28
	2,000 × 2	0/10
	2,000 × 3	0/10

TABLE 4. Local control of 8-mm fibrosarcoma in normal mice or in mice given glucan i.v. when the fibrosarcoma was 5 mm in size

	No. control/no. treated (at 31 days)				
	Radiation dose (rad)				
Treatment	0	1,500	2,500	3,750	4,500
γRT[a] @ 8 mm 2 mg glucan i.v. @ 5 mm	0/6[b]	1/6	2/6	6/6	9/9
γRT @ 8 mm	0/6	2/10	2/10	9/9	—

Glucan was from Batch 3.
[a] RT, radiation therapy.

no indication of an improved cure rate for glucan combined with radiation as compared to radiation alone.

DISCUSSION

These experiments provide clear encouragement regarding glucan; using glucan from our batch 1 (one of the three batches tested) 20 to 30% of mice bearing 5-mm fibrosarcoma isotransplants were cured by single or multiple i.v. injections of 1,000 μg of glucan. Glucan at that dose level is nontoxic, viz., there are no gross reactions and no fatalities. However, work with two other glucan preparations failed to cure a single mouse out of a total of 80 receiving doses in the range of 350 μg × 1 to 2,000 μg × 3, indicating to us that a serious effort to improve the technical aspects of preparing the glucan is warranted.

Also of interest was the observation that although 2,000 μg of glucan batch 3 caused a splenomegaly comparable to that following 350 μg of C. parvum, there was an enormous difference in the proportion of mice cured of their 5-mm fibrosarcoma, viz., $\simeq$ 40 vs. 0% for C. parvum and glucan, respectively. Although the splenomegaly produced by the immunopotentiators in this model system was great, that in vivo end point did not correlate with the antitumor effect. From this experience we would favor an antitumor effect as the end point in quality control during production of the glucan that is intended to be used as a potentiator of the immune reaction against tumor.

Glucan treatment of fibrosarcoma hosts with 2,000 μg (batch 3) was without apparent effect on the response of tumor to local irradiation. In earlier work (3) 350 μg C. parvum given when the fibrosarcoma was 5 mm and radiation applied to the 8-mm tumor resulted in a dramatic increase in cure rate. Namely, at 800 rads the cure frequency was $\simeq$ 75% in the combined treatment group but only 5% in the radiation alone group, viz., a very large shift upward of the low end of the dose-response curve. In this present study, dose levels of 1,500 and 2,500 rads were employed with 10 mice per group; there was no hint of a better response in the glucan-treated mice, even though this same dose level of 2,000 μg did achieve a definite slowing of tumor growth (no radiation). Thus, despite the fact that the glucan treatment was capable of inducing marked splenomegaly and a modest reduction of growth, tumor control rate by radiation was not improved. Thus, in this system and for this study, splenomegaly, growth delay, and tumor destruction were not obviously interrelated.

SUMMARY

The effectiveness of glucan in producing splenomegaly and in causing delay in growth or permanent regression of an isotransplanted fibrosarcoma is described. The results achieved varied markedly between the three batches of glucan employed. Glucan given i.v. caused a dose- and time-dependent splenomegaly. Spleen weights at 10 days after 2,000 μg glucan and after 350 μg of C. parvum were 16.0 and 15.3 mg/10 g (for batch 3 of glucan), respectively; spleen weight in control (untreated) mice was 3.5 mg/g body weight. The extent of delay in tumor growth or the proportion of mice cured of their fibrosarcoma following i.v. glucan given when the tumor was 5 mm varied sharply between batches 1, 2, and 3. Namely, three of 15 and five of 15 mice were cured by a single i.v. dose of 1,000 μg or three doses of 1,000 μg, respectively, from batch 1. No cures were obtained among 80 mice injected with 350 μg × 1 up to 2,000 μg × 3 glucan from batches 2 and 3. The proportions of mice cured after 350 μg C. parvum or after 2,000 μg glucan (batch 3) were 40/90 and 0/28, respectively; these doses yielded comparable degrees of splenomegaly. Further, 2,000 μg of glucan i.v. (batch 3) to mice with 5-mm fibrosarcoma did not improve results of local irradiation of 8-mm fibrosarcoma.

ACKNOWLEDGMENTS

This work was supported in part by NIH grants no. CA13311 and no. CA19415.

H. D. Suit is the Andres Soriano Director of Cancer Management at Massachusetts General Hospital.

REFERENCES

1. Hranitsky, E. B., Almond, P. R., Suit, H. D., and Moore, E. B. (1973): A Cesium-137 irradiator for small laboratory animals. Radiology, 107:641–644.
2. Suit, H. D., Sedlacek, R., Wagner, M., and Orsi, L. (1975): Radiation response of C3H fibrosarcoma enhanced in mice stimulated by Corynebacterium parvum. Nature, 255:493.
3. Suit, H. D., Sedlacek, R., Wagner, M., Orsi, L., Silobrcic, V., and Rothman, K. (1976): Effect of Corynebacterium parvum on the response to irradiation of a C3H fibrosarcoma. Cancer Res. 36:1305–1314.
4. Suit, H. D., Sedlacek, R. S., Silobrcic, V., and Linggood, R. M. (1976): Radiation therapy and Corynebacterium parvum in the treatment of murine tumors. Cancer, 37:2573–2579.
5. W. D. Terry (editor) (1976): Symposium on Immunotherapy in Malignant Disease. The Medical Clinics of North America, Vol. 60, No. 3, pp. 387–651. Saunders, Philadelphia.

Immune Modulation and Control of Neo-plasia by Adjuvant Therapy, edited by M. A. Chirigos. Raven Press, New York, 1978.

Tumoricidal Effect *In Vitro* of Peritoneal Macrophages from Mice Treated with Glucan

Richard M. Schultz, Joseph D. Papamatheakis, and Michael A. Chirigos

Lab of RNA Tumor Viruses, National Cancer Institute, National Institutes of Health, Bethesda, Maryland 20014

Recent successes using purified naturally occurring polysaccharides to enhance host resistance against neoplasia have stimulated research on the mechanism of their protective effect. The most beneficial antitumor activity has been demonstrated by structures containing chains of β-(1 → 3)-linked D-glucose residues such as yeast-derived glucan (4,9,10), scleroglucan (11,14), and lentinan (2,3,7,8). The antitumor activity of these glucans has been found to be host mediated, since no direct cytotoxicity was manifested for tumor cells *in vitro* (7,9). Di Luzio et al. have reported phagocytic hyperfunction and hyperplasia of the reticuloendothelial system (RES) following glucan administration (4). Furthermore, the most effective antitumor therapy with glucan has been intralesional treatment where dissolution of the tumor mass was correlated with macrophage content (9). In view of our recently developed techniques to measure macrophage tumoricidal function (12,13), studies were undertaken to evaluate the effect of glucan on both specific and nonspecific macrophage-mediated cytotoxicity.

MATERIALS AND METHODS

Mice

Male BALB/c and CD2F1 mice, 6 to 8 weeks old, were obtained from the Mammalian Genetics and Animal Production Section, National Institutes of Health, Bethesda, Md. Male athymic nude mice were supplied by the Animal Breeding Farms at the Frederick Cancer Research Center, Frederick, Md.

Cell Cultures

Established cell lines of MBL-2 (H2^b[C57B1/6]) murine leukemia and M109 (H2^d[BALB/c]) murine alveolar carcinoma cells were maintained in RPMI-1640 medium supplemented with 20% heat-inactivated (56°C, 30 min) fetal calf serum, 100 μg/ml gentamicin solution, 0.075% NaHCO$_3$, and 10 mM

HEPES buffer (RPMI-FCS). Other BALB/c lines, including the J774 reticulum cell sarcoma, CoCa26 colonic carcinoma, and 3T3 embryonic fibroblasts, were tested as specificity controls. These cells were similarly cultured in RPMI-FCS.

Drugs

Glucan, a purified polysaccharide from the outer membrane of *Saccharomyces cerevisiae,* was received as a sterile suspension in distilled water from N. R. Di Luzio, Department of Physiology, Tulane University School of Medicine, New Orleans, La. Lentinan, extracted from the edible mushroom *Lentinus edodes,* was kindly supplied by G. Chihara, National Cancer Center Research Institute, Tsukiji, Tokyo, Japan. Scleroglucan was obtained from the National Cancer Institute, Drug Research and Development Section, Bethesda, Md. Scleroglucan and lentinan were suspended in distilled water and sterilized at 120°C for 15 min prior to use. Pyran copolymer (NSC-46015), a copolymer of divinyl ether and maleic anhydride, was supplied by D. Breslow, Hercules Research Center, Wilmington, Del. Pyran was dissolved in phosphate-buffered saline and adjusted to pH 7.2 by the addition of 1N NaOH.

Preparation of Peritoneal Macrophages

Noninduced peritoneal exudates were harvested from mice by intraperitoneal injection of 5 ml of Hank's balanced salt solution containing 2 U heparin/ml. Within 10 min after injection, the mice were sacrificed and the peritoneal exudate was collected by paracentesis. Macrophages were purified by adherence as previously described (13) and kept in an ice bath prior to use to prevent adherence. Representative preparations of purified peritoneal adherent cells were stained with Giemsa stain; $> 95\%$ of the cells had morphologic characteristics of macrophages.

Chromium-51 Release Test for Macrophage-Mediated Cytotoxicity

For target cell labeling, 1.0×10^7 viable cells were resuspended in 2 ml of RPMI-FCS containing 200 μCi of $Na_2{}^{51}CrO_4$. The mixture was then incubated at 37°C in a CO_2 incubator for 90 min with occasional shaking. After incubation, the cells were pelleted by centrifugation and washed four times with 30-ml volumes of medium. Specific activity was maintained between 0.1 and 0.3 cpm/cell.

Suspensions of ^{51}Cr-labeled target cells were diluted to contain 1.0×10^5 cells/ml. In 100-μl aliquots, 10^4 cells were plated into wells of no. 3040 Microtest II Plates (Falcon Plastics, Oxnard, Cal.). One hundred microliter aliquots containing 5.0×10^5 peritoneal macrophages were added to quadruplicate wells. Effector-to-target cell ratios were maintained at 50:1. The plates were incubated at 37°C for 16 hr in a 5% CO_2-in-air atmosphere. Following this incubation, the plates were centrifuged (1,000 rpm for 10 min), and radioactivity was measured in the cell-free supernatant.

$$\text{Percent specific } {}^{51}\text{Cr release} = \frac{\text{cpm}_E - \text{cpm}_N}{\text{cpm}_M} \times 100$$

where cpm_E = counts per minute released in the presence of test effector cells — spontaneous release, cpm_N = counts per minute released in the presence of normal mouse effector cells — spontaneous release, and cpm_M = maximum release — spontaneous release.

Inhibition of DNA Synthesis Assay for Macrophage-Mediated Cytostasis

Macrophage-mediated cytostasis of the target cells was measured by inhibition of DNA synthesis as previously described (12). Target cells were trypsinized from exponentially growing cultures and resuspended at 5.0×10^4 cells/ml RPMI-FCS, and 2 ml were placed in 30-mm tissue culture dishes. Purified peritoneal macrophages were adjusted to 1.0×10^6 cells/ml RPMI-FCS, and 1 ml was added to the target cell cultures; the effector: target cell ratio was, therefore, 10:1. The DNA synthesis of the target cells was assessed after 20 hr of incubation at 37°C. The percent specific inhibition of DNA synthesis was calculated by the formula:

$$\text{Percent specific inhibition} = \frac{\text{cpm}_N - \text{cpm}_E}{\text{cpm}_N} \times 100$$

where cpm_N = counts per minute in cultures containing effector cells from normal control mice, and cpm_E = mean counts per minute in cultures containing test effector cells. P values were calculated by Student's t-test.

RESULTS

Influence of Glucan Treatment on Macrophage-Mediated Cytotoxicity

We have previously reported that specifically cytotoxic macrophages can be obtained from mice bearing MBL-2 leukemia allografts (13). To test whether alloimmune macrophage cytotoxicity could be enhanced by glucan therapy, CD2F1 mice were treated intraperitoneally 6 days after MBL-2 allograft inoculations, and macrophages were harvested 6 days later. Pyran copolymer was incorporated in the study as a positive control. Both glucan and pyran markedly potentiated specific macrophage reactivity ($p < 0.001$) (Fig. 1A). Lentinan, scleroglucan, dextrose, and phosphate-buffered saline were without significant effect.

We also studied the effect of glucan therapy on macrophage reactivity from nonsensitized mice. The drugs were administered intraperitoneally to CD2F1 mice, and 6 days later, the macrophages were tested for cytotoxic activity against

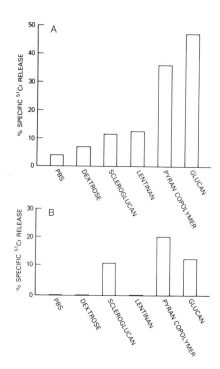

FIG. 1. A: Effects of various agents on the cytotoxic activity of purified peritoneal macrophages from MBL-2 tumor-bearing CD2F$_1$ mice to MBL-2 target cells. Mice were inoculated s.c. with 1.0×10^7 ascites tumor cells on day 0, and drugs were administered i.p. on day 6. Pyran was given at 25 mg/kg, whereas all other drugs were at 1 mg/kg. Peritoneal macrophages were subsequently harvested on day 12 after tumor inoculation and reacted against MBL-2 target cells. The values represent the means obtained from triplicate cultures. **B:** Effects of various agents on the cytotoxic activity of normal CD2F$_1$ peritoneal macrophages against MBL-2 target cells. Drugs were administered i.p. on day 0. Peritoneal macrophages were harvested on day 6 and reacted against MBL-2 target cells. The values represent the means obtained from triplicate cultures. PBS, phosphate-buffered saline.

MBL-2 cells. Only pyran copolymer ($p < 0.001$) and glucan ($p < 0.05$) stimulated macrophages to lyse MBL-2 targets (Fig. 1B). Lentinan, scleroglucan, and dextrose were without significant effect.

Influence of Glucan Treatment on Macrophage-Mediated Cytostasis

Peritoneal macrophages were harvested after glucan or pyran inoculation from normal BALB/c mice and tested *in vitro* for their ability to inhibit M109 cell DNA synthesis. Drugs were administered intraperitoneally at doses ranging

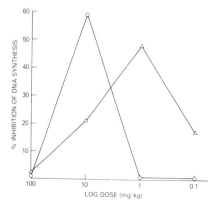

FIG. 2. Dose dependency of glucan- or pyran-induced macrophage activation to inhibit M109 cellular DNA synthesis. Drugs were administered i.p. to normal BALB/c mice at doses ranging from 100 to 0.1 mg/kg, and macrophages were harvested 6 days later. Experiments involved six mice per group, and values represent the means obtained from triplicate cultures. O, Pyran copolymer; Δ, glucan.

from 100 to 0.1 mg/kg. Macrophages were harvested on day 6. Activation by both glucan and pyran was sharply dose dependent (Fig. 2). Glucan treatment produced optimal stimulation at 1 mg/kg, whereas pyran required 10 mg/kg. Higher levels of drug were completely inhibitory.

Effect of Activated Macrophages on Proliferation of Normal and Tumor Target Cells

Using the inhibition of DNA synthesis assay, we have tested the ability of pyran- and glucan-activated macrophages to inhibit the proliferation of a number of syngeneic BALB/c target cell lines. Macrophages were harvested 6 days after a single i.p. treatment with either pyran (25 mg/kg) or glucan (1 mg/kg). Target cells included the M109 lung carcinoma, 3T3 embryonic fibroblasts, CoCa26 colonic carcinoma, and J774 reticulum cell sarcoma. All cell lines showed differential sensitivity to the presence of activated macrophages, but all were significantly inhibited (Fig. 3).

Thymus Independence of Cytostatic Effects by Glucan

We next studied the effect of glucan treatment on macrophages from nonsensitized, athymic nude mice. Drugs were administered intraperitoneally at 1 mg/

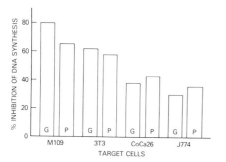

FIG. 3. Effects of activated macrophages on proliferation of various syngeneic target cell lines. Glucan (G) and pyran (P) were administered i.p. to normal BALB/c mice at 1 and 25 mg/kg, respectively. Macrophages were harvested 6 days later and tested for their ability to inhibit DNA synthesis of established BALB/c lines including M109 lung carcinoma, 3T3 embryonic fibroblasts, colonic carcinoma 26, and J774 reticulum cell sarcoma. The values represent the means obtained from triplicate cultures.

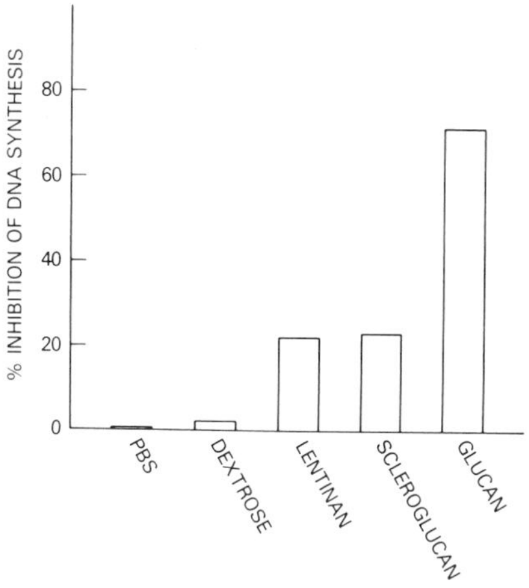

FIG. 4. Effects of various glucans on the cytostatic activity of purified normal macrophages from athymic nude mice for M109 target cells. Drugs were administered i.p. 6 days prior to harvesting the peritoneal exudates. Experiments involved six mice per group each, and values represent the means obtained from triplicate cultures. PBS, phosphate-buffered saline.

kg on day 0. Peritoneal macrophages were harvested on day 6 and tested for their ability to suppress M109 cell DNA synthesis. Glucan treatment greatly enhanced the cytostatic capacity of macrophages from athymic animals (Fig. 4), indicating that T-cell factors are not responsible for macrophage activation by glucan. Whereas scleroglucan and lentinan were marginally active, dextrose was without significant effect.

DISCUSSION

Glucan treatment has been shown to suppress the growth of solid tumors in both human (9) and murine (11) systems. This effect appears to be host mediated, since glucan exerts no direct toxicity for tumor cells *in vitro* (7,9, and R. M. Schultz, *unpublished observations*). The investigation reported here has established that the intraperitoneal inoculation of glucan into mice induces the appearance of macrophages capable of both cytocidal and cytostatic effects on tumor target cells. Macrophage activation by glucan was found to be sharply dose dependent and thymus independent. Although the mechanism of glucan stimulation of the RES is unknown, glucan particles, 3 to 4 μm in diameter, are known to be localized within macrophages and possibly exert their stimulatory effect as a result of solubilization (9).

In the past, the major emphasis has been placed on the role of the T-derived lymphocyte as the main effector of tumor cell cytotoxicity and cytostasis. However, increasing evidence is being provided that the critical determinant in tumor cell proliferation and dissemination is the functional activity and concentration of macrophages at the tumor site. In contrast to lymphocytes, activated macrophages can exert their cytotoxic effects on tumor cells at what can be considered physiologic concentrations (6). Furthermore, we have recently shown the positive correlation that exists between agents that stimulate reticuloendothelial function and agents that enhance antitumor resistance (13).

In many regards, glucan shares many properties with other nonspecific immunostimulants such as Bacillus Calmette-Guérin (BCG) and *Corynebacterium parvum;* they all have the ability to induce cytotoxic macrophages and when introduced intralesionally, lead to a histiocytic infiltrate into the tumor site (5,9). However, the histologic pattern of intralesional glucan differs from that of BCG-injected lesions in that glucan-injected lesions show no tuberculoid response and the monocytic response is more intense and distinctive (9). Glucan has the advantage of being a nontoxic, chemically defined agent that has the ability to be standardized for clinical trials and without complications due to infection or toxic metabolites.

Other structures closely related to glucan containing $\beta(1 \rightarrow 3)$-linked D-glucose residues such as lentinan and scleroglucan were without significant effects on macrophage activity. The mechanism by which lentinan exerts its antitumor activity is not clear. Maeda and Chihara showed that antitumor activity was lost in neonatally thymectomized mice, indicating that an intact T-cell system was a prerequisite for the antitumor effect of lentinan. Furthermore, Maeda et al. postulated that lentinan may exert its antitumor effect by stimulation of histamine and serotonin (8).

Glucan-activated macrophages were capable of effectively inhibiting proliferation in a number of syngeneic tumor cell lines. The supposedly "normal" BALB/3T3 cells were similarly inhibited and have recently been shown by Boone to be potentially malignant (1). In contrast to macrophages from glucan-treated animals, normal macrophages always exerted a weak and transient cytostatic effect. Keller showed that macrophages from mice treated with peptone were activated to inhibit the growth of rapidly replicating cell lines irrespective of whether they were of syngeneic, allogeneic, or xenogeneic origin, or whether they showed normal or neoplastic growth characteristics (6). He postulated that the mononuclear phagocyte system has a major role in surveillance against transformed cells and possibly a broader and more basic function in regulation of cell proliferation.

The further elucidation and characterization of nontoxic, pharmacologic agents capable of selectively enhancing reticuloendothelial function such as glucan may be useful both prophylactically and therapeutically in the control of malignant disease.

SUMMARY

Intraperitoneal glucan treatment rendered peritoneal macrophages both cytocidal and cytostatic for tumor target cells. Similar treatment of MBL-2 allograft-bearing mice acted synergistically to potentiate specific macrophage reactivity. However, enhanced cytotoxicity was not observed with other structures containing $\beta(1 \rightarrow 3)$-linked D-glucose residues such as lentinan and scleroglucan. Macrophages from glucan-treated animals suppressed DNA synthesis in a number of syngeneic (BALB/c) target cell lines; macrophage activation was sharply dose dependent and thymus independent. These functionally activated macrophages induced by glucan appear to have an important role in the enhancement of host resistance to neoplasia.

REFERENCES

1. Boone, C. W. (1975): Malignant hemangioendotheliomas produced by subcutaneous inoculation of BALB/3T3 cells attached to glass beads. *Science,* 188:68–70.
2. Chihara, G., Hamuro, J., Maeda, Y. Y., Arai, Y., and Fukuoka, F. (1970): Fractionation and purification of the polysaccharide with marked antitumor activity, especially lentinan, from *Lentinus edodes* (Berk.) Sing. (an edible mushroom). *Cancer Res.,* 30:2776–2781.
3. Dennert, G., and Tucker, D. (1973): Brief communication: Antitumor polysaccharide lentinan— a T cell adjuvant. *J. Natl. Cancer Inst.,* 51:1727–1729.
4. Di Luzio, N. R., Pisano, J. C., and Saba, T. M. (1970): Evaluation of the mechanism of glucan-induced stimulation of the reticuloendothelial system. *RES, J. Reticuloendothel. Soc.,* 7:731–742.
5. Hanna, M. G., Snodgrass, M. J., Zbar, B., and Rapp, H. J. (1972): Histopathology of *Mycobacterium bovis* (BCG)-mediated tumor regression. *Natl. Cancer Inst. Monogr.,* 35:345–357.

6. Keller, R. (1976): Cytostatic and cytocidal effects of activated macrophages. In: *Immunobiology of the Macrophage,* edited by D. S. Nelson, pp. 487–508. Academic Press, New York.
7. Maeda, Y. Y., and Chihara, G. (1973): The effects of neonatal thymectomy on the antitumor activity of lentinan, carboxymethylpachymaran and zymosan, and their effects on various immune responses. *Int. J. Cancer,* 11:153–161.
8. Maeda, Y. Y., Hamuro, J., Yamada, Y. O., Ishimura, K., and Chihara, G. (1973): The nature of immunopotentiation by the antitumor polysaccharide lentinan and the significance of biogenic amines in its action. In: *Immunopotentiation,* edited by G. E. W. Wolstenholme and J. Knight, pp. 259–285. Elsevier, New York.
9. Mansell, P. W. A., Ichinose, H., Reed, R. J., Krementz, E. T., McNamee, R., and Di Luzio, N. R. (1975): Macrophage-mediated destruction of human malignant cells *in vivo. J. Natl. Cancer Inst.,* 54:571–580.
10. Riggi, S. J., and Di Luzio, N. R. (1961): Identification of a reticuloendothelial stimulating agent in zymosan. *Am. J. Physiol.,* 200:297–300.
11. Sakai, S., Takada, S., Kamasuka, T., Momoki, Y., and Sugayama, J. (1968): Antitumor action of some glucans; especially on its correlation to their chemical structure. *GANN,* 59:507–512.
12. Schultz, R. M., Papamatheakis, J. D., Luetzeler, J., Ruiz, P., and Chirigos, M. A. (1977): Macrophage involvement in the protective effect of pyran copolymer against the Madison lung carcinoma (M109). *Cancer Res.,* 37:358–364.
13. Schultz, R. M., Papamatheakis, J. D., Stylos, W. A., and Chirigos, M. A. (1976): Augmentation of specific macrophage-mediated cytotoxicity: Correlation with agents which enhance antitumor resistance. *Cell. Immunol.,* 25:309–316.
14. Singh, P. P., Whistler, R. L., Tokuzen, R., and Nakahara, W. (1974): Scleroglucan, an antitumor polysaccharide from *Sclerotinium glucanicum. Carbohydr. Res.,* 37:245–247.

Immune Modulation and Control of Neoplasia by Adjuvant Therapy, edited by M. A. Chirigos. Raven Press, New York, 1978.

Treatment of Cutaneous and Subcutaneous Metastatic Tumors with Intralesional Glucan

Lucien Israel and Richard Edelstein

Centre Hospitalier Universitaire, Université Paris Nord, 93000 Bobigny, France

Glucan is a polysaccharide extract from the cell wall of the yeast *Saccharomyces cerevisiae* that has been shown to induce activation of the reticuloendothelial system and to cause tumor regressions in mouse and rat models (2). It has also been reported to cause tumor size reduction following intralesional injection in humans (4,5).

The purpose of this work was to determine the effect of intralesional glucan on metastatic skin nodules, both clinically and histologically, to monitor for a possible systemic effect when administered by this route and to study tolerance and side effects. No attempt was made to monitor any immunologic or other biologic parameters.

MATERIALS AND METHODS

Patient Population

Eleven patients were treated with intralesional glucan (kindly supplied by N. R. Di Luzio, Department of Physiology, Tulane University Medical School, New Orleans, La.) There were seven female patients and four male patients whose ages ranged from 29 to 80 years (mean, 55.8 years).

All these patients but one had accessible cutaneous and subcutaneous metastases from a previously resected primary malignant melanoma. The remaining patient had subcutaneous metastases from a thyroid carcinoma. The number of lesions ranged from one to 50.

Seven patients had lesions confined to the skin with no detectable visceral metastases, whereas four had both cutaneous and visceral involvement.

Of the 11 patients, six had no prior systemic or intralesional therapy, two had previously been treated with intralesional Bacillus Calmette-Guérin (BCG), and three had previously been treated with intralesional BCG and chemotherapy. In the five patients who had received prior intralesional BCG (with or without chemotherapy), the lesions injected with glucan were *new lesions* that appeared during or following prior therapy and had not been injected.

Seven patients were treated with intralesional glucan alone, whereas the four remaining patients, because of the extent of their disease, received concomitant chemotherapy or chemoimmunotherapy.

Glucan Administration

In all patients, all accessible lesions were injected once a week (except for a few control lesions left to monitor for a possible systemic effect) until the lesion was considered resolved or until there was evidence of progressing visceral disease. If new skin lesions appeared these were also injected. Glucan was injected directly into, under, and around the lesion using a 0.6×31 mm sterile disposable needle. In one patient with previously injected lesions (BCG) residual ulcerated lesions were treated with glucan-soaked dressings applied topically. In some patients, ethyl chloride was used as a spray-on local anesthetic to attenuate local pain associated with the injections. The dose injected into any single lesion depended on its size. Initially very low doses were used so that individual lesions received anywhere between 1 and 40 mg of glucan (180 in one particularly large lesion). The total dose administered during any one session depended on the number of lesions injected (1 to 25) and ranged from 4 to 560 mg.

The number of courses of intralesional therapy ranged from 2 to 19 (2 to 19 weeks) for a total cumulative dose of 60 to 2,700 mg.

RESULTS

Response of Injected Lesions

Local response was related to the dose injected and also appeared to differ according to individual sensitivity. With the initial dose of 1 to 2 mg per lesion, virtually no response was observed in four patients after four to six weekly injections.

Nine patients were treated with higher doses (seven from the outset, and two after first receiving low doses).

5 to 10 mg Per Lesion (One Patient)

This patient who had previously had a violent response to very low doses of BCG intralesionally also showed strong reactivity to glucan since, with 5 to 10 mg per nodule, intense inflammation occurred after only one injection, with necrosis and suppuration after the second and resolution of the injected nodules.

20 to 40 mg Per Lesion (Six Patients)

This was the most common dose used. Five of these patients had moderate inflammation of injected lesions after one to three weekly injections without decrease in size of injected lesions and without suppuration following 2, 4, 10, 11, and 19 injections, respectively.

The other patient who received this dose showed a strong inflammatory response after two injections, with suppuration and resolution of certain lesions after four injections.

80 to 190 mg (One Patient)

This dose produced intense inflammation after one injection, with ulceration after the second injection in an 80-year-old patient with a large (6 X 4 cm) lesion situated at the site of the initial resected lesion.

Topical Application

Topical weekly application of glucan-soaked dressings (380 mg) for 10 weeks in a patient with residual ulcerated lesions previously treated with BCG resulted in disappearance of all lesions and healing of the ulcers 2 months after the end of treatment.

Noninjected Lesions and New Lesions

Of the seven patients treated with intralesional glucan alone, five had nontreated lesions that served to monitor for a systemic effect. In one patient lesions progressed and new lesions appeared. Three patients had no change in existing nontreated lesions but had appearance of new lesions, and one patient had three untreated lesions that diminished in size by close to 50% with no new lesions during the 19 weeks of treatment.

Histologic Findings

Histologic examination of injected lesions was performed in two patients and a nontreated lesion from one of these patients (which diminished by close to 50%) was also examined.

In the first patient, the skin lesion removed for examination had been treated with four weekly injections of 20 mg each. The specimen was obtained 14 days after the last injection and proved to contain a residual metastatic nodule surrounded by inflammatory cell infiltrates containing predominantly macrophages with sparse lymphocytes and neutrophils.

In the second patient, the lesion examined was removed 7 days after the 19th weekly injection of 20 mg of glucan and revealed the presence of a large number of macrophages, many of which contained melanin, with no trace of tumor cells.

Examination of a noninjected lesion from this patient revealed no trace of tumor cells but large quantities of melanin, most of which was extracellular, between the collagen fibers of the dermis, some being seen in the cytoplasm of a few sparse macrophages.

SIDE EFFECTS AND TOXICITY

Local injections became increasingly painful as time went by, and in some cases this was a limiting factor for the number of lesions treated during any one session. The use of spray-on ethyl chloride helped to overcome local pain.

Systemic reactions were related to the total dose administered during any one session. In patients receiving glucan alone, no systemic reactions were seen at less than 20 mg per session. At doses above 100 mg, five out of six patients complained of moderate-grade fever. The severity of this symptom appeared to be dose related. The typical pattern was onset of fever 2 hr after injection, rising to a maximum of 39°C (and even 40 in one patient) in 6 to 12 hr and return to normal within 48 hr. Two patients out of six complained of headaches and asthenia. One patient exhibited no systemic reactions after 220 mg.

INFLUENCE OF GLUCAN ON THE GENERAL COURSE OF DISEASE

In six patients (three of whom were receiving chemotherapy) new lesions continued to appear during treatment with glucan.

One patient who developed regional cutaneous metastases 10 weeks after surgical removal of the primary lesion and had new lesions each week until the start of glucan therapy, had no new lesions for 19 weeks, and then new lesions appeared.

One patient had resolution of three lesions injected with glucan, but a new lesion appeared 3 weeks thereafter.

One patient with 20 residual ulcerated lesions previously treated with BCG had resolution and healing of her lesions after 10 weekly topical applications of glucan-soaked dressings with no new lesions since the end of treatment (2 months).

One patient on concomitant chemotherapy had a > 50% response that lasted about 3 months.

The last patient had a rapidly progressing recurrence at the site of the primary lesion. Injection of 190 mg of glucan weekly appeared to arrest the growth of this lesion for about 6 weeks, after which progression was seen.

CONCLUSION

Intralesional therapy of cutaneous metastases from malignant melanoma or other primary sites, whether using BCG, *Corynebacterium parvum,* or other agents has proved capable of destroying treated lesions but in our experience (3) has never shown systemic activity, in that distant and even neighboring lesions have always continued to grow uninhibited. Other authors have reported regression of uninjected nodules (1,6,7) although in these studies the lesions were superficial intradermal ones rather than subcutaneous and/or no biopsy specimens were obtained for histologic examination.

Glucan was administered intralesionally to 11 patients with cutaneous and subcutaneous metastases to test (a) the effect on injected lesions, (b) the effect on uninjected lesions, and (c) tolerance.

The response of injected lesions varied depending on the dose and individual sensitivity. Doses of 2 mg per lesion or less had little if any clinically detectable effect. At above 10 mg there was inflammation appearing after 1 to 4 weekly injections leading to suppuration and resolution of the lesion in some cases. When suppuration did not occur, it was difficult to ascertain whether the lesion had resolved or not. Surgical removal of one such lesion (after 19 weekly injections) showed no residual tumor cells and dense macrophage infiltrates, whereas a noninjected lesion, from this same patient, that had diminished in size by close to 50% proved to contain large amounts of melanin but no tumor cells.

Tolerance was satisfactory on the whole. Systemic reactions were less severe than with either BCG or *C. parvum,* two other agents we have used intralesionally. All but one patient receiving at least 100 mg per session complained of fever, and two patients complained of transient headaches and asthenia, but these reactions were never dose limiting.

The relatively good tolerance to glucan, its chemoattractant properties for macrophages, and the histologically confirmed disappearance of a noninjected lesion, the first to date in our experience, certainly warrant pursual of investigations on intralesional therapy with this agent.

SUMMARY

Glucan, a polysaccharide extract of yeast cell wall, was injected intratumorally in 11 patients with cutaneous and subcutaneous metastases, 10 from a malignant melanoma and one from a thyroid carcinoma.

Tolerance was satisfactory on the whole, and apart from local pain on injection, most patients complained of moderate-grade fever lasting 24 to 48 hr when the total dose injected during any one session exceeded 100 mg. Two patients complained of transient headache and asthenia.

No local response occurred at doses of 1 to 2 mg per lesion. At above 10 mg per lesion an inflammatory response leading to suppuration in some cases was seen after one to four weekly injections. Control lesions diminished by close to 50% in one patient. Clinical resolution of injected lesions was achieved in some but not all cases.

Two patients had lesions removed for histologic examination. In one case, after 19 weekly injections, no tumor cells were found in an injected lesion, *or in an uninjected lesion.* In our experience with intralesional BCG and *C. parvum,* this is the first documented case of resolution of a noninjected nodule.

In the other case, after four weekly injections, residual tumor cells were found. A prominent histologic finding in this study was the presence of dense macrophage infiltrates around the injected lesions suggesting that glucan is a potent macrophage chemoattractant.

REFERENCES

1. Bornstein, R. S., Mastrangelo, M. J., Sulit, D., Chee, D., Yarbro, J. W., Prehn, L., and Prehn R. T. (1973): Immunotherapy of melanoma with intralesional BCG. *Natl. Cancer Inst. Monogr.,* 39:213–220.
2. Di Luzio, N. R., McNamee, R., Jones, E., Cook, J. A., and Hoffmann, E. O. (1977): The employment of glucan and glucan activated macrophages in the enhancement of host resistance to malignancies in experimental animals. In: *Proceedings of the NCI Workshop—Role of Macrophages in Neoplasia (in press).*
3. Israël, L., Depierre, A., Edelstein, R., Cros-Decam, J., and Maury, P. (1975): Effect of intranodular BCG in 22 melanoma patients. *Panminerva Med.,* 17:187–188.
4. Mansell, P. W. A., Ichinose, H., Reed, R. J., Krementz, E. T., McNamee, R., and Di Luzio, N. R. (1975): Macrophage mediated destruction of human malignant cells *in vivo. J. Natl. Cancer Inst.,* 54:571–580.
5. Mansell, P. W. A., and Di Luzio, N. R. (1977): The *in vivo* destruction of human tumor by glucan activated macrophages. In: *Proceedings of the NCI Workshop—Role of Macrophages in Neoplasia (in press).*
6. Morton, D. L., Eilber, F. R., Malmgren, R. A., and Wood, W. C. (1970): Immunological factors which influence response in malignant melanoma. *Surgery,* 68:158–164.
7. Pinsky, C. M., Hirshaut, Y., and Oettgen, H. F. (1973): Treatment of malignant melanoma by intratumoral injection of BCG. *Natl. Cancer Inst. Monogr.,* 39:225–228.

Immune Modulation and Control of Neoplasia by Adjuvant Therapy, edited by M. A. Chirigos. Raven Press, New York, 1978.

Clinical Experiences with the Use of Glucan

*P. W. A. Mansell, G. Rowden, and C. Hammer

McGill University Cancer Research Unit Montreal; and Division of Oncology, Royal Victoria Hospital, Montreal, Canada

The use of glucan clinically in man is still largely confined to intralesional injections into easily accessible subcutaneous metastases, most often of malignant melanoma. The results of this form of treatment have been reported before (1–4) and have not varied in our further experience.

Glucan is a long-chain polyglucose, the individual units being linked by β1–3 glycosidic bonds (5,6). Its mode of action is entirely unknown but is thought to reside, in part at least, in the unique form of the chemical bonding and the steric configuration of the molecule. It is of interest to note that whereas glucan is one constituent of zymosan (7), the other constituent mannan (8–10) is entirely inactive as a macrophage activator (11).

Although it was originally thought that the action of glucan was entirely confined to macrophages, in the sense that it is chemotactic for these cells and also activates them (11,12), there are undoubtedly other aspects to its action that may be just as important and are certainly of very great interest. It will be shown that glucan acts on all the elements of cell-mediated immunity, both in man and in experimental animals (13,14). It appears that both B and T cells may be affected by glucan; however, at this stage in the experimental work, it is extremely difficult to work out the exact relationship between these cell types and their interactions when under the influence of glucan. It is worth noting here that the mode of action of the other, much more widely used nonspecific reticuloendothelial system (RES) stimulators, such as Bacillus Calmette-Guérin (BCG), *Corynebacterium parvum,* and levamisole, is also almost entirely unknown.

The other perplexing problem, and this is almost certainly true for all forms of immunotherapy, is that individual patients react differently, not only with respect to other patients with the same disease, but also at different stages in the evolution of their own disease. These differences are influenced by a wide variety of factors both in the host and in the tumor, and also resulting from concomitant treatment, so that the detailed analysis of the action of a single

---

* *Present address:* Comprehensive Cancer Center for the State of Florida, P.O. Box 520875, Biscayne Annex, Miami, Florida 33152

agent within an individual becomes exceedingly complex. Little, if anything, except broad principles can be learned from the random study of groups of patients, and it is depressing, but not surprising, to note that the great majority of such studies show little, if any, benefit from attempts at immunotherapy (15). Although Woglom's observation on immunity that "nothing may accordingly be hoped for at present in respect to a successful therapy from this direction" (16) is probably no longer true, it is obvious that much more attention needs to be paid to the modes of action of immunostimulants (17). This chapter and others in this volume attempt, in part, to answer these questions as applied to glucan.

One of the approaches described in this chapter is the investigation of the effect that glucan may have *in vitro* on various populations of peripheral blood leukocytes from healthy donors and from patients with a variety of neoplasms, either as a mitogen in its own right or as a costimulator in the presence of the conventional mitogens phytohemagglutinin (PHA), pokeweed mitogen (PWM), and concanavalin A (Con A), and on its ability to generate suppressor cells in man. These studies show, unequivocally, that glucan has an action, not only on macrophages, as was originally thought, but also on B lymphocytes and on suppressor T cells. Thus the beginnings of an understanding of the action of this substance may be appearing. By studying the ultrastructure of cellular interaction under the influence of glucan, it is also possible to begin to understand how this substance may work. Some such investigations have already been reported (2–18) but are expanded on here since recent studies shed important new light on this aspect of the subject.

MATERIALS AND METHODS

Glucan was originally prepared at a concentration of 100 mg/g of a lipid emulsion base and sterilized by autoclaving. Before use, this emulsion was mixed with sterile saline on a Vortex mixer to form a uniform suspension. By the use of this method, the glucan particles were approximately 3 to 4 μm in diameter. A recent modification in the method has allowed a much smaller particle size to be achieved (1 μm); this smaller particle does not require addition of lipid emulsion and can easily be injected through a 23-gauge needle.

Administration

Glucan can easily be given by percutaneous injection. No complications have occurred in the more than 50 patients to whom it has been given, except for the mild discomfort of the injection, followed by an erythematous reaction associated with mild local discomfort, which lasts up to 96 hr. In only two cases was any systemic reaction noted (mild fever); however, on previous and subsequent injections of glucan, no such reaction was experienced, so these isolated incidents could be attributed to some other cause.

Clinical

Patients in the trial were those with easily accessible subcutaneous tumor nodules. All had an extensive immunologic work-up and signed an informed consent. The tumors studied were malignant melanoma, breast cancer, and adenocarcinoma of the lung. Tumor nodules were injected with glucan; control nodules were injected with dextrose saline. At regular intervals after injection, the nodules were excised under local anesthesia and subjected to histologic examination. The slides were read blind.

Experimental

Peripheral blood lymphocytes were separated in a Ficoll gradient, washed three times, and plated on tissue culture plates at 2×10^5 cells per well in medium RPMI 1640 with 10% fetal calf serum (FCS) and 1% penicillin/streptomycin. Glucan was added at various doses. After 3 days at 37°C, cell proliferation was measured by ^{3}H-thymidine uptake.

In parallel experiments, PHA (5.0 μg/ml), PWM (20 μg/ml), and Con A (60 μg/ml) were added with glucan (0.4 μg). Cell proliferation was measured at day 4. Suppressor T cells were prepared from lymphocytes of healthy donors or cancer patients incubated with Con A, glucan, or both. Populations of these cells (1×10^5/well) were then examined on day 4 for their ability to suppress mitogen stimulation of untreated normal lymphocytes.

Electron Microscopy

Tissue blocks (1 mm^3) fixed for 1 hr at room temperature in half-strength Karnovsky fixative, washed in cacodylate buffer, and postfixed in s-collidine-buffered osmium tetroxide for 1 hr at room temperature. Specimens were stained *en bloc* with aqueous uranyl acetate for 1 hr at room temperature, followed by dehydration with ethanol and embedding in Spurr resin. Half micron sections were cut on a Reichert OMU3 ultramicrotome with diamond knives and stained with alkaline toluidine blue. Thin sections were contrasted with lead citrate and examined in a Philips EM301 microscope operating at 60 KeV. Areas of close contact/cytoplasmic continuity between host and tumor cells were studied by means of a goniometric stage for rotation and tilting, fitted to a Philips EM300. Micrographs were taken at magnifications between X20,000 and X30,000 of areas where distinct plasma membranes were not evident. Subsequent observations and photographs were made of the same areas after various degrees of tilt up to 60° in either direction. One-hundred interactions were analyzed by this method.

RESULTS

Clinical

As previously mentioned (1–4), the lesion consequent on the injection of glucan into a tumor nodule results from the accumulation within the nodule of very large numbers of macrophages. We have attempted to visualize the sequence of change that occurs in this process (Figs. 4 to 12). There is no doubt that the effect is dose dependent; in other words, if a large nodule is injected with a very small quantity of glucan, then relatively little effect, if any, is seen, whereas if a small nodule is injected, then the whole tumor may resolve completely, leaving in its place a small sterile abscess containing many mononuclear cells with some dead tumor cells, debris, and occasional polymorphs. The clinical time course of these events is variable, but in most cases an effect can be seen within 48 hr that appears to be maximal at approximately 5 days.

As far as the patient is concerned, there is little, if any, toxicity. In a small number of cases, local pain has been experienced while the injection is being made, but this soon passes off. In two cases, a transient febrile episode occurred within half an hour of the injection. In one of these cases, a total of 400 mg was given into 10 lesions (there can be no doubt that some of this material was given intravenously) and the fever subsided without treatment; the patient felt perfectly well an hour later. For the subsequent treatment this same patient was hospitalized as a precaution, and no such reaction was observed. The material was tested for endotoxin and was found to be negative. The second such case was similar and occurred when several large lesions were injected with a total of 300 mg of glucan; again the fever subsided within hours. In a small number of cases where large injections were given into superficial lesions, a sterile abscess formed and discharged for a short time. The material from these lesions has never become infected, and the condition resolves rapidly, never ulcerating.

A systemic effect for glucan has never been definitely established, even though it is our impression that distant metastases have slowed in their growth following its administration. It is probable that the best effect of glucan in this respect is seen when the material can be given either intravenously or intraperitoneally,

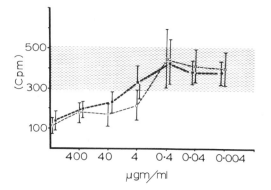

FIG. 1. Dose-response curve of glucan added to peripheral blood lymphocytes. The optimal dose lies at about 0.4 µg/ml. ■, Healthy ($N=15$); ○, patients ($N=87$).

as has been shown in a number of animal models (2,11,13,19–21). Preliminary results, in our hands, of the intraperitoneal administration of glucan in humans have shown, as in animals, that an exudate containing activated macrophages in very large numbers can be obtained; to date the local and systemic effect of this exudate has not been examined in detail; no toxic effects have been seen following the use of glucan in this manner.

There continues to be a remarkable consistency in the results seen. Providing a satisfactory injection can be given both into, and around, the lesion, 100% of treated lesions show the desired effect. Now that the material is better prepared, these injections can be simply done with fine gauge needles in the out-patient department.

Experimental

It was shown that glucan added in high concentrations to peripheral blood lymphocytes inhibited cell growth, whereas in a narrow range at the optimal amount of 0.4 to 0.2 μg/ml, a slight but significant stimulation was observed in healthy donors and patients (Fig. 1).

Glucan added to mitogens altered the proliferation considerably. Augmentation and depression were found in various degrees in both patients and controls (Table 1). In controls, glucan lowered the PHA response in 60% and augmented the response in 26% of the tested individuals. Cancer patients, however, showed a significantly higher degree of augmentation than suppression. The percentage of augmentation and suppression was approximately the same in cells stimulated with PWM in both patients and controls. In Con A-stimulated lymphocytes, T cells, the amount of augmentation and suppression was highest in cancer patients and lowest in healthy controls. Con A-stimulated cells seemed much more significantly affected, either positively or negatively, than those treated with PHA or PWM.

Further dissection of these results in groups of cancer patients are shown in the subsequent figures. In a group of 18 healthy donors, it can be seen that the addition of glucan to peripheral blood lymphocytes stimulated with PHA, PWM, and Con A causes both augmentation and suppression of response, the

TABLE 1. *Influence of glucan on mitogen-induced blastogenesis of peripheral lymphocytes in tumor patients and controls*

	Augmentation[a] (%)	Suppression[a] (%)	Unchanged (%)
	Controls (N = 14)		
PHA	26	60	14
PWM	33	46	21
Con A	27	46	27
	Tumor patients (N = 82)		
PHA	57	31	12
PWM	35	45	20
Con A	40	52	8

[a] Augmentation or suppression indicates a difference of at least 10% away from the mean.

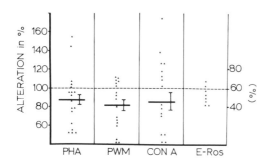

FIG. 2. Effect of cocultivation with glucan on the mitogen stimulation of peripheral blood lymphocytes from 18 healthy donors. In all cases, suppression can be seen; the numbers of E-rosettes are normal. The thick bar is the mean ± SEM.

mean not varying significantly from that seen in the same system without the addition of glucan (Fig. 2).

A group of 14 melanoma patients in stages II or III of their disease or stages III or IV with a bad prognosis is shown. As compared with controls, glucan augmented the responses in all three mitogen-stimulated populations. The number of E-rosettes determined in some of the patients showed low distribution values, particularly in those in the later stages of their disease (Fig. 3).

A group of sarcoma and lymphoma patients also showed a high degree of costimulation by glucan in the PHA and PWM population, whereas the response toward Con A was decreased, indicating that in this population suppressor T-cell production might be increased. This same phenomenon occurred in a group of 13 patients with metastatic breast carcinoma. In these patients, the number of T cells in terms of E-rosettes was well below normal values.

A group of 17 patients, mostly with advanced adenocarcinoma of colon or ovary, showed results in these costimulation experiments that approach the values of healthy blood donors.

These results on small numbers of patients, although not very significant in adenocarcinoma and breast carcinoma patients, indicate that this action may be due to the influence of suppressor-T-cell activity or a variation in the numbers of these regulator cells. The generation of such cells, acting as suppressor cells in mitogen stimulation, is time dependent, with an optimum between 48 and 72 hr of preincubation. Incubation with Con A stimulates the production of suppressor cells significantly, and even this can be augmented by adding glucan to the medium. Glucan alone is less effective than Con A, but induces higher suppression than is seen in untreated preparations.

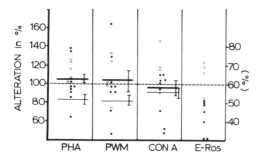

FIG. 3. Cocultivation with glucan in a group of 14 melanoma patients. Glucan augmented the response in all patients (thick bar) as compared to controls (thin bar). The numbers of E-rosettes was low, particularly in the patients with advanced disease (•) compared to those with early disease (o).

TABLE 2. *Generation of suppressor T cells*

Peripheral blood lymphocytes (%)	T-enriched lymphocytes (%)	Fe-treated lymphocytes (%)	B-enriched lymphocytes (%)	48-Hr incubation with:
75	46	81	138	No pretreatment
54	40	72	85	Con A
48	39	77	91	Con A & glucan
61	40	76	111	Glucan

Enrichment of T cells by eliminating adherent B cells amplifies suppression in healthy donors, whereas the withdrawing of phagocytic cells with carbonyl iron reduces this suppressive effect. An enriched B-cell fraction shows almost no suppression. Irradiation with 400 rads before and after the generation of suppressor cells did not alter their activity, whereas radiation with 800 rads at both time points eliminated this activity almost completely, thus showing that the suppressor cells are not macrophages (Table 2).

Similar experiments could not be done in cancer patients because of the large amounts of blood needed. However, from preliminary results it would seem that in cancer patients three different groups of reaction can be observed.

Group I: Where all parameters follow the values of healthy blood donors—however, with slightly decreased values of suppression.

Group II: Where only slight suppression is seen in the PHA-stimulated group, but significant stimulation over normal values is seen in the PWM and Con A response.

Group III: Where all three mitogen actions are significantly suppressed.

It is too early to make firm statements; it seems, however, that in these groups of patients, glucan balances these values in the direction of normal values.

The correlation of these results with the various clinical and therapeutic parameters of these patients is being undertaken and will be reported elsewhere.

MORPHOLOGY OF GLUCAN-INDUCED TUMOR REGRESSION

Histology

The pattern of tumor response to local injection of glucan has been briefly described previously (1–3). In essence, the response consisted of a transient inflammatory reaction at the site of injection with neutrophil immigration. This was followed within hours by the appearance of mononuclear phagocytes that engulfed large quantities of glucan. The glucan-laden macrophages permeated the sheets of tumor cells (Fig. 4) and rapidly induced local cellular destruction; giant cells are present; areas adjacent to deposits of glucan and glucan-laden macrophages also underwent destruction with the appearance of coagulative

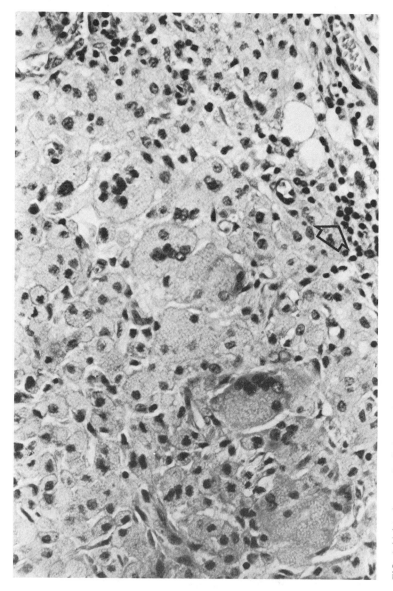

FIG. 4. Light micrograph of sheets of macrophages with foamy cytoplasm infiltrating into a tumor nodule. Some lymphocytic infiltrate is evident *(arrow)*. X712.

necrosis. Within 96 hr a large sterile "cold abscess" resulted from the influx of macrophages and their cytotoxic effects on the tumor. The abscess contained much cell debris of destroyed tumor cells and macrophages, plus fibrin and extravasated erythrocytes, as well as a second influx of neutrophils. Depending on the size of the injected nodules and the administered dose of glucan, areas were found in some specimens where apparently viable tumor cells were evident.

Ultrastructure

The immigrant macrophages were often grossly distorted with engulfed glucan. This material had a characteristic appearance (1). Various degrees of consolidation and rarification in the content of such vacuoles suggested that the glucan was metabolized by the phagocytes (Fig. 5). The population of mononuclear cells was, however, quite pleomorphic in that many monocytes were detected that had not, in the time period under observation, engulfed glucan. These may represent newly arrived elements of the host's cellular response. These cells contained significant numbers of lysosomes and were generally of the "activated" phagocyte form. The interaction of macrophages without obvious glucan content with a tumor cell is illustrated in Fig. 6.

Areas of the abscess contained abundant fibrin, polymorphonuclear leukocytes, and lakes of lipid (Fig. 7). It was evident that the residual macrophages present in such areas contained an abundance of phagocytosed cell debris; phagocytosis of whole tumor cells was also noted in the later stages (Fig. 8). Cell destruction, however, did not appear to result totally in the liberation of cell content. Examples of the formation of apoptotic bodies (22) of both nuclear and cytoplasmic forms were very obvious in the areas of cell destruction. However, in the associated areas of coagulative necrosis, adjacent to the major focus of macrophage activity, little evidence of this form of cell death was noted.

Viable tumor cells were seen at the edges of some of the abscess cavities. Areas of lymphocyte accumulation in structures resembling germinal centers were also noted in injected dermal nodules biopsied several weeks after injection (Fig. 9).

Nature of the Cell Contact

Very close approximation of the plasma membranes of the activated macrophages to those of tumor cells was a constant finding. This peripolesis involved an extensive increase in cell surface projections of both macrophage and tumor cell. No evidence was found for emperipolesis. No secretion of material between cells in close contact was evident, but membrane thickenings were noted on the cytoplasmic aspects of the plasma membranes of tumor cells in contact with macrophages and also with lymphocytes (Figs. 10 and 11).

Areas where there was apparent fusion, or continuity, of cytoplasm were, in fact, shown not to exist. Tilting of the specimen to angles of 30° in either direction brought the membranes perpendicular to the axis of observation and

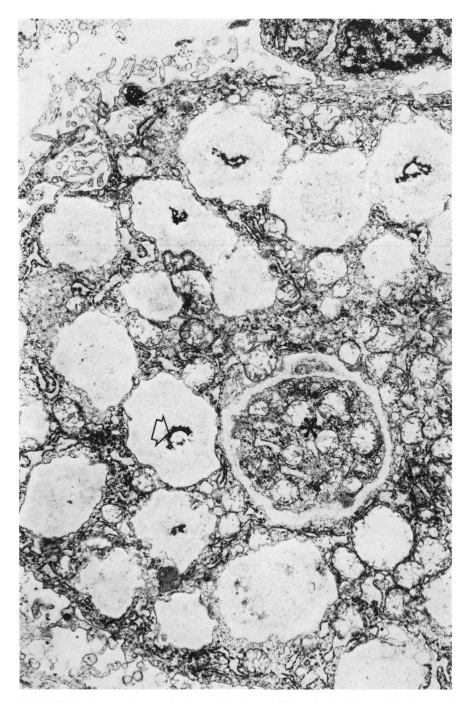

FIG. 5. TEM of macrophage cytoplasm with glucan within cytoplasmic vacuoles. Areas of granulating and fibrillar structure are evident. A central electron-dense structure is also present *(arrow)*. An autophagic vacuole or an engulfed apoptotic body is present (*). X11,250.

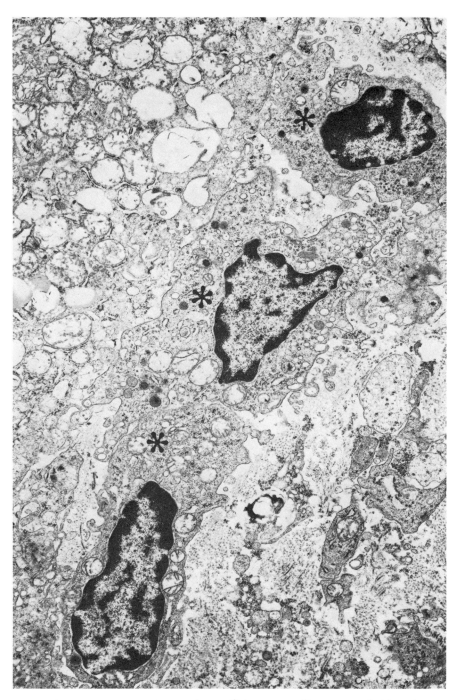

FIG. 6. TEM of activated macrophages (*) in contact with a tumor cell. X11,250.

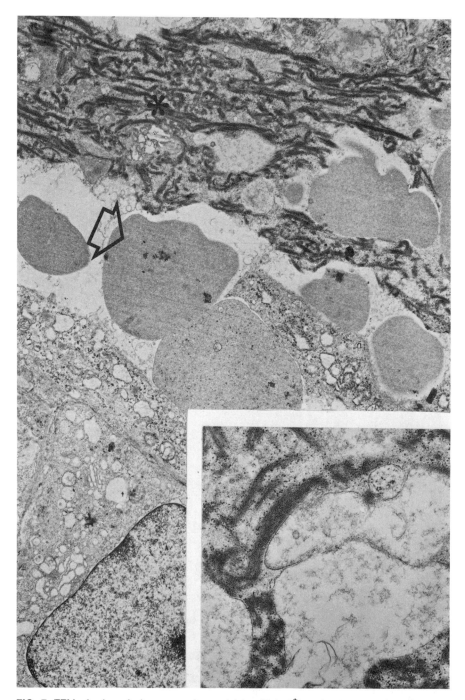

FIG. 7. TEM of edge of abscess cavity containing fibrin (*) and extravasated erythrocytes *(arrow).* A focus of viable tumor cells is present. X6,650. **Insert:** Detail of the fibrin meshwork showing periodicity. X22,750.

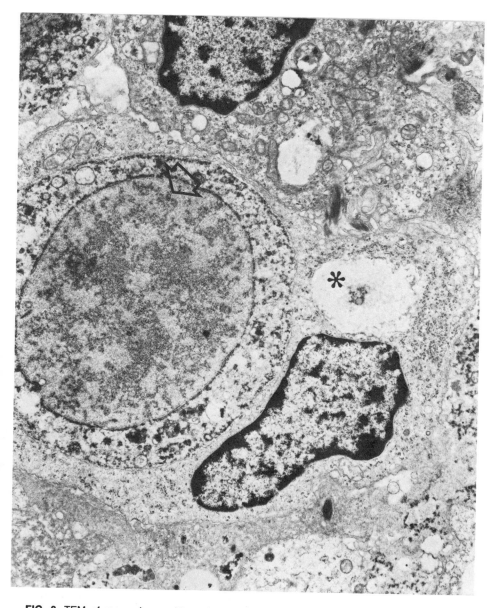

FIG. 8. TEM of macrophage with a glucan vacuole (*) containing an engulfed tumor cell *(arrow).* X8,748.

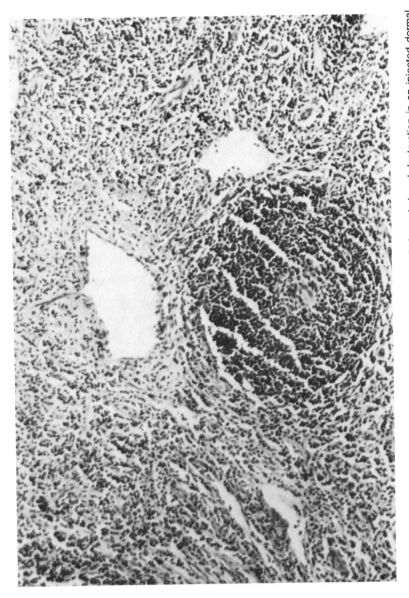

FIG. 9. Light micrograph of germinal center present near an area of glucan-induced destruction in an injected dermal nodule. ×782.

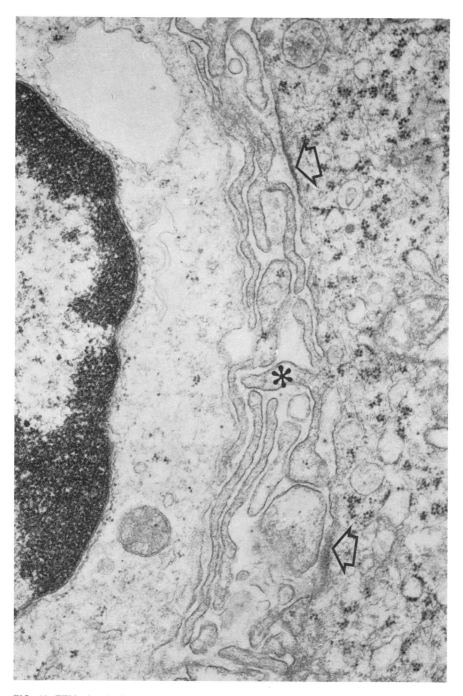

FIG. 10. TEM of peripolesis of a macrophage to a melanoma cell. Extensive increase in cell surface area via microvilli (*). Areas of density on the cytoplasmic aspect of the plasma membrane of the tumor cell *(arrows).* X36,500.

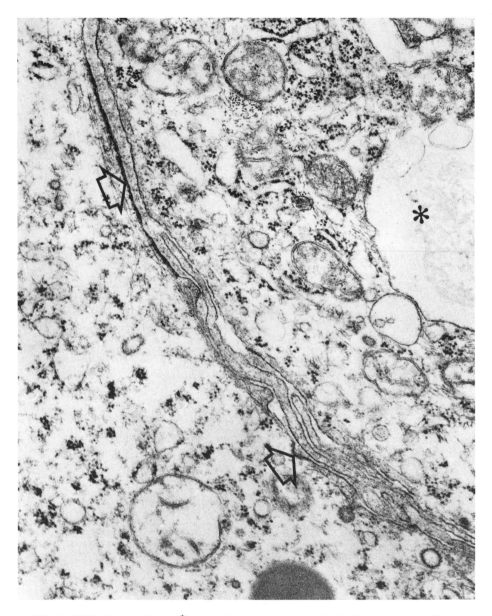

FIG. 11. TEM of glucan-laden (*) macrophage closely associated with a tumor cell. Dense deposits along the cytoplasmic leaflet of the plasma membrane of the melanoma cell *(arrows)*. X37,310.

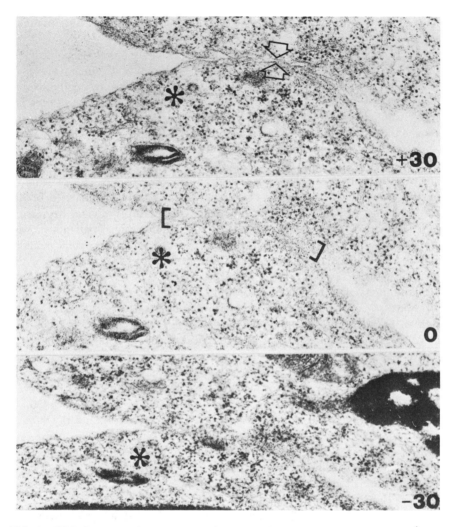

FIG. 12. TEM of an area of apparent cytoplasmic continuity between a macrophage (*) and a tumor cell ([]). Photographed at 0, +30°, and −30° tilt. Two distinct cell membranes visible at +30° tilt *(arrows)*. X32,550.

thereby demonstrated the existence of two intact membranes separated by a gap of approximately 20 to 30 nm in 98% of cases studied (Fig. 12).

DISCUSSION

Cellular Interaction

It has been found that all cell-mediated immunity in tumor bearing animals and man is moderately to severely depressed (23–27), therefore a clinical need exists for therapeutic agents designed to augment this immune response in tumor patients with deficient or depressed resistance mechanisms.

Glucan was found to be an effective drug in inducing macrophage-mediated destruction in malignant lesions in animals (11–13,19) and humans (1–4). In recent experiments, glucan was found to be engulfed also by peripheral mononuclear cells (14), a phenomenon that could even be increased by costimulating these lymphocytes with Con A. Extrapolation of these *in vitro* experiments leads to the suggestion that glucan is able to increase the activity of immunoregulating cells and may, therefore, be able to balance the action of regulator cells.

It has been possible to show that glucan has no significant direct mitogenic effect on the peripheral blood mononuclear cells in either cancer patients or healthy controls. The reactivity of standard mitogens was augmented or depressed by cocultivation with glucan. Although in healthy donors depression dominated in all three mitogen-stimulated populations, cancer patients showed a more marked augmentation of the mitogenic response. This apparent modulation of the lymphocyte response was found to increase with the stage of the tumor. Similar results have been found in experiments using levamisole (28).

The suppression of mitogen-induced proliferation and the numbers of T cells (E-rosettes) were found to correlate in healthy donors as compared to patients with an enhanced PHA and Con A response and a decrease of T cells. This action of glucan indicates a glucan-linked mechanism for influencing regulator T cells (suppressor T cells).

In animal models, many systems have been developed to study the action of suppressor cells (29). None of these methods is applicable to man. However, it was found that cells generated according to the methods used in mice (30,31) were able to suppress the mitogen response of lymphocytes from healthy donors. Suppressor cells, which decrease the *in vitro* PHA and Con A response and in most cases augment the PWM stimulation of peripheral lymphocytes, are present in each individual, healthy or tumor bearing (32,33).

Studies during the generation of these cells show this population is preexisting (33) and can be increased during the optimal incubation time of 48 to 72 hr. Stimulation with a specific T-cell mitogen increased this activity, and the addition of glucan to this system was able to amplify the effect in some cases. Glucan by itself had a stimulatory effect; however, the effect was less significant than that seen with Con A. Irradiation of the cells before and after generation with 400 rads did not influence the suppressive effect, whereas 800 rads abolished the suppression almost completely, indicating that these suppressor cells are not radioresistant, and therefore not macrophages (34).

Enrichment of T cells in the suppressor cell fraction increased the suppression, whereas enrichment with adherent cells (B cells) abolished suppression. This verifies that T cells play at least a major role in this system (35).

The decreased effect after carbonyl iron and magnet treatment indicates, however, that Con A and glucan-stimulated suppressor cells may also depend on the action of a third cell, the macrophage. The participation of such a cooperator cell would explain the action of the RES stimulator glucan as a regulator in this central mechanism; also, the increase in the B-cell mitogen response could explain the findings of higher antibody production in tumor-bearing (36) and normal animals treated with glucan (12,19).

Further stimulation of suppressor cells containing lymphocyte populations with PHA show that this action is not disturbed after the 2-day incubation period. The lower response in the PWM-stimulated groups indicates that these cells respond to signals from Con A-stimulated autologous suppressor T cells (37). The lack of such a mechanism could explain the difference of behavior between patient groups, where, in some cases, either the cooperator cells do not operate as such or the B cells are unable to answer such signals for other reasons. The possibility that the cooperator cells are defective in their action needs further investigation.

Nature of the Cytolytic Event

There have been numerous investigations of the interactions between host and tumor cells in an attempt to delineate the nature of the effector cells in cell-mediated immunity. These studies, which have been carried out mainly in *in vitro* systems, have a firm basis in the observation of dense mononuclear cell infiltrates present in many primary tumors.

In the main, the effector arm of the host's response to tumors may be summarized as follows (38): T-cell contact; diffusible products of T cells—lymphotoxins, etc.; antibody-dependent cytolysis mediated via lymphocytes bearing Fc receptors; armed macrophages (39,40), cytophilic antibody; and antibody and complement.

Concerning the role played by lymphocytes, it is generally agreed that close contact, or peripolesis (41), of effector cell to target cell is a necessary prerequisite for cytostasis and cytolysis of target cells. Close contact has been noted not only in tumors, but also in Hashimoto's thyroiditis (42) and in graft rejection (43). Similarly, *in vitro* in a variety of situations including mitogen-stimulated lymphocytes and lymphocytes exposed to specific antigenic stimulation, cell-to-cell contact has been noted (44–49). These studies have been confirmed by transmission electron microscopy (TEM) (50,51) and scanning electron microscopy (SEM) (52), also in autologous lymphocyte-tumor cell systems (53). The actual events leading to cell destruction still, however, remain a subject of much speculation. The suggestion has been made that peripolesis of lymphocytes to target cells results in the formation of sites of continuity of the cytoplasm of the two cells.

Cellular communication via intercellular bridges has been reported from morphologic studies (45,54,55) and from transfer of vital dyes (56). In most instances, however, it has not been possible to demonstrate clearly damage to, or deletions in, the apposed plasma membranes. Thus, although peripolesis undoubtedly plays an essential role in lymphocyte-mediated cytotoxicity, the situation is still unresolved. Biberfeld and Johansson (57) have recently demonstrated, by elegant tilting of TEM specimens, that apparent areas of cytoplasmic continuity, previously reported to exist in both mitogen-stimulated lymphocyte-target cells and antibody-mediated cytotoxic reactions, are the result of failure to take into account the influence of the plane of sectioning.

Despite the observation of Ferlunga and Allison (58) indicating that much of the cytotoxic effect of the T cell appears to reside in the plasma membranes themselves, alternative explanations have been proposed. Peripolesis of cells appears to be a primary event in target cell destruction, but the actual lytic event that appears to occur as a result of osmotic imbalances (58), may be mediated via soluble products secreted by the effector cells. Such lymphocytotoxins have been shown to be effective, if present in sufficiently high concentrations (59). It may well be that areas of close association of cells provide the environment for concentrating such an attack (60).

Reports have also appeared on the shedding of material from lymphocytes in contact with tumor cells (49,61). Immunoelectron microscopy demonstrated the transfer of immunoglobulin in this process. The shedding of the surface material and its penetration into target cells may have parallels with the high-affinity antibody released, suggested by Karush and Eisen (62) as being important in delayed hypersensitivity reactions.

Concerning the interaction of macrophages with tumor cells, much less has been achieved in analyzing either the in vitro or the in vivo situation. Undoubtedly, the recent studies of Evans et al. (40,63) and others (64,65) have focused attention on the macrophage as an important effector cell in the host's response to growing tumors.

Several ultrastructural studies both on tumors (66–68) and on grafts (69,70) have again illustrated the importance of the close contact of effector cell with target cell. These studies have, as in the lymphocyte investigations, led to numerous attempts to dissect the process in suitable in vitro models (19,71–73). A number of common observations have come from such studies. The macrophages involved have the morphologic appearance and biochemical characteristics associated with the activated form. Among these features are extensive surface projections and increased numbers of lysosomes (74). Although it is clear that macrophages make contact with the target cells, the subsequent cytotoxic events are as uncertain as they are in lymphocyte-mediated cytotoxicity. Chambers and Weiser (75,76) have stressed the importance of phagocytosis by macrophages. This type of activity, termed "piecemeal phagocytosis," has also been reported by others (77). Hanna (78) and associates (79,80), in investigations of BCG-mediated destruction by histiocytes of guinea pig hepatocarcinomatas, have suggested that fusion occurs between effector and tumor cells. Others have implicated a similar mechanism in other systems (81,82). Recently, Hibbs (83,84) has proposed that tumor cell destruction is brought about by heterocytolysis. In this case, macrophages activated by BCG appear to liberate lysosomes at areas of close contact (exocytosis). These are subsequently taken up by the tumor cells bringing about their destruction. Other workers have been unable to detect accumulation or transfer of lysosomes (85). The lysosome system may, however, not be the only one involved, since the antimicrobial myeloperoxidase system of macrophages has also been proposed as being important in tumor cell destruction (86).

An alternative proposal has been made which parallels that made for lympho-cytotoxicity, involving the effect of soluble factors synthesized by macrophages (87–89) that have been shown to be effective in inhibiting proliferation in lympho-cytes. Initial attempts to demonstrate the existence of such factors failed (90). Subsequent investigations have, however, demonstrated their existence (91,92), although their nature is far from clear.

It is clear from the present investigation, as in the studies of lymphocytotoxic-ity, that careful analysis of regions of suspected fusion that might indicate cyto-plasmic continuity between macrophage and tumor cell demonstrates that no such communication can be shown. Macrophages are apposed to tumor cells by both point and broad contact regions in which the plasma membranes are separated by gaps of less than 25 nm. No evidence was found for a clustering of lysosomes near such areas, nor were the plasma membranes morphologically altered. However, deposits of electron-dense material on the cytoplasmic aspect of the membranes of the melanoma cells were noted on occasions where macro-phages were in close contact. The significance of this observation is not clear; however, they were not seen in other tumor systems involved with glucan-laden macrophages. It may be significant that normal melanocytes have a somewhat similar modification of their plasma membranes adjacent to the basal lamina (93,94).

Similar accumulations of electron-dense material have been reported along the cytoplasmic aspect of the inner leaflet of the plasma membranes in both synthesizing fibroblasts (95) and macrophages near heterologous fibrillar protein (amyloid) (96). In both these instances, the dense plaques were not typical hemidesmosomes since they lacked anchoring filaments. These filaments are probably attachment devices for extracellular elements of a fibrous nature. It may be significant, therefore, that Colvin and Dvorak (97) have demonstrated the binding of components of the fibrinogen/fibrin system to the surface of macrophages. They suggest that adherence in macrophages in certain situations is mediated via activation of the clotting system.

The present study then demonstrates the involvement of activated glu-can-laden macrophages in tumor cell destruction. The destruction of tumor occurs as a result of the close apposition of the cell membranes of effector and target cells. No evidence was found to support the proposition that cytolysis occurs as a result of either fusion, transfer of lysosomes, or piecemeal phagocyto-sis. Phagocytosis, when it occurs, appears as a late phenomenon, perhaps in order to remove cell debris and apoptotic bodies. Whether the macrophage-mediated destruction of tumor cells results from plasma membrane contact or from secretion of soluble cytotoxins remains to be shown. Similarly, whether tumor cells are removed as a result of a direct lytic phenomenon, or because of their inability to withstand prolonged periods of cytostasis, cannot be determined from these studies.

Conclusion

Although the mechanism of action of glucan remains largely obscure, it does appear to have a multifactorial effect on both cell-mediated (14,98) and humoral immunity (12,19,36). The toxicity of other nonspecific immunotherapeutic agents, such as BCG, MER, and *C. parvum,* has been recognized for some time, but has received scant attention when considering the limitations of such agents for treating human disease (15,99–101). The most recently popular agent, levamisole, is also not without its severe complications (102–104), but again these have been largely ignored even though a significant proportion of the treated population are unable to continue the treatment because of them. Glucan has the advantage, if none other, of being virtually nontoxic, there having been only two transient episodes of possible side effects in over 50 patients in our hands.

Because of these facts, and the agent's undoubted and reproducible efficacy (1–4), there seems little excuse for not continuing with the further investigation of this agent as a nonspecific immune stimulant, either alone or in combination (105). The argument that its action is not understood is no reason for abandoning the investigation, since the same could well be said of other more "popular" agents (106,107).

ACKNOWLEDGMENTS

These studies were supported by grants from the Canadian National Cancer Institute and the Cancer Research Society of Montreal, Inc.

REFERENCES

1. Mansell, P. W. A., Ichinose, H., Krementz, E. T., McNamee, R., and Di Luzio, N. R. (1975): Glucan induced macrophage mediated destruction of human malignant cells *in vivo. J. Natl. Cancer Inst.,* 54:571–580.
2. Mansell, P. W. A., Di Luzio, N. R., McNamee, R., Rowden, G., and Proctor, J. W. (1976): Recognition factors and non specific macrophage activation in the treatment of neoplastic disease. *Ann. NY Acad. Sci.,* 277:20–44.
3. Mansell, P. W. A., and Di Luzio, N. R. (1976): The *in vivo* destruction of human tumour by glucan activated macrophages. In: *The Macrophage in Neoplasia,* edited by M. Fink, pp. 227–243. Academic Press, New York.
4. Mansell, P. W. A., and Di Luzio, N. R. (1976): Macrophages and neoplasia. In: *Immunocancerology in Solid Tumours,* edited by M. Martin and L. Dionne, pp. 51–61. Symposia Specialists, Miami.
5. Hassid, W. Z., Joslyn, M. A., and McCready, R. M. (1941): The molecular constitution of an insoluble polysaccharide from yeast *Saccharomyces cerevisiae. J. Am. Chem. Soc.,* 63:294–298.
6. Riggi, S. J., and Di Luzio, N. R. (1961): Identification of a reticuloendothelial stimulating agent in zymosan. *Am. J. Physiol.,* 200:297–300.

7. Benacerraf, B., and Sebestyen, M. M. (1957): Effect of bacterial endotoxins on the reticulo-endothelial system. *Fed. Proc.,* 16:860–867.
8. Northcote, D. H., and Horne, R. W. (1952): The chemical composition and structure of the yeast cell wall. *Biochem. J.,* 51:232–236.
9. Di Carlo, F. J., and Fiore, J. V. (1958): On the composition of zymosan. *Science,* 127:756–757.
10. Mundkur, B. (1960): Electron microscopical studies of frozen-dried yeast. *Exp. Cell Res.,* 20:28–42.
11. Di Luzio, N. R., Hoffmann, E. O., Cook, J. A., Browder, W., and Mansell, P. W. A. (1977): Glucan-induced enhancement in host resistance to experimental tumors. In: *Control of Neoplasia by Modulation of the Immune System (Progress in Cancer Research and Therapy, vol. 2),* edited by M. A. Chirigos, pp. 475–500. Raven Press, New York.
12. Di Luzio, N. R. (1975): Macrophages, recognition factors and neoplasia. In: *The Reticuloen-dothelial System,* edited by J. W. Rebuck, C. W. Berard, and M. R. Abell. Williams & Wilkins, Baltimore.
13. Proctor, J. W., Auclair, B. G., Stokowski, L., and Mansell, P. W. A. (1978): A comparison of the antitumor effects of glucan, BCG, and levamisole *(this volume).*
14. Hammer, C., Mansell, P. W. A., Lewis, M. G., Shibata, H. R., and Jerry, L. M. (1977): The role of glucan in immune regulation. *J. Reticuloendothel. Soc. (in press).*
15. Terry, W., and Windhorst, D. (Eds.) (1977): *Immunotherapy of Cancer: Present Status of Trials in Man (Progress in Cancer Research and Therapy, vol. 6).* Raven Press, New York *(in press).*
16. Woglom, W. H. (1929): Immunity to transplantable tumours. *Cancer Rev.,* 4:129–214.
17. Proctor, J. W., Lewis, M. G., and Mansell, P. W. A. (1976): Immunotherapy for cancer: An overview. *Can. J. Surg.,* 19:12–22.
18. Rowden, G., Proctor, J. W., and Mansell, P. W. A. (1977): Activation of macrophages by the polysaccharide glucan: TEM studies of tumor cell destruction in B16 melanoma and in humans. In: *Proc. 34th EMSA Mtg.,* edited by G. W. Bailey. Claiton's Publ. Div., Baton Rouge *(in press).*
19. Di Luzio, N. R., McNamee, R., Jones, E., Cook, J. A., and Hoffmann, E. O. (1976): The employment of glucan and glucan activated macrophages in the enhancement of host resistance to malignancies in experimental animals. In: *The Macrophage in Neoplasia,* edited by M. Fink, pp. 181–193. Academic Press, New York.
20. Silobrcic, V., Elman, A., Suit, H., and Steele, E. L. (1977): A comparison of the antitumour effect of *Corynebacterium parvum* and glucan in mice. *Proc. Am. Soc. Ther. Radio.,* (Abstr. 80) *(in press).*
21. Wainberg, M. (1976): *Personal communication.*
22. Kerr, J. R. R., Wyllie, A. H., and Currie, A. R. (1972): Apoptosis: A basic biological phenome-non with wide-ranging implications in tissue kinetics. *Br. J. Cancer,* 26:239–257.
23. Cohen, G., Douglas, D., König, E., and Brittinger, G. (1973): *In vitro* lymphocyte response to PHA and PWM in Hodgkin's disease. *Cancer,* 31:1346.
24. Sutherland, R. M., Inch, W. R., and McCredie, J. W. (1971): PHA induced transformation of lymphocytes from patients with cancer. *Cancer,* 27:574–578.
25. Herr, H. W., Beau, M. A., and Whitmore, W. F. (1976): Decreased ability of blood leukocytes from patients with tumours of the urinary bladder to act as stimulator cells in mixed leukocyte culture. *Cancer Res.,* 36:2754–2760.
26. Gatti, D. A., Garrioch, D. B., and Good, R. A. (1971): Depressed PHA responses in patients with non lymphoid malignancies. In: *Proc. Fifth Leukocyte Culture Conf.,* edited by J. Harris, p. 399. Academic Press, New York.
27. Adler, W. H., Takiguchi, H. T., and Smith, R. T. (1971): PHA unresponsiveness in mouse spleen cells induced by methylcholanthrene sarcomas. *Cancer Res.,* 31:864.
28. Sampson, D., and Lui, A. (1976): The effect of levamisole on cell mediated suppressor cell function. *Cancer Res.,* 36:952–955.
29. Dutton, R. W. (1975): Suppressor T-cells. *Transplant. Rev.,* 26:39–55.
30. Peavy, D. L., and Pierce, G. W. (1974): Cell mediated immune response *in vitro.* I. Suppression of the generation of cytotoxic lymphocytes by concanavalin A and concanavalin A-activated spleen cells. *J. Exp. Med.,* 140:356–368.
31. Rich, R. R., and Pierce, C. W. (1974): Biological expression of lymphocyte activation. II.

Suppression of plaque-forming cell response *in vitro* by supernatant fluids from concanavalin A-activated spleen cell cultures. *J. Immunol.,* 112:1360–1368.

32. Shou, L., Schwartz, S. A., and Good, R. A. (1976): Suppressor cell activity after concanavalin A treatment of lymphocytes from normal donor. *J. Exp. Med.,* 143:1100–1110.

33. Burns, F. D., Marrack, P. C., Kappler, J. W., and Janeway, C. A. (1975): Functional heterogeneity among the T-derived lymphocytes of the mouse. IV. Nature of spontaneously induced suppressor cells. *J. Immunol.,* 114:1345–1347.

34. Dutton, R. W. (1973): Inhibitory and stimulatory effects of concanavalin A on the response of mouse spleen cell suppressions to antigen. *J. Exp. Med.,* 138:1486–1505.

35. Rich, S. S., and Rich, R. R. (1976): Regulatory mechanisms in cell mediated immune response. *J. Exp. Med.,* 144:1214–1226.

36. Bitter-Suerman, H. (1976): *Personal communication.*

37. Kirchner, T. M., Chused, R. B., Herberman, R. B., Holden, H. T., and Lavrin, D. H. (1974): Evidence of suppressor cell activity in spleens of mice bearing tumours induced by Moloney sarcoma virus. *J. Exp. Med.,* 139:1473–1487.

38. Ginsberg, H., Naot, Y., and Hollander, N. (1976): Lysis and necrosis: Analysis of two cytotoxic phenomena mediated by lymphocytes. *Israel J. Med. Sci.,* 12:435–453.

39. Lohmann-Matthes, M., Schipper, H., and Fisher, H. (1972): Macrophage mediated cytotoxicity against allogenic target cells *in vitro. Eur. J. Immunol.,* 2:45–49.

40. Evans, R., and Alexander, P. (1972): Mechanism of immunologically specific killing of tumour cells by macrophages. *Nature,* 236:168–170.

41. Sharp, J. A., and Burwell, R. G. (1960): Interaction (peripolesis) of macrophages and lymphocytes after skin homografting or challenge with soluble antigens. *Nature,* 188:474–475.

42. Brandes, D., Antone, E., and Orbegoso, G. M. (1969): Hashimoto's thyroiditis ultrastructure and histology of the cellular infiltrate. *Johns Hopkins Med. J.,* 124:211–218.

43. Porter, K. A. (1965): Morphological aspects of renal homograft rejection. *Br. Med. Bull.,* 21:171–175.

44. Biberfeld, P., Holm, G., and Perlmann, P. (1968): Morphological observations on lymphocyte peripolesis and cytotoxic action *in vitro. Exp. Cell Res.,* 52:672–677.

45. Weiss, L. (1968): Interactions of sensitized lymphoid cells and homologous target cells in tissue culture and in grafts: An EM and immunofluorescence study. *J. Immunol.,* 101:1346–1362.

46. Rosenau, W., and Moon, H. D. (1961): Lysis of homologous cells by sensitized lymphocytes in tissue culture. *J. Natl. Cancer Inst.,* 27:471–483.

47. Perlmann, P., and Holm, G. (1969): Cytotoxic effect of lymphoid cells *in vitro. Adv. Immunol.,* 11:117–193.

48. Koran, H. A., Ax, W., and Freund-Moelbert, E. (1973): Morphological observations on the contact-induced lysis of target cells. *Eur. J. Immunol.,* 3:32–37.

49. Deodhar, S. O., Crile, G., and Esselstyn, C. B. (1975): Study of tumour cell-lymphocyte interaction in patients with breast cancer. *Cancer,* 29:1321–1325.

50. Mitchen, J. R., Moore, G. E., Gerner, R. E., and Woods, L. K. (1973): Interaction of human melanoma cell lines with autochthonous lymphoid cells. *Yale J. Biol. Med,* 46:669–680.

51. Kalina, M., and Ginsberg, H. (1975): Ultrastructural aspects of the adherence to target cells of *in vitro* differentiated lymphocytes. *Proc. Soc. Exp. Biol. Med.,* 149:796–799.

52. Lin, P. S., Tsai, S., Wallach, D. F. H., and Neurath, P. (1973): Membrane interaction between lymphocytes and monolayer cells *in vitro. Proc. ITTRI,* pp. 543–548.

53. Pihl, E., Nind, A. P. P., and Nairn, R. C. (1974): E.M. observations of the *in vitro* interaction between human leucocytes and cancer cells. *Aust. J. Exp. Biol. Med. Sci.,* 52:737–743.

54. Sura, S. N., Chernyakhovskaya, I. Y., Kodoghidze, Z. G., Fuks, B. B., and Svet-Moldovsky, G. J. (1967): Cytochemical study of interaction between lymphocytes and target cells in tissue culture. *Exp. Cell Res.,* 48:656–660.

55. Peters, J. H. (1972): Contact co-operation in stimulated lymphocytes. I. Influence of cell contact on unspecifically stimulated lymphocytes. *Exp. Cell Res.,* 74:179–186.

56. Sellin, D., Wallach, D. F., and Fischer, H. (1971): Intercellular communication in cell-mediated cytotoxicity. *Eur. J. Immunol.,* 1:453–458.

57. Biberfeld, P., and Johansson, A. (1975): Contact areas of cytotoxic lymphocytes and target cells. *Exp. Cell Res.,* 94:79–87.

58. Ferlunga, J., and Allison, A. C. (1971): Observation on the mechanism by which T-lymphocytes exert cytotoxic effects. *Nature,* 250:673–675.

59. Russel, S. W., Rosenau, W., and Lee, J. C. (1972): Cytosis induced by human lymphocytoxins. *Am. J. Pathol.,* 69:103–118.
60. Williams, T. W., and Granger, G. A. (1969): Lymphocyte *in vitro* cytotoxicity: Mechanisms of lymphocytotoxin-induced target cell death. *J. Immunol.,* 102:911–918.
61. Adelstein, E. H., Barrett, B. A. L., and Senhauser, D. A. (1976): Ultrastructure of lymphocyte-tumour cell interaction with localization of cell bound antibody by ferritin labelling. *Cancer Res.,* 36:302–308.
62. Karush, F., and Eisen, H. N. (1962): A theory of delayed hypersensitivity. *Science,* 131:1032–1039.
63. Eccles, S. A., and Alexander, P. C. (1974): Sequestration of macrophages in growing tumour and its effect on the immunological capacity of the host. *Br. J. Cancer,* 30:42–49.
64. Wood, G. W., and Gillespie, G. Y. (1975): Studies on the role of macrophages in regulation of growth and metastasis of murine chemically induced fibrosarcomas. *Int. J. Cancer,* 16:1022–1029.
65. Gauci, C. L. (1975): The macrophage content of human malignant melanoma. *Behring Inst. Mitt.,* 56:73–78.
66. Baum, M., Sumner, D., Edwards, H., and Smythe, P. (1973): Macrophage phagocytic activity in patients with breast cancer. *Br. J. Surg.,* 60:899–900.
67. Birbeck, M. S. C., and Carter, R. L. (1972): Observations on the ultrastructure of two hamster lymphomas in hamsters with particular reference to infiltrating monocytes. *Int. J. Cancer,* 9:249–257.
68. Vobrodt, A., Hliniak, A., Krzyzowska-Gruca, S., and Gruca, S. (1972): Ultrastructural studies on the behaviour of monocytes in the course of x-ray therapy of human skin cancer. *Acta Histochem. Jena,* 43:270–280.
69. Gershon, R. K., Carter, R. L., and Lane, N. J. (1967): Studies on homotransplantable lymphomas in hamsters. IV. Observations on macrophages in the expression of tumour immunity. *Am. J. Pathol.,* 51:1111–1133.
70. Journey, L. J., and Amos, D. D. (1962): An EM study of histicytic responses to ascites tumour homografts. *Cancer Res.,* 22:998–1001.
71. Kraehenbuhl, J. L., and Lembert, L. H. (1975): Cytokinetic studies of the effects of activated macrophages on tumour target cells. *J. Natl. Cancer Inst.,* 54:1433–1437.
72. Lejeune, F., and Evans, R. (1972): Ultrastructural cytochemical and biochemical changes occurring during syngeneic macrophage-lymphoma interaction *in vitro. Eur. J. Cancer,* 8:549–555.
73. Amos, D. B. (1960): Possible relationships between cytotoxic effects of isoantibody and host cell function. *Ann. NY Acad. Sci.,* 87:273–292.
74. Carr, I. (1967): The cellular basis of reticulo-endothelial stimulation. *J. Pathol. Bact.,* 94:323–330.
75. Chambers, V. C., and Weiser, R. S. (1969): The ultrastructure of target cells and immune macrophages during their interaction *in vitro. Cancer Res.,* 29:301–317.
76. Chambers, V. C., and Weiser, R. S. (1971): The ultrastructure of target L cells and immune macrophages during their interactions *in vivo. Cancer Res.,* 31:2059–2066.
77. Bennett, B., Old, L. J., and Boyse, E. A. (1964): The phagocytosis of tumour cells *in vitro. Transplantation,* 2:183–202.
78. Hanna, M. G., Jr. (1974): Immunologic aspects of BCG-mediated regression of established tumours and metastases in guinea pigs. *Semin. Oncol.,* 1:319–335.
79. Snodgrass, M. J., and Hanna, M. G., Jr. (1973): Ultrastructural studies of histiocyte-tumour cell interactions during tumour regression after ultralesional injection of *Mycobacterium bovis. Cancer Res.,* 33:701–716.
80. Snodgrass, M. J., Morahan, P. S., and Kaplan, A. M. (1975): Histopathology of the host response to mouse lung carcinomata: Modulation by pyran. *J. Natl. Cancer Inst.,* 55:455–462.
81. Vobrodt, A., Grabska, A., and Krzyzowska-Gruca, S. (1973): Cytochemical and ultrastructural studies on the contact formation between macrophages and irradiated cancer cells *in vitro. Folia Histochem. Cytochem. (Krakow),* 11:357–358.
82. Vobrodt, A., Grabska, A., Krzyzowska-Gruca, S., and Gruca, S. (1973): The formation of contacts between macrophages and neoplastic cells. *Folia Histochem. Cytochem. (Krakow),* 11:185–190.

83. Hibbs, J. B. (1974): Heterocytolysis by macrophages activated by bacillus Calmette-Guerin. Lysosome exocytosis into tumour cells. *Science,* 184:468–471.

84. Hibbs, J. B., Jr., Lambert, L. H., Jr., and Remington, J. S. (1972): Control of carcinogenesis: A possible role for the activated macrophage. *Science,* 177:998–1000.

85. Puvion, F., Fray, A., and Halpern, B. (1976): A cytochemical study of the *in vivo* interaction between normal and activated mouse peritoneal macrophages and tumour cells. *J. Ultrastruct. Res.,* 54:95–108.

86. Clark, T. S., Klebanoff, S. J., Einster, A. B., and Fefer, A. (1975): Peroxidase-H_2O_2 halide system; cytotoxic effect on mammalian tumour cells. *Blood,* 45:161–170.

87. Keller, R. (1975): Major changes in lymphocyte proliferation evoked by activated macrophages. *Cell. Immunol.,* 17:542–551.

88. Keller, R. (1976): Susceptibility of normal and transformed cell lines to cytostatic and cytocidal effects exerted by macrophages. *J. Natl. Cancer Inst.,* 56:369–374.

89. Calderon, J., Williams, R. T., and Unanue, E. R. (1974): An inhibitor of cell proliferates released by cultured macrophages. *Proc. Natl. Acad. Sci. USA,* 71:4273–4277.

90. Evans, R., and Alexander, P. (1971): Endotoxin and double stranded RNA render macrophages cytotoxic. *Nature [New Biol.],* 232:76–79.

91. Currie, G. A., and Basham, C. C. (1975): Activated macrophages release a factor which lyses malignant cells but not normal cells. *J. Exp. Med.,* 142:1600–1605.

92. Melstrom, H., Kearny, G., Gruca, S., and Seljelid, R. (1974): Evidence for a cytolytic factor released by macrophages. *J. Exp. Med.,* 140:1085–1096.

93. Odland, G. F. (1958): The fine structure of inter-relationships of cells in the human epidermis. *J. Biophys. Biochem. Cytol.,* 4:529–538.

94. Tarnowski, W. M. (1970): Ultrastructure of the epidermal melanocyte dense plate. *J. Invest. Dermatol.,* 55:265–268.

95. Porter, K. R. (1964): Cell fine structure and biosynthesis of intercellular macromolecules. *Biophys. J.,* 4(suppl.):167–196.

96. Shirahama, R., and Cohen, A. (1970): The association of hemi desmosome-like plaques and dense coating with the pinocytotic uptake of a heterologous fibrillar protein (amyloid) by macrophages. *J. Ultrastruct. Res.,* 33:587–597.

97. Colvin, R. B., and Dvorak, H. F. (1975): Fibrinogen/fibrin on the surface of macrophages. *J. Exp. Med.,* 142:1377–1390.

98. Cook, J. A., Taylor, D., Cohen, C., Rodrigue, J., Malshet, V., and Di Luzio, N. R. (1978): A comparative evaluation of the role of macrophages and lymphocytes in mediating the antitumor action of glucan *(this volume).*

99. Sparks, F. C., Silverstein, M. J., Hunt, J. S., Haskell, C. M., Pilch, Y. H., and Morton, D. L. (1973): Complications of BCG immunotherapy in patients with cancer. *N. Engl. J. Med.,* 289:827–830.

100. Mansell, P. W. A., and Krementz, E. T. (1973): BCG and its complications. *JAMA,* 226:1560–1561.

101. Schwarzenberg, L., Simmler, M. C., and Pico, J. L. (1976): Human toxicology of BCG applied in cancer immunotherapy. *Cancer Immunol. Immunother.,* 1:69–76.

102. Parkinson, D. R., Cano, P., and Jerry, L. M. (1977): Complications of levamisole therapy; a case report of agranulocytosis occurring during levamisole therapy with demonstration of levamisole dependent leucoagglutinins and a review of side effects encountered in 58 patients with malignant melanoma receiving levamisole immunotherapy. *Lancet (in press).*

103. Jerry, L. M., Lewis, M. G., Shibata, H. R., Mansell, P. W. A., Capek, A., and Marquis, G. (1978): Combination immunotherapy with levamisole, BCG, and tumor vaccines: Toward a rationale *(this volume).*

104. Ruuskanen, O., Reemes, M., Mäkelä, A.-L., and Toivanen, A. (1976): Agranulocytosis in two children taking levamisole. *Lancet,* 2:958.

105. Di Luzio, N. R., Cook, J. A., Cohen, C., Rodrigue, J., Kokoshis, P., and McNamee, R. B. (1978): Enhancement of the inhibitory effect of cyclophosphamide on experimental acute myelogenous leukemia by glucan immunopotentiation and response of serum lysozyme *(this volume).*

106. Florentin, I., Hachet, R., Bruley-Rosset, M, Halle-Pannenko, O., and Mathé, G. (1976): Studies on the mechanisms of action of BCG. *Cancer Immunol. Immunother.,* 1:31–39.

107. Geffard, M., and Orback-Arbouys, S. (1976): Enhancement of T suppressor activity in mice by high doses of BCG. *Cancer Immunol. Immunother.,* 1:41–43.

Immune Modulation and Control of Neoplasia by Adjuvant Therapy, edited by M. A. Chirigos. Raven Press, New York, 1978.

Recent Developments in the Chemistry and Biology of Thymosin

A. L. Goldstein, T. L. K. Low, J. L. Rossio, J. T. Ulrich, P. H. Naylor, and G. B. Thurman

Division of Biochemistry, University of Texas Medical Branch, Galveston, Texas 77550

A functioning thymus gland is necessary for the development and regulation of cell-mediated immunity. Those functions under thymic control in mammals include primary transplant and tumor immunity as well as viral, mycobacterial, fungal, and protozoal immunity. Thymic-dependent lymphocyte populations directly involved in these functions are collectively termed T cells. It is now recognized that subpopulations of T cells (e.g., helper cells, suppressor cells, effector cells, etc.) may also influence activity of B-cell populations that produce antibodies. Little knowledge exists at the cellular and molecular level about how the thymus gland exerts this control over T-cell development.

As indicated in Fig. 1, it is clear, however, that a vital part of the thymic-dependent process occurs via a hormonal mechanism. The thymus produces thymosin (5,7,10), and perhaps a whole spectrum of other thymic hormones and/or factors (17) that play an important role in the differentiation of precursor T cells, both *in situ* and at sites far removed from the thymus, to maintain a normal immune balance. Ongoing studies suggest that an immune imbalance resulting from deficiency in thymic factors due to genetic, viral, chemical, or radiation damage is expressed in T- and B-cell deficiency and can result ultimately in a number of serious disease states including autoimmune diseases, cancer, and infectious diseases.

For the past 13 years our laboratory has investigated the endocrine role of the thymus in the development, growth, and function of lymphoid tissue. Using a partially purified thymosin preparation thymosin fraction 5, we have established in a number of animal models (8), as well as in humans with primary immunodeficiency diseases (4,9,18) and most recently in immunosuppressed cancer patients (2,14), that thymosin can correct some of the deficiencies resulting from lack of thymic function. The clinical studies with thymosin are presented elsewhere in this volume.

Our studies indicate that a number of biologically active peptides are present in the partially purified fraction 5 that contribute to its biological activity. In this chapter we summarize the results of our ongoing chemical studies of the characterization of these polypeptides along with the progress we are making to increase our understanding of the early molecular events leading to the activa-

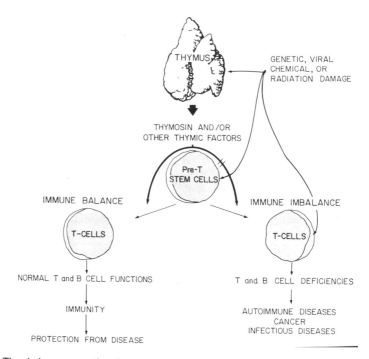

FIG. 1. Thymic hormone action. Lack of normal hormone production results in immune imbalance leading to disease.

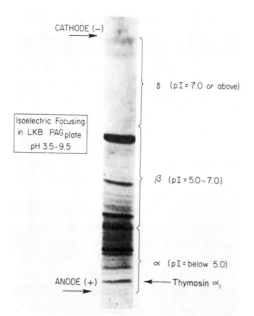

FIG. 2. Suggested nomenclature for thymosin polypeptides. Isoelectric focusing gel of thymosin fraction 5 at pH 3.5 to 9.5.

tion of T cells. In addition, we discuss development of two new functional assays designed to determine the efficacy of thymosin in the induction of T cells capable of immune function.

FURTHER CHEMICAL CHARACTERIZATION OF THYMOSIN

Nomenclature of Thymosin Polypeptides and
Sequence Analysis of Thymosin α_1

To facilitate the identification and comparison of thymic polypeptides from one laboratory to another, a nomenclature has been devised based on the isoelec-

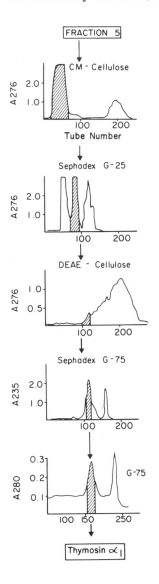

FIG. 3. Flow diagram of the fractionation of thymosin α_1 from bovine thymosin fraction 5. Shaded areas in elution profiles indicate fractions pooled for purifying thymosin α_1. In these profiles, the abscissa is the tube number and the ordinate absorption. For details, see ref. 6.

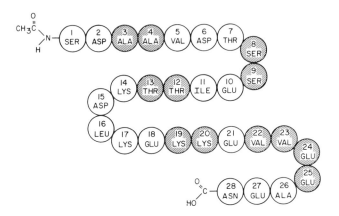

FIG. 4. Amino acid sequence of thymosin α_1. The shaded areas indicate repeating amino acid residues along the polypeptide chain.

tric focusing pattern of thymosin fraction 5 in the pH range 3.5 to 9.5 (6). As indicated in Fig. 2, the separated polypeptides are divided into three regions based on their migration patterns. The regions are identified by the Greek letters α, β, and γ. The α region consists of the polypeptides with isoelectric points below 5.0 (highly acidic), the β region 5.0 to 7.0 (acidic), and the γ region above 7.0 (basic). Subscript numbers α_1, α_2, α_3, etc., are used to identify the polypeptides from the region in the order of their isolation and sequence determination.

The isolation and total purification of the first thymosin polypeptide, termed thymosin α_1, is illustrated in Fig. 3. The amino acid sequence of thymosin α_1 has been determined (6). This polypeptide, shown in Fig. 4, consists of 28 amino acid residues and has a molecular weight of 3,108 as calculated from the established structure. The sequence of this polypeptide was determined by manual sequence analysis of peptides isolated from the various enzymatic digests. The enzymes used included trypsin, chymotrypsin, thermolysin, α-protease, and subtilisin. As illustrated in Fig. 5, we have now purified to homogeneity or

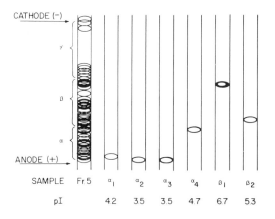

FIG. 5. Drawing of isoelectric focusing gels (LKB PAG plate, pH 3.5 to 9.5) of isolated thymosin polypeptides and fraction 5 showing the relative locations of the various components of fraction 5 thus far isolated.

near homogeneity five additional polypeptides termed α_2, α_3, α_4, β_1, and β_2. The isoelectric points are 3.5, 3.5, 4.7, 6.7, and 5.3, respectively.

THYMOSIN-INDUCED CHANGES IN CYCLIC NUCLEOTIDES

One of the first detectable effects of thymosin fraction 5 on thymocytes is the increase of intracellular cyclic GMP levels (13). Using a radioimmunoassay for the determination of adenosine 3'5' cyclic monophosphate (cyclic AMP) and an acetylation RIA procedure to measure guanosine 3'5' cyclic monophosphate (cyclic GMP), we have observed that after *in vitro* incubation with thymosin cyclic GMP levels, but not cyclic AMP levels, are significantly elevated in murine thymocytes (Table 1). As shown in Fig. 6, stimulation of intracellular cyclic GMP levels is seen as early as 1 min after incubation with thymosin

TABLE 1. *Murine thymocyte cyclic nucleotide levels determined after 15 min incubation at 37°C with the agents indicated*

	cyclic AMP (pmoles/10⁷ cells)	cyclic GMP (fmoles/10⁶ cells)
Medium control[a]	1.70 ± 0.17[b]	2.70 ± 0.63
100 µg Thymosin fraction 5	1.38 ± 0.03 (NS)[c]	7.55 ± 0.07 ($p < 0.001$)
100 µg Spleen fraction 5	0.81 ± 0.03 ($p < 0.005$)	1.57 ± 0.21 (NS)

[a] RPMI-1640, HEPES buffered.
[b] Standard deviation for independent triplicate samples.
[c] Statistical significance based on Student's t-test. (NS = not significant, $p > 0.05$.)

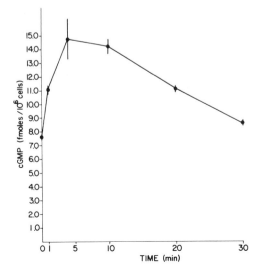

FIG. 6. Cyclic GMP levels in murine thymocytes incubated with 100 µg/ml of thymosin fraction 5. The increase is detectable at 1 min (11.13 ± 28 fmoles/10⁶ cells). The value for the cells at zero time is computed from the average and standard error for the control cells at 0, 10, 20, and 30 min. There is no significant shift in the values of cyclic GMP in the nonstimulated cells over the 30-min incubation period.

fraction 5 and is maximal between 5 and 10 min. Dose-response studies indicate an optimal stimulation of cyclic GMP with a thymosin fraction 5 concentration of 100 μg/ml. Control extracts of spleen fraction 5, prepared under conditions similar to that of thymosin, did not stimulate cyclic GMP levels. In contrast to our findings with thymosin, Kook and Trainin using THF (11) and Scheid et al. (15) with thymopoietin and ubiquitin have reported that these thymic factors increase cyclic AMP levels. We have used several different assays for cyclic AMP, including the RIA, kinase binding, and an assay utilizing the prelabeling of intracellular adenine pools, and are unable to demonstrate a statistically significant stimulatory effect of thymosin on cyclic AMP levels in either spleen or thymic cells (Table 1 and *unpublished observations*). This certainly does not eliminate cyclic AMP as an important second messenger for specific T-cell responses since cyclic AMP can mimic thymosin in some *in vitro* systems, such as the induction of spontaneous rosette-forming cells in the adult thymectomized spleen (1) and appearance of TL and thy-1 in pre-T-cell-enriched bone marrow (15). Thus this information and our observations appear to provide additional evidence for the hypothesis that there is a family of thymic polypeptides. Their influence over T-cell development could be via several different mechanisms, some of which may include changes in cyclic GMP or cyclic AMP, and others of which may not directly involve cyclic nucleotides in their mode of action.

THYMOSIN-INDUCED FUNCTIONAL CHANGES IN LYMPHOCYTES

Stimulation of Macrophage Migration Inhibitory Factor Production and Increased Production of Plaque-Forming Cells

Field and Shenton (3) have reported that thymectomy of guinea pigs sensitized 10 days before to tuberculin purified protein derivative (PPD) causes a rapid loss of the reactivity of peripheral blood lymphocytes (PBL) to PPD as measured by the microphage electrophoretic mobility test. The reactivity could be restored *in vitro* by the addition of small amounts of serum from the thymus-bearing guinea pig and also by human serum. Serum from a thymectomized animal could not restore reactivity of the PBL to PPD. They suggested the substance in the normal serum that allows for reconstitution of this system is thymosin, although thymosin was not utilized in their system. Based on their observations, we have developed an assay for studying the effects of thymosin and purified thymosin peptides on migration inhibitory factor (MIF) production *in vitro*. This assay is illustrated in Fig. 7. As shown in Table 2, thymosin fraction 5 at 50 and 100 μg/ml was sufficient to restore the thymectomized guinea pigs response to PPD. Addition of the purified thymosin polypeptide termed thymosin α_1 at a concentration as low as 10 ng/ml is enough to significantly induce MIF production. Another thymosin polypeptide termed thymosin α_3 at concentrations as high as 1,000 ng/ml did not induce MIF production.

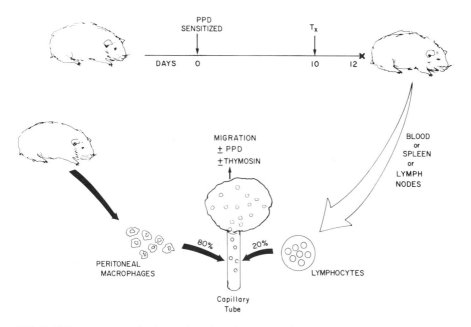

FIG. 7. MIF assay system for thymosin activity. Peripheral blood cells of guinea pigs thymecto- mized 10 days after tuberculin PPD sensitization respond to thymosin *in vitro* by producing MIF in the presence of PPD. For details, see ref. 16.

As diagrammed in Fig. 8, we are developing an assay to measure the effect of thymosin on plaque-forming cells (19S) *in vitro* using a modified Mishell- Dutton procedure (12) with normal, thymectomized, and shammed animals. As indicated in Table 3, thymosin fraction 5 at a concentration of 100 μg/ml in tissue culture stimulates an increase in plaque-forming cells of normal and

TABLE 2. *Reconstitution of the specific inhibition of macrophage migration in response to PPD by the addition of thymosin to the PBL of thymectomized guinea pigs*

Chamber contents	Concentration	Specific inhibition (%)
Thymosin fraction 5	10 μg/ml	−24.5
	50 μg/ml	20.8
	100 μg/ml	34.6
Thymosin α_1	1 ng/ml	12.6
	10 ng/ml	26.5
	100 ng/ml	54.5
	1,000 ng/ml	−38.2
Thymosin α_3	1 ng/ml	−29.9
	10 ng/ml	−47.8
	100 ng/ml	−36.7
	1,000 ng/ml	− 6.9

From Thurman et al., ref. 16.

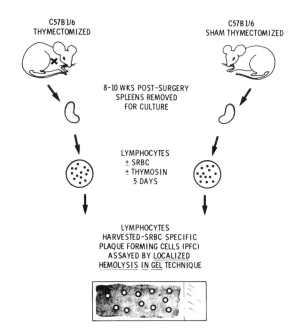

FIG. 8. *In vitro* antibody-producing cell assay for thymosin activity. Spleen cells from thymecto-mized, sham-thymectomized, or normal mice are cultured in the presence of SRBC antigen; thymosin increases the production of plaque-forming cells from thymectomized animals.

TABLE 3. *Thymosin-induced increase in plaque-forming cells of C57B1/6 spleen cells from normal, sham-thymectomized, and thymectomized mice*

Animals	Fraction (μg/ml)	No. of positive expts/total expts	Increase in plaque-forming cells	% Range
Normal	Thymosin fr. 5 (100)	3/3	+ 34	+12 to + 53
Sham thymec-tomized	Thymosin fr. 5 (100)	5/8	+ 44	−30 to +146
Thymectomized [a]	Thymosin fr. 5 (100)	8/8	+244	+57 to +758
Normal	Spleen fr. 5 (100)	1/1	+119	—
Sham thymec-tomized	Spleen fr. 5 (100)	2/2	+ 66	+12 to +120
Thymectomized [a]	Spleen fr. 5 (100)	1/2	+ 28	+ 3 to + 53

[a] Greater than 2 weeks post-adult thymectomy.

sham-thymectomized mice as does a similar preparation of spleen fraction 5. It is not presently understood why a spleen fraction 5 is stimulatory to lympho-cytes derived from mice with intact thymus glands. However, following thymec-tomy (greater than 2 weeks postthymectomy), the ability of thymosin fraction 5 to stimulate this increase is significantly enhanced whereas the ability of spleen fraction 5 is somewhat reduced.

DISCUSSION

As summarized in Table 4, the observation that thymosin α_1 is more potent than fraction 5 in enhancing some T-cell responses (E-rosettes, lymphokines, mitogen) but is not active in triggering other lymphocyte responses, such as the mixed lymphocyte reactivity (MLR) and antibody production, suggests that more than one peptide component is necessary to elicit full immunological responsivity. Preliminary studies with some of the other recently purified thymosin polypeptides support the conclusion that there are a family of biologically active polypeptides within fraction 5. These polypeptides may act in concert, sequentially, or separately on pre-T and T-cell populations to maintain normal immunological reactivity.

The observation that thymosin fraction 5 stimulates cyclic GMP but not cyclic AMP is of great interest in terms of increasing our understanding of early molecular events leading to activation of T cells. A major difficulty in accurately measuring cyclic nucleotide changes induced by thymosin is the large heterogeneity of lymphocyte populations and the possibility that only a small population of cells is responding. Cell separation experiments are presently being used in our laboratory to investigate whether thymosin induces changes in cyclic AMP levels in T-cell subsets and to determine which T-cell subsets are responsibile for responding to thymosin by increasing intracellular cyclic GMP. The probability that we are measuring an increase in one or more T-cell populations is suggested by the fact that spleen cells respond as do those of the thymus *(unpublished observation)*. It is possible that in the more immature cell populations, cyclic AMP is involved in an initial commitment to differentiate along the thymocyte pathway, whereas cyclic GMP is more important in the later stages of maturation and final differentiation. Thus, thymosin, in its multipotential role, might modulate cyclic AMP levels in more immature T-cell populations such as exist in nude mouse spleens or the bone marrow.

The thymosin-induced changes in functional response of lymphocytes, namely stimulation of MIF production, enhancing plaque-forming cell production, and induction of MLR of thymocytes with some but not all of the biologically active polypeptides found within fraction 5, strongly support the developing

TABLE 4. *Thymosin activity in various* in vitro *and* in vivo *bioassays*

	MLR (μg)	MIF (μg)	E-rosette (μg)	Mitogen[a] (μg)	Antibody (μg)	Lymphotoxin[a] (μg)
Thymosin fraction 5	1–10	1–5	1–10	1–10	1–10	100–500
Thymosin α_1	NA[b]	0.01–0.1	0.001–0.01	0.01–0.1	NA	50

[a] *In vivo* treatment with thymosin.
[b] Not active at any concentration tested.

concept that thymic control is exerted by a family of polypeptides perhaps acting at discrete points in the differentiation of T cells. This observation is obviously of major importance clinically where it is possible that a particular immunodeficiency disease is due to a block in the maturation pathway of a particular subset of T cells.

SUMMARY

One of the most potentially important advances in medical research in the past decade has been our understanding of the role played by the thymic-dependent immune system in various diseases including the primary immunodeficiency diseases—cancer and autoimmune disease. Major research thrusts as presented in this volume have capitalized on this new information, and studies designed to unravel the various components and maturational sequence involved in the development and maintenance of immunological competence have resulted in our appreciation of the importance of learning how to manipulate the immune system in the treatment of disease.

Our ongoing studies on the endocrine role of the thymus gland strongly support the existence of a family of polypeptide hormones from the thymus gland that carry out many of the functions ascribed to the intact thymus. Recent studies indicate that these polypeptides act either individually or in concert on subsets of T cells to induce the functional maturation and maintenance of the immune system. The first thymosin polypeptide to be totally purified and sequenced, thymosin α_1, has some but not all of the biological potency of fraction 5. Studies are continuing to establish the chemical and biological properties of the other biologically active components within fraction 5.

REFERENCES

1. Bach, M-A., Fournier, C., and Bach, J-F. (1975): Regulation of θ-antigen expression by agents altering cyclic AMP level and by thymic factor. *Ann. NY Acad. Sci.,* 249:316–327.
2. Costanzi, J. J., Gagliano, R. G., Loukas, D., Delaney, F., Sakai, H., Harris, N. S., Thurman, G. B., and Goldstein, A. L. (1977): The effect of thymosin on patients with disseminated malignancies: A Phase I study. *Cancer (in press).*
3. Field, E. J., and Shenton, B. K. (1975): Assay of thymosin in blood. *Lancet,* 1:49.
4. Goldstein, A. L., Cohen, G. H., Rossio, J. L., Thurman, G. B., Brown, C. N., and Ulrich, J. T. (1976): Use of thymosin in the treatment of primary immunodeficiency diseases and cancer. *Med. Clin. North Am.,* 60:591–606.
5. Goldstein, A. L., Guha, A., Hardy, M. A., and White, A. (1972): Purification and biological activity of thymosin, a hormone of the thymus gland. *Proc. Natl. Acad. Sci. USA,* 69:1800–1803.
6. Goldstein, A. L., Low, T. L. K., McAdoo, M., McClure, J., Thurman, G. B., Rossio, J. L., Lai, C-Y., Chang, D., Wang, S-S., Harvey, C., Ramel, A. H., and Meienhofer, J. (1977): Thymosin α_1: Isolation and sequence analysis of an immunologically active thymic polypeptide. *Proc. Natl. Acad. Sci. USA,* 74:725–729.
7. Goldstein, A. L., Slater, F. D., and White, A. (1966): Preparation, assay and partial purification of a thymic lymphocytopoietic factor (thymosin). *Proc. Natl. Acad. Sci. USA,* 56:1010–1017.
8. Goldstein, A. L., Thurman, G. B., Cohen, G. H., and Hooper, J. A. (1975): Thymosin: Chemistry, biology and clinical applications. In: *The Biological Activity of Thymic Hormones,* edited by D. W. van Bekkum, pp. 173–197. Kooyker Sci. Publ., Rotterdam.

9. Goldstein, A. L., Wara, D. W., Ammann, A. J., Sakai, H., Harris, N. S., Thurman, G. B., Hooper, J. A., Cohen, G. H., Goldman, A. S., Costanzi, J. J., and McDaniel, M. C. (1975): First clinical trial with thymosin: Reconstitution of T cells in patients with cellular immunodeficiency diseases. *Transplant. Proc.,* 7:681–686.

10. Hooper, J. A., McDaniel, M. C., Thurman, G. B., Cohen, G. H., Schulof, R. S., and Goldstein, A. L. (1975): The purification and properties of bovine thymosin. *Ann. NY Acad. Sci.,* 249:125–144.

11. Kook, A. J., and Trainin, N. (1974): Hormone-like activity of a thymus humoral factor on the induction of immune competence in lymphoid cells. *J. Exp. Med.,* 139:193–207.

12. Mishell, R. I., and Dutton, R. W. (1967): Immunization of dissociated spleen cell cultures from normal mice. *J. Exp. Med.,* 126:423–442.

13. Naylor, P. H., Sheppard, H., Thurman, G. B., and Goldstein, A. L. (1976): Increase of cyclic GMP induced in murine thymocytes by thymosin fraction 5. *Biochem. Biophys. Res. Commun.* 73:843–849.

14. Schafer, L. A., Goldstein, A. L., Gutterman, J. U., and Hersh, E. M. (1976): *In vitro* and *in vivo* studies with thymosin in cancer patients. *Ann. NY Acad. Sci.,* 277:607–620.

15. Scheid, M. P., Goldstein, G., Hammerling, U., and Boyse, E. A. (1975): Induction of T and B lymphocyte differentiation *in vitro.* In: *Membrane Receptors of Lymphocytes,* edited by M. Seligmann, J. L. Preudhomme, and F. M. Kourilsky, pp. 353–359. Elsevier, New York.

16. Thurman, G. B., Rossio, J. L., and Goldstein, A. L. (1977): Thymosin-induced enhancement of MIF production by peripheral blood lymphocytes of thymectomized guinea pigs. In: *Regulatory Mechanisms in Lymphocyte Activation,* edited by D. O. Lucas, pp. 629–631. Academic Press, New York.

17. Trainin, N. (1974): Thymic hormones and the immune response. *Physiol. Rev.,* 54:272–315.

18. Wara, D. W., Goldstein, A. L., Doyle, W., and Ammann, A. J. (1975): Thymosin activity in patients with cellular immunodeficiency. *N. Engl. J. Med.,* 292:70–74.

Immune Modulation and Control of Neo-plasia by Adjuvant Therapy, edited by M. A. Chirigos. Raven Press, New York, 1978.

Maturation of Thymus-Derived Cells Under the Influence of Thymosin

Aftab Ahmed, Allan H. Smith, and Kenneth W. Sell

Cellular Immunology Division, Clinical and Experimental Immunology Department, Naval Medical Research Institute, Bethesda, Maryland 20014

It is generally believed that hemopoietic stem cell migration to the primary lymphoid organs precedes differentiation along the lymphoid cell lines. Thus it is under the influence of the thymus gland that stem cells mature into the thymus-derived or T cells, generally believed to be mediators of cellular immunity. Although the precise chain of events in the development and maturation of T cells has been the subject of considerable investigation, the number of differentiation steps is, at present, unknown. However, in considering the process of T-cell maturation we can envision three distinct phases. The first involves the commitment of a stem cell to the thymus-derived pathway (precursor T), which does not require an intact thymus since it can occur in athymic (Nu/Nu) mice. The second phase characterized by the metamorphosis of precursor T cells into immature T cells is most likely triggered by a factor or inducer released by the thymus gland. It is during this period that the acquisition of phenotypic T-cell markers such as TL, theta, and Ly occurs. The third phase involves the changes through which the T cell becomes mature and immunocompetent, and it is as yet unclear whether a thymic factor is involved at this stage.

The concept that thymic factors can influence the differentiation and maturation of T cells led numerous investigators to the extraction, purification, and characterization of products of the thymus (7), which possesses such biological activity, including thymosin (9,10), thymic humoral factor (12), thymin or thymopoietin (5), and thymic factor (4). In the course of these studies it became apparent that a convenient and reliable assay for T-cell maturation was needed. We previously reported that augmentation of the response of bone marrow cells to the T-cell mitogen phytohemagglutinin (PHA) and concanavalin A (Con A) occurs following *in vitro* incubation of the cells in crude dialyzed extracts of thymus tissue (23) and subsequently found a similar augmentation of the Con A response of lymph node, but not spleen cells, following *in vivo* administration of thymosin fraction 5 (7,22). It is the purpose of this study to extend our observations on the utility of these procedures as assays for thymic hormonal activity. In addition, we report a novel approach to the problem of elucidating the process of helper-cell maturation and describe our initial investigations in the phenotypic acquisition of T-cell surface markers *in vitro*.

MATERIALS AND METHODS

Mice

Normal adult BALB/c and C56BL/6 mice were obtained from the Jackson Laboratory, Bar Harbor, Maine. We are deeply grateful to M. Cherry, Jackson Laboratory, for the Ly congenic mice.

Immunodeficient Mice

Athymic Nu/Nu mice and their normal littermates +/Nu were obtained through the courtesy of the Small Animal Production Unit, Division of Research Services, National Institutes of Health, Bethesda, Maryland. Thymectomized irradiated and anti-theta and complement-treated bone marrow cell reconstituted (T X Bm) mice were prepared as described previously (18). (CBA/N X DBA/2)F_1 male and female mice were obtained from the National Institutes of Health. Groups of BALB/c mice were treated since birth with either goat antimouse IgM (heavy chain specific) or normal goat serum (NGS), as described previously (19) for the depletion of B cells. Asplenic mice were obtained through the courtesy of E. Di Luzio, University of Tennessee.

Thymosine Fraction 5

Thymosin fraction 5 was prepared as described previously (8,9) and was the generous gift of A. L. Goldstein.

DNP$_5$-Thymosin

Thymosin fraction 5 was coupled with DNP by the method of Little and Eisen (13) and used as described in detail elsewhere (3). The degree of haptenation was determined as described (13), and an average molecular weight of 10,000 daltons/thymosin polypeptide was used in the calculations.

Cell Suspensions

Spleen, bone marrow, and lymph node cells were prepared as previously described (2).

Mitogens and Mitogen Cultures

The ability of the various cell populations to respond to the T-cell mitogens PHA-P and Con A, and to the B-cell mitogens *Escherichia coli* lipopolysaccha-

TABLE 1. *Strain combinations for the production of anti-Ly*

Specificity	Donor	Recipient	Titer
Ly 1.1	B6 · PL Ly 1	(B6A)F$_1$	1/128
Ly 1.2	CE/J	(C3H/He X DBA/2)F$_1$	1/256
Ly 2.1	CE/J	B10 · Br/SgSn	1/512
Ly 2.2	B10 · Y/Sn	(C3H/He X BDP)F$_1$	1/64
Ly 3.1	C58	(CBA/H-T6T6J X SJL)F$_1$	1/256
Ly 3.2	CE/J	C58/J	1/128

ride (LPS) and polyriboinosinic-polyribocytidylic acid (poly I · C) has been described in detail elsewhere (19–21). For reasons of clarity and conciseness, only the optimum responses are reported in this communication. A range of both cell concentration and mitogen dilutions were used in these experiments.

Antisera

Anti-theta serum was prepared by the hyperimmunization of AKR mice with CBA/J thymocytes. Anti-Ly 1.1, 1.2, 2.1, 2.2, 3.1, and 3.2 antisera were prepared as described above (Table 1). The antisera were always absorbed with recipient thymocytes in efforts to remove autoantibody, and each assay was performed using anti-Ly sera of the opposite allele along with Ly congenic mice as controls with each experiment.

Plaque Assay

Direct (19S) and indirect (7S) plaque-forming cells (PFC) were assayed as previously described (18).

RESULTS

Splenic Dependence of the Thymosin-Induced Augmentation of the Con A Response

As we have previously shown, lymph node cells, but not spleen cells, exhibit an augmented Con A response following administration of thymosin *in vivo* (7,22). Although we feel this phenomenon reflects a stimulus toward T-cell maturation, it could also be argued that the effect is due to changes in cell traffic. This latter possibility was explored by repeating these experiments in adult BALB/c mice—thymectomized, splenectomized, or both. The groups were then subdivided and received either saline or 100 μg thymosin fraction 5, i.p., every other day for a total of 400 μg. Twenty-four hours following the last injection, the lymph node cells were removed and assayed for the response to T-cell and B-cell mitogens. As seen from the data, lymph node cells from thymec-

TABLE 2. Effect of thymosin on the response of lymph node cells from normal, adult thymectomized, and adult splenectomized mice to polyclonal T-Cell and B-Cell mitogens

Mitogens	Normal adult		Adult thymectomized		Adult splenectomized	
	Saline	Thymosin	Saline	Thymosin	Saline	Thymosin
Control	227 ± 21	353 ± 82	344 ± 13	289 ± 22	128 ± 37	298 ± 89
PHA-P	7,829 ± 349	10,041 ± 668	2,021 ± 352	9,988 ± 1,026	2,814 ± 301	1,926 ± 47
Con A	12,411 ± 806	70,152 ± 3,210	3,956 ± 379	126,142 ± 8,954	3,115 ± 254	3,499 ± 68
LPS	744 ± 48	1,222 ± 67	1,551 ± 42	1,359 ± 62	2,957 ± 497	1,828 ± 111
poly I·C	1,012 ± 54	2,145 ± 102	1,432 ± 59	2,007 ± 127	1,146 ± 186	1,596 ± 134

TABLE 3. *Effect of thymosin on the response of lymph node cells from normal adult, splenectomized, and thymectomized mice to the polyclonal T-cell and B-cell mitogens*

Mitogens	Normal Adult		Adult splenectomized and thymectomized	
	Saline	Thymosin	Saline	Thymosin
Control	331 ± 51	446 ± 28	248 ± 41	186 ± 24
PHA-P	7,004 ± 359	12,418 ± 739	3,142 ± 142	2,010 ± 135
Con A	14,186 ± 792	94,417 ± 4,541	6,418 ± 339	7,535 ± 691
LPS	854 ± 46	1,056 ± 108	2,846 ± 137	2,118 ± 129
poly I · C	1,600 ± 83	2,057 ± 139	3,010 ± 111	3,256 ± 156

tomized mice do exhibit the increased response to Con A (Table 2), whereas those cells from splenectomized and thymectomized-splenectomized mice (Tables 2 and 3) do not. These results suggest that either the spleen is important as a source of precursor T cells, as a reserve pool of Con A-responsive cells that can migrate to the lymph node following thymosin administration, or the enhanced Con A response is sensitive to surgical trauma.

In order to further explore these possibilities, similar experiments were carried out with congenitally asplenic mice and their normal littermates. As seen in Table 4, absence of an intact spleen resulted in only a modest increase in Con A responsiveness following thymosin administration. Although this experiment does not allow a decision between the first two possibilities, it does rule out surgical trauma.

Further studies of this system in B-cell-deficient mice, however, revealed that the splenic-dependent character of the augmented Con A response is not due to the spleen acting as a pool of Con A-reactive T cells. BALB/c mice chronically treated from birth with goat antimouse IgM serum (anti-μ) were used as a source of B-cell-deficient mice (14). Controls were mice similarly treated with NGS. As seen in Table 5, the control mice exhibited the increased response after fraction 5 treatment as described above, whereas the anti-μ-treated mice (less than 1% Ig$^+$ cells) showed a slightly reduced response to Con A. We

TABLE 4. *Effect of thymosin on the response of lymph node cells from congenitally asplenic mice and their normal littermates to respond to the polyclonal T-cell and B-cell mitogens*

Mitogens	Normal +/+ littermate		Asplenic	
	Saline	Thymosin	Saline	Thymosin
Control	337 ± 44	289 ± 21	536 ± 29	418 ± 56
PHA-P	5,895 ± 246	8,487 ± 505	8,554 ± 337	9,545 ± 513
Con A	9,448 ± 407	118,439 ± 4,136	9,217 ± 419	14,618 ± 748
LPS	756 ± 32	898 ± 38	1,276 ± 132	1,517 ± 89
poly I · C	1,205 ± 66	1,407 ± 79	899 ± 101	1,255 ± 69

TABLE 5. *Effect of thymosin on the response of lymph node cells from anti-μ treated mice to the polyclonal T-cell and B-cell mitogens*

Mitogens	NGS		Anti-μ serum	
	Saline	Thymosin	Saline	Thymosin
Control	337 ± 21	581 ± 49	132 ± 20	249 ± 73
PHA-P	4,945 ± 283	9,254 ± 404	7,792 ± 623	8,295 ± 455
Con A	7,338 ± 354	110,289 ± 4,283	16,337 ± 511	15,384 ± 7,212
LPS	2,216 ± 137	1,821 ± 209	289 ± 47	332 ± 126
poly I · C	1,598 ± 112	1,552 ± 127	117 ± 32	144 ± 29

TABLE 6. *Effect of thymosin on the response of lymph node cells from thymectomized (CBA × DBA/2)F$_1$ female and male mice to polyclonal T-cell and B-cell mitogens*

Mitogens	F$_1$♀		F$_1$♂	
	Saline	Thymosin	Saline	Thymosin
Control	428 ± 32	486 ± 41	228 ± 11	741 ± 18
PHA-P	8,014 ± 349	12,412 ± 789	9,336 ± 406	12,992 ± 563
Con A	12,339 ± 609	136,432 ± 6,332	18,442 ± 2,121	22,295 ± 1,323
LPS	1,024 ± 86	1,139 ± 241	129 ± 39	158 ± 14
poly I · C	2,215 ± 118	3,418 ± 132	246 ± 22	211 ± 18

feel this is strong evidence that a B cell, null cell, or yet another type of cell is involved in this phenomenon since no abnormalities in T-cell function have been associated with chronic anti-μ treatment (14).

We have also pursued these studies in an X-linked B-deficient mouse strain—the CBA/N. Parental and (CBA/N ♀ × DBA/2 ♂) F$_1$ male mice show a decreased number of Ig$^+$ lymphocytes, do not respond to certain thymic-independent antigens such as DNP-lys-Ficoll, and respond relatively poorly to B-cell mitogens, the response of F$_1$ female being normal (1,16,18).

This B-cell defect has been attributed to a stem cell deficiency in B-cell maturation (17). Groups of adult thymectomized (CBA/N × DBA/2)F$_1$ male and female mice[1] were treated with thymosin fraction 5 as described and their lymph node cells assayed for response to Con A. As seen in Table 6, the thymosin-treated F$_1$ female lymph node cells exhibited a markedly augmented Con A response, whereas the increase in the response of the thymosin-treated male cells was minimal. These data provide further evidence that the spleen is important as a source of a precursor cell that responds to thymosin stimulation, and is not acting as a reserve pool of Con A-responsive cells, since gross T-

---

[1] Thymectomy was performed on these mice in order to ensure a rise in Con A responsiveness would be observed following thymosin treatment.

cell defects are not evident in the F_1 male mice (16). Interestingly, however, the data also indicate that it is either a B cell or an as-yet-not-characterized cell that is deficient in the F_1 male that is the target of the thymosin activity leading to the augmented Con A response.

Concurrent Hormonal and Antigenic Activity of DNP$_5$-Thymosin

In the course of these studies, we became interested in the possibility that injection of thymus-deficient mice with haptenated derivatives of thymosin followed by subsequent assay for antihapten PFC could serve as an assay for the maturation of T-helper cells. Thus a number of such experiments were performed with Nu/Nu mice and control Nu/+ littermates, and a representative sample of the results is shown in Table 7. From this experiment, it is clear that the DNP$_5$-thymosin is a potent immunogen for both 19S and 7S responses in normal and athymic mice. We have recently confirmed this data in AT X Bm mice, and subsequent studies have shown that the response is not polyclonal nor is it T independent, but rather reflects T-cell maturation. Thus in Nu/Nu mice haptenated thymosin preparations can act antigenically and also induce T-cell maturation.

Induction of Cell Surface Markers *In Vitro*

In view of our previously published results where *in vitro* incubation of bone marrow cells with a thymus preparation led to the acquisition of T-cell mitogen responsiveness, we anticipated a need for a similar *in vitro* system to investigate maturation of T-cell surface markers. Therefore we began a series of experiments utilizing the system of Komura and Boyse (11) to look for per cent increase in θ^+ and Ly$^+$ phenotypes following incubation with thymosin. Bone marrow cells from Nu/Nu mice and their normal littermates were separated on discontinuous BSA gradients as described and incubated with thymosin, but for reasons unclear at the present time, it was difficult to demonstrate an increase in per cent θ^+ cells. In other experiments with C57BL/6 spleen cells, however, phenotypic conversion of Ly$^-$ to Ly$^+$ was observed. As seen in Table 8, the cells in layers A and B show increases in Ly 1^+ and Ly 2^+, 3^+ cells in response to thymosin, but not to the spleen extract. That this increase is not cumulative (% Ly 1^+ + % Ly 2^+, $3^+ \neq$ % Ly 1^+ + Ly 2^+, 3^+) probably reflects conversion of the majority of the cells to the Ly 1^+, 2^+, 3^+ phenotype, which has been postulated by Cantor to precede the Ly 1^+ and Ly 2^+, 3^+ phenotype in T-cell ontogeny (6). The changes occurring in layers C and D as a result of incubation in thymosin do not, however, conform to his model of T-cell maturation, i.e., Ly 1^-, 2^-, $3^- \rightarrow$ Ly 1^+, 2^+, $3^+ \rightarrow$ either Ly 1^+, or Ly 2^+, 3^+. Rather it seems that conversion of Ly $1^+ \rightarrow$ Ly 1^+, 2^+, 3^+ occurs. We have repeated this experiment several times, and the data have been consistent with that shown in Table 8. Therefore we are pursuing these studies further in an effort to resolve this apparent conflict.

TABLE 7. Kinetics of the response of Nu/+ and Nu/Nu mice to DNP-thymosin

Days after immunization	D-PFC/spleen		I-PFC/spleen	
	Nu/+	Nu/Nu	Nu/+	Nu/Nu
Saline control	900 ± 220	1,093 ± 633	281 ± 191	493 ± 377
Day 3	9,581 ± 4,290	6,575 ± 2,057	4,162 ± 1,599	2,293 ± 1,164
Day 4	30,287 ± 4,191	39,225 ± 2,216	19,893 ± 2,419	20,737 ± 1,434
Day 5	67,700 ± 7,801	35,200 ± 8,742	35,475 ± 2,933	17,750 ± 1,087
Day 6	61,012 ± 7,083	38,131 ± 11,318	36,750 ± 6,001	24,375 ± 3,326
Day 7	22,087 ± 2,676	28,631 ± 4,993	29,850 ± 3,486	20,437 ± 203

TABLE 8. *Differentiation of C57BL/6 splenic T lymphocytes into Ly phenotypes by incubation with thymosin (fraction 5)*

	Antisera C+	Gradient layers			
		A	B	C	D
	Anti-Ly 1.2	3.8	4.4	41.5	37.7
Thymosin	Anti-Ly 1.2	21.1	25.6	43.0	46.8
Spleen extract	Anti-Ly 1.2	1.6	4.2	38.6	45.4
	Anti-Ly 2.2 or 3.2	1.5	3.2	12.4	6.9
Thymosin	Anti-Ly 2.2 or 3.2	22.7	25.9	46.0	49.1
Spleen extract	Anti-Ly 2.2 or 3.2	0.8	2.8	10.1	7.4
	Anti-Ly 1 + Anti-Ly 2, 3	3.4	5.3	40.7	49.1
Thymosin	Anti-Ly + Anti-Ly 2, 3	24.4	29.4	39.2	51.4
Spleen extract	Anti-Ly 1 + Anti-Ly 2, 3	2.6	1.4	38.6	48.9

DISCUSSION

The primary feature of any assay procedure used to detect thymic hormonal activity must be that the activity actually detected by the assay is indeed compatible with that specified by the properties of the hormone. Our present studies of the augmented lymph node cell response to Con A following thymosin treatment therefore shed some doubt about the utility of this procedure alone as an assay for thymic hormonal activity. The data clearly indicate that a functional spleen is necessary for the increased Con A response following thymosin administration (Tables 2 and 3) and that, furthermore, another type of stem cell or mature lymphoid cell that is not a T cell is required. This latter conclusion is supported by the data obtained with the anti-μ-treated (Table 5) and (CBA/N $\times$ DBA/2)F_1 male mice (Table 6). Both groups of mice are clearly deficient in B-cell function (14,16,18), and at present we are unaware of any evidence suggesting that either their mature or precursor T cells are abnormal. In terms of the level of maturity at which their respective immune deficiencies are evident, it seems that those of the CBA/N appears earlier in lymphocyte development. We base this conclusion on the following observations: (a) bone marrow reconstitution of irradiated male or female F_1 hosts with F_1 male cells produces mice that are phenotypically male (I. Scher, *personal communication,* 18); (b) X-irradiated male or female F_1 mice reconstituted with female bone marrow are phenotypically female (I. Scher, *personal communication*); and (c) irradiated mice reconstituted with syngeneic bone marrow from chronically anti-μ-treated mice are phenotypically normal (15).

These observations also indicated that splenic functions in F_1 male mice are normal, and therefore are not the cause for their unaugmented lymph node cell response to Con A. Since the effects of chronic anti-μ treatment on splenic function are not well characterized, it is possible that some loss of this organ's integrity associated with anti-μ treatment is responsible for the refractory lymph node cell response to Con A, although at present we favor the alternative explanation that the B-cell defect *per se* is responsible.

The dependence of the thymosin-induced augmentation of the lymph node cell response to Con A on an intact spleen is shown by the experiments with splenectomized (Tables 2 and 3) and congenitally asplenic (Table 4) mice. Furthermore, it seems that it is the microenvironmental aspects of the spleen that are important. If the spleen were serving as a storage depot for cells that become Con A responsive following thymosin treatment, one would expect that splenectomized mice could then be reconstituted by intravenous injection of normal spleen cells; however, in a preliminary experiment, we found such treatment did not enhance the Con A response. Thus we believe that some form of processing by the spleen is necessary for the cell to be induced by thymosin.

If, as has been suggested by these experiments, thymosin has the capacity to convert B cells into Con A-responsive cells, it may be that commitment of stem cells into B-lymphocyte development is not an irreversible step. Before such a notion can be seriously entertained, however, it is important to establish that other T-cell characteristics are acquired by lymph node cells following thymosin treatment and that such acquisition is sensitive to splenectomy and anti-μ treatment and does not occur in asplenic or (CBA/N $\times$ DBA/2)F_1 male mice.

The studies of the response of Nu/Nu mice to DNP_5-thymosin imply that this antigen can be used to investigate maturation of helper T cells *in vivo,* provided that the response to DNP_5-thymosin is truly T dependent. Thus far our data from subsequent studies support this proposition. Both male and female (CBA/N $\times$ DBA/2)F_1 mice respond vigorously to DNP_5-thymosin in anti-DNP plaque assays, whereas it has previously been shown that the F_1 male mice are very deficient in their response to T-independent antigens (18). In addition, this preparation is not mitogenic for normal spleen cells *in vitro* and does prime for a secondary response in both Nu/Nu and Nu/+ mice. Therefore we feel that experiments performed with this antigen may be useful in elucidating the mechanism of helper T-cell maturation.

Our results obtained in the conversion of Ly phenotype *in vitro* agree with those reported by Komuro and Boyse (11) in describing their system of T-cell surface marker maturation, in that for layers A and B of the gradient, roughly 20% of the cells become Ly 1$^+$. However, although they did not report data for the C and D gradient layers, we found an increase in the percentage of cells sensitive to anti-Ly 2, 3, but no increase in the percentage of cells sensitive to anti-Ly 1 or in the cumulative percentage (Ly 1 + Ly 2, 3). This result can only be interpreted in terms of a conversion from Ly 1$^+$, 2$^-$, 3$^-$ to Ly 1$^+$, 2$^+$, 3$^+$. Such a conversion is inconsistent with the system of Ly maturation described by Cantor (6, see results) and can only be reconciled with his model by postulating that a dedifferentiation of Ly 1$^+$ cells occurs. At present we feel further investigation of this system is needed before it can be applied to general studies of T cell maturation, particularly with regard to changes in Ly phenotype.

ACKNOWLEDGMENTS

We wish to gratefully acknowledge the expert technical assistance of Robert Etter, the excellent editorial assistance of Betty J. Sylvester, and the gift of thymosin fraction 5 by Dr. A. L. Goldstein.

This work was supported by the Naval Medical Research and Development Command, Work Unit Nos. MR041.02.01.0034 and MR041.02.01.0039. The opinions or assertions contained herein are the private ones of the authors and are not to be construed as official or reflecting the views of the U.S. Navy Department or the naval service at large. The experiments reported herein were conducted according to the principles set forth in the *Guide for the Care and Use of Laboratory Animals,* Institute of Laboratory Animal Resources, National Research Council, DHEW Pub. No. (NIH) 74–23.

REFERENCES

1. Ahmed, A., and Scher, I. (1976): Studies on non-H-2 linked lymphocyte activating determinants. II. Non-expression of Mls determinants in a mouse strain with an X-linked B-lymphocyte immune defect. *J. Immunol.,* 117:1922–1926.
2. Ahmed, A., Scher, I., and Sell, K. W. (1977): Studies on non-H-2 linked lymphocyte activating determinants. IV. Ontogeny of the Mls product on murine B cells *(submitted for publication).*
3. Ahmed, A., Smith, A. H., Sell, K. W., Gershwin, M. E., Steinberg, A. D., and Goldstein, A. L. (1977): Thymic-dependent anti-hapten response in congenitally athymic (nude) mice immunized with DNP thymosin *(submitted for publication).*
4. Bach, J. F., and Dardenne, M. (1973): Studies on thymus products. II. Demonstration and characterization of a circulating thymic hormone. *Immunology,* 25:353–366.
5. Basch, R. S., and Goldstein, G. (1974): Induction of T-cell differentiation *in vitro* by thymin, a purified polypeptide hormone of the thymus. *Proc. Natl. Acad. Sci. USA,* 71:1474–1478.
6. Cantor, H., and Boyse, E. A. (1975): Functional classes of T lymphocytes bearing different Ly antigens. I. The generation of functionally distinct T cell subclasses is a differentiative process independent of antigen. *J. Exp. Med.,* 141:1376–1389.
7. Friedman, H. (editor) (1975): *Ann. N.Y. Acad. Sci.,* 249:1–547.
8. Gershwin, M. E., Ahmed, A., Steinberg, A. D., Thurman, G. B., and Goldstein, A. L. (1974): Correction of T cell function by thymosin in New Zealand mice. *J. Immunol.,* 113:1068–1071.
9. Goldstein, A. L., Slater, F. D., and White, A. (1966): Preparation, assay, and partial purification of a thymic lymphocytopoietic factor (thymosin). *Proc. Natl. Acad. Sci. USA,* 56:1010–1017.
10. Goldstein, A. L., and White, A. (1973): Thymosin and other thymic hormones: Their nature and roles in the thymic dependency of immunological phenomena. In: *Contemporary Topics in Immunobiology,* Vol. 2, edited by A. J. S. Davies and R. L. Carter, pp. 339–350. Plenum Publ., New York.
11. Komuro, K., and Boyse, F. A. (1973): *In vitro* demonstration of thymic hormone in the mouse by conversion of precursor cells into lymphocytes. *Lancet,* 1:740–743.
12. Kook, A. I., and Trainin, N. (1974): Hormone-like activity of a thymus humoral factor on the induction of immune competence in lymphoid cells. *J. Exp. Med.,* 139:193–207.
13. Little, J. R., and Eisen, H. N. (1967): Preparation of immunogenic 2,4-dinitrophenyl and 2,4,6-trinitrophenyl proteins. In: *Methods in Immunology and Immunochemistry. Vol. I. Preparation of Antigens and Antibodies,* edited by C. A. Williams and W. C. Merrill, pp. 128–132. Academic Press, New York.
14. Manning, D. D. (1975): Heavy chain isotype suppression: A review of the immunosuppressive effects of heterologous anti-Ig heavy chain antisera. *J. Reticuloendothel. Soc.,* 18:63–86.
15. Manning, D. D., and Jutila, J. W. (1972): Immunosuppression of mice injected with heterologous anti-immunoglobulin heavy chain antisera. *J. Exp. Med.,* 135:1316–1333.
16. Scher, I., Ahmed, A., Strong, D. M., Steinberg, A. D., and Paul, W. E. (1975): X-linked B-

lymphocyte immune defect in CBA/HN mice. I. Studies of the function and composition of spleen cells. *J. Exp. Med.,* 141:788–803.

17. Scher, I., Sharrow, S. O., and Paul, W. E. (1976): X-linked B-lymphocyte defect in CBA/N mice. III. Abnormal development of B-lymphocyte populations defined by their density of surface immunoglobulin. *J. Exp. Med.,* 144:507–518.

18. Scher, I., Steinberg, A. D., Berning, A. K., and Paul, W. E. (1975): X-linked B-lymphocyte immune defect in CBA/N mice. II. Studies of the mechanisms underlying the immune defect. *J. Exp. Med.,* 142:637–650.

19. Scher, I., Strong, D. M., Ahmed, A., Knudsen, R. C., and Sell, K. W. (1973): Specific murine B-cell activation by synthetic single- and double-stranded polynucleotides. *J. Exp. Med.,* 138:1545–1563.

20. Selgrade, M. K., Ahmed, A., Sell, K. W., Gershwin, M. E., and Steinberg, A. D. (1976): Effect of murine cytomegalovirus on the *in vitro* responses of T and B cells to mitogens. *J. Immunol.,* 116:1459–1465.

21. Strong, D. M., Ahmed, A., Scher, I., Knudsen, R. C., and Sell, K. W. (1975): Specificity of *in vitro* murine B cell activation by protein and polysaccharide polymers. *J. Immunol.,* 113:1429–1437.

22. Thurman, G. B., Ahmed, A., Strong, D. M., Gershwin, M. E., Steinberg, A. D., and Goldstein, A. L. (1975): Thymosin-induced increase in mitogenic responsiveness of lymphocytes of C57BL/6J, NZB/W, and nude mice. *Trans. Proc.,* 7(Suppl. 1):299–303.

23. Woody, J. N., Ahmed, A., Strong, D. M., and Sell, K. W. (1972): Effect of calf thymus extracts on mouse bone marrow cells. In: *Proc. 7th Leukocyte Culture Conf.,* pp. 513–522. Academic Press, New York.

Immune Modulation and Control of Neoplasia by Adjuvant Therapy, edited by M. A. Chirigos. Raven Press, New York, 1978.

In Vitro and *In Vivo* Studies with Thymosin

Michael A. Chirigos

Laboratory of RNA Tumor Viruses, National Cancer Institute, National Institutes of Health, Bethesda, Maryland 20014

In recent years, the application of nonspecific immune stimulators, when used alone or combined with other forms of therapy to augment host immunity, suggests that immunological control measures are valuable adjuncts to the control of neoplasia.

Bacillus Calmette-Guérin affords protection against tumors induced with chemicals or viral-transplantable cells and inhibits viral oncogenesis. Bacillus Calmette-Guérin has also been reported effective in controlling human leukemias and malignant melanomas.

The use of chemicals known to stimulate cellular or humoral immune responses (1,6,7,13) has not been investigated to a great extent to determine the effect of the chemicals when used in concert with chemotherapy in the treatment of leukemia. Levamisole (LMS) reportedly has a stimulatory effect on antibacterial immunization (8), on antibody-forming cells (10), and in enhancing the graft-versus-host reaction (9). Of particular significance are the reports of LMS acting as an immunostimulant in man (2,5,12,14). We recently reported the beneficial effect of LMS when used in concert with an effective remission-inducing drug (3,4). The results of these studies showed that with the murine LSTRA and MCAs-10 transplantable lymphoid leukemias, when LMS was used following one administration of 1,3-bis (2-chloroethyl)-1-nitrosourea (BCNU), a significantly higher percentage of long-term survivors was attained.

In the present study we employed the LSTRA lymphoid leukemia and determined the effect of thymosin when used in combination with BCNU or cyclophosphamide (Cytoxan®).

MATERIALS AND METHODS

Animals

Adult BALB/c $\times$ DBA/2 (hereafter called CD2F$_1$) male mice, 6 to 8 weeks old, were supplied by the Mammalian Genetics and Animal Production Section, Division of Cancer Treatment, National Cancer Institute, NIH, Bethesda, Md. The animals were housed in plastic cages and fed Purina laboratory chow with water *ad libitum*. All animals weighed at least 23 g before they were used for experimentation.

Tumor

A Moloney lymphoid leukemia (LSTRA), originally induced in BALB/c mice by the Moloney murine leukemia virus, has been maintained and passaged routinely in our laboratory as a transplantable tumor line for over 320 generations in $CD2F_1$ mice. The ascitic tumor is serially transplanted intraperitoneally at weekly intervals.

Drugs

BCNU and cyclophosphamide were kindly supplied by The Drug Synthesis and Chemistry Branch, Division of Cancer Treatment, National Cancer Institute, NIH, Bethesda, Md. BCNU was dissolved in hydroxypropyl cellulose (0.3% solution), and cyclophosphamide was dissolved in phosphate-buffered saline and administered intraperitoneally in a constant volume of 0.01 ml/g of body weight.

Thymosin (calf thymus extract, fraction 5) was kindly supplied by A.L. Goldstein, University of Texas Medical Branch, Galveston, Tex.

Macrophage-Mediated Cytoxicity

The method for measuring the cytotoxic activity of purified peritoneal macrophages has been previously reported (11). Briefly, 10^4 labeled target cells in 100 μl aliquots were plated into wells of no. 3040 Microtest II Plates (Falcon Plastics, Oxnard, Cal.). One hundred microliter aliquots containing 5.0×10^5 peritoneal macrophages were added to quadruplicate wells; effector-to-target cell ratios were therefore 50:1. Spontaneous release was determined from wells that contained only target cells. The plates were incubated at 37°C for 16 hr in a 5% CO_2-in-air atmosphere. Following this incubation, the plates were centrifuged (1,000 rpm for 10 min), and radioactivity was measured in the cell-free supernatant. One hundred microliters of supernatant fluid from each well was placed into a disposable vial and counted in a Beckman Biogamma Spectrometer.

RESULTS

Table 1 contains the results when thymosin was combined with a single or two-drug combination. All nontreated tumor control mice died with a median survival time (MST) of 12 days. Treatment with BCNU resulted in a 100% increase in MST and a 10% survival rate. Cyclophosphamide treatment alone resulted in only a 40% increase in MST. Combined treatment with BCNU and cyclophosphamide provided a substantially higher number of survivors and

TABLE 1. *Response of LSTRA to multiple drug treatment and thymosin*

Group no.	LSTRA[a] (1 × 10⁴)	BCNU[b] (30 mg/kg)	Cyclophosphamide[b] (100 mg/kg)	Thymosin[c]		MST (days)	Range of death	Survival[d] (%)
				10 µg	50 µg			
1	D0	—	—	—	—	12	12–13	0
2	D0	D10	—	—	—	24	20 > 60	10
3	D0	—	D14	—	—	17	14–19	0
4	D0	D10	D14	—	—	28	22 > 60	25
5	D0	D10	D14	D19	—	32	24 > 60	36
6	D0	D10	D14	—	D26	36	26 > 60	38
7	D0	D10	D14	D19 & D26	—	37	28 > 60	32
8	D0	D10	D14	—	D19 & D26	60	29 > 60	50

D, day; MST, median survival time.
[a] LSTRA tumor cells injected s.c. in the right inguinal area.
[b] Administered i.p.
[c] Administered i.p., dose per mouse.
[d] Survival based on 60-day observation period.

a 133% increase in MST indicating the effectiveness of combined drug treatment. Employing the combined drug treatment, thymosin at two doses and at different time intervals was tested for its adjuvant effect. In every case where thymosin was employed, an enhanced MST and survival rate was achieved. The most significant effect occurred when thymosin was administered at the 50 μg dose on days 19 and 26. Considering the fact that treatment with BCNU and/or cyclophosphamide was withheld until systemic leukemia was established and that death, in untreated controls, occurred within 2 to 3 days after chemotherapy, the combined chemotherapy-adjuvant effect was impressive.

It was anticipated that if a lower inoculum of tumor cells were employed the chemoimmunoadjuvant effect could be enhanced since there would be a lower tumor burden present at the time of treatment (Table 2). Indeed, a higher percentage of cures and a longer MST was attained than in previous experiments when a 1×10^4 inoculum was used (Table 1). Thymosin adjuvant provided a higher percentage of long-term survivors and a significant increase in MST. It was particularly interesting that thymosin was effective when administered as late as 8 days after chemotherapy. It appears that if thymosin treatment is delayed longer than 8 days, a decrease in effectiveness occurs. There was only a 15% increase in survival over the BCNU-treated controls when thymosin treatment was delayed until 11 days after chemotherapy.

Results in Table 3 show the effect of different regimens of thymosin treatment in animals bearing different tumor burdens. In each case, 10^4 or 10^5 cell inoculum BCNU treatment was withheld until systemic leukemia was established. As the result of BCNU treatment, 30% survival rate occurred in mice inoculated with 10^4 cells in contrast to only a 10% survival rate in mice inoculated with 10^5 cells. Accordingly, a much better response was achieved with thymosin adjuvant treatment in mice with the initial lower tumor burden (10^4). Several deaths were attributable to toxicity in animals receiving daily or every-other-day treatment of thymosin. The most effective thymosin regimen in animals inoculated with 10^4 tumor cells receiving initial BCNU treatment was when thymosin was administered every 3 or 4 days (groups 9–12) for a total of five treatments. However, a single treatment was also effective (group 13). A clear

TABLE 2. *Effect of combined single treatment with thymosin and BCNU—low tumor load*

Group	LSTRA (1×10^3)	BCNU (30 mg/kg)	Thymosin (μg/kg)	Survival[a] (%)	MST (days)
1	D0			0	14
2	D0	D7		40	35
3	D0	D7	100, D8	60	>70
4	D0	D7	100, D11	70	>70
5	D0	D7	100, D13	70	>70
6	D0	D7	100, D15	70	>70
7	D0	D7	100, D18	55	>70

[a] Survival based on 70-day observation period.

TABLE 3. *Relationship of LSTRA tumor load and BCNU treatment to regimen of thymosin treatment*

Group no.	Dose (μg/mouse)	Thymosin[a] regimen	No. of treatment	10⁴ Cell inoculum			10⁵ Cell inoculum		
				Toxicity death	Tumor death	Survival (%)	Toxicity death	Tumor death	Survival (%)
1					100[b]	0		100[b]	0
2					70[c]	30		90[c]	10
3	10	ED	5	10	80	10	20	40	40[d]
4	25	ED	5	—	90	10	20	70	10[d]
5	50	ED	5	—	100	0	30	60	10
6	100	ED	5	10	80	10	10	90	0
7	50	EOD	5	20	60	20[d]	30	40	30[d]
8	100	EOD	5	10	90	0[d]	10	80	10
9	50	E3D	5	0	70	30[d]	30	60	10
10	100	E3D	5	0	60	40[d]	20	70	10
11	50	E4D	5	0	20	80[d]	30	70	10[d]
12	100	E4D	5	10	20	70[d]	20	80	0
13	100	1×wk	1	0	70	30[d]	0	100	0

[a] Thymosin treatment began on D12 (5 days after BCNU); ED, every day; EOD, every other day; E3D, every third day; E4D, every fourth day; 1×wk, once a week.
[b] Untreated tumor controls.
[c] Tumored mice receiving BCNU treatment alone 7 days after tumor inoculation (D7).
[d] Median survival time greater than controls (25% or greater).

TABLE 4. *Measurement of macrophage-mediated cytotoxicity by ^{51}Cr release*

Host injection		Percent specific ^{51}Cr release
Tumor (1×10^7)	Thymosin $(\mu g/kg)$	
+	—	6
—	100	2
—	50	0
+	100	48
+	50	37

Macrophage: target cell ratio of 50 : 1.

distinction cannot be drawn between the 50 or 100 μg doses employed. It appears that each was equally effective. Both the chemotherapeutic and adjuvant effects were sharply diminished when a greater tumor burden was present (10^5). It appears that although there were a greater number of toxicity deaths occurring with the multiple thymosin treatment schedules (groups 3 to 12), treatment with thymosin every day or every other day (groups 3, 4, and 7) was more beneficial. Despite the toxicity observed with multiple thymosin treatments in both the 10^4 or 10^5 inoculated groups, a significant increase in survival and MST was achieved than attained with BCNU treatment alone.

It has been reported that several immunoadjuvants augment specific macrophage-mediated cytotoxicity. Results in Table 4 show that when macrophages were harvested from nontumored mice receiving 100 or 200 μg/kg of thymosin no enhanced macrophage cytotoxicity was observed. However, in tumored mice that received thymosin 6 days after tumor inoculation, enhanced macrophage cytotoxicity was attained. These results indicate that thymosin markedly potentiated the specific tumoricidal action of armed macrophages from a value of 6 to 37 through 48%.

DISCUSSION

In all studies where thymosin was employed as an adjuvant to chemotherapy, a prolongation of life-span and increase in the survival rate were attained. Considering that chemotherapeutic agents are immunosuppressive and treatment with immunoadjuvants when administered too soon after chemotherapy may be counterproductive, the present experimental results indicate that thymosin was maximally effective when administered 4 to 5 days after chemotherapy and effective as late as 8 days after.

Employing three different tumor cell inoculum levels, the present results indicate that the tumor burden present in the host at the time of adjuvant treatment may be critical. This is understandable in that if the cellular immune response is responsible for the prolongation in survival time and higher percent of survivors, the responding immune cells are better capable of eliminating a smaller number of cells. This can be accomplished only by decreasing the number of tumor cells through chemotherapy, as demonstrated in the present studies, or through surgery or irradiation.

The observation that macrophages from tumored animals treated with thymosin demonstrated enhanced tumoricidal activity implies that thymosin was causing activation of macrophages. However, a ratio of 50 macrophages to 1 target tumor cell was required to produce the 37 to 48% cytolysis.

Of particular interest is the observation that thymosin was an effective adjuvant when combined with one or two chemotherapeutic drugs, because chemotherapy regimens for cancer treatment consist of two-to four-drug combinations.

SUMMARY

Thymosin was found to enhance the chemotherapeutic response attained in leukemic mice. When used in concert with one or two chemotherapeutic agents, significant increases in survival rate and life prolongation were attained. Thymosin was found to be most beneficial when the tumor burden was significantly reduced and when used within 5 to 7 days after chemotherapy. When used in different treatment regimens and different doses, the results indicate that a single treatment may be as effective as multiple treatment and that thymosin is effective at a dose of 100 μg/kg.

REFERENCES

1. Braun, W., Regelson, W., Yajima, T., and Ishizuka, M. (1970): Stimulation of antibody formation by pyran copolymer. *Proc. Soc. Exp. Biol. Med.,* 133:171–175.
2. Brugmans, J., Schuermans, V., De Cock, W., Theinpoint, D., Janssen, P., Verhaegen, H., Van Nimmer, L., Louewagie, A. C., and Stevens, E. (1973): Resistance of host defense mechanisms in man by levamisole. *Life Sci.,* 13:1499–1504.
3. Chirigos, M. A., Pearson, J. W., and Pryor, J. (1973): Augmentation of chemotherapeutically induced remission of a murine leukemia by a chemical immunoadjuvant. *Cancer Res.,* 33:2615–2618.
4. Chirigos, M. A., Fuhrman, F., and Pryor, J. (1975): Prolongation of chemotherapeutically induced remission of a syngeneic murine leukemia by L-2, 3, 5, 6-tetrahydro-6-phenylimidazo [2,1-b]thiazole hydrochloride. *Cancer Res.,* 35:927–931.
5. Churchill, W. H., and David, J. R. (1973): Editorial: Levamisole and cell-mediated immunity. *N. Engl. J. Med.,* 289:375–379.
6. Kapila, K., Smith, D., and Rubin, A. A. (1971): Effect of pyran copolymer on phagocytosis and tumor growth. *RES J. Reticuloendothel. Soc.,* 9:447–450.
7. Munson, A. E., Munson, J. A., Regelson, W., and Wampler, G. L. (1974): Effects of tilorone hydrochloride and congeners on reticuloendothelial system, tumors, and the immune response. *Cancer Res.,* 32:1397–1403.
8. Renoux, G., and Renoux, M. (1971): Immunologie. Effect immunstimulant d'un imidothiazole dans l'immunisation des souris contre l'infection par Brucella abortus. *Compt. Rend.,* 272:349–350.
9. Renoux, G., and Renoux, M. (1972): Action du phynylimidothiazole (tetramisole) sur la reaction du graffon contre l'hote. Role des macrophages. *Compt. Rend.,* 274:3320–3323.
10. Renoux, G., and Renoux, M. (1972): Immunologie. Action Immunostimulant de derives du phynylimidothiazole sur le cellules splenigues tormatrices d'anticorps. *Compt. Rend.,* 274:756–757.

11. Schultz, R. M., Papamatheakis, J. D., Stylos, W. A., and Chirigos, M. A. (1976): Augmentation of specific macrophage-mediate cytotoxicity: Correlation with agents which enhance antitumor resistance. *Cell. Immunol.,* 25:309–316.

12. Tripodi, D., Parks, L. C., and Brugmans, J. (1973): Drug induced restoration of cutaneous delayed hypersensitivity in anergic patients with cancer. *N. Engl. J. Med.,* 289:354–358.

13. Turner, W., Chan, S. P., and Chirigos, M. A. (1970): Stimulation of humoral and cellular antibody formation in mice with Poly I:C. *Proc. Soc. Exp. Biol. Med.,* 133:334–338.

14. Verhaegen, H., DeCree, J., De Cock, W., and Verbruggen, F. (1973): Lavamisole and the immune response. *N. Engl. J. Med.,* 289:1148–1149.

Immune Modulation and Control of Neoplasia by Adjuvant Therapy, edited by M. A.
Chirigos. Raven Press, New York, 1978.

Thymocyte-Mitogen Bioassay for Thymosin

Patrick W. Trown, Carol Lewinski, Phyllis L. Meyer, Alicia V.
Palleroni, and Oksana Krochak

Department of Chemotherapy, Hoffmann-La Roche Inc., Nutley, New Jersey 07110

Extracts of the thymus gland have been shown to act on thymus-derived cells (T cells) in their early stages of maturity and confer on them an increased capacity to participate in immune reactions (2,6). One manifestation of this increased T-cell function is a greater ability to react to T-cell mitogens, such as phytohemagglutinin (PHA) and concanavalin A (Con A). An increased response to Con A and PHA has been reported after exposure of lymphoid cells to thymic humoral factor (5), the Bach thymic factor (3), and thymopoietin (1). This phenomenon is also observed with thymosin, as shown in Fig. 1. In this case, the cells were rat thymocytes that had been preincubated with thymosin for 24 hr prior to a 48-hr incubation with Con A at various concentrations. The mitogenic activity was quantitated via a ^{3}H-thymidine pulse during the last 24 hr of the incubation. A stimulation of the incorporation of ^{3}H-thymidine into the DNA of thymocytes preincubated with thymosin compared to controls was observed over a wide range of concentrations of Con A. Maximum incorporation of ^{3}H-thymidine was observed at 20 μg/ml Con A, which was chosen as the standard concentration for development of an assay.

The assay, which we have named the thymocyte-mitogen (or TM) assay, is sufficiently reliable for use in quality control of thymosin for clinical trials. The TM assay procedure is outlined in Fig. 2 and described below.

ASSAY PROCEDURE

The thymus gland is removed aseptically from a 30 to 50 g, male, Fischer F-344 rat (Charles River). A cell suspension is prepared by forcing the gland through a 140-μm stainless steel screen (Cistron Corp., Elmsford, N.Y.) into a Petri dish containing RPMI 1640 (Flow Laboratories, Rockville, Md.) supplemented with 2% human A (Rh$-$) heat-inactivated serum, 25 mM N-2-hydroxyethylpiperazine-N'-2-ethanesulfonic acid (HEPES: Calbiochem., La Jolla, Cal.), 6 mM glutamine, 0.06% NaHCO$_3$, 100 IU/ml penicillin, 100 μg/ml streptomycin, and 25 μg/ml amphotericin B (Fungizone®) (RPMI-2%). The suspension is filtered by gravity through a Swinnex filter holder (Millipore Corp., Bedford, Mass.), containing a 105-μm stainless steel screen, attached to a 10-ml syringe.

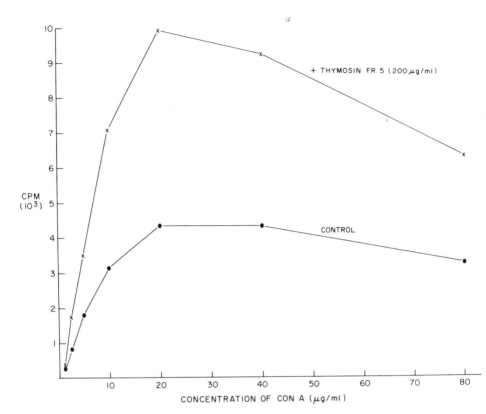

FIG. 1. Effects of thymosin on response of rat thymocytes to Con A.

The filtered suspension, in a 15-ml conical tube, (Corning, Corning, N.Y.) is brought to 10 ml with RPMI-2%, and 0.15 M mercaptoethanol is added to a final concentration of 3×10^{-4}M.

The cells are centrifuged at 500 g for 5 min in a GLC-1 centrifuge (Sorvall, Norwalk, Conn.). The pelleted thymocytes are resuspended in 10 ml of RPMI-2% and counted in a Coulter Counter (Model ZBI, Coulter Electronics, Inc., Hialeah, Fla.). The suspension is adjusted with RPMI-2% to 1×10^7 cells/ ml, aliquoted into 16×125-mm tissue culture tubes (Corning), and pelleted as above.

Thymocytes in one tube are resuspended in RPMI modified as above but containing 10% human A (Rh—) serum (RPMI-10%) for a control, and the remaining cells are resuspended in solutions (in RPMI-10%) of a standard lot of thymosin and of test samples. The tubes are then incubated at 37°C for 24 hr in a 5% CO_2-air atmosphere.

After the incubation period, the thymocytes are pelleted, washed once with RPMI-10%, and resuspended in the original volume of medium. Then, 1×10^6 cells (in 100 μl) are dispensed into each well of a Microtest II plate (Falcon,

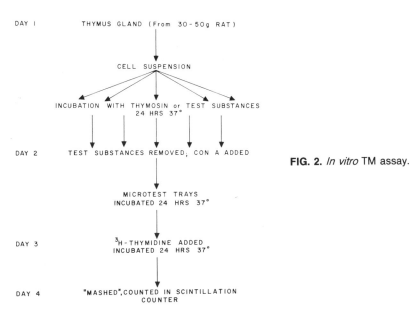

DAY I   THYMUS GLAND (From 30-50g RAT)

CELL SUSPENSION

INCUBATION WITH THYMOSIN or TEST SUBSTANCES
24 HRS 37°

DAY 2   TEST SUBSTANCES REMOVED; CON A ADDED

MICROTEST TRAYS
INCUBATED 24 HRS 37°

DAY 3   ³H-THYMIDINE ADDED
INCUBATED 24 HRS 37°

DAY 4   "MASHED", COUNTED IN SCINTILLATION
COUNTER

FIG. 2. *In vitro* TM assay.

Oxnard, Cal.) using a repeating dispenser (Hamilton, Reno, Nev.). Six replicates are done for each unknown; 12 for the control. A solution of Con A (Pharmacia, Inc., Piscataway, N.J.; 100 μl, 40 μg/ml in RPMI-10%) is added to each well (final concentration, 20 μg/ml), except three of the control wells, which receive 100 μl RPMI-10%. The trays are again incubated, and 24 hr later, 1 μCi of ³H-thymidine (40 to 60 Ci/mmole, New England Nuclear, Boston, Mass.) in 50 μl RPMI-10% is added to each well and the trays incubated for 24 hr.

The cells are harvested with 0.15 M NaCl onto glass fiber filters (934 AH, Reeve Angel, Clifton, N.J.) using the Multiple Automatic Sample Harvester (MASH II, Microbiological Associates, Bethesda, Md.). The filters are dried at 70°C, and the discs are put into scintillation vials containing 3 ml of 0.05% Butyl PBD (Yorktown Research, New Hyde, N.Y.) in toluene, and counted in a liquid scintillation counter.

ASSAY RESULTS

The increased capacity of rat thymocytes to respond to Con A following incubation with thymosin for 24 hr is expressed as a ratio of the mean cpm for the six wells treated with thymosin (T) divided by the mean cpm for the nine control wells (C). This ratio is called a stimulation index or T/C ratio. Results of a typical assay are shown in Table 1. BPM 390, a standard lot of thymosin, gave T/C ratios of 5.71, 4.52, and 2.33 at 200, 100, and 50 μg/ml, respectively. Unknown samples are always compared with the standard lot of thymosin in the same assay because the stimulation index for a standard lot of thymosin is variable from one assay to another. An empirical set of criteria

TABLE 1. *Results of a typical TM assay*

Sample	Concentration (μg/ml)	Mean cpm	Standard deviation	T/C ratio	Activity
Medium controls		242			
Con A controls		6,512 (C)	1,012		
BPM 390	200	35,685 (T)	2,295	5.71	
BPM 390	100	28,254 (T)	1,818	4.52	++
BPM 390	50	14,548 (T)	1,323	2.33	
Unknown 1	200	23,956 (T)	2,178	3.83	
Unknown 1	100	17,537 (T)	2,057	2.86	+
Unknown 1	50	16,282 (T)	1,964	2.60	
Unknown 2	200	6,076 (T)	1,044	0.97	
Unknown 2	100	7,669 (T)	1,547	1.22	−
Unknown 2	50	6,553 (T)	1,078	1.20	

T, treated; C, control.
Note: Criteria for Determination of Activity

1. The assay is acceptable only if the T/C value of BPM 390 at 200 μg/ml (defined as A) is >2.
2. The minimum T/C value for activity is 1.5, or 0.5A, whichever is greater.
3. Degree of activity of unknowns is determined as follows:

T/C		Activity
200 μg/ml	100 μg/ml	
<0.5A	<0.5A	−
0.5–0.9A	<0.5A	±
0.5–0.9A	>0.5A	+
>0.9A	>0.5A	++

BPM 390 is, by definition, ++ in every assay.

4. If the requirements for ++ in (item 3 above) are met at lower levels than described in (3), the unknown is rated +++.

has been established to judge the potency of an unknown preparation relative to the standard lot (see *Note* to Table 1). For example, in the assay shown in Table 1, *A,* the T/C ratio for the standard lot of thymosin, BPM 390 at 200 μg/ml, is 5.71. Therefore, unknown 1 is rated + because the T/C ratio at 200 μg/ml is 3.83, i.e., in the range 0.5 to 0.9*A* (2.86 to 5.14), and the T/C ratio at 100 μg/ml is 2.86, i.e., $\geq$ 0.5A (2.86). Unknown 2 is inactive because the T/C ratio at 200 μg/ml is less than 0.5*A* (2.86).

PARAMETERS AFFECTING THE RESPONSE OF THE ASSAY

The response of the TM assay to thymosin fraction 5 is dependent on the type of serum employed. Thus far we have not been able to obtain a stimulation of Con A responsiveness by thymosin using any of the commonly available animal sera. Only human sera support the thymosin stimulation, and the ability

TABLE 2. *Effects of different lots of serum on the response of the TM assay to thymosin (BPM 390)*

Donor	Blood type	Stimulation index (T/C) for BPM 390 at:		
		200 μg/ml	100 μg/ml	50 μg/ml
T. U.	A (Rh−)	2.1	1.8	
N. P.	O (Rh−)	1.7	1.5	
T. U.	A (Rh−)	2.2	2.5	
J. C.	A (Rh−)	1.5	1.1	
T. U.	A (Rh−)	2.6	1.9	
R. W.	B (Rh−)	1.6	1.4	
P. S.	A (Rh−)	2.5	2.0	1.9
M. F.	A (Rh−)	4.3	2.9	1.8
P. S.	A (Rh−)	3.0	2.6	2.3
T. S.	A (Rh−)	1.7	1.7	1.6
P. S.	A (Rh−)	5.1	4.3	3.0
R. D. S.	A (Rh−)	2.7	2.3	2.0

Note: Each donor's serum was tested against reference serum T.U. or P.S. using a single rat for the test. One lobe of the thymus was used for the reference serum and the other lobe for the test serum.

to do so seems to depend on the blood type of the donor (Table 2). On the basis of the data currently available, it appears that the sera of donors whose blood type is A (Rh−) most often support thymosin stimulation of Con A responsiveness in rat thymocytes. Not all A (Rh−) sera work; each lot of serum is, therefore, screened using a standard active lot of thymosin fraction 5 before being used in an assay. A T/C ratio of at least 2.0 at 200 μg/ml of the standard lot of thymosin is required before the lot is acceptable.

The results obtained in a given TM assay are also dependent on the particular rat used as the source of thymocytes (Table 3). The reasons for variability in response between individual rats are unknown and are under investigation.

The response of thymocytes to Con A in this assay is highly stimulated by endotoxin (lipopolysaccharide). A T/C ratio greater than 2 can be obtained with as little as 1 ng/ml. Therefore, test samples are routinely assayed for endotoxin content using the limulus lysate bioassay (4) and only tested in the

TABLE 3. *Variable responses of individual rats in TM assay*

Animal number	Stimulation index (T/C) for BPM 390 at:	
	200 μg/ml	100 μg/ml
1	3.2	2.9
2	2.1	2.5
3	2.8	2.3
4	5.6	5.3

Note: These four assays were carried out on the same day using the same batches of serum, medium, BPM 390, and Con A.

TM assay if the final concentration of endotoxin in the assay is less than 0.1 ng/ml.

REPRODUCIBILITY OF THE ASSAY

Only the standard lot of thymosin fraction 5, BPM 390 has been tested enough times to produce data on reproducibility of the assay. These results are shown in Table 4. The stimulation index for the standard lot is dependent on the particular donor used, and the standard deviations for the three levels of BPM 390 are high. This may be a result of the dependence of assay response on the particular rat used as the source of thymocytes. Nevertheless, the responses observed are clearly dose related, and useful data are obtainable from the assay.

TABLE 4. *Reproducibility of the TM assay with the standard lot of thymosin BPM 390*

Donor	Blood type	No. of assays	Stimulation index (T/C) at:		
			200 µg/ml	100 µg/ml	50 µg/ml
T.U.	A (Rh−)	9	2.46 (±0.89)[a]	2.02 (±0.55)	1.79 (±0.70)
P.S.	A (Rh−)	13	4.12 (±1.14)	3.21 (±0.82)	2.42 (±0.64)
T.U. + M.F.	A (Rh−)	7	4.04 (±2.11)	4.06 (±2.56)	2.23 (±1.31)
R.D.S. + P.S.	A (Rh−)	6	2.27 (±0.71)	1.82 (±0.15)	1.55 (±0.14)
Totals		35	3.36 (±1.50)	2.83 (±1.48)	2.07 (±0.83)

[a] ± Standard Deviation.

REFERENCES

1. Basch, R. S., and Goldstein, G. (1975): Thymopoietin-induced acquisition of responsiveness to T cell mitogens. *Cell. Immunol.,* 20:218–228.
2. Goldstein, A. L., and White, A. (1973): Thymosin and other thymic hormones. Their nature and roles in the thymic dependency of immunological phenomena. *Contemp. Top. Immunobiol.,* 2:339–350.
3. Kruisbeek, A. M. (1974): Summary of the results of the workshop. In: *Biological Activity of Thymic Hormones,* edited by D. W. van Bekkum, pp. 209–211. Kooyker Sci. Publ., Rotterdam.
4. Leven, J., and Bang, F. B. (1968): Clottable protein in Limulus; its localization and kinetics of its coagulation by endotoxin. *Thromb. Diath. Haemorrh.,* 19:186.
5. Rotter, V. (1974): The effect of THF on the reactivity of lymphoid cells to PHA and Con A. In: *Biological Activity of Thymic Hormones,* edited by D. V. van Bekkum, pp. 227–228. Kooyker Sci. Publ., Rotterdam.
6. Trainin, N. (1974): Thymic hormones and the immune response. *Physiol. Rev.,* 54:272–315.

Immune Modulation and Control of Neoplasia by Adjuvant Therapy, edited by M. A. Chirigos. Raven Press, New York, 1978.

In Vitro Induction of Human T-Cell Differentiation

Sheldon Horowitz

Division of Immunology, Department of Pediatrics, University of Wisconsin Center for Health Sciences, Madison, Wisconsin 53706

Various thymic factors have been reported to influence T-lymphocyte differentiation. Such factors include thymopoietin (10), thymosin (15), thymus humoral factor (21), and thymic factor (2). Incubation of putative stem cells with these thymus-derived factors has led to the appearance of T-cell surface markers (2,3,15,27) and/or T-cell functional responses (3,15,21,27). These thymic factors differ in their molecular weight, chemical composition, and potency. The best defined of these agents, thymopoietin, is a 49 amino acid polypeptide (28) that induces the rapid appearance of T-cell markers *in vitro*. The mode of action of these thymic factors has not been completely worked out; however, many studies suggest that these factors induce T-cell differentiation by activation of membrane adenyl cyclase via specific or nonspecific T-cell surface receptors leading to increased intracellular cyclic AMP (22,26,27).

In normal humans incubation of bone marrow cells with thymosin (18,31) or conditioned thymic medium (24) resulted in increased numbers of cells bearing T markers. In addition, putative stem cell fractions from normal human peripheral blood showed increased E-rosette formation following exposure to thymosin (32). Increased active rosette formation has also been noted following incubation of normal peripheral blood lymphocytes with thymosin (35). In some patients with immunodeficiency diseases, increased numbers of cells bearing T-cell markers were noted following incubation of peripheral blood or bone marrow cells with thymic factors (17,30,33).

The present experiments were undertaken to study the effect of various agents, including thymosin and cyclic nucleotides, on human lymphocyte differentiation. I found that the number of E-rosette-forming lymphocytes was significantly increased by incubation with thymosin or dibutyryl cyclic AMP in individuals with T-cell defects. In addition, these agents induced increased responsivity to phytohemagglutinin (PHA) in a child with a significant B- and T-cell defects. These studies also showed that putative stem cell fractions of normal peripheral blood form E-rosettes and display T-cell functional responses following incubation with thymosin or agents that increase cyclic AMP.

MATERIALS AND METHODS

Separation of Lymphocytes

Lymphocytes were separated from heparinized peripheral blood of normal adult human donors and immunodeficient patients by centrifugation on a Ficoll-Hypaque density gradient (4,29).

Fractionation of Cells on Bovine Serum Albumin Gradients

Gradients were prepared by modification of the method of Dicke as described by August et al. (1). Nine fractions were obtained—fraction 1 represented cells of the interface between 17 and 19% albumin, and fraction 9 those between 33 and 35% albumin.

In Vitro Incubation of Lymphocytes with Various Agents

Mononuclear cells obtained by Ficoll-Hypaque density gradient separation with or without subsequent bovine serum albumin (BSA) gradient fractionation were incubated with various agents for 90 min to 24 hr at 37°C, 5% CO_2 in air. These cells were then washed, the cell concentration adjusted, and B- and T-cell surface markers and T-cell functional responses studied.

The agents tested included calf thymosin fraction 5, kindly provided by Allan Goldstein, U. of Texas Medical Branch—Galveston, and cyclic AMP, O_2-dibutyryl-adenosine 3',5'-cyclic monophosphoric acid (DB cyclic AMP), guanosine 3',8 bromoguanosine 3',5' cyclic monophosphoric acid (8 Br cyclic GMP), aminophylline, L-isoproterenol, and bovine albumin, fraction 5, all provided by Sigma Chemical Co., St. Louis, Mo.

Identification of Cells

T lymphocytes were defined as those forming spontaneous rosettes with sheep red blood cells according to modifications of the methods of Jondal et al. (total E-rosettes) (20) and Wybran et al. (active E-rosettes) (34) as has been previously described (16). The mean value for total E-rosette-forming cells was $68.4 \pm 2.4\%$ and the mean for active E-rosette-forming cells was $24.3 \pm 4.8\%$.

B lymphocytes were defined by surface markers, including surface immunoglobulin and the Fc and C3 receptor. Surface immunoglobulin was detected by direct immunofluorescence using heavy (γ,μ,α) chain antisera prepared in our laboratory (16). The Fc receptor was detected by direct immunofluorescence using aggregated gamma globulin prepared according to the method of Dickler and Kunkel (8). Cells carrying receptors for complement were detected by the erythrocyte-antibody complement (EAC) rosette assay (25).

Monocytes were defined by morphology, latex uptake, and peroxidase staining

(23). Approximately 5 to 20% of the mononuclear cells were monocytes as defined by latex uptake and peroxidase staining. Null cells were defined as cells that did not bear B or T surface markers and were not monocytes.

In Vitro Lymphocyte Responses

The proliferative response of lymphocytes following PHA stimulation was evaluated by measuring [³H]thymidine incorporation. Following a 3-day incubation with PHA, lymphocytes were pulsed with [³H]thymidine (1 μCi/0.05 ml), harvested 12 hr later, and counted in a Packard 3375 liquid scintillation spectrometer.

The one-way mixed leukocyte culture (MLC) assay was performed according to the micromethod of Hartzman et al. (12). Stimulator cells were treated with mitomycin C; the proliferative response was measured by [³H]thymidine incorporation following a 5-day culture period.

Subjects

Patients with various immunodeficiency diseases were studied; individuals with no B- or T-cell function were defined as having combined immunodeficiency ($N = 4$), patients with no T-cell function but secreted (nonfunctional) immunoglobulin were defined as having cellular immunodeficiency with immunoglobulin ($N = 2$), patients with no or decreased T-cell function but relatively normal B-cell function were defined as having isolated T-cell deficiency ($N = 5$), patients with no functional antibody but normal T-cell function were defined as having B-cell deficiency ($N = 3$), and healthy adults were used as controls ($N = 10$).

RESULTS

Effect of Agents on Peripheral Blood Cells from Patients with Immunodeficiency Diseases

Peripheral blood mononuclear cells obtained by Ficoll-Hypaque density gradient separation from patients with immunodeficiency disease were incubated with various agents for 90 min at 37°C, 5% CO_2 in air (Fig. 1). In five patients with isolated T-cell defects (V. H., G. D., T. M., T. C., and J. H.) a significant increase of total E-rosette-forming cells (associated with a proportionate decrease of null cells) was noted following incubation with thymosin or DB cyclic AMP; no change in B cells or monocytes was detected. Four patients with combined immunodeficiency, two patients with cellular immunodeficiency with immunoglobulin, and three patients with agammaglobulinemia demonstrated no change in the number of T cells, B cells, or monocytes following incubation with any of these agents. Incubation with these agents did not affect cell viability or cell number.

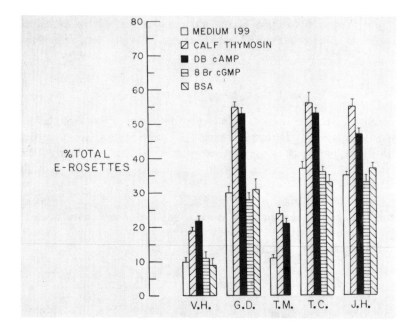

FIG. 1. Effect of agents on cells from T-deficient patients. Control values: V. H. 10% T cells, 64% B cells, 2% monos, 24% null cells; G. D. 30% T cells, 37% B cells, 10% monos, 23% null cells; T. M. 12% T cells, 15% B cells, 13% monos, 60% null cells; T. C. 37% T cells, 26% B cells, 12% monos, 25% null cells; J. H. 35% T cells, 29% B cells, 8% monos, 28% null cells. Cells were incubated with medium 199, 250 µg/ml calf thymosin fraction 5, 5×10^{-4}M DB cyclic AMP, 5×10^{-4}M 8 Br cyclic GMP, or 10 mg/ml BSA for 90 min at 37°C, 5% CO_2 in air. Incubation with 10^{-3} to 10^{-9}M 8 Br cyclic GMP gave similar results.

In patient J. C. (Table 1) with common variable immunodeficiency with significant B- and T-cell defects, no change in the number of total E-rosettes, B cells, or monocytes was observed following incubation with any agent. However, active E-rosette formation increased significantly after incubation of the cells with thymosin ($p < 0.001$) or DB cyclic AMP ($p < 0.001$) for 90 min. An increased proliferative response to PHA was also observed following incubation with thymosin ($p < 0.001$) or DB cyclic AMP ($p < 0.05$) (Table 1), due not only to a decreased base-line response but also to a significantly increased PHA response. In normals ($N = 5$), incubation of peripheral blood mononuclear cells with these agents did not have a significant effect on the base-line or PHA proliferative response.

Effect of Agents on Peripheral Blood Cells from Normals

Mononuclear cells obtained by Ficoll-Hypaque gradient separation of peripheral blood were incubated with the various agents (Table 2). Significant inhibition of total E-rosette formation was observed following exposure to isoproterenol

TABLE 1. *Effect of agents on patient J. C.'s cells*

Agent	Total E-rosettes[a] (%)	Active E-rosettes[a] (%)	B cells (%)	Monocytes (%)	Nulls (%)	Base line[b] (cpm)	PHA[b] (cpm)	SI[c]
Media	43 ± 0.7	7 ± 0.7	21	31	5	668 ± 119	862 ± 163	1
Calf thymosin fraction 5	42 ± 2.8	12 ± 0.7[e]	20	30	8	45 ± 5	2,587 ± 290[e]	57
Human thymosin fraction 5	44 ± 2.8	16 ± 1.8[e]	18	32	6	—	—	—
Calf spleen fraction 5	41 ± 1.0	8 ± 1.1	23	30	6	714 ± 10	810 ± 180	1
DB cyclic AMP 10^{-3} M	39 ± 0.7	8 ± 2.8	23	32	6	88 ± 67	186 ± 30	2
10^{-4} M	46 ± 4.6	19 ± 1.2[e]	21	28	5	47 ± 8	1,396 ± 142[f]	30
8 Br cyclic GMP 10^{-4} M[d]	41 ± 2.1	8 ± 1.1	20	32	7	—	—	—

[a] The values represent the mean ± SD of triplicate determinations.
[b] [3H]thymidine incorporation after 72-hr incubation. The values represent the mean ± SD of triplicate determinations.
[c] SI = stimulation index.
[d] 10^{-3} to 10^{-9} M 8 Br cyclic GMP gave similar results.
[e] Different from control group by Student's t-test $p < 0.001$.
[f] Different from control group by Student's t-test $p < 0.05$.

TABLE 2. *Effect of agents on total E-rosette formation of normal peripheral blood separated on Ficoll-Hypaque gradient*

Agent	90-Min incubation		24-Hr incubation	
	% Total E-rosettes[a]	% Inhibition[b]	% Total E-rosettes[a]	% Inhibition[b]
Media	53.7 ± 2.3	—	50.0 ± 2.7	—
Thymosin (250 μg/ml)	51.8 ± 2.1	4	46.4 ± 2.4	7
DB cyclic AMP (5×10^{-4}M)	52.7 ± 0.6	2	27.0 ± 3.6^e	46
Aminophylline (5×10^{-4}M)	51.0 ± 2.7	5	34.7 ± 3.2^d	31
Isoproterenol (5×10^{-4}M)	44.2 ± 2.5^d	18	38.1 ± 2.1^d	24
8 Br cGMP (5×10^{-4}M[c])	56.5 ± 2.1	0^c	49.4 ± 3.1	1

[a] Results from a representative experiment are expressed as mean ± SD of triplicate determinations ($N=5$).

[b] % inhibition $= 100 - \frac{\% \text{ total E-rosettes }_{\text{reagent}}}{\% \text{ total E-rosettes }_{\text{control}}}$.

[c] 10^{-3} to 10^{-9}M 8 Br cyclic GMP gave similar results.

[d] Different from control group by Student's *t*-test $p < 0.01$.

[e] Different from control group by Student's *t*-test $p < 0.001$.

TABLE 3. *Effect of agents on percent of total E-rosette formation of BSA gradient-separated cells*

Fraction no.	Control	Thymosin (250 µg/ml)	DB cyclic AMP (5×10^{-4}M)	Aminophylline (5×10^{-4}M)	8 Br cyclic GMP (5×10^{-4}M)[b]	BSA (10 mg/ml)
				Total E-rosettes (%)[a]		
1–2	6	25	24	22	7	5
3	28	27	30	26	22	25
4	63	58	57	57	60	61
5	18	16	14	15	19	17
6	4	3	2	3	6	4
7	2	2	1	2	3	2
8–9	3	2	2	3	3	4

[a] Results from a representative experiment ($N = 10$). Percentage in each case represents the mean of two determinations; variability of two determinations was always less than 4%.
[b] 10^{-3} to 10^{-9}M 8 Br cyclic GMP gave similar results.

TABLE 4. Effect of agents on PHA response of BSA gradient-separated cells

	PHA response (24-hr incubation)											
Fraction	Control[a]		Thymosin (250 µg/ml)		DB cyclic AMP (5 × 10⁻⁴M)		Aminophylline (5 × 10⁻⁴M)		8 Br cyclic GMP[c] (5 × 10⁻⁴M)		BSA (10 mg/ml)	
1–2	12,000[a] 4,128 48,760	2.9[b]	32,416[d] 2,634 52,492	12.3	30,040[d] 2,518 50,185	11.9	24,720[d] 3,010 47,200	8.2	14,444 3,621 55,204	4.0	13,600 4,440 49,376	3.1
3	5,138 93,200	9.5	4,946 90,150	10.6	3,915 94,108	12.8	4,320 92,000	10.9	4,637 94,860	11.9	5,014 92,816	9.9
4	885 86,500	109.5	806 85,010	111.9	910 84,203	103.4	810 87,204	113.6	858 86,503	110.6	870 87,310	106.7
5	750 18,093	115.3	803 19,550	105.9	759 19,066	111.0	695 17,803	125.5	710 19,540	121.9	694 19,001	125.8
6	840 10,889	21.5	816 9,548	23.2	715 11,001	26.7	811 9,666	22.0	791 10,120	24.7	815 11,063	23.3
7	890 9,450	12.2	860 10,011	11.1	911 9,050	12.1	865 8,850	11.2	785 8,631	12.9	781 9,305	14.2
8–9	765	12.4	705	14.2	901	10.0	815	10.9	701	12.3	740	12.6

[a]Stimulated cpm/base-line cpm. Results from a representative experiment ($N = 10$) are expressed as [³H]thymidine incorporation, mean cpm of triplicate cultures; 1 SD was always less than 15% of the mean.

[b]Stimulation index = stimulated cpm/base-line cpm.

[c]10^{-3} to 10^{-9}M 8 Br cyclic GMP gave similar results.

[d]Different from control group by Student's t-test $p < 0.001$.

TABLE 5. *Effect of agents on MLC response of BSA gradient-separated cells*

		MLC response (24-hr incubation)									
Fraction	Control		Thymosin (250 µg/ml)		DB cyclic AMP (5×10^{-4}M)		Aminophylline (5×10^{-4}M)		8 Br cyclic GMP[e] (5×10^{-4}M)		BSA (10 mg/ml)	
1–2[a]	$\dfrac{7,080^{b}}{4,250}$	1.7[c]	$\dfrac{15,341^{d}}{2,411}$	6.4	$\dfrac{16,100^{d}}{2,610}$	6.2	$\dfrac{14,860^{d}}{2,550}$	5.8	$\dfrac{7,548}{4,110}$	1.8	$\dfrac{6,963}{3,922}$	1.7

[a] No change in proliferative response of fractions 3–9.
[b] Stimulated cpm/base-line cpm. Results from a representative experiment ($N = 10$) are expressed as [^{3}H]thymidine incorporation, mean cpm; 1 SD was always less than 15% of the mean. Stimulator cells were obtained by Ficoll-Hypaque separation of normal peripheral blood and used at a concentration of 1×10^5 cells per well. Responder cells, obtained by BSA gradient separation, were incubated with the various agents, washed ×3, and used at a concentration of 1×10^5 cells per well.
[c] Stimulation index = stimulated cpm/base-line cpm.
[d] Different from control group by Student's *t*-test $p < 0.001$.
[e] 10^{-3} to 10^{-9}M 8 Br cyclic GMP gave similar results.

for 90 min ($p < 0.01$) and DB cyclic AMP ($p < 0.001$), aminophylline ($p < 0.01$), or isoproterenol ($p < 0.01$) for 24 hr ($N = 5$). These agents did not affect cell viability or the number of B cells or monocytes.

The effect of these agents on peripheral blood cells obtained by Ficoll-Hypaque and subsequent BSA gradient separation was studied next. In normal subjects ($N = 10$), significantly increased total E-rosette formation was demonstrated in cells from fraction 1–2 following incubation with thymosin, DB cyclic AMP, or aminophylline for 90 min (Table 3). Significantly increased proliferation following PHA or allogeneic cell stimulation was also seen after incubation of cells from fraction 1–2 with thymosin ($p < 0.001$), DB cyclic AMP ($p < 0.001$), or aminophylline ($p < 0.001$) for 24 hr (Tables 4 and 5). There was no change in the number of B cells or monocytes in any fraction following incubation with these agents. Incubation with the various reagents did not alter total E-rosette formation or *in vitro* proliferative responses of fractions 3 to 9; cell viability was not affected.

DISCUSSION

In this study, increased numbers of E-rosette-forming lymphocytes were demonstrated *in vitro* in patients with T-cell deficiency following incubation of peripheral blood mononuclear cells with thymosin or DB cyclic AMP; these agents did not affect the number of B cells or monocytes, the cell viability, or the cell number. In one child with a profound defect of B- and T-cell function, exposure to thymosin or DB cyclic AMP *in vitro* led to increased active E-rosette formation associated with increased proliferation following stimulation with PHA. In patients with combined immune deficiency, cellular immunodeficiency with immunoglobulin and agammaglobulinemia, no change in the number of E-rosette-forming cells was observed following incubation with thymosin, DB cyclic AMP, or 8 Br cyclic GMP. Previous studies have reported increased numbers of cells with T surface markers in children with immunodeficiency after exposure of peripheral blood or bone marrow cells to thymosin (33), thymopoietin (19), human thymus monolayer (24), or theophylline (13).

Incubation of normal peripheral blood mononuclear cells, obtained by Ficoll-Hypaque density gradient centrifugation, with thymosin or agents that increase intracellular cyclic AMP, inhibited E-rosette formation. These results are similar to those previously reported by Chesari and Edington (5), Galant et al. (9), and Greico et al. (11). However, exposure of normal peripheral blood putative stem cell fractions (fraction 1–2), obtained by BSA density gradient separation, to thymosin or agents that increase cellular cyclic AMP resulted in increased total E-rosette formation and increased proliferation following PHA or allogeneic cell stimulation. Previous studies (6,7) indicate that under the conditions utilized in this experiment proliferation following PHA or allogeneic cell stimulation is a T-cell response. Incubation with thymosin or agents that increase cyclic AMP appeared to induce real T-cell differentiation in cells from fraction 1–2 as there was no change in cell number or viability and there was no selective loss of B cells or monocytes. In addition, a loss of T suppressor cell activity as the basis for the induction seems unlikely in view of increased E-rosette formation and decreased base-line proliferation following incubation with thymosin or agents that increase cyclic AMP.

In mice, Scheid et al. (26,27) showed that the differentiation of prothymocytes to thymocytes was mediated by factors that increased cellular cyclic AMP including thymosin, thymopoietin, and "non-specific" inducers such as ubiquitin, theophylline, and DB cyclic AMP. The induction of T-cell differentiation by factors that increase cyclic AMP in T-cell-deficient patients and normals described in this chapter is consistent with Scheid's findings (26,27).

It is possible that patients with immunodeficiency with circulating "null" cells that are inducible *in vitro* by agents that increase cyclic AMP (eg., aminophylline) may also respond to such agents *in vivo*. In addition, there are a number of patients with serious immune deficiency who have large numbers of circulating "null" cells that are not inducible *in vitro* by agents that affect cyclic AMP or cyclic GMP. Other inductive signals may be required for differentiation of stem cells arrested at a very early stage of maturation. In some children with combined immune deficiency, significant B- and T-cell reconstitution has been demonstrated following cultured thymus epithelium transplantation although no effect of thymosin or agents that affect cyclic AMP or cyclic GMP could be shown *in vitro* (14). Study of the effect of cultured thymus epithelium and fractionated supernatants obtained from these cultures on putative stem cell fractions may help define other important mediators of lymphocyte differentiation.

ACKNOWLEDGMENT

This work has been supported in part by National Institutes of Health grants HD-07778, CA-14520, and AI-11576.

REFERENCES

1. August, C. S., Merler, E., Lucas, D. O., and Janeway, C. A. (1970): The response *in vitro* of human lymphocytes to phytohemagglutinin and to antigens after fractionation on discontinuous density of gradients of albumin. *Cell. Immunol.,* 1:603–618.
2. Bach, J. F., Dardenne, M., Pleau, J. M., and Bach, M. A. (1975): Isolation, biochemical characteristics, and biological activity of a circulating thymic hormone in the mouse and in the human. *Ann. NY. Acad. Sci.,* 249:186–210.
3. Basch, R. S., and Goldstein, G. (1974): Induction of T cell differentiation *in vitro* by thymin, a purified polypeptide hormone of the thymus. *Proc. Natl. Acad. Sci. USA,* 71:1474–1478.
4. Boyum, A. (1968): Isolation of mononuclear cells and granulocytes from human blood. Isolation of mononuclear cells by one centrifugation, and of granulocytes by combining centrifugation and sedimentation at 1 g. *Scand. J. Clin. Lab. Invest.* 21(Suppl. 97):9–50.
5. Chesari, F. V., and Edington, T. S. (1974): Human T lymphocyte "E" rosette function. I. A process modulated by intracellular cyclic AMP. *J. Exp. Med.,* 140:1122–1126.
6. Chess, L., MacDermott, R. P., and Schlossman, S. F. (1974): Immunologic functions of isolated

human lymphocyte subpopulations. I. Quantitative isolation of human T and B cells and response to mitogens. *J. Immunol.,* 113:1113–1121.

7. Chess, L., MacDermott, R. P., and Schlossman, S. F. (1974): Immunologic functions of isolated human lymphocyte subpopulations. II. Antigen triggering of T and B cells *in vitro. J. Immunol.,* 113:1122–1127.

8. Dickler, H. B., and Kunkel, H. L. (1972): Interaction of aggregated γ-globulin with B lymphocytes. *J. Exp. Med.,* 136:191–196.

9. Galant, S. P., Lundak, R. L., and Eaton, L., (1976): Enhancement of early human E-rosette formation by cholinergic stimuli. *J. Immunol.,* 117:48–51.

10. Goldstein, G. (1974): Isolation of bovine thymin: A polypeptide hormone of the thymus. *Nature,* 247:11–14.

11. Grieco, M. H., Siegel, I., and Goel, Z. (1976): Modulation of human T lymphocyte rosette formation by autonomic agonists and cyclic nucleotides. *J. Allergy Clin. Immunol.,* 58:149–159.

12. Hartzman, R. M., Segall, M., Bach, M. L., and Bach, F. H. (1971): Histocompatibility matching. VI. Miniaturization of the mixed leukocyte culture test: A preliminary report. *Transplantation,* 11:268–273.

13. Hayward, A. R., and Graham, L. (1976): Increased E-rosette formation by foetal liver and spleen cells incubated with theophylline. *Clin. Exp. Immunol.,* 23:279–284.

14. Hong, R., Santosham, M., Schulte-Wissermann, H., Horowitz, S., Hsu, S. H., and Winkelstein, J. A. (1976): Reconstitution of B and T lymphocyte function in severe combined immunodeficiency disease following transplantation with thymic epithelium. *Lancet,* ii:1270–1272.

15. Hooper, J. A., McDaniel, M. C., Thurman, G. B., Cohen, G. H., Schulof, R. S., and Goldstein, A. L. (1975): Purification and properties of bovine thymosin. *Ann. NY Acad. Sci.,* 249:125–144.

16. Horowitz, S., Groshong, T., Albrecht, R., and Hong, R. (1975): The "active" rosette test in immunodeficiency diseases. *Clin. Immunol. Immunopathol.,* 4:405–414.

17. Horowitz, S., and Hong, R. (1974): *In vitro* effects of various agents on B and T lymphocyte markers and function. *J. Clin. Invest.,* 54:34a.

18. Incety, G. S., L'Esperance, P., and Good, R. A. (1975): *In vitro* differentiation of human marrow cells into T lymphocytes by thymic extracts using the rosette technique. *Clin. Exp. Immunol.,* 19:475–483.

19. Incefy, G. S., Grimes, E., Kagan, W. A., Goldstein, G., Smithwick, E., O'Reilly, R., and Good, R. A. (1976): Heterogeneity of stem cells in severe combined immunodeficiency. *Clin. Exp. Immunol.,* 25:462–471.

20. Jondal, M., Holm, G., and Wigzell, H. (1972): Surface markers on human B and T lymphocytes. I. A large population of lymphocytes forming non-immune rosettes with sheep red blood cells. *J. Exp. Med.,* 136:207–215.

21. Kook, A. I., and Trainin, N. (1974): Hormone-like activity of a thymus humoral factor on the induction of immune competence in lymphoid cells. *J. Exp. Med.,* 139:193–207.

22. Kook, A. I., and Trainin, N. (1975): Intracellular events involved in the induction of immune competence in lymphoid cells by a thymus humoral factor. *J. Immunol.,* 114:151–157.

23. Preud'Homme, J. L., and Flandrin, G. (1974): Identification by peroxidase staining of monocytes in surface immunofluorescence tests. *J. Immunol.,* 113:1650–1653.

24. Pyke, K. W., and Gelfand, E. W. (1974): Morphological and functional maturation of human thymic epithelium in culture. *Nature,* 251:421–423.

25. Ross, G. D., Rabellino, E. M., Polley, M. J., and Grey, H. M. (1973): Combined studies of complement receptor and surface immunoglobulin bearing cells and sheep erythrocyte rosette-forming cells in normal and leukemic human lymphocytes. *J. Clin. Invest.,* 52:377–385.

26. Scheid, M. P., Goldstein, G., Hammerling, U., and Boyse, E. A. (1975): Lymphocyte differentiation from precursor cells *in vitro. Ann. NY Acad. Sci.,* 249:531–540.

27. Scheid, M. P., Hoffman, M. K., Komuro, K., Hammerling, U., Abbott, J., Boyse, E. A., Cohen, G. H., Hooper, J. A., Schulof, R. S., and Goldstein, A. L. (1973): Differentiation of T cells induced by preparations from thymus and by non-thymic agents. *J. Exp. Med.,* 138:1027–1032.

28. Schlesinger, D. H., and Goldstein, G. (1975): The amino acid sequence of thymopoietin II. *Cell,* 5:361–365.

29. Thorsby, E., and Bratlie, A. (1970): A rapid method for preparation of pure lymphocyte suspen-

sions. In: *Histocompatability Testing,* edited by P. Terasaki, pp. 655–656. Williams & Wilkins, Baltimore.

30. Touraine, J. L., Incefy, G. S., Touraine, F., L'Esperance, P., Siegal, F. P., and Good, R. A. (1974): T-lymphocyte differentiation *in vitro* in primary immunodeficiency diseases. *Clin. Immunol. Immunopathol.,* 3:228–235.
31. Touraine, J. L., Incefy, G. S., Touraine, F., Rho, Y. M., and Good, R. A. (1974): Differentiation of human bone marrow cells into T lymphocytes by *in vitro* incubation with thymic extracts. *Clin. Exp. Immunol.,* 17:151–158.
32. Vogel, J. E., Incefy, G. S., and Good, R. A. (1975): Differentiation of population of peripheral blood lymphocytes into cells bearing sheep erythrocyte receptors *in vitro* by human thymic extract. *Proc. Natl. Acad. Sci. USA,* 72:1175–1178.
33. Wara, D. W., Goldstein, A. L., Doyle, N. E., and Ammann, A. J. (1975): Thymosin activity in patients with cellular immunodeficiency. *N. Engl. J. Med.,* 292:70–74.
34. Wybran, J., Carr, M. C., and Fudenberg, H. H. (1972): The human rosette-forming cell as a marker of a population of thymus-derived cells. *J. Clin. Invest.,* 51:2537–2543.
35. Wybran, J., Levin, A. S., Fudenberg, H. H., and Goldstein, A. L. (1975): Thymosin: Effects on normal human blood T-cells. *Ann. NY Acad. Sci.,* 249:300–307.

Immune Modulation and Control of Neoplasia by Adjuvant Therapy, edited by M. A. Chirigos. Raven Press, New York, 1978.

In Vitro and *In Vivo* Effects of Thymosin on T-Lymphocyte Function in Primary Immunodeficiency Disease

Diane W. Wara, Alan C. Johnson, and Arthur J. Ammann

Department of Pediatrics, Immunology Section and Pediatric Clinical Research Center, University of California, San Francisco, San Francisco, California 94143

The mechanism by which the thymus gland regulates the development and maintenance of cell-mediated immunity remains poorly understood. Recognition of the thymus as an endocrine gland that produces humoral factors followed the observation that cellular immunity was restored in thymus-deprived mice by either thymus implants in cell-impermeable chambers (11) or the injection of extracts from thymic tissue (8,21). Both methods of reconstitution prevent clinical disease in the mice and restore lymphocyte numbers and function.

Since these early observations, multiple thymic humoral factors have been evaluated for their ability to reconstitute cellular immunity (T-cell immunity) or to interact with B cells (bone marrow-derived lymphocytes) in providing a normal antibody response in thymic-deprived mice (18). The humoral factors include thymosin (4), thymic humoral factor (17), thymic factor (5), thymopoietin (9), and T-cell-replacing factor (14). Other antibody-enhancing factors produced by the thymus have been described. The studies suggest that the thymus produces multiple humoral agents, in addition to or included within thymosin, that enhance the expression of T-cell immunity. Thymosin's effects on cellular and humoral immunity in animals have been extensively investigated. Thymosin decreases the incidence of wasting disease in thymus-deprived mice, stimulates lymphoid tissue regeneration, and restores the capacity of host cells to elicit a normal graft-versus-host reaction and to reject histoincompatible skin grafts (4). Both in newborn and adult normal mice, thymosin injections promote the development of cellular immunity and the normal *in vitro* response of lymphocytes to T-cell mitogens, such as Concanavalin A, or to allogeneic cells, or both (6,7). The dose and route of thymosin injection influence the biological effects observed (A. Goldstein, *personal communication).* The precise mechanism by which thymosin enhances cellular and humoral immunity in various animal models is not completely understood. Komuro and Boyse (10) first demonstrated that thymosin, when incubated *in vitro* with mouse bone marrow or spleen cells, induces cells bearing T-lymphocyte surface antigens.

Armeding and Katz (3) induced antibody formation by spleen cells from athymic nude mice when the cells were cultured with thymosin and specific antigen. Thymosin also enhanced the one-way mixed lymphocyte culture (MLC) reaction by spleen cells obtained from athymic mice. The observations taken together suggest that thymosin acts on precursor and/or more fully matured T cells responsible for providing helper function to B cells in one instance, and on T cells participating in the mixed lymphocyte reaction in a second instance. Thymosin is currently being characterized biochemically. It is now known that thymosin fraction 5 contains 12 polypeptides, each of which may have a unique role in the maintenance of normal immunity.

The first convincing evidence of a thymic humoral substance in humans was provided by Steele et al. (15); a 10-week-old female infant with cellular immunodeficiency and hypoparathyroidism (DiGeorge syndrome) received a transplant of a fetal thymus in a millipore diffusion chamber. Within 6 hr following transplantation, an increase in the peripheral blood lymphocyte response to phytohemagglutinin (PHA) was demonstrated. The effect was most probably a result of activation of the patient's T cells by a thymic factor.

We and others have now documented that peripheral blood human lymphocytes obtained from patients with immunodeficiency disease, when incubated in vitro with thymosin, form increased numbers of T-cell rosettes (1,16,19,20). This phenomenon has been observed in primary immunodeficiency disease, various malignancies (12), systemic lupus erythematosus (13), and viral syndromes. Recently, we have demonstrated that lymphocytes obtained from a subpopulation of patients with immunodeficiency have an enhanced response to allogeneic cells [mixed lymphocyte culture (MLC)] when incubated with thymosin. The majority of children with primary immunodeficiency disease and significant abnormalities of their cellular immune function have both decreased numbers of T cells and abnormal T-cell function. Until recently, successful reconstitution of immunity in these patients has been limited to bone marrow transplantation from a donor compatible for HLA or MLC, or both. Compatible bone marrow donors are rarely available, and children with severe disease generally die by age 1 year with overwhelming infection. Children with milder forms of cellular immunodeficiency were treated with supportive therapy with only limited success. Therefore, after demonstrating that thymosin incubation in vitro could enhance T-cell rosette formation or lymphocyte response to allogeneic cells, or both, and following exhaustive studies by others on the purity and safety of the product, we began to administer thymosin in vivo to a subpopulation of our patients with primary immunodeficiency disease.

We have treated 11 patients with cellular immunodeficiency disease with thymosin injections. All patients have been evaluated immunologically prior to the initiation of therapy and at regular intervals thereafter. Prior to therapy, enhancement of T-cell rosette formation and of in vitro lymphocyte response to allogeneic cells by thymosin incubation has been evaluated. An effort has been made to correlate *in vitro* enhancement of T-cell number and function by thymosin incubation with patient response following *in vivo* therapy.

METHODS

In Vitro Lymphocyte Stimulation with PHA or in MLC, or Both

Peripheral blood lymphocytes are isolated by Ficoll-Hypaque gradient. The cell suspension is adjusted to 2×10^6 lymphocytes/ml utilizing RPMI-1640 (25 mmoles HEPES buffer) with 15% human plasma. PHA is added in concentrations varying from 0.5 to 10.0 μg/ml cell suspension. The cell suspensions are immediately aliquoted into microtiter plates—0.2 ml cell suspension per well. The microtiter plates are incubated at 37°C for 96 hr in a 5% CO_2 incubator. Each cell culture is pulsed with 0.5 μCi (^{3}H-methyl-thymidine) for 4.5 hr in the incubator. The cells are then harvested utilizing the multiple automated sample harvester, and counted in a scintillation counter. Normal maximum *in vitro* lymphocyte stimulation with PHA in microculture is greater than 42,000 cpm (includes two standard deviations from the mean). For stimulation of lymphocytes by allogeneic cells, each patient's cells are stimulated by lymphocytes from a single nonrelated adult control or by pooled lymphocytes obtained from three unrelated adult controls, or both. Stimulating cells are treated with 3,000 rads. Two hundred thousand responding cells from the patient are incubated with 200,000 lymphocytes from the control in 0.2 ml of media at 37°C, in 5% CO_2 for 144 hr. Following the incubation period, the cells are labeled, harvested, and counted in a manner identical to that used for lymphocyte stimulation with PHA. Normal stimulated *in vitro* lymphocyte response in MLC is greater than 7,000 cpm.

Percent T-Cell Rosette Formation

Peripheral blood lymphocytes are isolated by Ficoll-Hypaque gradient as described above. The cells are adjusted to 4×10^6 cells per ml in Hank's balanced salt solution (HBSS) supplemented with 10% sheep red blood cell absorbed fetal calf serum. Sheep red blood cells (GIBCO) are washed twice and adjusted to a 1% suspension in fetal calf serum-supplemented HBSS. A 0.25-ml aliquot of the lymphocyte suspension is incubated with 0.25 ml of the sheep red blood cell suspension at 37°C for 5 min, centrifuged at 200 g for 5 min, and then incubated at 4°C for 18 hr. Cell suspensions are observed under phase microscopy and percentage of spontaneous rosette-forming cells determined. A rosette-forming cell is defined as a lymphocyte with three or more adherent sheep red blood cells. Normal mean spontaneous rosette-forming cells ± one standard deviation equals 73 ± 7%. Greater than 59% spontaneous rosette-forming cells is considered normal by current methodology.

Thymosin Incubation Studies

Bovine thymosin fraction 5, supplied by Hoffmann-LaRoche Pharmaceutical Co., is added to cell suspensions in concentrations varying from 50 to 500 mcg per ml. When enhancement of T-cell rosette formation is being determined, after the addition of thymosin, the suspensions are incubated for 5 min at 37°C, centrifuged for 5 min at 200 g, and then incubated for 18 hr at 4°C. Determination of T-cell rosettes is as described above. When enhancement of lymphocyte response to allogeneic cells is being determined, thymosin is added to the lymphocyte suspensions at the initiation of the incubation period and to both resting cells and cells undergoing stimulation.

Thymosin Administration

All thymosin is obtained from Hoffmann-LaRoche, and thymosin fraction 5 is utilized.

After an initial dose of thymosin (1 mg) given intradermally, thymosin (1 mg/kg given subcutaneously) is administered each day for 2 weeks. Subsequently, thymosin is given once each week in a dose that varies with each patient from 1 to 5 mg/kg weekly. An immunological evaluation is performed at 3-month intervals. The evaluation includes quantitative immunoglobulins, specific antibody production, T-cell rosettes, lymphocyte response to PHA, allogeneic cells, specific antigen when appropriate, B cells as identified by surface immunoglobulin or EAC rosettes, or both, and a total white blood cell count with differential. Intradermal skin tests are placed prior to the initiation of therapy, 2 weeks after completion of daily injections, and then at 3-month intervals. Antigens are injected in 0.1-ml volume; antigens utilized include *Candida,* streptokinase-streptodornase, mumps when available, and trichophyton when appropriate.

RESULTS

As we reported earlier (19,20), *in vitro* incubation of thymosin in concentrations varying from 50 to 500 μg/ml of cell suspension increased the percent T-cell rosettes *in vitro* in patients with certain cellular immunodeficiency disorders. Enhancement of T-cell rosette formation occurred in four patients with cellular immunodeficiency and immunoglobulin synthesis (Nezelof's syndrome), four with Wiskott-Aldrich syndrome, and two with ataxia-telangiectasia. Four patients with the DiGeorge syndrome were evaluated. Two patients with depressed T-cell rosettes (20 to 30%) responded to thymosin incubation with a greater than 50% increase over base-line values. Two patients with the DiGeorge syndrome had no significant increase in T-cell rosettes following thymosin incubation. In one patient the initial percent of T-cell rosettes was 41%, and the incubation was performed at a time when a graft-versus-host reaction was in progress. In the other patient the baseline percent of T-cell rosettes were less than 10%, and a graft-versus-host reaction was in progress at the time the study was performed. Both patients subsequently died with graft-versus-host reactions and gram-negative sepsis. Six patients with severe combined immunodeficiency disease and base-line T-cell rosettes of less than 10% have had no *in vitro* response to thymosin incubation. It is possible that the two patients with DiGeorge syndrome and the six with severe combined immunodeficiency disease in whom thymosin did not enhance T-cell rosette formation *in vitro,* have in common a lack of prethymic cells capable of responding to thymosin incubation.

Eleven patients with various forms of immunodeficiency disease were selected for *in vivo* treatment with thymosin. None of the patients treated had a suitable histocompatible and/or MLC identical donor for bone marrow transplantation. Other appropriate therapeutic measures, such as antibiotic treatment, transfer factor, or fetal thymus transplantation, had not resulted in complete reconstitution of cell-mediated immunity and/or improvement in clinical status. In all cases, the patients selected for treatment had some evidence *in vitro* of enhanced lymphocyte formation of T-cell rosettes or enhanced lymphocyte function as assayed by response to allogeneic cells, or both, following incubation with thymosin (Table 1). Of the patients treated (Table 2), one (no. 5, N. F.) expired within 3 weeks after the initiation of therapy, one (no. 2, L. M.) may have become sensitized to thymosin fraction 5, and two (no. 1, H. G.; no. 10, M. O.) had no improvement in *in vitro* lymphocyte function although their percent T-cell rosettes increased following therapy. These same two patients continued to have increased clinical infections, and it became necessary to utilize other methods for reconstitution. The remainder of the patients had both clinical improvement and *in vitro* evidence of reconstitution of cellular immunity.

Two patients with thymic hypoplasia and immunoglobulin synthesis (Nezelof's syndrome) have received thymosin therapy. H. G. (no. 1) was a 4-year-old girl who was treated for 33 months (19,20). She improved clinically for approximately 28 months while receiving thymosin and had weight gain (26 to 42 lbs) as well as decreased numbers and severity of infections and diarrhea. Between 28 and 33 months following the initiation of thymosin therapy, she deteriorated clinically with increasing numbers of infections (skin, otitis media, pneumonia). Following 1 month of thymosin therapy she had a conversion of her delayed hypersensitivity skin tests for mumps and *Candida* and an increase in absolute numbers of lymphocytes (400 to 1,400/mm³) and percent T-cell rosettes (10 to 60%). Intermittently, the patient's *in vitro* lymphocyte response to PHA improved but never became normal. Her *in vitro* lymphocyte response to allogeneic cells always remained markedly abnormal; *in vitro* incubation of her cells with thymosin did not increase the response. Over the same time period the patient's IgG increased from 220 to 1,220 mg/dl. However, she remained unable to produce specific antibody. Following 33 months of therapy, a monoclonal peak in the beta region of her protein electrophoresis was noted; on immunoelectrophoresis this proved to be IgA, predominantly kappa chain. She was evaluated thoroughly for a malignancy of the gastrointestinal tract,

TABLE 1. Correlation between in vitro and in vivo lymphocyte response to thymosin

Patient	Disorder	In vitro TCR—TCR + THY F5 (%)	In vivo TCR after Rx (%)	In vitro MLR—MLR + THY F5	In vivo MLR after Rx	Clinical improvement
1. H. G.	Thymic hypoplasia	10–45	58	295 (2.8)—302 (2.9)	1,600 (1.6)	Yes
2. L. M.	Thymic hypoplasia w. nucleoside phosphorylase deficiency	13–55	63	537 (7.8) not done	4,000 (8.5)	Yes
3. D. A.	Wiskott-Aldrich	21–45	59	909 (1.7) not done	14,568 (13.5)	Yes
4. J. M.	Wiskott-Aldrich	32–65	58	2,248 (2.3) not done	21,836 (8.2)	Yes
5. N. F.	DiGeorge	<10–<10	<10	234 (4) not done	490 (2)	No
6. M. S.	DiGeorge	18–64	60	105 (1.2)—4,964 (4.4)	14,986 (65)	Yes
7. P. T.	Chronic candidiasis	43–70	62	4,024 (5.4) not done	6,474 (42)	Yes
8. G. G.	Chronic trichophyton	45–80	67	43,061 (68)—68,681 (108)	24,370 (80)	Yes
9. M. O.	Severe combined immunodeficiency	92–92	88	869 (1.5)—902 (1.6)	3,477 (1.4)	No
10. L. N.	Acquired hypogammaglobulinemia	85–92	82	1,554 (15.5)—6,484 (65)	7,265 (70)	Yes (?)
11. K. J.	Ataxia-telangiectasia	62–78	66	638 (1.0)—10,705 (17.5)	Too early to evaluate	Too early to evaluate

MLR, mixed lymphocyte reaction = maximum stimulation (stimulation index); TCR, % T-cell rosettes; THY F5, thymosin fraction 5.

TABLE 2. *Patients treated with thymosin*

Patient	Disorder	Increase in T-cell number with Rx[a]	Increase in T-cell function with Rx[b]	Improved B-cell function with Rx[c]	Clinical Improvement
1. H. G.	Thymic hypoplasia	Yes	No	Yes	Yes
2. L. M.	Thymic hypoplasia w. nucleoside phosphorylase deficiency	Yes	Yes	Unchanged	Yes
3. D. A.	Wiskott-Aldrich	Yes	Yes	No	Yes
4. J. M.	Wiskott-Aldrich	Yes	Yes	No	Yes
5. N. F.	DiGeorge	No	No	Unchanged	No
6. M. S.	DiGeorge	Yes	Yes	Unchanged	Yes
7. P. T.	Chronic candidiasis	Yes	Yes	Unchanged	Yes
8. G. G.	Chronic trichophyton	Yes	Unchanged	Unchanged	Yes
9. M. O.	Severe combined immunodeficiency	Unchanged	No	No	No
10. L. N.	Acquired hypogammaglobulinemia	Unchanged	Yes	No	Yes (?)
11. K. J.	Ataxia-telangiectasia	Unchanged	Too early to evaluate	Too early to evaluate	Too early to evaluate

[a] T-cell rosettes.
[b] Lymphocyte response to PHA or allogeneic cells, or both.
[c] Normalization of quantitative immunoglobulins.

but none was detected. Patient no 2. (L. M.), a 5-year-old girl with normal B-cell immunity but thymic hypoplasia and nucleoside phosphorylase deficiency, improved significantly following the initiation of thymosin, with a reduction in number of respiratory infections. Quantitative immunoglobulins and her ability to form specific antibody remained normal. Percent T-cell rosettes increased from 13 to 63% within 1 month following therapy, and delayed hypersensitivity skin test conversion to mumps occurred. The patient's *in vitro* lymphocyte response to PHA (maximum response 3,000 increasing to 28,000 cpm) and to allogeneic cells (maximum response 537 increasing to 4,000 cpm) improved slowly over a 6-month period. Prior to the initiation of therapy, the patient's lymphocytes had not been incubated *in vitro* with thymosin to evaluate enhanced response to allogeneic cells. After 6 months of therapy, the patient became sensitized to thymosin and developed urticaria at the site of injection associated with respiratory wheezing. Therapy was discontinued. Within 1 month the patient's T-cell rosettes decreased to previously observed abnormal levels, and the *in vitro* response of lymphocytes to PHA and to allogeneic cells returned to her base-line abnormal values.

Two patients with the Wiskott-Aldrich syndrome have been treated. The first (no. 3, D. A.), a 10-year-old boy, showed significant clinical improvement following the initiation of thymosin therapy. Eczema became less extensive, and recurrent herpes stomatitis resolved. The patient's quantitative immunoglobulins remained stable, and he had no increment in ability to respond to immunization with specific polysaccharides. However, within 1 month following initiation of thymosin, his T-cell rosettes increased from 21 to 59%. Over the course of 6 months of therapy his *in vitro* lymphocyte response to PHA increased from a maximum of 499 to 62,367 cpm. The patient's *in vitro* lymphocyte response to allogeneic cells was normal 1 year following the initiation of therapy (14,568 cpm) but has fluctuated since that time. A 2½-year-old boy (no. 4, J. M.) with Wiskott-Aldrich syndrome, severe eczema, and recurrent infections has been receiving thymosin therapy for 10 months. He has had moderate clinical improvement but continues to have eczema, occasional otitis media, and pneumonia. Following the initiation of therapy, percent T-cell rosettes increased from 32 to 58% and *in vitro* lymphocyte response to PHA remained normal at 42,000 cpm and to allogeneic cells increased from 2,248 to 21,836 cpm. Again, percent T-cell rosettes became normal within approximately 1 month after the initiation of therapy, whereas *in vitro* lymphocyte response to allogeneic cells required 6 months of therapy before normalizing. Conversion of skin tests in the two patients with Wiskott-Aldrich syndrome was not evaluated; the patients bled into their skin test sites, preventing adequate evaluation.

Two patients with the DiGeorge syndrome have been treated with thymosin. Both infants were diagnosed within 3 days following birth because of congenital heart disease involving the ascending aortic arch, persistent and severe hypocalcemia, and lymphopenia for age. The first infant (no. 5, N. F.) had total lymphocytes varying between 1,900 and 2,300/mm^3 and percent T-cell rosettes on three occasions less than 10% that were not increased *in vitro* with thymosin incubation. The patient's *in vitro* lymphocyte response to PHA was abnormal on three occasions (less than 500 cpm), and response to allogeneic cells likewise was abnormal (234 cpm). There was no evidence of *in vitro* thymosin enhancement of lymphocyte response to allogeneic cells. However, because a fetal thymus gland was not available for transplantation, thymosin therapy was begun. The infant received 2 weeks of therapy. At the end of that time she still had less than 10% T-cell rosettes, and no improvement of *in vitro* lymphocyte response to PHA or to allogeneic cells was noted. At age 10 days she developed a fine maculopapular rash that was evanescent and felt to be consistent with a graft-versus-host reaction; we were unable to confirm the diagnosis by demonstrating HLA chimerism. Approximately 1 week later, following a stormy clinical course, she expired with *Pseudomonas sepsis* and peritonitis. The second patient (no. 6, M. S.) with DiGeorge syndrome who received thymosin, had no evidence of a graft-versus-host reaction and no significant infections. On day 3 of life the patient had a total lymphocyte count of 2,200 and T-cell rosettes of 18% that increased with *in vitro* thymosin incubation to 64%. *In vitro* lymphocyte response to PHA was 50% of normal at 20,533 cpm and to allogeneic cells 2% of normal at 105 cpm. When the patient's lymphocytes were incubated *in vitro* with thymosin, their response to allogeneic cells increased to 4,964 cpm. Again, because a fetal thymus gland was not available for transplantation, the infant was begun on thymosin therapy on day 5 of life. He received 14 daily injections, and at the end of this time his percent of T-cell rosettes had increased to 60%, *in vitro* lymphocyte response to PHA was 49,579 cpm (normal), and *in vitro* lymphocyte response to allogeneic cells had increased to 9,117 cpm. It was elected to discontinue thymosin therapy and to follow the infant. He received no thymosin for 1 month, remained clinically well, and when evaluated immunologically continued to have normal cell-mediated immunity. At age 3 months, he expired following open heart surgery.

Two patients with chronic fungal skin disease have been treated with thymosin therapy. The first (no. 7, P. T.) has classic chronic mucocutaneous candidiasis. Prior to initiation of therapy at age 12, she had diffuse skin and mucous membrane involvement with *Candida,* external otitis media secondary to *Candida,* and chronic pulmonary disease. Total lymphocyte count was 1,335, 43% forming T-cell rosettes and 24% with surface immunoglobulins. When the patient's lymphocytes were incubated with thymosin the percent T-cell rosettes increased from 43 to a maximum of 70%. Prior to the initiation of therapy, the patient's *in vitro* lymphocyte response to PHA was normal (40,327 cpm) and to allogeneic cells was only slightly decreased (4,024 cpm). She had no *in vitro* lymphocyte response to *Candida* antigen and was anergic to all skin tests prior to treatment. She has now received thymosin therapy for approximately 1 year and has had marked clearing of her cutaneous lesions. Within 2 months following the initiation of therapy, her old lesions began to desquamate, and normal skin appeared underneath. Approximately 9 months after the initiation of therapy, her nails began to fall off, normal skin was seen underneath, and nail regrowth appeared normal. Prior to therapy she weighed 19 kg (no weight gain for approximately 4 years); she now weighs 23.5 kg. Her bilateral draining external otitis has cleared, and examination of her tympanic membranes is entirely normal. Auscultation of her lungs is now normal. At present, percent T-cell rosettes are normal at 73%, B cells by surface immunoglobulin are 20%, *in vitro* lymphocyte response to PHA remains normal, and *in vitro* lymphocyte response to allogeneic cells has improved slightly. At this point, 1 year following initiation of therapy, *in vitro* lymphocyte response to allogeneic cells can be enhanced by incubation with thymosin from 6,474 to 11,539 cpm. There is still no enhancement by thymosin of *in vitro* lymphocyte response to *Candida* antigen and no evidence of reconstitution of T-cell response to *Candida* by *in vitro* lymphocyte stimulation, migration inhibition factor quantitation, or skin test positivity. A second patient with diffuse cutaneous trichophyton has been started on thymosin (no. G. G.). The patient is 48 years old, has had disseminated trichophyton for 20 of those years, and has received oral griseofulvin during this entire time without improvement of the lesions. He has no evidence of pulmonary disease. Three months following the initiation of therapy, his skin lesions began to improve. Prior to therapy the patient had a normal total lymphocyte count on two occasions, 45% T-cell rosettes that increased to 80% with thymosin incubation, and 9% B cells by surface immunoglobulin. *In vitro* lymphocyte response to PHA and to allogeneic cells was normal. On two occasions, the patient had enhancement of *in vitro* lymphocyte response to allogeneic cells; however, on both occasions, base-line response to allogeneic cells was within our normal range (greater than 8,000 cpm).

A patient with severe combined immunodeficiency disease (no. 9, M. O.) received 4 months of *in vivo* thymosin therapy. At age 1 month he had received a fetal thymus transplant intraperitoneally with subsequent demonstration of cell chimerism, normal percent T-cell rosettes, and normal *in vitro* T-cell function (2). At approximately age 3 years he began to deteriorate clinically with chronic diarrhea and malabsorption, recurrent otitis media, pneumonia, and finally bronchiectasis. Simultaneously, although his *in vitro* percent T-cell rosettes remained greater than 80%, *in vitro* T-cell function as assayed by lymphocyte response to PHA and to allogeneic cells had deteriorated. Cell chimerism, as determined by HLA typing, persisted. Although *in vitro* thymosin incubation with his lymphocytes failed to enhance any cell function, a trial of thymosin was begun when he was 5 years old. After 5 months of therapy, there was no evidence of clinical improvement or normalization of *in vitro* T-cell function. Thymosin was discontinued, and a cultured thymus epithelial transplant was performed.

Patient L. N. (no. 10) is a 34-year-old man with acquired hypogammaglobulinemia, recurrent infections, diarrhea, 20-lb weight loss in 1 year, hepatomegaly, and premalignant cells on liver biopsy. T-cell rosettes increased only from 52 to 60% with thymosin incubation, but the patient's *in vitro* lymphocyte response to allogeneic cells increased from 1,554 to 6,484 cpm following thymosin incubation. Nine months following the initiation of therapy, the patient maintained his weight at 75 kg and had decreased diarrhea, decreased hepatomegaly, and return of liver function studies to near normal (alkaline phosphatase 348 decreasing to 255, SGOT 160 decreasing to 49, LDH 325 decreasing to 101). Repeat biopsy of the patient's liver has not been performed. The patient continues to have hypogammaglobulinemia of the acquired type with 13% circulating lymphocytes bearing surface immunoglobulin. T-cell rosettes remain normal at 86%. *In vitro* lymphocyte response to PHA and to allogeneic cells remains depressed. A final patient, with ataxia-telangiectasia (no. 11, K. J.), has received thymosin therapy for 2 weeks. Clinically and immunologically, it is too soon in the patient's course to evaluate response to thymosin therapy. Prior to therapy the patient's total lymphocyte count was 1,280, 62% T-cells with an increase to 78% following *in vitro* thymosin incubation, and 17% B cells. *In vitro* lymphocyte stimulation by PHA was 4,422 (10% of normal) and by allogeneic cells 638 cpm (10% of normal) with an increase to 10,705 cpm following thymosin incubation *in vitro*. Thymosin therapy was begun and T-cell rosettes increased to 66%.

DISCUSSION

The response by patients to *in vivo* thymosin therapy, both clinically and in the laboratory, has been variable. Of 10 patients evaluated, eight patients have shown evidence of clinical improvement that includes decreased numbers and severity of infections, decreased diarrhea, and weight gain (Table 2). Patients 5 and 9 showed no evidence of clinical improvement following initiation of therapy, no evidence of *in vitro* enhancement of T-cell number or function prior to thymosin incubation, and none of reconstitution of cellular immunity following initiation of therapy. Patients 1, 2, 3, 4, 6, 7, and 8, which included those with diagnoses of thymic hypoplasia, Wiskott-Aldrich syndrome, DiGeorge syndrome, and chronic fungal infection, had decreased numbers of T-cell rosettes prior to the initiation of therapy, evidence of *in vitro* enhancement of T-cell rosette formation following thymosin incubation, and marked improvement in T-cell rosette numbers within 1 month following initiation of therapy (Table 1). Patient no. 5, with DiGeorge syndrome, had T-cell rosettes of less than 10% and no evidence of enhancement *in vitro* with thymosin incubation; following therapy there was no evidence of increased T-cell rosette formation. The remainder of the patients had T-cell rosettes of greater than 60% prior to the initiation of thymosin, little or no response *in vitro* following thymosin incubation, and only minimal changes following the initiation of therapy. Patients 6, 10, and 11 with diagnoses of DiGeorge syndrome, acquired hypogammaglobulinemia, and ataxia-telangiectasia showed evidence prior to thymosin therapy of *in vitro* enhancement of lymphocyte response to allogeneic cells by thymosin incubation. Following the initiation of therapy, these patients, in addition to patients 2, 3, and 4 (thymic hypoplasia, Wiskott-Aldrich) showed improvement in *in vitro* lymphocyte response to allogeneic cells. Enhanced lymphocyte response to allogeneic cells by thymosin incubation *in vitro* in patients 2, 3, and 4 was not evaluated prior to the initiation of thymosin. Patients 1 and 9 (thymic hypoplasia, severe combined immunodeficiency) showed no evidence *in vitro* of enhanced cell function with thymosin incubation. Following prolonged periods of therapy, there was no evidence of improvement in cell function. It is interesting that clinical improvement appears to correlate best with normalization of lymphocyte function. Normalization of percent and total T-cell rosettes did not necessarily correlate with marked clinical improvement. Further, although percent T-cell rosettes and total lymphocyte count improved within 1 month following the initiation of *in vivo* thymosin, normalization of cell function often required 4 to 6 months of therapy.

It is clear, even from the limited number of patients we have treated with thymosin, that they respond in varying degrees and over varying time periods to therapy. Enhancement of T-cell rosette formation *in vitro* with thymosin incubation predicts which patients will have increased percent T-cell rosettes following the initiation of therapy. Further, enhancement of a patient's *in vitro* response to allogeneic cells may predict whether the patient will respond to therapy with improved lymphocyte function.

Variation in response to thymosin therapy most likely reflects a variation in the thymic defect present in our patient population. It is interesting that even patients with the same diagnosis (DiGeorge syndrome) may respond differently to thymosin; our findings in two patients treated with thymosin and in two additional patients evaluated *in vitro* support recent clinical evidence that the DiGeorge syndrome is composed of a spectrum of deficiencies ranging from severe depletion of cell-mediated immunity to a more classic picture, responsive to humoral therapy. Patients with the DiGeorge syndrome may be deficient in an epithelial-enhancing factor or in a cell population; interpreted differently, patients with DiGeorge syndrome may have varying severities in abnormal formation of thymic tissue.

The variation in response to thymosin therapy between patients with different forms of thymic abnormalities may represent deficiencies of different thymic humoral factors. It has recently been appreciated that thymosin Fraction 5 contains 12 polypeptides; the first has been isolated and amino acid sequenced. It is probable that patients with similar but not identical clinical and laboratory syndromes are deficient in different factors. Isolation of these specific factors with subsequent evaluation in biological systems may result in the treatment of patients with the specific factor(s) they lack. A specific approach to replacement therapy in patients with adequate populations of prethymic cells should result in the specific and complete reconstitution of their immune systems.

ACKNOWLEDGMENT

This research was supported by the Pediatric Clinical Research Center, NIH, 5M01-RROO79-15, The John A. Hartford Foundation, Inc., and the National Foundation, March of Dimes.

REFERENCES

1. Aiuti, F., Schirrmacher, V., Ammirati, P., and Fiorilli, M. (1975): Effect of thymus factor on human precursor T-lymphocytes. *Clin. Exp. Immunol.,* 20:499–503.
2. Ammann, A. J., Wara, D. W., and Salmon, S. (1973): Thymus transplantation. Permanent reconstitution of cellular immunity in a patient with sex-linked combined immunodeficiency. *N. Engl. J. Med.,* 289:5–9.
3. Armerding, D., and Katz, D. H. (1975): Activation of T and B lymphocytes *in vitro.* IV. Regulatory influence on specific T-cell functions by a thymus extract factor. *J. Immunol.,* 114:1248–1254.
4. Asanuma, Y., Goldstein, A. L., and White, A. (1970): Reduction in the incidence of wasting disease in neonatally thymectomized CBA-W mice by the injection of thymosin. *Endocrinology,* 86:600–610.
5. Bach, J. F., and Dardenne, M. (1973): Studies on thymus products. II. Demonstration and characterization of a circulating thymic hormone. *Immunology,* 25:353–366.
6. Cohen, G. H., Hooper, J. A., and Goldstein, A. L. (1975): Thymosin-induced differentiation of murine thymocytes in allogeneic mixed lymphocyte cultures. *Ann. NY Acad. Sci.,* 249:145–153.
7. Goldstein A. L., Asanuma, Y., Battisto, Hardy, M. A., Quint, J., and White, A. (1970): Influence of thymosin on cell-mediated and humoral immune responses in normal and in immunologically deficient mice. *J. Immunol.,* 104:359–366.
8. Goldstein, A. L., Guha, A., Zatz, M. M., Hardy, M. A., and White, A. (1972): Purification and biological activity of thymosin, a hormone of the thymus gland. *Proc. Natl. Acad. Sci. USA,* 69:1800–1803.
9. Goldstein, G., and Schlesinger, D. H. (1975): Thymopoietin and myasthenia gravis: Neostigmine-responsive neuromuscular block produced in mice by a synthetic peptide fragment of thymopoietin. *Lancet,* 2:256–259.
10. Komuro, K., and Boyse, E. A. (1973): *In vitro* demonstration of thymic hormone in the mouse by conversion of precursor cells into lymphocytes. *Lancet,* 1:740–743.
11. Osoba, D., and Miller, J. F. A. P. (1963): Evidence for a humoral thymus factor responsible for the maturation of immunological faculty. *Nature,* 199:653.
12. Sakai, H., Costanzi, J., Loukas, D., Gagliano, R. G., Ritzmann, S. E., and Goldstein, A. L. (1975): Thymosin-induced increase in E-rosette-forming capacity of lymphocytes in patients with malignant neoplasms. *Cancer,* 36:974–976.
13. Scheinberg, M. A., Cathcart, E. S., and Goldstein, A. L. (1975): Thymosin induced reduction of "null cells" in peripheral blood lymphocytes of patients with systemic lupus erythematosus. *Lancet,* 1:424–428.
14. Schimpl, A., and Wecker, E. (1973): Stimulation of IgG antibody response *in vitro* by T-cell replacing factor. *J. Exp. Med.,* 137:547–552.
15. Steele, R. W., Limas, C., Thurman, G. B., Schuelein, M., Bauer, H., and Bellanti, J. A. (1972): Familial thymic aplasia. Attempted reconstitution with fetal thymus in a millipore diffusion chamber. *N. Engl. J. Med.,* 287:787–791.
16. Touraine, J. L., Incefy, G. S., Touraine, F., L'Esperance, P., Siegal, F. P., and Good, R. A. (1974): T-lymphocyte differentiation *in vitro* in primary immunodeficiency diseases. *Clin. Immunol. Immunopathol.,* 3:228–235.
17. Trainin, N., and Small, M. (1970): Studies on some physiochemical properties of a thymus humoral factor conferring immunocompetence on lymphoid cells. *J. Exp. Med.,* 132:885–897.
18. Trainin, N. (1974): Thymic hormones and the immune response. *Physiol. Rev.,* 54:272–315.

19. Wara, D. W., and Ammann, A. J. (1975): Activation of T-cell rosettes in immunodeficient patients by thymosin. *Ann. NY Acad. Sci.,* 249:308–315.
20. Wara, D. W., Goldstein, A. L., Doyle, N. E., and Amman, A. (1975): Thymosin activity in patients with cellular immunodeficiency. *N. Engl. J. Med.,* 292:70–74.
21. Zisblatt, M., Goldstein, A. L., Lilly, F., and White, A. (1970): Acceleration by thymosin of the development of resistance to murine sarcoma-induced tumor in mice. *Proc. Natl. Acad. Sci. USA,* 66:1170–1174.

Immune Modulation and Control of Neoplasia by Adjuvant Therapy, edited by M. A. Chirigos. Raven Press, New York, 1978.

Lymphocyte Response to Thymosin *In Vitro* in Cancer Patients: Correlation with Initial T-Cell Levels

Daniel E. Kenady, Claude Potvin, and Paul B. Chretien

Surgery Branch, National Cancer Institute, National Institutes of Health, Bethesda, Maryland 20014

Thymosin fraction 5 (7) improves cellular immunity in children with thymic deficiencies (6,14). Similarities of cellular immune defects in these children and cancer patients provoke speculation about whether thymosin would improve cellular immunity in cancer patients. Prior to a clinical assessment of the effects of thymosin in cancer patients, it appears prudent to assess its effect *in vitro* on percent peripheral blood T-cell levels as a measure of potential responsiveness *in vivo,* since the results of this assay correlated with thymosin's beneficial effect in children with cellular defects due to thymic deficiency. Prior to treatment with thymosin, in patients who improved, T-cell levels were low and increased *in vitro* after incubation with thymosin. After treatment, T-cell levels increased and other parameters of cellular immunity improved, but T-cell levels no longer increased *in vitro* after incubation with thymosin. We determined the effect of thymosin *in vitro* on peripheral blood T-cell levels in normals, patients with solid malignancies who were studied prior to and during treatment with radiation therapy or chemotherapy, and patients who had surgical removal of solid malignancies 5 or more years beforehand and who had no evidence of residual tumor. This report reviews the major findings (9–11) of this investigation thus far.

MATERIALS AND METHODS

Populations Studied

Concurrently, we studied:

1. Three hundred fifty patients with previously untreated solid malignancies, in whom the tumor was clinically confined to the primary site or did not extend beyond the regional lymph nodes. Patients with disseminated tumor were excluded. The histologic classifications of the tumors were squamous carcinomas (*N*-67), adenocarcinomas (*N*-63), melanomas (*N*-101), sarcomas (*N*-77), and undifferentiated carcinomas, transitional cell carcinomas, and testicular carcinomas (*N*-42).

TABLE 1. *Distribution of determinations in the study for each radiation portal and cumulative radiation dose*

Cumulative radiation dose (rads)	Portal		
	Head and neck	Mediastinal	Pelvic
0	[22]	[22]	[30]
<1,000	21[a](17%)	23 (15%)	20 (17%)
1,000–2,000	20 (17%)	23 (15%)	18 (16%)
2,000–3,000	23 (19%)	32 (21%)	20 (17%)
3,000–4,000	21 (17%)	30 (20%)	19 (17%)
4,000–5,000	20 (17%)	28 (18%)	24 (31%)
5,000–6,000	15 (13%)	17 (11%)	14 (12%)
Totals[b]	120	153	115

Figures in brackets represent untreated patients. Figures in parentheses indicate percent of the total number of determinations for each portal during radiation therapy.

[a] Number of patients studied who had received the cumulative radiation dose given.

[b] Total numbers of determinations during radiation therapy. Some patients were studied at more than one treatment interval during therapy.

2. One hundred fifty-seven patients with no evidence of tumor 5 or more years after surgical treatment for the histologic types of tumors in the untreated patients.

3. Three hundred forty patients with malignancies clinically confined to the head and neck, mediastinal-hilar, or pelvic regions who were receiving radiation therapy via portals encompassing the tumors. Similar percentages of patients were studied at each cumulative radiation dose level (Table 1). A total of 388 determinations were performed in these patients at intervals during radiation therapy.

4. Eighty tumor-bearing patients with solid malignancies who were studied while receiving chemotherapy, usually consisting of multiple-drug regimens. Although patients in this group had systemic tumor dissemination, all were fully ambulatory and were being treated in the out-patient clinic. Excluded from this group were patients who had signs or symptoms of impaired function of central organs.

5. Four hundred twenty-seven healthy volunteers. Fifty-seven percent were male and 80% were Caucasian, and their mean age was 41 with a range of 18 to 85. By these parameters they did not differ from any of the patient groups studied. Volunteers with a history of malignancy, systemic disease, or recent viral infections were excluded. In all populations, subjects with total leukocyte counts above 10,000 were excluded from study.

Spontaneous Lymphocyte Rosette (T-Cell) Assay

Peripheral blood thymus-derived lymphocytes (T cells) were quantitated by the formation of spontaneous rosettes when mixed with sheep erythrocytes by a technique previously described (10). Briefly, triplicate samples were prepared for T-cell determination, and three additional samples were prepared in an identical fashion with the addition to each tube of 0.1 ml of phosphate-buffered saline containing 100 μg of thymosin fraction 5 (7) (provided by Allan Goldstein and by Jack Snyder, Hoffmann-LaRoche Laboratories) prior to incubation. The tubes were coded so as to prevent identification of the blood donor or of the tubes containing thymosin by the person performing the T-cell determinations. The effect of thymosin (ΔT) was determined by subtracting the mean of the triplicate samples without thymosin from the mean of the triplicate samples with thymosin.

Statistical Methods

Comparisons of parameters among groups of individuals were performed using Student's *t*-test (2). The statistical significance of the correlations between T-cell response to thymosin and initial percent T-cell level was evaluated using the Kendall-Stuart linear regression procedure when both variables are measured with error (12). The error in the measurement of the percentage of T cells without thymosin was estimated from 100 sets of triplicate determinations. This regression procedure evaluates the strength of the correlation above that expected by chance from the regression toward the mean phenomenon. All *p* values correspond to two-tailed statistical tests.

RESULTS

The mean percent T-cell level in normals was higher than in untreated patients ($p < 0.001$) and cured patients ($p < 0.005$). Compared to normals, the mean total T-cell levels in untreated and cured patients did not differ, but cured

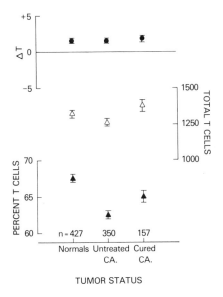

FIG. 1. Mean percent and total T-cell levels and the effect of thymosin *in vitro* in normals, untreated, and cured patients.

patients had a higher level than untreated patients ($p < 0.025$). After incubation with thymosin *in vitro,* the mean percent T-cell levels increased (ΔT) significantly in normals, untreated patients, and cured patients (Fig. 1).

Analysis of untreated patients by histology indicated that patients with melanomas had percent T-cell levels higher than patients with squamous carcinomas, adenocarcinomas, or sarcomas ($p < 0.025$). However, there were no differences in total T-cell levels or in ΔT among untreated patient groups. Comparison of cured patients by histology showed no differences by these three parameters. Comparison of untreated and cured patient groups within each histology revealed percent T-cell levels higher in cured patients than in untreated patients with squamous carcinomas and adenocarcinomas ($p < 0.05$). However, there were no differences in total T-cell levels among these groups. Cured melanoma patients had a higher ΔT than untreated melanoma patients ($p < 0.05$) (Fig. 2).

Regression analysis was used to investigate the relationship between the effect of thymosin on T-cell levels and initial percent T cells. Correction was made for artificial correlation induced by the inherent error in measurement in both variables. There was a significant ($p < 0.001$) inverse relationship between initial percent T cells and effect of thymosin *in vitro* on percent T cells in normals, untreated cancer patients, and cured patients (Fig. 3). These regressions show a similar progressively greater increase in T-cell levels after incubation with thymosin among subjects with low T-cell levels and a progressively lower T-cell level after incubation with thymosin in subjects with high T-cell levels.

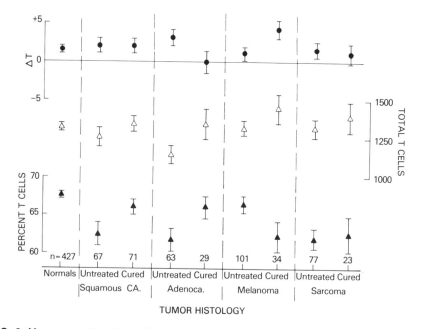

FIG. 2. Mean percent and total T-cell levels and the effect of thymosin *in vitro* in patients with solid malignancies grouped by tumor histology and clinical status.

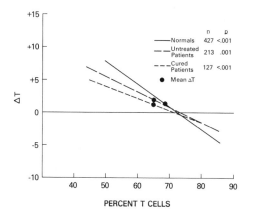

FIG. 3. Correlation of initial T-cell level and the effect of thymosin *in vitro* in normals, untreated, and cured patients.

We next further analyzed the relationship of initial T-cell levels to ΔT in patients receiving radiation therapy. The untreated patients were subdivided into those with tumors corresponding to the three radiation treatment portals used—head and neck, mediastinal-hilar, and pelvic—and by tumor histology. They were compared to their respective counterparts receiving irradiation and to normals. The mean percent T-cell level in normals (68.4%) was higher than in each untreated group ($p < 0.025$–0.005) and in each group during radiotherapy ($p < 0.001$). The mean percent T-cell level in patients with head and neck irradiation did not differ from that in their untreated counterparts. However, the levels in patients with mediastial-hilar and pelvic carcinomas during irradiation were lower than in their respective untreated counterparts ($p < 0.01$ and $p < 0.005$, respectively) and did not differ from each other. Among untreated patients, only in those with mediastinal-hilar malignancies was the mean total T-cell level lower than in normals ($p < 0.05$). During radiation therapy, the mean total T-cell level in each group was lower than in normals ($p < 0.001$) and also lower than in each corresponding untreated group ($p < 0.001$). Total T-cell levels in patients during mediastinal-hilar and pelvic irradiation were also significantly lower than in patients with head and neck irradiation ($p < 0.001$) and were similar to each other. After incubation with thymosin, the mean T-cell level in normals increased significantly ($p < 0.005$). In untreated patients with head and neck and pelvic malignancies, the levels also increased significantly ($p < 0.01$ and < 0.005, respectively). These increases did not differ from the increase in normals. In untreated patients with mediastinal-hilar malignancies, however, the increase was not significant. Mean T-cell levels in patients with head and neck and pelvic malignancies during irradiation did not change significantly after incubation with thymosin, and in patients with pelvic malignancies the change was less than in untreated patients ($p < 0.025$). However, in patients with mediastinal-hilar malignancies, during irradiation the mean level increased ($p < 0.001$), and the increase was greater than in normals ($p < 0.05$) (Fig. 4).

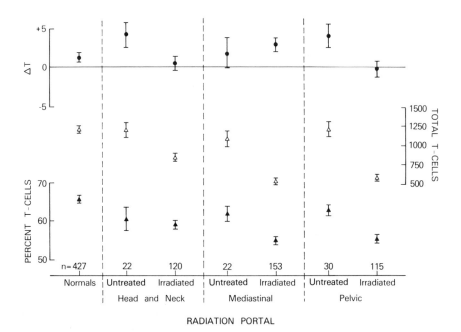

FIG. 4. Mean percent and total T-cell levels and the effect of thymosin *in vitro* in patients prior to and during radiation therapy—correlation with radiation portal and treatment status.

Investigation of the three portal groups by regression analysis showed a relationship similar to that defined for normals, total untreated patients, and cured patients. A significant inverse relationship existed between initial T-cell level and ΔT for each group tested ($p < 0.001$). At a given initial T-cell level, patients receiving mediastinal-hilar irradiation had a mean increase in T-cell levels similar to their untreated counterparts (Fig. 5). Patients receiving head and neck or pelvic irradiation, however, had lesser mean increases in T-cell levels after incubation with thymosin for a given initial T-cell level (Figs. 6 and 7). Thus, the

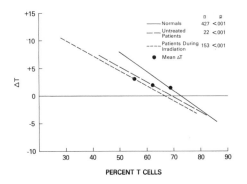

FIG. 5. Patients with mediastinal-hilar carcinomas—correlation of initial T-cell level and the effect of thymosin *in vitro* before and during radiation therapy.

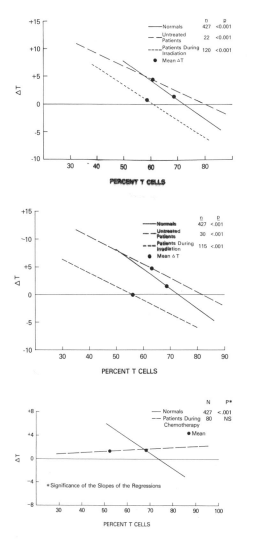

FIG. 6. Patients with head and neck carcinomas—correlation of initial T-cell level and the effect of thymosin *in vitro* before and during radiation therapy.

FIG. 7. Patients with pelvic carcinomas—correlation of initial T-cell level and the effect of thymosin *in vitro* before and during radiation therapy.

FIG. 8. Patients receiving chemotherapy—correlation of initial T-cell level and the effect of thymosin *in vitro*.

effect of thymosin was not a generalized increase of T cells; rather, at low T-cell levels, the effect was that of reconstitution, and at high T-cell levels, that of modulation toward a lower level.

Among patients receiving chemotherapy, mean percent T-cell level was significantly lower than in normals ($p < 0.005$) as was mean total T-cell level ($p < 0.001$). There was a significant mean response to thymosin ($p < 0.05$). However, regression analysis did not show a significant correlation between initial T-cell level and response to thymosin (Fig. 8).

DISCUSSION

In these studies, we found correlations of change in T-cell levels after incubation with thymosin *in vitro* with initial T-cell levels among normals, untreated cancer patients, cured cancer patients, and cancer patients during radiation therapy. Although there were differences among these groups in mean percent and total T-cell levels, in each group there was a similar increase in mean T-cell level after incubation with thymosin as well as a similar correlation of change in T-cell level with initial T-cell level.

Other investigators have demonstrated an increase in T-cell levels after incubation of lymphocytes from cancer patients with thymosin *in vitro* (8,13), and the increases were greater than that obtained in this study. These previous studies were conducted in patients with advanced or disseminated malignancies, whereas our study was confined to patients whose tumors clinically did not extend beyond the regional lymph nodes, with the exception of the patients receiving chemotherapy. The studies of T-cell levels (4) and the other methods of assessing cellular immunity (3,5) showing a progressive decrease in these parameters with increasing tumor burden and the present data showing a progressively greater increase in T-cell levels after incubation with thymosin in patients with progressively lower initial T-cell levels explain an apparent discrepancy and show correlations between findings in previous studies (8,13) and those of the present one.

The results of the present study suggest that administration of thymosin produces an increase in T-cell levels in cancer patients with low T-cell levels regardless of tumor histology or clinical tumor burden and has a similar effect in normals with low T-cell levels. Also, they suggest that a similar effect could be obtained in patients receiving radiation therapy. The results also raise speculation about whether, in subjects with high T-cell levels, the administration of thymosin has a reverse effect, i.e., that of lowering T-cell levels.

In patients with chemotherapy the finding that the increase in T-cell levels after incubation with thymosin was independent of the initial T-cell level suggests that, in such patients as a group, thymosin has the greatest efficacy because suppression of T-cell levels in subjects with high levels does not occur. Additional studies of large numbers of patients receiving homogenous chemotherapy regimens are needed to determine whether the relationship demonstrated in this study is applicable to all chemotherapy regimens that suppress parameters of cellular immunity.

The results of this study correlate with those studies of levamisole's effects on immune responses showing that the agent has a reconstituting effect on suppressed cell-mediated immune responses but a modulating effect at high levels of cellular immunity (1). These combined data indicate that the predominant effect of these two agents is reconstitution of defects of cellular immunity, in contrast to the effects of immune-reactive agents such as Bacillus Calmette-Guerin (BCG), *Corynebacterium parvum,* and MER, which may increase intact

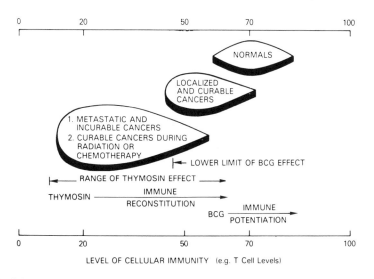

IMMUNE RECONSTITUTION AND IMMUNE POTENTIATION

FIG. 9. Schematic representation of the differing effects on immune reactivity of thymosin and BCG.

cellular immunity above normal levels. Thus, these immune-reactive agents appear to form two groups, those that reconstitute cellular immune defects due to tumor burden or the effects of conventional therapy and those that augment or potentiate cellular reactivity above normal levels. Tentatively at least, this grouping provides a basis for the selection of immune-reactive agents and design of clinical trials that evaluate their effectiveness as adjuvants for treatment of cancer. For example, the available information concerning the effects of thymosin and BCG in experimental animal systems and in humans can be assembled as in Fig. 9 to provide a schema for evaluation of their effectiveness as immunoadjuvants in cancer therapy.

SUMMARY

The effect of thymosin *in vitro* on T-cell levels was determined in blood specimens from normal volunteers, from patients with local-regional solid malignancies prior to treatment, from patients clinically cured of these malignancies, and from patients receiving either radiation therapy or chemotherapy. With the exception of patients receiving chemotherapy, there was a significant inverse relationship between T-cell levels after incubation with thymosin *in vitro* and initial T-cell levels in the groups studied. In patients receiving chemotherapy, T-cell levels increased independently of initial T-cell levels. These results parallel other findings indicating that the predominant effect of thymosin is an increase in low T-cell levels rather than a generalized increase in T-cell levels regardless of the initial T-cell level.

REFERENCES

1. Amery, W. K. (1976): Levamisole (NSC-177023) in clinical immunotherapy. *Cancer Treat. Rep.,* 60:217.
2. Armitage, P. (1971): *Statistical Methods in Medical Research,* p. 119. Blackwell, Oxford.
3. Cheema, A. R., and Hersh, E. M. (1971): Patient survival after chemotherapy and its relationship to *in vitro* lymphocyte blastogenesis. *Cancer,* 28:851–855.
4. Dellon, A. L., Potvin, C., and Chretien, P. B. (1975): Thymus-dependent lymphocyte levels in bronchogenic carcinoma: Correlations with histology, clinical stage, and clinical course after surgical treatment. *Cancer,* 35:687–694.
5. Eilber, F. R., Nizze, J. A., and Morton, D. L. (1975): Sequential evaluation of general immune competence in cancer patients: Correlation with clinical course. *Cancer,* 35:660–665.
6. Goldstein, A. L., Cohen, G. H., Rossio, J. L., Thurman, G. B., and Ulrich, J. T. (1976): Use of thymosin in the treatment of primary immunodeficiency diseases and cancer. *Med. Clin. North Am.,* 60:591–606.
7. Goldstein, A. L., Slater, F. D., and White, A. (1966): Preparation, assay, and partial purification of a thymic lymphocytopoietic factor (thymosin). *Proc. Natl. Acad. Sci. USA,* 56:1010–1017.
8. Hardy, M. A., Dattner, A. M., Sarkar, D. K., Stoffer, J. A., and Friedmann, N. (1976): The effect of thymosin on human T-cells from cancer patients. *Cancer,* 37:98–103.
9. Kenady, D. E., Chretien, P. B., Potvin, C., Simon, R. M., Alexander, J. C., Jr., and Goldstein, A. L. (1977): Effect of thymosin *in vitro* on T-cell levels during radiation therapy: Correlations with radiation portal and initial T-cell levels. *Cancer,* 39:642–652.
10. Kenady, D. E., Potvin, C., Simon, R. M., and Chretien, P. B. (1977): *In vitro* effect of thymosin on T-cell levels in cancer patients receiving radiation therapy. In: *Control of Neoplasia by Modulation of the Immune System,* edited by M. A. Chirigos, pp. 305–313. Raven Press, New York.
11. Kenady, D. E., Potvin, C., Simon, R. M., and Chretien, P. B. (1977): Thymosin reconstitution of T-cell deficits *in vitro* in cancer patients. *Cancer,* 39:575–580.
12. Kendall, M. G., and Stuart, A. (1973): *The Advanced Theory of Statistics,* Vol. 2, p. 397. Charles Griffin & Co. Ltd., London.
13. Sakai, H., Costanzi, J. J., Loukas, D. F., Gagliano, R. G., Ritzmann, S. E., and Goldstein, A. L. (1975): Thymosin-induced increase in E-rosette forming capacity of lymphocytes in patients with malignant neoplasms. *Cancer,* 36:974–976.
14. Wara, D. W., Goldstein, A. L., Doyle, N. E., and Ammann, A. J. (1975): Thymosin activity in patients with cellular immunodeficiency. *N. Engl. J. Med.,* 292:70–74.

Immune Modulation and Control of Neoplasia by Adjuvant Therapy, edited by M. A. Chirigos. Raven Press, New York, 1978.

Clinical and Immunological Evaluation of the Use of Thymosin Plus BCG ± DTIC in the Adjuvant Treatment of Stage 3B Melanoma

Yehuda Z. Patt, Evan M. Hersh, Larry A. Schafer, *Lance K. Heilbrun, Marvette L. Washington, Jordan U. Gutterman, Giora M. Mavligit, and **Allan L. Goldstein

*Section of Immunology, Department of Developmental Therapeutics and * Section of Biometrics, Department of Biomathematics, The University of Texas System Cancer Center, M. D. Anderson Hospital and Tumor Institute, Houston, Texas 77030; and the ** Division of Biochemistry, University of Texas Medical Branch, Galveston, Texas 77050*

The concept of adjuvant chemotherapy and immunotherapy is based on the existence of micrometastases following surgical removal of all obvious disease and on the need for systemic treatment for these (20).

Bacillus Calmette-Guerin (BCG) was shown to delay the progression of micrometastases into evident disease in several studies (1,9,13,17). Thus, high-dose BCG (6×10^8 viable organisms) applied by scarification close to regional draining lymph nodes prolonged the median disease-free interval in stage 3B melanoma (10).

Since the protective effect of BCG was demonstrated primarily in immunocompetent melanoma patients (10), and there is definite evidence for a decline in both cell-mediated and humoral immunity in cancer patients with progressive disease (11), it seemed reasonable to add an immunorestorative agent such as thymosin to the adjuvant treatment with BCG with or without DTIC.

Thymosin (7,8) increases the percent E-rosette-forming cells in patients with Hodgkin's disease, lung carcinoma, melanoma, and leiomyosarcoma (6). Also, thymosin reversed the decrease in E-rosette-forming cells created by irradiation in lung cancer patients (15).

The purpose of this study was:

1. To determine the efficacy of thymosin in combination with BCG or BCG + DTIC in prolonging disease-free interval in stage 3B melanoma patients,
2. To determine the optimal dose of thymosin, and
3. To correlate clinical response with the patients' cell-mediated immunity.

Material and Methods

Forty-five consecutive patients with melanoma stage 3B and 3AB (16) were entered into the study. Patients with a primary melanoma removed from a limb or the trunk and subsequent recurrence in regional lymph nodes (stage 3B), or in both lymph nodes and metastases *en route* to the regional lymph node (stage 3AB) were examined and included. The patients underwent a regional lymph node dissection and rendered free of evident disease (NED). The lymph nodes removed were counted, and the proportion of involved nodes was calculated.

Patients were evaluated for residual disease with the following tests before therapy—history, physical examination, and blood chemistry including liver and spleen scan, brain scan, EEG, and a bone marrow aspiration.

Immunological Evaluation

An immunological evaluation was carried out prior to initiation of chemotherapy and immunotherapy, following completion of thymosin treatment and prior to the second cycle of therapy. This consisted of a battery of delayed hypersensitivity skin tests to recall antigens and included dermatophytin, *Candida,* streptokinase-strephodornase, mumps, and intermediate strength purified protein derivative (9). The average diameter of induration obtained by two right-angle measurements at 24 and 48 hr was recorded in millimeters.

Absolute lymphocyte count and relative enumeration of E-rosette-forming cells using permanently fixed slides (21) were performed prior to initiation of therapy.

Patients' peripheral blood lymphocytes (PBL) were separated by layering the defibrinated buffy coat on an 8-ml 8% Ficoll and 2-ml 50% Hypaque gradient as previously described (2). Cells were washed twice in minimum essential medium (MEM), counted, and brought to a concentration of 0.75×10^6 cells/ml in RPMI + 10% autologous human serum, of which 0.2 ml (1.5×10^5 cells) was plated in each well, of a flat bottom microculture Linboro plate.

Cells were stimulated with 0.02 parts of Difco phytohemagglutinin (PHA) M 1:10 dilution per well, or with Concavavalin A (Con A) 1.6 mg in 0.02 ml RPMI per well. The cultures were incubated for 5 days. Eight hours prior to harvesting 1 mc of ^{3}H-thymidine (^{3}H TdR) was added to each well, in 0.02 ml of RPMI. After the 8-hr period has elapsed cells were harvested with a multiple automatic sample harvester (MASH) using saline to deposit the well content onto $9\frac{1}{2}'' \times 1''$ strip of glass fiber filter paper (Reeve Angel #934AH). Filter discs were dried, placed in vials containing 10 ml of liquid scintillation cocktail, and then counted.

Results were expressed as a stimulation index (SI) of the counts per minute (CPM) of the PHA- or Con A-stimulated cells over CPM of nonstimulated cells.

The number of PBL-stimulated with allogeneic cells in a mixed lymphocyte culture (MLC) was 1.5×10^5/well in 0.1 ml of RPMI supplemented with 10% autologous human serum. For stimulator cells PBL were drawn from normal donors, frozen in 10% DMSO, and stored in liquid nitrogen. Before use cells were rapidly thawed in a 37°C water bath, immediately washed twice in MEM supplemented with 10% heat-inactivated pooled normal serum, and resuspended in RPMI with 10% of the culture serum counted for viability, and concentration adjusted to 1.5×10^6 cells/ml. Stimulator cell were irradiated at 4,000 rads using a cesium source irradiator in 12×75 mm plastic Falcon tubes, then 1.5×10^5 cells in 0.1 ml were added to each well of responding cells. Mononuclear cells from a single donor were repeatedly used as stimulator cells.

Cultures were left for 7 days in a highly humidified 5 or 7% CO_2 atmosphere at 37°C. Tritiated thymidine incorporation was determined as for the PHA- and the Con A-stimulated cultures (see above).

Results were expressed as cpm of stimulated cells over cpm of irradiated cells.

Immunological evaluation by the above-mentioned parameters was performed prior to initiation of therapy, following completion of the first thymosin course, and prior to second cycle of therapy.

Chemo and Immunotherapy

Forty-five sequential patients were entered on the study between December 31, 1975 and August 31, 1976. They were divided into two groups according to the number of involved nodes. Thirty patients who had one to four involved regional nodes (3B $<$ 5) were treated with BCG and thymosin. The thymosin was given daily for the first 14 days subcutaneously, 4 mg/m² for the first 10 patients and 40 mg/m² to subsequent patients. In addition patients received 6×10^8 viable organisms of fresh frozen BCG on day 1 and at weekly intervals thereafter by scarification (Table 1). BCG and thymosin were administered on different limbs.

Fifteen patients who had five or more involved regional nodes (3B $>$ 5) or who had a metastases in transit from the primary lesion to the regional lymph-node (3AB) were treated with DTIC 250 mg/m² on day 1 through day 5 of each cycle of chemoimmunotherapy. Thymosin 4 mg/m² for the first 10 patients and 40 mg/m² for the following ones was administered subcutaneously daily beginning on day 7 until day 17, on the first cycle, and on day 7, 12, and 17 on the subsequent cycles. Fresh frozen BCG (6×10^8 viable organisms) was administered by scarification on days 7, 12, and 17 of each cycle. These cycles were repeated every 21 days (Table 1).

The efficacy of the treatment was evaluated by the duration of the disease-free interval. Recurrence was defined as local or distant reappearance of disease. The response to this mode of treatment was compared to the response of histori-cally matched patients treated with BCG alone.

TABLE 1. Adjuvant postsurgical treatment plan for stage 3AB and 3B melanoma patients, using thymosin and BCG with or without DTIC

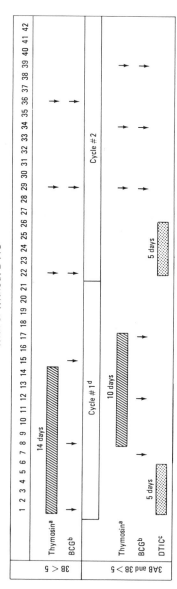
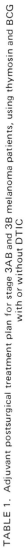

a. Thymosin dose: 4 mg/M² for the first 10 patients of each category, 40 mg/M² for the subsequent patients.
b. BCG: 6 × 10⁸ viable organisms of fresh frozen pasteur BCG administered by scarification, weekly for 12 doses and every other week thereafter, for 3B < 5 patients, and on days 7, 12 and 17 of each cycle for 3AB and 3B > 5 patients.
c. DTIC: 250 mg/M² I.V. on days 1 through 5 of each cycle.
d. Cycles were repeated every 21 days.

Statistics

The statistical methods used included a generalized two-tailed Wilcoxon test for differences between remission or survival curves (5) and the method of Kaplan and Meier (14) for calculating and plotting such curves. The life-table regression model of Cox (4) was used in a stepwise fashion for the multivariate analysis of time to recurrence and how it was affected by the various immunological variables.

Results

Table 2 shows the accrual rate and the evaluability on each arm of the study. Of the 45 patients, 30 were entered on the 3B < 5 arm and 15 on the 3AB and 3B ≥ 5 arm. Only 20 3B < 5 patients were evaluable for clinical response, and only 19 of these had a complete initial immunological evaluation, the other patients being inevaluable due to short follow-up (three patients), ineligibility, having stage 4 disease at the time of registration (two patients), nonadherence to protocol (four patients), or protocol violation (one patient). There were nine evaluable patients of the 15 entered on the 3AB and 3B ≥ 5 arm. Five were ineligible (stage 4 disease), and one had too short a follow-up.

Clinical Response

This is shown in Table 3 for the 29 evaluable patients. A total of 6/20 recurrences were observed in the 3B < 5 group, or 2/7 and 4/13 for the 4 mg/m² and 40 mg/m² treated patients, respectively. In the 3AB and 3B ≥ 5 group, 5/9 patients have recurred. There were 2/6 and 3/3 recurrences for the 4 mg/m² and 40 mg/m² patients, respectively.

The disease-free interval of the BCG- and thymosin-treated groups, compared to historical controls treated with BCG alone, is plotted in Figs. 1, 2, and 3.

TABLE 2. Distribution of patients entered to the adjuvant stage 3AB and 3B melanoma postsurgical treatment study

Clinical Stage	3B < 5 Nodes	3AB & 3B > 5 Nodes	Total
Total number of patients entered	30	15	
Too early to evaluate	3	1	
Ineligible	2	5	
Inevaluable	4		
Protocol violation	1		
Evaluable patients	20	9	29
Evaluable patients for clinical response and immunological workup	19	9	28

TABLE 3. Clinical course of evaluable stage 3AB and 3B melanoma patients with thymosin and BCG with or without DTIC

Clinical Stage	3B < 5 Nodes		3AB & 3B > 5 Nodes	
Thymosin Dose	4 mg/M^2	40 mg/M^2	4 mg/M^2	40 mg/M^2
Total number evaluable patients	20	7	13	9	6	3
NED*	14	5	9	4	4	0
Relapsed	6	2	4	5	2	3

* NED = No Evident Disease

Figure 1 depicts the disease-free interval of the stage 3B melanoma patients with < 5 involved nodes. The median duration of the disease-free interval has not been reached yet, but the 75th percentile is 36 weeks for the BCG-treated group, 18 weeks for the low-dose thymosin + BCG, and 15 weeks for the high-dose thymosin + BCG. The differences are not statistically significant (all $p > 0.20$). The disease-free interval of the 3B $\geq$ 5 and 3AB group treated with BCG + low-dose thymosin (4 mg/m^2) is shown to be similar to BCG alone (Fig. 2). The median disease-free interval was 40 weeks for the BCG-treated historical controls. Although the median has not been reached for the low-dose thymosin + BCG group, ($p = 0.11$), all three patients treated with high-dose thymosin *have* relapsed at 18 weeks ($p = 0.11$). It was noted that these three patients had a pretreatment PHA SI of > 50 and were treated with BCG, DTIC, and high-dose (40 mg/m^2) thymosin. This observation stimulated an

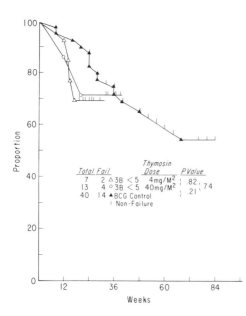

FIG. 1. Disease-free interval of stage 3B melanoma patient with 1 to 4 involved nodes. Correlation with thymosin dose compared to BCG-treated historical controls.

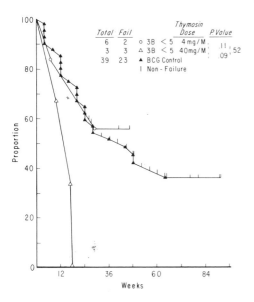

FIG. 2. Disease-free interval of stage 3AB and 3B melanoma patient with > 5 involved nodes. Correlation with thymosin dose compared to BCG-treated historical controls.

analysis of the interrelation between pretreatment, immunocompetence, thymosin dose, and recurrence rate. Figure 3 compares disease-free intervals for the total 3B and 3AB group compared to BCG-treated controls. The patients treated with low-dose thymosin had longer time to recurrence than the high-dose patients, but not statistically so ($p = 0.31$). This seems to further substantiate the above-mentioned observation.

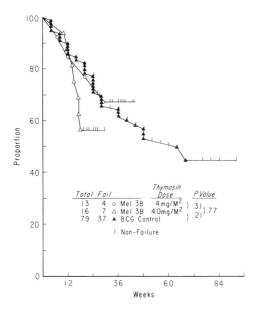

FIG. 3. Disease-free interval of the total group of stage 3AB and 3B melanoma patients. Correlation with thymosin dose compared to BCG-treated historical controls.

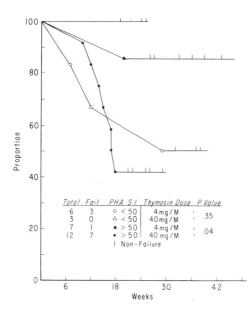

FIG. 4. Disease-free interval of stage 3AB and 3B melanoma patients. Correlation with pretreatment PHA SI and thymosin dose.

Total	Fail	PHA S.I.		Thymosin Dose	P Value
6	3	○	< 50	4 mg/M	.35
3	0	△	< 50	40 mg/M	
7	1	▲	> 50	4 mg/M	.04
12	7	●	> 50	40 mg/M	
			Non-Failure		

Univariate Analyses

An attempt was made therefore to correlate clinical response with initial immunological evaluation. Figures 4 through 7 correlate this with individual immunological parameters and thymosin dose. The following cut-off points were arbitrarily chosen to create two categories for each immunological variable—dermatophytin skin test response (≥ 10 mm), percent rosettes (≥ 40), initial MLC (SI ≥ 20), Con A (SI ≥ 10), and PHA (SI ≥ 50).

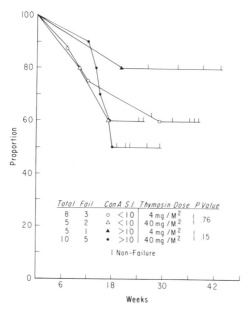

FIG. 5. Disease-free interval of stage 3AB and 3B melanoma patients. Correlation with pretreatment Con A SI and thymosin dose.

Total	Fail	Con A S.I.		Thymosin Dose	P Value
8	3	○	< 10	4 mg/M^2	.76
5	2	△	< 10	40 mg/M^2	
5	1	▲	> 10	4 mg/M^2	.15
10	5	●	> 10	40 mg/M^2	
			Non-Failure		

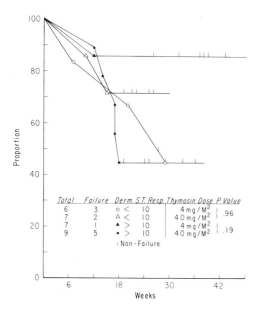

FIG. 6. Disease-free interval of stage 3AB and 3B melanoma patients. Correlation with pretreatment dermatophytin skin test response and thymosin dose.

The striking feature of Fig. 4 is a recurrence of 7/12 of the patients who had a PHA SI > 50 who received 40 mg/m² thymosin versus 1/7 of these patients who received 4 mg/m² thymosin ($p = 0.04$ when time to recurrence is compared by a two-tailed Wilcoxon).

Patients who had a Con A SI ≥ 10 and were treated with 40 mg/m² of thymosin had a higher recurrence rate than those treated with 4 mg/m²— 5/10 versus 1/5 ($p = 0.15$ in Fig. 5). Also 5/9 patients who had a high derma-

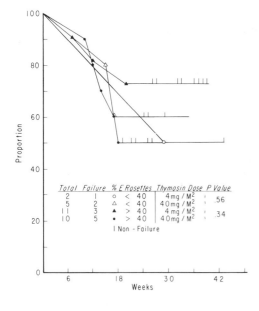

FIG. 7. Disease-free interval of stage 3AB and 3B melanoma patients. Correlation with pretreatment percent E-rosette-forming cells and thymosin dose.

TABLE 4. Recurrence rate in stage 3AB and 3B melanoma patients treated with thymosin and BCG with or without DTIC: Correlation with thymosin dose and immune status prior to treatment

	Immunological Parameters	Thymosin Dose	
		4 mg/M²	40 mg/M²
Immuno-competent	PHA S.I. ⩾ 50	1/7[a]	7/12
	Con A S.I. ⩾ 10	1/5	5/10
	Dermatophytin Response ⩾ 10 mm	1/7	5/9
	E Rosettes ⩾ 40%	3/11	5/10
Immuno-incompetent	PHA S.I. < 50	3/6	0/3
	Con A S.I. < 10	3/8	2/5
	Dermatophytin < 10 mm	3/6	2/7
	E Rosettes < 40%	1/2	2/5

[a] Number of patients with tumor recurrence/Total

S.I. = Stimulation Index

tophytin skin test response ($\geq$ 10 mm) and were treated with 40 mg/m² of thymosin recurred versus 1/7 on the low dose ($p = 0.19$ in Fig. 6). In Fig. 7 it is shown that 5/10 patients whose percent E-rosette-forming cells was ≥ 40 were treated with 40 mg/m² of thymosin experienced recurrence versus 3/11 who received 4 mg/m² of thymosin ($p = 0.34$). There was no correlation between a high MLC SI (≥ 20), high-dose thymosin, and relapse rate (3/7 relapsed on high dose versus 2/6 on low dose, $p = 0.71$). Cut-off points for the various analyses were chosen either for their demonstrated prognostic value, as for dermatophytin (12) or by arbitrary choice according to patients' disease-free interval distribution.

Table 4 summarizes the correlation between "immunocompetence" as derived from this univariate approach, thymosin dose, and clinical response. It excludes the parameters that do not substantiate this concept (eg., MLC).

Multivariate Analyses

The time to recurrence of the melanoma patients has been analyzed using the life-table regression model of Cox (5) in a stepwise fashion. The simultaneous prognostic influence of five immunological parameters (PHA SI, MLC SI, percent rosettes, dermatophytin response, and Con A SI) plus thymosin dose and age was investigated. These seven variables were selected for inclusion into the model in decreasing order of relative importance as shown in Table 5.

Unfortunately, none of these variables was significantly (all $p > 0.10$) related to time to recurrence. It should be emphasized that this is a multiple-variable procedure executed in a stepwise fashion that can yield much more informative results than univariate analysis. The favorable (but not statistically significant)

TABLE 5. Simultaneous prognostic influence of the seven parameters
analyzed in state 3AB and 3B melanoma patients treated with BCG
and thymosin with or without DTIC

Step	Variable	Significance level
1	MLC	0.113
2	Thymosin dose	0.287
3	Derm response	0.512
4	% Rosettes	0.559
5	PHA	0.418
6	Con-A	0.412
7	Age	0.690

At each step in the use of Cox's (1972) model, this reflects
whether the variable included adds any additional prognostic
information, given the other variables already in the model.

characteristics related to a longer time to recurrence are high MLC SI and
low-dose thymosin.

DISCUSSION

BCG alone or in combination with DTIC has been shown to increase the
disease-free interval in stage 3B melanoma patients (12,15,19). Thymosin fraction
5 increased the level of E-rosette-forming cells in cancer patients, therefore it
was felt that the combination of BCG and thymosin might further increase
survival and disease-free interval in this setting. This study was initiated in an
attempt to further improve the adjuvant treatment of stage 3B melanoma
patients.

Our results suggest that high-dose thymosin when added to BCG or to
BCG + DTIC was detrimental (Figs. 1, 2, and 3). Thymosin in low dose (4
mg/m^2) combined with BCG is similar to BCG alone (Figs. 2 and 3). Although
it is still too early there is a suggestion that thymosin in low dose when added
to BCG benefits the responding patients by prolonging their disease-free interval.
Due to the small number of patients and short follow-up time, these statements
are not significant at the 5% level.

In an attempt to explain these findings, we examined the initial immunological
evaluation of these patients in a univariate and multivariate analysis. In the
univariate analysis the disease-free interval was correlated with each of the
immunological parameters separately. It could be shown that immunocompetent
patients who received the high thymosin dose had a higher relapse rate. Only
the correlation between a high PHA SI (≥ 50), high thymosin dose, and shorter
time to recurrence was statistically significant ($p = 0.04$) (Fig. 4). In a decreasing
order of significance this was also suggested by the initial Con A SI ($p = 0.15$)
(Fig. 5), dermatophytin skin test response ($p = 0.19$) (Fig. 6), and percent
E-rosette-forming cells (Fig. 7) ($p = 0.34$). The initial MLC SI did not confirm
this observation in this form of analysis.

The multivariate analysis has investigated the simultaneous prognostic influence of the five immunological parameters, using Cox's life-table regression model (4). This mode of analysis has selected MLC SI as the most important variable related to time to recurrence, although this was not statistically significant ($p = 0.113$). A multivariate analysis is a more powerful approach to a clinical study of this type since it takes into consideration each parameter analyzed in the presence of the others, and it avoids arbitrary selection of cut-off points for the immune parameters analyzed. Unfortunately, owing to the small sample size, none of the results obtained from the multivariate analysis is statistically significant. This type of approach to immunological analysis should be extended to a larger group of patients in order to select the most informative test.

The only statistically significant correlation was the high recurrence rate in patients having a high PHA SI who were treated with high-dose thymosin + BCG. Renoux et al. (19) found that cancer patients treated with levamisole who had a decrease in the percent of transformed lymphocytes in response to PHA stimulation had a survival time of <6 months, whereas those who had an increase in blastogenesis following levamisole treatment survived >6 month. These findings were observed in patients who had either a low or a high PHA stimulation. Although the data presented here show that the high recurrence rate was primarily in patients who had a high PHA SI initially, or as we named them the Immunocompetent group, nevertheless both these independent observations tend to incriminate an immunomodulator such as levamisole or thymosin for decreasing the time to recurrence in certain groups of patients.

We have observed an increase in the lung colony-forming efficiency of intravenously injected tumor cells to mice receiving local thoracic irradiation (24), following thymosin and levamisole administration in very high doses (200 mg/kg of thymosin and 10 mg/kg levamisole). Thymosin and levamisole have not only caused tumor enhancement but also abolished the protective effect of *Corynebacterium parvum* (Y. Z. Patt and L. Peters, *unpublished data*). The tumor enhancement that occurs in these animals following local thoracic irradiation appears not to be due to specific or nonspecific immunosuppression (18,24). This situation might therefore be analogous to our immunocompetent melanoma patients treated with high-dose thymosin who had an earlier recurrence. A. Barker *(personal communication)* had observed tumor enhancement in AKR mice with leukemia, following treatment with high-dose thymosin. This leukemia is however a T-cell leukemia, and the tumor enhancement was observed in thymoma-bearing animals.

Data supporting possible tumor enhancement with high-dose thymosin or levamisole seem to accumulate. The data presented in this study tend to identify a group of patients at risk of tumor enhancement when exposed to thymosin in combination with BCG, namely, the immunocompetent patients. Possible benefits for the immunoincompetent group are not yet obvious due to the short follow-up. Also, the fact that a combination of thymosin and BCG was used in this study question any extrapolation to the use of thymosin alone.

The mechanism by which such an enhancement occurs is subject to speculation. Compromise of T-cell function due to continuous presence of thymic humoral factor in MLC has been observed by Trainin et al. (22) and attributed to inhibitory effect of adenylate cyclase accumulation on DNA synthesis. There is doubt whether thymosin activity is adenylate cyclase mediated (A. L. Goldstein, *this volume*). Generation of immunocompetence by thymosin happens according to Cohen et al. (3) by conversion of immunologically immature cell populations (T_1 cells) into immunocompetent lymphocytes (T_2 cells). An optimal T_1 to T_2 ratio may be needed for the optimal immune response. Overstimulation with thymosin, particularly in an immunocompetent patient or one whose immunocompetence has been already restored, might turn on a feedback mechanism that would shut off $T_1 \rightarrow T_2$ maturation (3) and reverse the direction to T_2 to T_1. Shutting off of killer cells by excessive thymosin might turn on suppressor cell and hence compromise the ability to eliminate tumor cells, thus causing tumor enhancement. Indeed, thymectomy has been shown to reduce the number of T cells with suppressor activity (A. Barker, *personal communication*). It could then be extrapolated that excessive thymosin increases suppressor T-cell proportion.

We have presented the phenomenon of tumor enhancement in humans following perturbation of the immune system with thymosin primarily in the immunocompetent patient. Our recommendation calls for a meticulous monitoring of the immune competence prior to the use of immunomodulators. It is our assumption that a dose should be tailored for each patient according to the immune competence. Moreover we intend to select immunoincompetent cancer patients for treatment with immunomodulators such as thymosin assuming they would be most likely to benefit from such an intervention.

SUMMARY

To improve results of adjuvant BCG + DTIC therapy in stage 3B melanoma patients, we have added thymosin in a low dose of 4 mg/m^2 and high dose of 40 mg/m^2. Twenty-eight patients were clinically and immunologically evaluable. Pretreatment immunological evaluation consisted of determination of delayed type hypersensitivity to recall antigens and E-rosettes in blood and response of blood lymphocytes to PHA, Con A, and allogeneic lymphocytes in MLC. Preliminary analysis based on median follow-up time of 24 weeks (range 7 to 43 weeks) suggests a shorter disease-free interval in patients with a PHA SI > 50 treated with high dose than those treated with low dose (7/12 versus 1/7 relapses, $p = 0.04$). Among patients with Con A SI $\geq$ 10 5/10 relapsed on 40 mg/m^2 versus 1/5 on 4 mg/m^2 ($p = 0.15$). Patients with a dermatophytin response $\geq$ 10 mm had a recurrence rate of 5/9 when treated with 40 mg/m^2 and 1/7 when treated with 4 mg/m^2. Five of 10 patients with $\geq$ 40% rosettes recurred on 40 mg/m^2 versus 3/11 on 4 mg/m^2 ($p = 0.34$). The simultaneous prognostic influence of the five immunological parameters, thymosin dose, and age was analyzed using Cox's life-table regression model. Although MLC, SI, and thymosin were the most important variables, none of them affected time to recurrence significantly (all $p > 0.10$). Immune modulators such as thymosin may have tumor-enhancing properties and should not be used indiscriminately. Monitoring of immune competence is required prior to their application.

ACKNOWLEDGMENT

This work has received support from contract no. NOI-CB 33888 and grants CA-05831 and CA-14984, from the National Cancer Institute, National Institutes of Health, Bethesda, Md. 20014, and from a grant from Hoffman-LaRoche Inc., Nutley, New Jersey 07110. Drs. Gutterman and Mavligit are recipients of Public Health Research Career Development Awards no. 1-K04-CA-71007 and no. 1-K04-CA-00130, respectively, from the National Institutes of Health, Bethesda, Md. 20014.

REFERENCES

1. Bluming, A. Z., Vogel, C. L., and Zigler, J. L. (1972): Immunological effects of BCG in malignant melanoma: Two modes of administration compared. *Ann. Intern. Med.,* 76:405–411.
2. Boyum, A. (1968): Separation of lymphocytes and erythrocytes by centrifugation. *Scand. J. Clin. Lab. Invest.,* 21:77.
3. Cohen, G. H., Hooper, J. H., and Goldstein, A. L. (1975): Thymosin induced differentiation of murine thymocytes in allogeneic mixed lymphocyte cultures. *Ann. NY Acad. Sci.,* 249:145–153.
4. Cox, D. R. (1972): Regression models and life tables. *J. R. Stat. Soc. (B),* 34:187–220.
5. Gehan, E. A. (1965): A generalized Wilcoxon test for comparing arbitrarily singly-censored samples. *Biometrika,* 52:203–223.
6. Goldstein, A. L., Cohen, G. H., Rossio, J. L., Thurman, G. B., Brown, C. N., and Ulrich, J. T. (1976): Use of thymosin in the treatment of primary immunodeficiency and cancer. *Med. Clin. North Am.,* 60:591–606.
7. Goldstein, A. L., Slater, F. D., and White, A. (1966): Preparation, assay, and partial purification of a thymic lymphocytopoietic factor (thymosin). *Proc. Natl. Acad. Sci. USA,* 56:1010–1017.
8. Goldstein, A. L., Thurman, G. B., Cohen, G. H., and Hooper, J. A. (1974): Thymosin: Chemistry, biology, and clinical application. In: *Biological Activity of Thymic Hormones,* edited by D. W. Van Beakuum, pp. 173–197. Kooyker Sci. Publ., Rotterdam.
9. Gutterman, J. U., McBride, C., Freireich, E. J., Mavligit, G., Frei, E., III, and Hersh, E. M. (1973): Active immunotherapy with BCG for recurrent malignant melanoma. *Lancet,* 2:1208–1212.
10. Gutterman, J. U., Mavligit, G. M., Kennedy, A., McBride, C. M., Burgess, M. A., and Hersh, E. M. (1976): Immunotherapy for malignant melanoma. In: *Neoplasms of the Skin and Malignant Melanoma,* pp. 497–531. Year Book Medical Publishers, Chicago.
11. Hellstrom, I., Hellstrom, K. E., Sjogren, H. O., and Warner, G. A. (1971): Demonstration of cell mediated immunity to human neoplasms of various histological types. *Int. J. Cancer,* 7:1.
12. Hersh, E. M., Gutterman, J. U., Mavligit, G. M., McBride, C. M., and Burgess, M. A. (1976): Immunocompetence, immunodeficiency, immunopotentiation and prognosis in malignant melanoma. In: *Neoplasms of the Skin and Malignant Melanoma,* pp. 331–344. Year Book Medical Publishers, Chicago.
13. Ikonopisov, R. L. (1975): The use of BCG in the combined treatment of malignant melanoma. *Behring. Inst. Mitt.,* 56:206–214.

14. Kaplan, E. L., and Meier, P. (1958): Nonpazametric estimation from incomplete observations. *J. Am. Stat. Assoc.,* 53:457–481.
15. Kenady, D. L., Chretien, M. D., Potvin, C., Simon, R. M., Alexander, J. C., and Goldstein, A. L. (1977): Effect of thymosin *in vitro* on T cell levels during radiation therapy: Correlation with radiation portal and initial T cell levels. *Cancer,* 39:642-652.
16. McBride, C. M. (1970): Advanced melanoma of the extremities: Treatment by isolation-perfusion with triple drug combination. *Arch. Surg.,* 101:122–126.
17. Morton, D. L., Eilber, F. R., Holmes, E. C., Hunt, J. S., Ketcham, A. S., Silverstein, M. J., and Sparks, F. C. (1974): BCG immunotherapy of malignant melanoma: Summary of seven-years experience. *Ann. Surg.,* 180:635–643.
18. Peters, L., McBride, C. M., and Mason, K. A. (1976): T cell depletion and tumor metastasis. *Int. J. Radiat. Biol. Oncol. Phys.,* Suppl. 1:106.
19. Renoux, G., and Renoux, M. (1976): Influence de l'administration de Levamisole sur la reactivite des lymphocytes T de cancereux avances. *Nouv. Presse Med.,* 5:67–70.
20. Schabel, F. M., Jr. (1975): Concepts for systemic treatment of micrometastases. *Cancer,* 35:15–24.
21. Schafer, L. A., Gutterman, J. U., Mavligit, G. M., Reed, R. C., and Hersh, E. M. (1975): Permanent slide preparation of T lymphocyte-sheep red blood cell rosettes. *J. Immunol. Methods,* 8:241–250.
22. Trainin, N., Kook, A. I., Umiel, T., and Albala, M. (1975): The nature and mechanism of stimulation of immune responsiveness by thymus extracts. *Ann. NY Acad. Sci.,* 249:349–361.
23. Wara, D. W., Goldstein, A. L., Doyle, N. E., and Ammann, A. J. (1975): Thymosin activity in patients with cellular immunodeficiency. *N. Engl. J. Med.,* 292:70–74.
24. Withers, M. R., and Milars, L. (1973): Influence of preirradiation of lung on development of artificial pulmonary metastases in mice. *Cancer Res.,* 33:1931–1936.

Immune Modulation and Control of Neoplasia by Adjuvant Therapy, edited by M. A. Chirigos. Raven Press, New York, 1978.

Thymosin in Patients with Disseminated Solid Tumors: Phase I and II Results

John J. Costanzi, *Nick Harris, and **Allan Goldstein

Department of Medicine, and Divisions of *,** Biochemistry and * Surgery, University of Texas Medical Branch, Galveston, Texas 77550

The key role of the thymus in the development and maintenance of cellular immune competence in animals and man is well established. The consequence of thymectomy in animals or the failure of the thymus to develop normally in man have shown that this organ has an important influence on tissue and organ transplantation (19,20) and on the development of autoimmune diseases (6,9), immune tolerance (3,16), immunologic deficiency states (11), and resistance to tumor induction by malignant cells or oncogenic viruses (7,17,21,23).

Defective cell-mediated immunity appears to be a general phenomenon in patients with far advanced malignancy (1,8,14,18). The degree of immunodeficiency may be correlated inversely with favorable prognosis (6,26). Those patients whose immunocompetence is restored following measures that reduce tumor bulk (14) or by the administration of immunostimulants have prolonged survival compared to those who remain immunoincompetent (12,13).

Thymosin has been shown to improve certain parameters of cell-mediated immunity in patients with primary immunodeficiency diseases or advanced malignancies. Thymosin has been shown to increase *in vitro* the "total" E-rosettes (28) and "active" rosettes (29) of patients with primary or secondary immunodeficiency disease *in vitro* (4). Thymosin administered *in vivo* to a single patient with thymic hypoplasia has been shown to cause an increase in E-rosettes and development of positive delayed hypersensitivity skin tests (28). Thymosin incubation *in vitro* has also been shown to cause a significant increase in E-rosettes in patients with advanced malignancies (25). Preliminary clinical trials conducted by Costanzi et al. (5) and Shafer et al. (27) have shown that thymosin administration was followed by partial cellular immune reconstitution, viewed as increased delayed hypersensitivity skin test reactivity and increased E-rosette-forming capacity in some immunodeficient cancer patients. The present report extends the preliminary observations on toxicology (phase I study, 4a) and effects on immune testing in patients with far advanced malignancy receiving thymosin *in vivo.*

MATERIAL AND METHODS

Preparation of Thymosin

Thymosin fraction 5 was prepared from calf thymus by the method of Goldstein et al. (10) with the recent modifications of Hooper et al. (15).

Patient and Treatment Characteristics

Ten patients with various widely disseminated malignancies received 12 courses of thymosin. Thymosin was administered intramuscularly daily for 7 days at a dose range of 10 to 250 mg/m^2. The dose of thymosin administration per course ranged from 105 to 3,500 mg. All patients had received extensive prior therapy and were at least 4 weeks post prior therapy. Eight patients had prior surgery, nine patients had major prior chemotherapy, and five patients had prior radiotherapy. None of the patients had prior hormonal therapy, and two patients received prior immunotherapy. A patient with adenocarcinoma of the lung received intralesional lymphokines into subcutaneous nodules, and a patient with melanoma had received Bacillus Calmette-Guérin vaccination prior to thymosin. Three patients also received weekly injections of thymosin at a dose of 75 mg/m^2 following their initial course for a period of 5 weeks.

A phase II study was performed on 15 patients with various disseminated solid tumors. These patients were composed of carcinoma of lung—5, hypernephroma—3, breast carcinoma—2, colon—2, melanoma—1, sarcoma—1, and seminoma—1. These patients received a dose of 10 mg/m^2 daily for 5 days i.m., then were maintained on a similar dose every 2 weeks.

Toxicity Parameters

Physical examination, tumor measurements, performance status (Karnofsky scale), complete blood count, serum electrolytes, blood urea nitrogen, serum creatinine, bilirubin, alkaline phosphatase, transaminases, prothrombin time, serum protein electrophoresis, chest X-ray, urinalysis, and electrocardiogram were performed pretreatment and on days 4,7,14, and 21. Bone marrow aspiration was performed pretreatment.

Lymphocyte Preparation

Peripheral blood lymphocytes were obtained by the method of Boyum (2) in which heparinized (50 μg/ml) blood was carefully layed over lymphoprep (Nyegaard & Company A/S, Oslo, Norway) and centrifuged at 400 $\times$ g for 40 min at 20°C. The mononuclear cells were aspirated from the plasma-gradient interface with a pasteur pipette and washed twice with HEPES-buffered RPMI-1640 media (H-RPMI, Gibco, Grand Island, New York) by centrifugation at

180 X g. The cells were then resuspended in H-RPMI, counted using a Coulter Counter, and the cell concentration adjusted to 4 X 10⁶ cells/ml.

E-Rosette Formation (22,30)

Blood lymphocytes and sheep red blood cells (SRBC) were washed separately three times in RPMI-1640. A suspension of 5% SRBC was then mixed with 1×10^6 lymphocytes and incubated for 5 min at 37°C. This cell mixture was centrifuged at 100 rpm for 5 min and subsequently incubated at 4°C for 1 hr. The excess supernate was removed; the remaining cells were resuspended by gently rocking for 5 to 10 sec. The resuspended cells were then transferred to clean glass slides and counted with the aid of a Reichert Zetopan interference contrast (nomarski) microscope. Lymphocytes with four or more SRBC on their surface were considered rosettes. At least 100 lymphocytes were counted in each of these preparations. Three milliliters of scintillation cocktail made with toluene and liquiflour (New England Nuclear, Boston, Mass.) was added, and the vials were capped and placed in lidless polyethylene scintillation vials (Packard Instrument Co., Downers Grove, Ill.). Tritiated thymidine incorporation was determined by a Packard 2450 liquid scintillation spectrophotometer.

Delayed Hypersensitivity Skin Testing

A battery of seven skin test antigens plus a saline control and a thymosin skin test were administered pretreatment and on days 4,7,14, and 21. The antigens were administered intradermally in a volume of 0.1 ml. Skin test antigens were as follows—*Candida* 1:1000 (Hollister-Stier), dermatophyton 1:1000, mumps (Lilly), streptokinase-streptodornase (SK-SD) 1:100 (Lederle), purified protein derivative (PPD) 5 U (Conaught), histoplasmin (Parke-Davis), coccidioidin 1:100 (Cutter), and thymosin fraction 5, 0.1 mg. Skin tests were measured by two right-angle measurements at 24 and 48 hr. A positive skin test was defined as being equal to or greater than 5×5 mm induration.

Other Immunologic Parameters

The harvested lymphocytes were also studied by the one-way mixed lymphocyte culture, mitogen stimulation (phytohemagglutinin, pokeweed, and Concanavalin A), and surface immunoglobulins on days 0,7,14, and 21. Serum immunoglobulins were similarly studied.

RESULTS

Toxicity

In the phase I study, a patient with stage IVB lymphocyte-depleted Hodgkin's disease developed a generalized urticarial rash on the seventh day of thymosin administration at a dose of 50 mg/m². The rash began 12 hr after thymosin administration and subsided over 24 hr with no treatment. Two patients developed low-grade fever (99–100°F) during the 7-day course of thymosin administration. One patient developed pain at the injection site. No evidence of parenchymal organ dysfunction related to thymosin administration was seen in any patient, and no hematopoietic or CNS toxicity was encountered. No toxicity was noted in the phase II study.

Skin Testing

Pretreatment (in the phase I study), 10 patients had 23 positive recall skin tests. One new positive skin test developed on day 4, two on day 7, two on day 14, and three on day 21. A total of eight new skin tests developed over the 21-day observation. One patient developed a positive skin test reaction to thymosin (20 X 15 mm) after the second course of thymosin administration.

In the phase II study, 13 new positive skin tests developed. These are tabulated by type and days on Table 1.

TABLE 1. *Development of new positive skin tests*

Test	Day				Total
	0	7	14	21	
Mumps	12	1	1		2
Candida	3	1	1		2
PPD	4				
Thymosin	2		1	1	2
Histo	4				
SK-SD	7	2	2		4
Cocci	1		1	2	3
	33	4	6	3	

Thirteen "new" positive skin tests ($\geq 5 \times 5$ mm) developed.

E-Rosettes

Table 2 shows the mean percent E-rosettes in normal subjects and cancer patients before and after the addition of *in vitro* thymosin in the phase I study. Thymosin added *in vitro* did not cause a significant increase in E-rosettes in normal subjects with normal percent E-rosettes, but the increase in E-rosettes in cancer patients with low E-rosettes was significant ($p = 0.04$). Table 3 shows that *in vivo* thymosin administration caused a statistically significant increase in mean percent E-rosettes on days 4,7,14, and 21 compared to day 0 (pretreatment). Figure 1 illustrates the changes in percent E-rosettes in three patients who received weekly injections of thymosin as maintenance therapy. It can be seen that all three patients had E-rosettes below the lower limit of the normal

TABLE 2. *Mean percent E-rosettes in normal subjects and cancer patients with and without thymosin* in vitro

	N	E-rosettes	p
Normal subjects			
(−) Thymosin	52	59.8 ± 8.5	NS
(+) Thymosin	52	55.8 ± 12.0	
Cancer patients			
(−) Thymosin	12	37.8 ± 10.8	0.04
(+) Thymosin	12	29.1 ± 12.5	

± (Standard deviation). (−) Is without. (+) Is with.

range prior to the initiation of thymosin therapy and that weekly injections maintained the E-rosette level of each patient in the normal range.

Table 4 shows the mean E-rosettes in normal subjects and cancer patients with and without thymosin in the phase II study. The nonsignificance of the change in the cancer patients may be attributed to the fact that this group of patients had less tumor load than the phase I patients and were more immunocompetent. Table 5 shows the mean E-rosettes in these patients following thymosin, by day. A significant increase was noted on days 14 and 21, and the overall increase was also significant.

TABLE 3. *Mean E-rosettes in cancer patients following thymosin* in vivo

Day	N	E-rosette	p Value vs. day 0
0	12	29.1 ± 12.5	
4	3	42.7 ± 3.1	0.04
7	11	38.6 ± 12.9	0.04
14	10	43.0 ± 15.5	0.01
21	6	47.8 ± 14.1	0.01

± (Standard deviation).

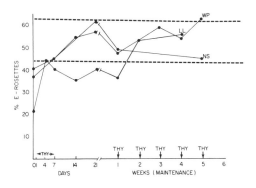

FIG. 1. Percent E-rosettes following weekly maintenance thymosin treatments in three cancer patients.

TABLE 4. *Mean percent E-rosettes in normal subjects and cancer patients with and without* thymosin in vitro

| | | E-rosettes | | |
	N	Mean	SE	p Value
NORMAL SUBJECTS				
(+) Thymosin	52	59.8	1.2	
(−) Thymosin	52	55.8	1.7	NS
CANCER PATIENTS				
(+) Thymosin	15	40.1	4.3	
(−) Thymosin	15	33.1	4.6	NS ($p \sim 0.20$)

SE, standard error.

TABLE 5. *Mean E-rosettes in cancer patients following* thymosin in vivo

| | | E-rosettes | | |
Day	N	Mean	SE	p Value vs. day 0
0	15	33.1	4.6	
4	3	42.7	1.8	0.17
7	14	37.1	3.6	0.24
14	11	44.6	4.5	0.04
21	7	49.1	5.0	0.02
4 + 7 + 14 + 21	35	42.6	2.4	0.02

SE, standard error.

Other Immunologic Parameters

No significant changes were noted in the one-way mixed lymphocyte cultures, mitogen assays, surface immunoglobulins, and serum immunoglobulins.

DISCUSSION

Bovine thymosin fraction 5 (10,15) was administered (in a phase I study) to 10 patients with far advanced disseminated malignancies and varying degrees of immunoincompetence as defined by impaired reactivity to recall skin test antigens and low total E-rosettes.

Toxicity observed with the doses and schedule employed was minimal. No parenchymal organ toxicity was encountered. Thymosin administration resulted in the increased skin test reactivity to recall skin test antigens. Thymosin further increased low E-rosettes of cancer patients but not normal E-rosettes of controls *in vitro*. Significant increases in E-rosettes occurred following thymosin administration *in vivo*. Weekly thymosin administration "maintained" the E-rosettes of three cancer patients in the normal range. This effect of thymosin *in vitro* is compatible with previously published data (24) and may allow prediction of which cancer patients are most likely to benefit from thymosin immunotherapy. This observation is also compatible with the proposed mechanism of action of thymosin, i.e., production of an increase in mature lymphocytes (T_2) where immature (T_0 or T_1) lymphocytes predominate (21).

In a phase II study, 15 patients with a variety of disseminated solid tumors were studied. Thirteen new positive skin tests to recall antigens developed, and this was associated with a significant increase in E-rosettes after *in vivo* thymosin. In this group of patients, the E-rosettes did not increase after thymosin was added *in vitro*, reflecting perhaps the fact that these patients were probably more immunocompetent than those in the phase I study.

In summary, the *in vivo* use of thymosin fraction 5 is safe and has minimal toxicity. Skin test and E-rosette changes probably reflect its immunostimulant capability. It should be studied in specific tumors in a randomized fashion to determine its ability to increase response rate and survival.

ACKNOWLEDGMENT

This work was supported in part by grants from the National Cancer Institute (CA 16964 and CA 17701) and the Clinical Study Center, R-73.

REFERENCES

1. Aisenberg, C. A. (1962): Studies on delayed hypersensitivity in Hodgkin's disease. *J. Clin. Invest.,* 41:1964–1970.
2. Boyum, A. (1968): Isolation of mononuclear cells and granulocytes from human blood. *Scand. J. Clin. Lab. Invest.,* 21:(97):87–89.
3. Burnet, M. (1962): Role of the thymus and related organs in immunity. *Br. Med. J.,* 2:807–811.
4. Cohen, G. H., Hooper, J. A., and Goldstein, A. L. (1975): Thymosin-induced differentiation of murine thymocytes in allogenic mixed lymphocyte culture. *Ann NY Acad. Sci.,* 249:145–153.
4A. Costanzi, J. J., Gagliano, R. G., Delaney, F., Cohen, G., and Thomson, P. D. (1977): The effect of thymosin on patients with disseminated malignancies: A Phase I study. *Cancer,* 40:14–19.
5. Costanzi, J., Gagliano, R., Loukas, D., Sakai, H., Thurman, G., Harris, N., and Goldstein, A. (1975): The use of Thymosin (THY) in patients with disseminated neoplasia: Toxicity and immunological correlation. *AACR,* 16:135.
6. Eiber, F. R., and Morton, D. L. (1970): Impaired immunologic reactivity and recurrence following cancer surgery. *Cancer,* 25:362–367.
7. Furth, J. (1946): Prolongation of life with prevention of leukemia by thymectomy in mice. *J. Gerontol.,* 1:46–52.
8. Gatti, R. A., Garrioch, D. B., and Good, R. A. (1970): Depressed responses in patients with non-lymphoid malignancies. In: *Proc. 5th Leucocyte Culture Conf.,* edited by J. E. Harris, pp. 339–358. Academic Press, New York and London.
9. Goldstein, G. (1966): Thymitis and myasthenia gravis. *Lancet* 2:1164–1167.
10. Goldstein, A. L., Guha, A., Zatz, M. M., Hardy, M. A., and White, A. (1972): Purification and biological activity of thymosin, a hormone of the thymus gland. *Proc. Natl. Acad. Sci. USA,* 69:1800–1803.
11. Good, R. A., Dalmasso, A. P., Martinez, C., Archer, O. K., Pierce, J. C., and Papermaster, B. W. (1962): The role of the thymus in the development of immunologic capacity. *J. Exp. Med.,* 116:773–795.

12. Gutterman, J. U., Mavligit, G., Gottlieb, J. A., Burgess, M. A., McBride, C. E., Einhorn, L., Freirich, E. J., and Hersh, E. M. (1974): Chemoimmunotherapy of disseminated malignant melanoma with Dimethyl Triazeno Imidazole Carboxamide and Bacillus Calmett-Guerin. *N. Engl. J. Med.,* 291:592–597.

13. Gutterman, J. U., Rodriguez, V., Mavligit, G., Burgess, M. A., Gehan, E., Hersh, E. M., McCredie, K. B., Reed, R., Smith, T., Body, G. P., and Freireich, E. J. (1974): Chemoimmuno-therapy of adult acute leukemia: Prolongation of remission in myeloblastic leukemia with B.C.G. *Lancet,* 2:1405–1409.

14. Hersh, E. M., Whitecar, J. P., McCredie, K. B., Bodey, G. P., and Freireich, E. J. (1971): Chemotherapy, immunocompetence, immunosuppression and prognosis in acute leukemia. *N. Engl. J. Med.,* 285:1211–1216.

15. Hooper, J. A., McDaniel, M. C., and Thurman, G. B. (1975): Purification and properties of bovine thymosin. *Ann. NY Acad. Sci.,* 249:125.

16. Iskovic, J., Smith, S. B., and Waksman, B. H. (1965): Immunologic tolerance in thymectomized, irradiated rats grafted with thymus from tolerant donors. *Science,* 148:1333–1335.

17. Law, L. W. (1966): Studies of thymic function with emphasis on the role of the thymus in oncogenesis. *Cancer Res.,* 26:551–574.

18. Levin, A. G., McDonough, E. F., Miller, D. G., and Southam, C. M. (1964): Delayed hypersensi-tivity response to DNFB in sick and healthy persons. *Ann. NY Acad. Sci.,* 120:400–409.

19. Martinez, C., Kersey, J., Papermaster, B. W., and Good, R. A. (1962): Skin homograft survival in thymectomized mice. *Proc. Soc. Exp. Biol. Med.,* 109:41–43.

20. Miller, J. F. A. P. (1961): Immunologic function of the thymus. *Lancet,* 2:748–749.

21. Miller, J. F. A. P. (1967): The thymus in relation to neoplasia. In: *Modern Trends in Pathology,* Vol. 2, edited by T. Crawford, pp.140–175.

22. Minowada, J., Ohnuma, T., and Moore, G. E. (1972): Rosette-forming human lymphoid cell lines. I. Establishment and evidence for origin of thymus-derived lymphocytes. *J. Natl. Cancer Inst.,* 49:891.

23. McEndy, D. P., Boon, M. C., and Furth, J. (1944): On the role of thymus, spleen and gonads in the development of leukemia in a high-leukemia stock of mice. *Cancer Res.,* 4:377–383.

24. Osba, D., and Miller, J. F. A. P. (1964): The lymphoid tissues and immune responses of neonatally thymectomized mice bearing thymus in millipore diffusion chambers. *J. Exp. Med.,* 119:177–194.

25. Sakai, H., Costanzi, J. J., Loukas, D. F., Gagliano, R. G., Ritzmann, S. E., and Goldstein, A. L. (1975): Thymosin induced increase in E-rosette-forming capacity of lymphocytes in patients with malignancy. *Cancer,* 36:974–976.

26. Sokla, J. E., and Aungust, C. W. (1969): Response to BCG vaccination and survival in advanced Hodgkin's disease. *Cancer,* 24:128–134.

27. Shafer, L. A., Washington, M. L., and Goldstein, A. L. (1975): Thymosin immunotherapy— A phase I study. *ASCO,* 16:233.

28. Wara, D. W., Goldstein, A. L., Doyle, N. E., and Ammann, A. J. (1975): Thymosin activity in patients with cellular immunodeficiency. *N. Engl. J. Med.,* 292:70–74.

29. Wara, D. W., and Ammann, A. J. (1975): Activation of T-cell rosettes in immunodeficient patients by thymosin. *Ann NY Acad. Sci.,* 249:308–315.

30. Wybran, J. H., Fudenberg, H. H., and Sielsinger, M. H. (1971): Rosette formation, a test for cellular immunity. *Clin. Res.,* 19:568.

*Immune Modulation and Control of Neo-
plasia by Adjuvant Therapy,* edited by M. A.
Chirigos. Raven Press, New York, 1978.

Immunoadjuvant and Antitumor Properties of Amphotericin B

* J. R. Little, ** T. J. Blanke, † F. Valeriote, and * G. Medoff

** Departments of Medicine, ** Surgery, † Radiology, and * Microbiology and
Immunology, Washington University School of Medicine, St. Louis, Missouri 63110*

AmB[1] is a polyene macrolide antibiotic that has been used extensively in the treatment of systemic fungal infections in man. It belongs to a group of structurally related compounds with similar biological effects produced by several *Streptomyces* species (Fig. 1). The toxic biological activities of the antifungal polyenes are the result of binding to membrane sterols (6). The selective effects of amphotericin B on fungi are related to a greater stability of binding to ergosterol, found in the membranes of fungi, than to cholesterol, the principal sterol of animal cell membranes. The cell permeability effects of AmB are dose dependent and cause both ion and molecular losses from cells as well as enhanced uptake of certain drugs and macromolecules (6,7,11). This AmB-induced uptake by eukaryotic cells of constituents in the medium has led to the demonstration of synergistic effects on fungi of AmB in combination with other antibiotics (10). This synergy has also been shown with actinomycin D-resistant tumor cells (9).

Our interest in the immunological properties of AmB was stimulated by the dramatic effects of combination chemotherapy with AmB and BCNU in the treatment of a transplantable murine leukemia (12). About 20 to 80% of AKR mice bearing an advanced syngeneic leukemia were cured by treatment with AmB and BCNU. Neither drug alone induced cures, and the survivors of the drug combination therapy were found to be solidly resistant to rechallenge with 10[6] leukemia cells. Spleen colony assays for leukemia cells recently showed *(unpublished results)* that mice treated with the optimal regimen of AmB and BCNU harbored viable leukemia cells for up to 8 days following treatment (Table 1). The few surviving mice that had detectable leukemia cells after 4 weeks of observation had them restricted to the central nervous system.

Because the cured mice were resistant to rechallenge and since tumor resistance

---

[1] Abbreviations used in this chapter are **AmB,** amphotericin B; **AME,** amphotericin methyl ester; **BCG,** Bacillus Calmette-Guerin; **BCNU,** 1,3-bis(2-chloroethyl)-1-nitrosourea; **GVH,** graft-versus-host; **LCFU,** leukemia colony-forming unit; **PFC,** plaque-forming cells; **SRBC,** sheep erythrocytes; **TNP,** the 2,4,6-trinitrophenyl group; **TNP-HSA,** trinitrophenylated human serum albumin; **TNP-SRBC,** trinitrophenylated sheep erythrocytes.

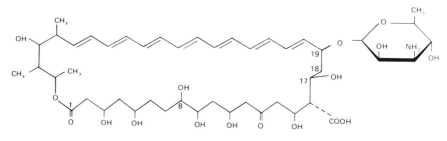

FIG. 1. The structural formula of AmB.

could be adoptively transferred to virgin **AKR** mice with spleen cells from cured mice, this led to examination of the possible immunological adjuvant properties of AmB. Recently published studies from other laboratories have shown that AmB can augment the *in vitro* murine immune response to SRBC (4) and that AmB is a polyclonal murine B-cell activator (3). The following studies describe some of the effects of AmB on the humoral and the cell-mediated immune responses of mice to several defined antigens. Initial studies made use of commercially available AmB (Fungizone®, E. R. Squibb and Sons, Inc.,

TABLE 1. *Femoral marrow LCFU following AmB and/or BCNU treatment of AKR transplantable leukemia*

Day	Group			
	Control	AmB alone	BCNU alone	AmB + BCNU
4	$5.7(\pm0.7) \times 10^4$ [a]	$3.2(\pm0.4) \times 10^4$		
	15 [b]	14		
5	$1.9(\pm0.3) \times 10^5$	$1.6(\pm0.2) \times 10^5$	$8.1(\pm1.1) \times 10^3$	$9.3(\pm2) \times 10^3$
	16	15	19	19
6	All dead	All dead	$1.0(\pm0.3) \times 10^5$	$4.8(\pm1.4) \times 10^4$
			5	5
7			$1.2(\pm0.2) \times 10^5$	$1.4(\pm0.3) \times 10^5$
			10	14
8			All dead	$2.4(\pm0.4) \times 10^5$
				14
10				$4.1(\pm1.2) \times 10^4$
				1/15 [c]
11				$1.2(\pm1.1) \times 10^4$
				3/14 [c]
12				$3.0(\pm1.2) \times 10^0$
				10/14 [c]
14				—
				10/10 [c]

Adult female AKR mice received 10^6 leukemia cells on day 0, 0.5 mg/mouse AmB (as Fungizone®) on days 1 through 4, and 0.2 mg/mouse BCNU on day 4.
[a] Values represent the mean and standard error of individual mouse assays.
[b] Number of mice in group.
[c] This fraction of assayed mice had no detectable LCFU (i.e., <1 LCFU/femur).

Princeton, N.J.), but more recently water-soluble AME has been found to produce equivalent results with less toxicity.

Humoral immunostimulation by AmB (or AME) has been observed consistently in mice immunized with the hapten-protein conjugate TNP-HSA. Quantitative comparisons between mice that received antigen plus AmB or antigen alone have been obtained by the enumeration of splenic antibody-forming cells (PFC) from immunized mice. Early studies showed that the maximum number of direct (IgM) PFC occurred 7 to 9 days after primary antigenic stimulation and 4 to 6 days after secondary stimulation with the same antigen (8). Indirect IgG PFC were observed in significant numbers only after secondary stimulation, and all assays were made specific for anti-TNP antibody-secreting cells by the use of TNP-SRBC as target cells in the homolysin in gel assay of Jerne and Nordin (5).

The immunoadjuvant effects of AmB in adult BALB/c mice are shown in Table 2. These results indicate that neither AmB alone nor antigen alone induced the formation of any detectable IgG antibody-producing cells in the secondary response to TNP-HSA. However, IgG antibody-producing cells were consistently observed in the spleens of mice that received a single dose of AmB along with the primary antigenic stimulation. All mice received the same "secondary" stimulus of 100 μg TNP-HSA in saline solution. Table 2 also shows a consistently augmented IgM response in the groups of animals that received antigen plus

TABLE 2. *Effect of AmB on the secondary response in BALB/c mice*

1° Immunization	2° Immunization [b]	Days after 1°	Days after 2°	PFC/1 $\times$ 10⁶ spleen cells [c]	
				IgM	IgG
AmB + TNP-HSA	TNP-HSA	20	7	25.1 ± 6.1	6.8 ± 12.0
TNP-HSA	TNP-HSA	20	7	18.0 ± 2.9	0
AmB	TNP-HSA	20	7	11.0 ± 4.3	0
AmB + TNP-HSA	TNP-HSA	27	7	30.2 ± 8.1	12.7 ± 8.8
TNP-HSA	TNP-HSA	27	7	21.6 ± 6.7	0
AmB	TNP-HSA	27	7	20.3 ± 6.0	0
AmB + TNP-HSA	TNP-HSA	34	7	37.4 ± 9.2	18.1 ± 11.6
TNP-HSA	TNP-HSA	34	7	20.6 ± 4.9	0
AmB	TNP-HSA	34	7	12.1 ± 4.3	0

[a] All mice were 7 to 8-week-old BALB/c males immunized by separate i.p. injections of each agent. Groups of mice were given either 300 μg AmB in 0.2 ml 5% dextrose solution and 100 μg TNP-HSA in 0.2 ml saline, 100 μg TNP-HSA in 0.2 ml saline and 0.2 ml dextrose solution, or 300 μg AmB in 0.2 ml 5% dextrose solution.

[b] At intervals of 13, 20, and 27 days after primary immunization, all mice received 100 μg TNP-HSA in 0.2 ml saline solution i.p.

[c] Spleens from each group of three mice were pooled and made in single-cell suspensions. The values given represent the arithmetic mean (±1 SD) of six separate PFC assays for each spleen cell suspension using TNP-SRBC as target cells. Parallel control PFC assays performed with unconjugated SRBC were done routinely and never yielded greater than three direct PFC or one indirect (IgG) PFC per 1 $\times$ 10⁶ spleen cells. No correction was made in the data shown for the control assays.

AmB. These results and many similar experiments show clearly that amphotericin has potent humoral immunostimulant effects in mice. They also indicate that AmB enhances the switching of lymphoid cells from IgM to IgG antibody production, a physiological step known to be dependent on stimulation by helper T cells.

Similar experiments have been performed in AKR mice as well as several other mouse strains and in every experiment AmB administration has induced some degree of enhancement in the frequency of splenic IgG anti-TNP antibody-producing cells in the anamnestic response to TNP-HSA. Similar but less dramatic results have been observed in the humoral response to SRBC. The format of these experiments has been similar to those with TNP-HSA except that groups of mice were injected with SRBC plus AME or with SRBC (or AME) alone. Table 3 shows that by using a very small dose of SRBC the primary PFC response is abrogated, but amphotericin-induced augmentation is observed by the greater frequency of IgM and IgG splenic PFC following a second small dose of SRBC. These data indicate that the immunostimulant effects of amphotericin are not limited to soluble antigens (i.e., TNP-HSA) nor are they restricted to a single antigenic specificity.

Further evidence of the immunostimulant properties of AmB in mice was provided by the data in Table 4 showing augmentation of the GVH reaction in a particular mouse strain pair. The numerical values given in the table (splenic indices) provide a quantitation of the intensity of the rejection reaction in the recipient neonatal F_1 mice (2). The experiments in Table 4 were performed with donor parental thymocytes derived either from adult normal donors or from adult mice of the same strain that had received AmB 48 hr before sacrifice and preparation of the thymocyte suspensions. As expected, there is a cell dose-response effect observed in the intensity of GVH reactions induced in F_1 neonates by normal thymocytes of each parental strain. It was unexpected, however, that AmB administration would augment the intensity of the GVH reaction

TABLE 3. *Effect of AME on splenic primary and secondary PFC responses to SRBC*

Mouse strain	AME	SRBC	1° Response[a]	2° Response[a]		Days after 1°
			IgM PFC	IgM PFC	IgG PFC	
BALB/c	+	1×10^6	0.89 ± 1.9	54.6 ± 12.5	18.2 ± 4.1	
	−	1×10^6	1.8 ± 2.7	16.2 ± 5.4	5.34 ± 3.0	27
	+	—	2.9 ± 6.4	10.7 ± 3.8	0.06 ± 0.22	

Male mice 5½ to 6½ weeks old were injected i.p. with 300 μg AME or with 1×10^6 washed SRBC through a separate i.p. injection site, or both. Splenic PFC assays were performed on groups of three mice from each injection group at each time point. The secondary stimulation was 1×10^6 SRBC i.p. for all mice.

[a]The primary response assay was performed 6 days after the primary stimulus, and the secondary response assay was done 6 days after the secondary injection (1×10^6 SRBC per mouse). The values given are average PFC/1×10^6 spleen cells ± 1 SD.

TABLE 4. *GVH reactions induced by parental thymocytes*

Donor thymocytes	Splenic index[a]		
	Exp. 1	Exp. 2	Exp. 3
Untreated A-$T1a^b$	3.80 ± 0.62 (1.0)	4.22 ± 0.62 (1.1)	4.91 ± 0.59 (1.6)
AmB-treated A-$T1a^b$	6.80 ± 3.25 (1.8)	7.20 ± 2.46 (1.9)	9.83 ± 2.56 (2.6)
Untreated C57BL/6	4.68 ± 0.81 (1.2)	3.20 ± 0.75 (0.85)	—
AmB-treated C57BL/6	3.95 ± 1.02 (1.0)	3.18 ± 0.90 (0.84)	—

Host mice for all experiments were (C57BL/6 X A-$T1a^b$)F_1. Donor parental thymocytes were injected i.p. into 7-day-old recipients. Each litter of recipients was divided such that half received thymocytes from AmB-treated donors and half received control thymocytes (either from F_1 donors or from untreated parental donors).

[a] Splenic index = spleen weight/body weight X 10^3. Also shown in parentheses is the ratio of spleen weight : body weight of experimental animals to the spleen weight : body weight of control animals. Values are expressed as arithmetic mean ± SEM. F_1 neonates received 3×10^7 thymocytes per mouse (Exp. 1), 4×10^7 (Exp. 2), or 5×10^7 (Exp. 3). Mean control splenic index ($F_1 \rightarrow F_1$) was 3.77 ± 0.42.

produced by the thymocytes from one parental strain (A-Tla^b) but not the other (C57BL/6). This experiment when repeated gave identical results indicating that not all mouse strains respond in an equivalent manner to AmB. The augmentation of the GVH reaction produced by A-Tla^b thymocytes obtained from AmB-treated mice show that amphotericin can lead to stimulation of a T-cell immune response in addition to the earlier demonstration of enhanced responses expressed by splenic B cells.

The asymmetry of the AmB-induced effect on the GVH reaction suggested that similar mouse *strain-specific* effects could be observed in a parallel fashion in assays of humoral immunity. The particular strains used in the GVH assays had not been studied in their responses to TNP-HSA, but these experiments were completed and showed that both A-Tla^b and A strain mice responded with a vigorous adjuvant effect to AME, whereas C57BL/6 mice were almost unresponsive (Fig. 2). In Fig. 2 the difference is shown in PFC/10^6 spleen cells (augmentation index) between the IgG response to antigen alone and the IgG response to antigen plus AME. The IgG augmentation index therefore represents a quantitative expression of the response to the adjuvant. Also shown in Fig. 2 is the parallel pattern of responses of these two mouse strains to an unrelated adjuvant—BCG. With each a relatively weak adjuvant effect (augmentation index) was observed in F_1 progeny of the high and low responders (Fig. 2). This pattern of responses is probably *not* a reflection of the genetic control of the response to the immunogen (TNP-HSA) since most immune response gene control displays dominant inheritance of the high-responder state (1). Also the parallelism in mouse strain pattern of responses to immunization with TNP-HSA (Fig. 2) and with the H-2 alloantigens that determine GVH reactions (Table 4) argue that mouse strains differ in their ability to respond to the immunostimulant effects of amphotericin, of BCG, and perhaps of other adjuvants

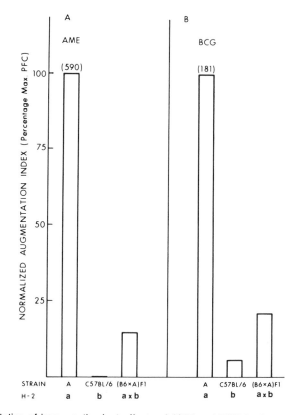

FIG. 2. Quantitation of immunostimulant effects of AME and BCG in different mouse strains. Primary and secondary immunization with TNP-HSA were performed as outlined in the legend to Table 2 except that experimental mice received primary i.p. injections consisting of 300 μg AME in 0.2 ml 5% dextrose **(A)** or 1×10^7 BCG (Trudeau strain) in 0.2 ml **(B)** in addition to 100 μg TNP-HSA in 0.2 ml. Control mice received separate i.p. injections of 5% dextrose and of TNP-HSA. Secondary immunization of all mice was 100 μg TNP-HSA i.p. Indirect (IgG) PFC were scored on TNP-SRBC 6 days after secondary and 34 days after primary immunization. The augmentation index was calculated by subtraction of the mean number of indirect PFC/ 10^6 spleen cells in control mice from the mean number of indirect PFC/10^6 spleen cells in experimental mice. The augmentation indices were normalized to the mean number of PFC/ 10^6 spleen cells given by the A strain. The number of IgG PFC in each experiment is shown in parentheses over the A strain bar in each panel.

as well. These data suggest that there is a consistent genetic control of the intensity of immunoadjuvant responsiveness in mice. In other experiments it has been shown that AKR is a relatively high-responder strain to the humoral immunostimulant effects of amphotericin. This supports the possibility that an immunological adjuvant mechanism is a major important factor in the induction of AKR transplantable leukemia cures by combination chemotherapy with AmB and BCNU. A genetic control of adjuvant responsiveness in mice also suggests that similar genetic regulation occurs in man. If this is so, it may help to explain some of the variability observed in immunotherapy with adjuvants such as BCG in the treatment of human malignancy.

ACKNOWLEDGMENT

This work was supported by NIH grants nos. CA 15665, 1 RO1 CA20168, and 1 PO2CA 13053–05, and by an NCI contract no. N01-CB-43872.

AME was a generous gift from Dr. W. E. Brown, E. R. Squibb and Sons, Inc. We are also indebted to Dr. C. P. Schaffner for his advice and assistance regarding the use of AME.

REFERENCES

1. Benacerraf, B., and Katz, D. H. (1975): The nature and function of histocompatibility-linked immune response genes. In: *Immunogenetics and Immunodeficiency*, edited by B. Benacerraf, pp. 117–178. Univ. Park Press, Baltimore.
2. Grebe, S. C., and Streilein, J. W. (1976): Graft-versus-host reactions. *Adv. Immunol.,* 22:120–221.
3. Hammarström, L., and Smith, E. (1976): Mitogenic properties of polyene antibiotics for murine B cells. *Scand. J. Immunol.,* 5:37–43.
4. Ishikawa, H., Narimatsu, H., and Saito, K. (1975): Adjuvant effect of nystatin on *in vitro* antibody response of mouse spleen cells to heterologous erythrocytes. *Cell. Immunol.,* 17:300–305.
5. Jerne, N. K., and Nordin, A. A. (1963): Plaque formation in agar by single antibody producing cells. *Science,* 140:405.
6. Kinsky, S. C. (1970): Antibiotic interactions with model membranes. *Annu. Rev. Pharmacol.,* 10:119–142.
7. Kumar, B. V., Medoff, G., Kobayashi, G., and Schlessinger, D. (1974): Uptake of *Escherichia coli* DNA into HeLa cells enhanced by amphotericin B. *Nature,* 250:323–325.
8. Mauch, P., Bridges, S. H., Little, K. D., and Little, J. R. (1974): The IgM and IgA immune response to the TNP determinant group in BALB/c mice. *J. Immunol.,* 112:812–821.
9. Medoff, J., Medoff, G., Goldstein, M. N., Schlessinger, D., and Kobayashi, G. S. (1975): Amphotericin B-induced sensitivity to actinomycin D in drug-resistant HeLa cells. *Cancer Res.,* 35:2548–2552.
10. Medoff, G., Kobayashi, G. S., Kwan, C. N., Schlessinger, D., and Venkov, P. (1972): Potentiation of rifampicin and 5-fluorocytosine as antifungal antibiotics by amphotericin B. *Proc. Natl. Acad. Sci. USA,* 69:196–199.
11. Medoff, G., Kwan, C. N., Schlessinger, D., and Kobayashi, G. S. (1973): Permeability control in animal cells by polyenes: A possibility. *Antimicrob. Agents Chemother.,* 3:441–443.
12. Medoff, G., Valeriote, F., Lynch, R. G., Schlessinger, D., and Kobayashi, G. (1974): Synergistic effect of amphotericin B and 1,3-bis(2-chloroethyl)-1-nitrosourea against a transplantable AKR leukemia. *Cancer Res.,* 34:974–978.

Immune Modulation and Control of Neoplasia by Adjuvant Therapy, edited by M. A. Chirigos. Raven Press, New York, 1978.

BM 06 002: A New Immunostimulating Compound

U. Bicker

Medical Research, Boehringer Mannheim GmbH, 6800 Mannheim 31, Federal Republic of Germany

Although several hundred aziridines with various substituents have been prepared and tested in animal experiments because of their potential cancerostatic action (9), compounds with an electron-attracting nitrile group on the carbon atom of the aziridine-3 ring were unknown until recently. Bicker was able to show in animal experiments (1–4) that these 2-cyan-substituted aziridines exhibited a good cancerostatic action in a syngenic tumor model in rats, in spite of the absence of alkylating action and low toxicity. The finding that this cancerostatic action was also observed if the compounds were administered several days before the inoculation of the tumors (4) indicated that systemic or immunological phenomena must be responsible for the action of these compounds.

The 4-imino-1,3-diazobicyclo-(3.1.0)-hexan-2-one (chemical structure [II.])(5), which is at present being tested clinically under the designation BM 06 002 (proposed INN Imexon) (13–15) is an isomer of the 1-carboxamido-2-cyan-aziridine (chemical structure [I.]) (1,2,16), the simplest representative of the two cyan-aziridines.

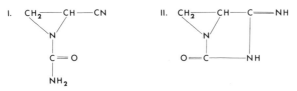

BM 06 002 (chemical structure [II.]) was developed for galenical reasons, but exhibits similar pharmacodynamic properties to those of the unstable 1-carboxamido-2-cyan-aziridine (chemical structure [I.]).

The carrying out of immunostimulating measures as an adjuvant to cancer therapy has gained increasing importance in recent years, especially for the prophylaxis of metastases and relapses, but also as an additional treatment to chemotherapeutic measures with cytotoxic compounds. As the immunosuppressive action of the cytostatics so far known is the limiting factor in cancer chemotherapy, recent efforts have been made to find means of compensating for the immunosuppression of these cytostatics without losing the cancerostatic effect. As the main substances used so far, i.e., the bacterial vaccines Bacillus Calmette-Guerin and *Corynebacterium parvum,* are accompanied by marked side effects and are also difficult to standardize, an intense search has been made for defined chemical compounds capable of producing immunomodulation or immunorestoration, or both.

The anthelmintic levamisol (11) was the first "antianergic" chemotherapeutic agent attributed with such an immunomodulating action.

BM 06 002 (chemical formula [2]) showed in various investigations that cell-mediated immune procedures are stimulated (P. G. Munder, *personal communication,* and refs. 4 and 8). The cancerostatic action of these compounds is attributed to such an immune stimulation.

In this chapter, we report on the cancerostatic action of BM 06 002 on various transplantation tumors in mice and rats, on the potentiation of delayed type hypersensitivity reaction in mice, on the influencing of the primary humoral immune response in the mouse, and on the potentiation of resistance to infection in mice. A possible alkylating action of BM 06 002 was tested for with the aid of the color test with 4-(4-nitrobenzyl)-pyridine.

MATERIALS AND METHODS

Compounds

BM 06 002 was manufactured according to (5) and prepared for intravenous administration in physiological saline and for oral administration was administered as a solution in 0.5% tylose. Cyclophosphamide (Endoxan® from Asta-Werke AG, Chemische Fabrik, 4812 Brackwede) and hydrocortisone acetate EP in micronized form (from Synochem-Präparate, Apotheker Fritz Zimmermann, 2000 Barsbüttel-Hamburg) were used as comparative preparations.

Animals

Female NMRI mice (randomly bred stains from S. Ivanovas GmbH & Co., Kisslegg/Allgäu) weighing 16 to 21 g, female inbred C 57 Bl 6 mice (Zentralinstitut für Versuchstierzucht, Hannover-Linden) weighing 20 to 25 g, and female Sprague-Dawley rats (S. Ivanovas GmbH & Co., Kisslegg/Allgäu) weighing 88 to 115 g were used for the experiments.

Methods

Tumor Experiments

Solid, Heterologous Tumors

The transplantation-ripe tumors were obtained under sterile conditions from sacrificed animals of the tumor-maintaining strain and were crushed in an embryo crusher. The tumor mass was triturated in a mortar with 8 ml physiological saline per g tumor. The suspension was injected into the animals in the individual experimental groups in a quantity of 0.5 ml/animal subcutaneously in the nape of the neck. When clear tumor growth was seen in the controls (7 to 14 days after tumor transplantation), the animals were killed and the tumors were removed, weighed, and the weights of those from the treated group compared with those from the control group.

Friend Virus Leukemia

The transplantation-ripe spleen was removed from sacrificed animals of the tumor-maintaining strain, and a suspension was prepared in a mortar by the addition of 25 ml physiological saline. A 0.2-ml-aliquot of this suspension was administered to each animal intraperitoneally. After 20 days, the animals were killed, the tumors removed, weighed, and the weights of the treated group were compared with those from the control group.

Lewis Lung Tumor

The tumor was removed from sacrificed animals of the tumor-maintaining strain under sterile conditions and crushed. One gram crushed tumor was mixed with 50 ml saline solution buffered to pH 7.3 (PBS), and this was stirred for 7 to 8 min. The supernatant was drawn off, and 40 ml of an 0.25% trypsin solution was added to the sediment. This was stirred for 10 min, mixed with 50 ml PBS, and allowed to settle. The sediment was subsequently mixed with 40 ml 0.25% trypsin solution and kept at 37°C for 30 min with stirring. Subsequently, it was filtered through sterile gauze, and the filtrate was mixed with 100 ml Eagle's + H medium. After centrifugation (1,000 rpm, 0°, 10 min), the sediment was taken up in 120 ml medium, and then the tumor cell count determined with the aid of trypan blue staining and the desired tumor cell dilution prepared with the medium.

Evaluation

The means and standard deviations were calculated for the tumor weights of the individual experimental groups. Student's t-test was used to determine significance, the significance limit being set at $p < 0.05$.

MacKaness' Delayed Type Hypersensitivity Reaction (12)

Technique. Five mice per experimental group were injected intravenously with 10^7 sheep erythrocytes in 0.5 ml buffered saline (PBS). The sheep erythrocytes were prepared as follows. Blood was taken from the carotid vein of an adult, male sheep with the aid of a Biopack® ACD (Biotest-Seruminstitut GmbH, Frankfurt). Two milliliters of the blood was diluted with 8 ml of a buffered physiological saline solution (pH 7.2). The PBS solution was prepared from 87.7 g sodium chloride, 2.6 g sodium dihydrogen phosphate $\cdot$ 2 H_2O and 23.9 g sodium hydrogen phosphate $\cdot$ 2 H_2O dissolved in 10 l distilled water and filtered sterile. The blood-saline solution is centrifuged at 15,000 rpm at room temperature, and the supernatant pipetted off, the residue again diluted with PBS to 10 ml and then again centrifuged. The erythrocytes were washed under the same conditions three times. Subsequently, the concentration of the erythrocytes to 10^7 per 0.5 ml PBS was adjusted with the aid of a Coulter counter. Two, one, and zero days before immunization, groups of five mice were injected with 250 mg/kg (group 1), 25 mg/kg (group 2), and 2.5 mg/kg (group 3) BM 06 002 dissolved in 10 ml PBS by intravenous injection into the tail vein. A fourth group of five mice (group 4) was injected with 10 ml/kg PBS and used as controls. On the fourth day after immunization, a dose of 1×10^8 sheep erythrocytes in 0.04 ml PBS was injected into the left hindpaw, and after 24 and 48 hr the diameter of both the left and right hindpaws was measured with the aid of the Odi test (skin thickness measure from H. C. Kroeplin GmbH, Schlüchtern). If the factor for the increase in the difference of the diameter between left and right paws of the BM 06 002-treated animals compared with the difference of the diameter between left and right paws of the control animals is greater than 1.2, then a relevant potentiation of the delayed type hypersensitivity reaction is said to have occurred (14).

INFLUENCE OF BM 06 002 ON PRIMARY IMMUNE RESPONSE IN MICE

Female NMRI mice (S. Ivanovas, Kisslegg/Allgäu) weighing 18 to 22 g were used. The mice were fed Ssniff pellets (from the Intermast Co., Soest), provided with water *ad lib.,* and kept under constant conditions at $23 \pm 1°C$ and $55 \pm 5\%$ relative humidity with a 12 hr day/night rhythm. The determination of the primary immune response was determined as follows in a manner based on Jerne and Nordin (10).

Groups of five mice were immunized intraperitoneally with 10^7 sheep erythrocytes in 0.5 ml PBS. BM 06 002 dissolved in 10 ml PBS/kg was administered intravenously on days -2, -1, 0, $+1$, $+2$, $+3$, and $+4$ of the immunization. On days $+4$ and $+5$, the animals were gassed with nitrogen, the spleens removed, and each spleen was homogenized in 2 ml medium with the aid of a Potter homogenizer. The medium was prepared as follows: 500 ml of an Eagle's and Dulbeccos' modified solution with a pH of 7.2 (GIBCO Co., Biocult, Glasgow, Scotland) was mixed with 1.2 g Hepes (from Serva Co., Heidelberg), 250 IU penicillin, and 250 μg streptomycin (Flow Laboratories Co.).

A 0.1-ml aliquot of the homogenisate was mixed with 5 ml Pibu (Pillemner buffer: stock solution: 42.5 g NaCl, 2.87 g 5,5-diethyl barbituric acid, 1.87 g barbital sodium, 2.5 ml of a 1 M $MgCl_2$ solution, and 0.75 ml of a 1 M $CaCl_2$ solution are dissolved in 750 ml hot distilled water with stirring, cooled, and the volume is made up to 1,000 ml with distilled water. The solution has a pH of 7.4; working solution: one part of the stock solution is diluted with four parts distilled water). Then 0.1 ml of the suspension is mixed with 0.1 ml Pibu and 0.1 ml 6% sheep erythrocyte solution in Pibu and 0.1 ml lyophilized guinea pig complement (from the Behring Co., Marburg). Of this mixture 200 μl is filled into a special chamber that is closed with paraffin and incubated for 1 hr at 37°C.

The special chambers are prepared as follows. Microscope slides (53 to 76 mm long, 1 mm thick) are cleaned in an ultrasound bath, rinsed for 10 min under flowing water, washed in distilled water, and dried in an incubating oven at 50°C. Two such microscope slides, displaced length-wise by 2 to 4 mm, are divided into two halves with double-sided tape and stuck together.

After incubation, the plaques formed by lysis of the erythrocytes are counted with a magnifying glass. The number of plaques in both chambers is multiplied by 500 so that the number of plaques per spleen can be calculated. The means and standard deviations are calculated from the individual values of the experimental and control animals.

EXAMINATION FOR ALKYLATED METABOLITES IN RAT SERUM AFTER ADMINISTRATION OF BM 06 002

Experimental Procedure

This investigation was carried out by the method described by N. Brock et al. (7).

Each of five male Sprague-Dawley rats (breeder, S. Ivanovas) weighing 180 to 220 g was injected with 200 mg/kg BM 06 002 dissolved in 10 ml distilled water (group 1), 10 ml/kg distilled water (controls: group 2), and 200 mg/kg cyclophosphamide (group 3), also dissolved in 10 ml distilled water. The solutions were injected intravenously into a tail vein. After 1, 2, 4, 6, and 24 hr, 3 to 5 ml blood were withdrawn from each animal in groups 1 to 3 from the retroorbital venous plexus, and the blood was centrifuged for 20 min at 2,300 g. Each milliliter of the serum was deproteinized with 2 ml 96% ethanol and was again centrifuged in the cold. Two nitrobenzylpyridine (NBP) determinations were carried out on the serum ethanol mixture for each individual animal, and the arithmetic mean was determined. Two-tenths of a milliliter of the serum mixture was pipetted into test tubes with ground glass stoppers and diluted with water to 2.1 ml. For each test solution a blank containing 2.1 ml distilled water instead of serum was prepared. The tubes were placed in an ice bath, and each was mixed with 0.7 ml acetate buffer (0.025 M, pH 4.6) and 0.28 ml NBP reagent (5% 4-(4-nitrobenzyl)-pyridine in acetone A.R.) and then placed in the closed state for 20 min in boiling water. Subsequently, the test tubes were cooled in ice water. After cooling, 1.4 ml acetone absolutely pure (A.P.), 3.5 ml ethyl acetate A.P., and 1.0 ml NaOH (0.25 N) were added consecutively.

From this point on, the procedure must be carried out speedily as the color produced on addition of the NaOH is not stable. The tubes were briefly shaken and centrifuged. The upper organic layer was pipetted off and put into cuvettes. The extinction was then measured photometrically against the reagent blank. Approximately 90 min were needed from the time of blood collection to photometric measurement. The measurement of the extinction was carried out at 546 nm in an Eppendorf photometer.

INFECTION EXPERIMENTS

Female NMRI mice (breeder, Wiga, Gassner, Sulzfeld) weighing 28 to 30 g were used for the experiment. The animals were fed on Ssniff-Standard-Diät R pellets (supplier, Intermast GmbH, Soest/Westfalen). Water was available *ad lib.* from drinking bottles. The animals were kept in fully air-conditioned laboratories with a room temperature of 22°C.

The yeast strain *Candida albicans* (219) used for the infection was maintained on sabouraud-maltose-agar plates. On the day before the infection, sabouraud fluid medium (Oxoid Co.) was inoculated with the yeast strain and incubated at 37°C for 18 hr. Immediately before infection, the inoculated culture was centrifuged and washed twice with physiological saline. The sediment was resuspended in physiological saline and diluted according to the desired infecting dose. The animals were infected with 0.2 ml of such a diluted inoculum intravenously.

RESULTS AND DISCUSSION

Figure 1 shows that BM 06 002 has a good cancerostatic action on various transplantation tumors.

At a dose of 5 mg/kg i.v. it was definitely superior to 125 mg/kg cyclophosphamide in Friend virus leukemia in mice. Both compounds were equally active at 125 mg/kg orally in Walker carcinoma of rats, whereas cyclophosphamide was slightly superior to BM 06 002 in the Ehrlich ascites carcinoma.

Figure 2 shows the dose-response relationship of BM 06 002 in rats with Walker carcinosarcoma. An optimum decrease in tumor size was obtained with 10 mg/kg intravenously. In contrast to alkylating agents, the effect decreased when subtoxic doses were used. The decreased effectiveness with sublethal doses was also observed in other experimental models such as the Ridgeway osteosarcoma in mice. The optimum dose of 10 mg/kg BM 06 002 was less than 2% of the median lethal dose, whereas more than 50% of the median lethal dose of cyclophosphamide has to be given to obtain a significant reduction in tumor size.

The most striking difference between BM 06 002 and cyclophosphamide was their effect on leukocytes (Fig. 3). A single intravenous injection of as little as 20 mg/kg cyclophosphamide produced the well-known leukocyte depression

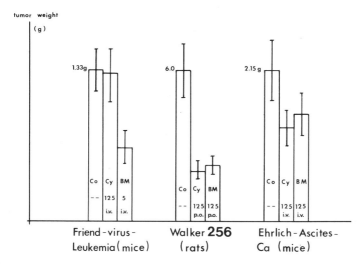

FIG. 1. Antitumor effect of BM 06 002 and cyclophosphamide. Co, control; Cy, cyclophosphamide; BM, BM 06 002.

in rats. The same dose of BM 06 002, however, produced leukocytosis on the fourth and sixth days.

Leukopenia is an inevitable side effect of all alkylating agents. This experiment suggests that the antitumor activity of BM 06 002 cannot be explained by alkylation.

No alkylation or cytotoxic effect could be found *in vitro*.

To exclude the formation of alkylating metabolites, the serum of rats treated with BM 06 002 was tested for alkylating metabolites by the NBP method.

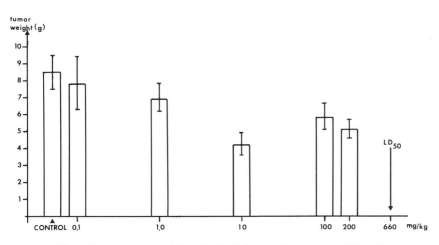

FIG. 2. Dose-response relationship in Walker carcinosarcoma 256 (rat).

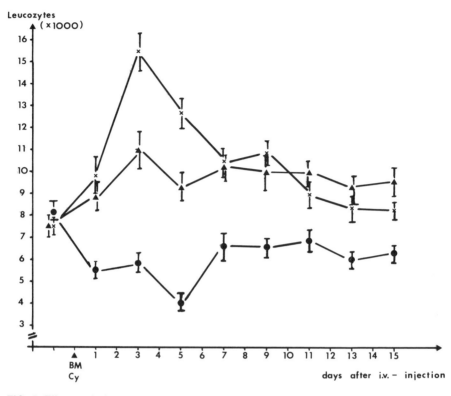

FIG. 3. Effect on leukocytes counts in rats. x———x, BM 06 002 (20 mg/kg, i.v.); ●———●, cyclophosphamide (20 mg/kg, i.v.); ▲———▲, control.

Cyclophosphamide gave the well-known color reaction 1 and 2 hr after the injection. BM 06 002 was negative up to 24 hr (Table 1).

The leukocytosis described suggested to us that the antitumor effect of BM 06 002 was due to immunostimulation rather than depression.

Stimulation of the immune system takes several days to develop. For this reason, BM 06 002 was injected 6 days before inoculation (with 5×10^5 tumor cells per mouse) (Table 2). Only four out of 30 controls survived without tumor. One milligram per kilogram BM 06 002 was without effect; 10 mg/kg BM 06 002 protected 23 out of 30 mice, and the number could not be increased by

TABLE 1. *Alkylating metabolites in rat serum—NBP-method*

Compound	1 hr	2 hr	4 hr	6 hr	24 hr
BM 06.002	0.003−	0.002−	0.007−	0.000−	0.001−
Cyclophosphamide	0.054+	0.020+	0.001−	0.000−	0.002−
Control	0.002−	0.000−	0.000−	0.004−	0.003−

200 mg/kg BM 06.002 or cyclophosphamide i.v.

TABLE 2. *Prevention of Lewis lung tumors in $C_{57}Bl_6$ mice*

Compound	mg/kg	Number of animals without tumor
Control	—	4/30
Levamisol	1	6/30
Levamisol	5	7/30
BM 06 002	1	8/30
BM 06 002	10	23/30
BM 06 002	50	20/30

I.v. injection 6 days before inoculation.

raising the dose to 50 mg/kg. The syngenic Lewis lung tumor was chosen as a model in order to exclude possible immunostimulating effects of BM 06 002 on H2 antigens.

The effects of BM 06 002 on cell-mediated immunity were tested in mice according to the system described by Mackeness. Various doses of BM 06 002 were injected 2 days before the sheep erythrocytes. A booster dose was given 7 days after the primary injection of SRBC. Twenty-four and 48 hr later the reaction was measured in both hindpaws. There was a clear-cut increase in the footpad swelling in the treated animals (Fig. 4). The figures on the ordinate

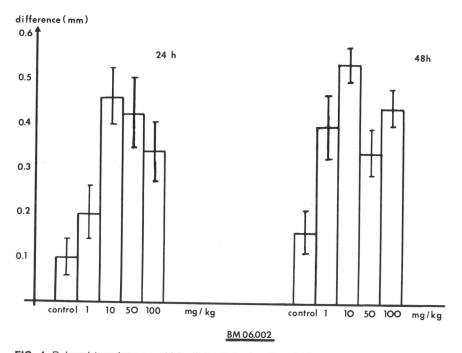

FIG. 4. Delayed type hypersensitivity C 57-Bl-6-mice ($N = 5$). BM 06 002 was given 2 days before immunization boosts, 7 days after immunization.

show the differences in the diameters of the boostered and the control paws. This enhancement of delayed type hypersensitivity was the first indication of stimulation of cellular immunoreactivity.

BM 06 002 had no mitogenic activity *in vitro,* but investigations by Cerni et al. (8) showed that an increased transformation of lymphocytes was observed when mice were pretreated *in vivo* with BM 06 002. The mice were injected intravenously with 20 mg/kg of BM 06 002. Spleen cells from mice treated only once with BM 06 002 incorporated consistently more H³-thymidine than cells from control animals (Fig. 5). This increased incorporation of H³-thymidine was observed after incubation with both phytohemagglutinin and concanavalin A.

The effect of BM 06 002 on the humoral immunoresponse was tested in Jerne's plaque test. BM 06 002 was injected on the day of immunization or 1 to 2 days afterward. The number of plaque-forming cells per spleen was determined on days 4 and 5. A slight stimulation was seen only when BM 06 002 was given together with the antigen (Fig. 6). These results have been confirmed by several other independent groups. It therefore appears that BM 06 002 stimulates mainly the cellular immune response.

It is conceivable that the stimulation of the cellular defense mechanism is also effective against certain infections.

Figure 7 shows the survival of mice infected with spores of *Candida albicans.* Four intraperitoneal injections of 20 mg/kg BM 06 002 6 to 0 days before infection significantly prolonged the survival.

BM 06 002 is also able to restore immunity. Mice pretreated with 120 mg/ kg hydrocortisone die after infection with *Candida albicans* at a dose that does not kill untreated animals. Pretreatment with BM 06 002 markedly prolonged the survival (Fig. 8).

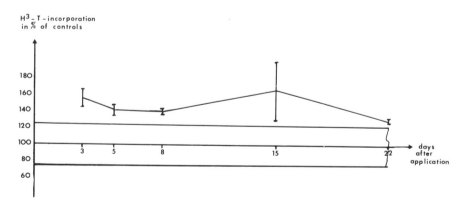

FIG. 5. Stimulation of the lymphocyte transformation to phytohemagglutinin after application of BM 06 002, 20 mg/kg i.p. (From ref. 8.)

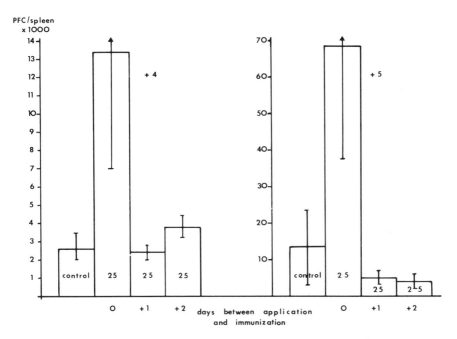

FIG. 6. Jerne test. NMRI mice (*N* = 7). BM 06 002, i.v., 25 mg/kg.

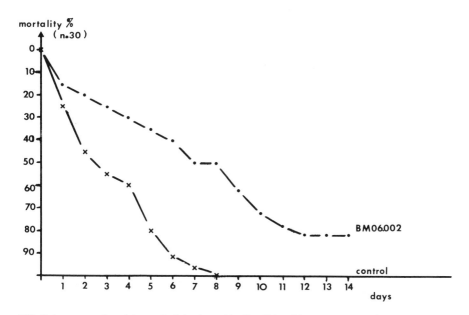

FIG. 7. Increase of resistance to infection with *Candida albicans* (mice). BM 06 002 (4 × 20 mg/kg i.p.) 6, 4, 2, and 0 days before i.v. infection. Infection-dose, 9.6 × 10⁵ germs/mouse.

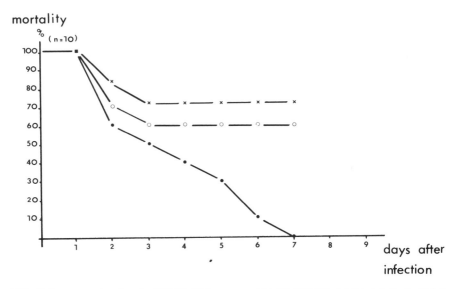

FIG. 8. Immunorestoration by BM 06 002. ○——○, BM 06 002 (25 mg/kg p.o. 6, 4, and 2 days before infection); ●——●, hydrocortisone (120 mg/kg i.p., 5, 3, and 1 days before infection); x——x, control. Infection dose, 2.7×10^5 germs/mouse.

These findings indicate that BM 06 002 exerts its antitumor activity via immunological routes. Further investigations show that BM 06 002 has an influence on cell-mediated immune procedures.

After the general pharmacological and toxicological investigations had been carried out, it was found in a preliminary clinical trial in tumor patients that BM 06 002 also had such an immune-stimulating action in man, so that, in principle, the findings obtained from animal experiments with regard to immune stimulation are transferable to man also.

BM 06 002 is the first representative of a new class of substances with immune-modulating properties. In the meantime, other active compounds have been found that have the advantages of better stability and higher oral activity. Reports on the biological properties of these subsequent compounds will be made in the near future.

REFERENCES

1. Bicker, U. (1974): Verfahren zur Herstellung zytostatisch wirksamer 2-Cyanaziridine. D.D.R.-WP 110.492.
2. Bicker, U. (1975): N-(2-cyanethylen-)urea—an asparagine analogous cytostatic compound? *Exp. Pathol. Jena,* 10:106–108.
3. Bicker, U., and Fuhse, P. (1975): Carcinostatic action of 2-cyanaziridines against a sarcoma in rats. *Exp. Pathol. Jena,* 10:279–284.
4. Bicker, U., and Hebold, G. (1977): Verstärkung der zellvermittelten Immunreaktivität durch BM 06.002 (Prop. INN Imexon) bei Mäusen. *Exp. Pathol. Jena (in press).*
5. Bicker, U., Kampe, U., and Steingross, W., (1975): Organische Verbindung. Deutsche Patentanmeldung P 25.30.3984.

6. Bicker, U. and Hebold, G. (1977): Antitumorwirksamkeit der immunstimulierenden Verbindung 4-Imino-1,3-diazabicyclo-(3.1.0)-hexan-2-on (BM 06.002, Prop. INN Imexon). *Exp. Pathol. Jena (in press).*

7. Brock, N., Hoefer-Janker, H., Hohorst, H. J., Scheef, W., Schneider, B., and Wolf, H. C. (1973): Die Aktivierung von Ifosfamid an Mensch und Tier. *Arzneim. Forsch.,* 23:1–14.

8. Cerni, E. M., Rella, U. A., and Bicker, U. (1977): Immunstimulation durch BM 06.002. *Oncology (in press).*

9. Dermer, O. C., and Ham, G. E. (1969): *Ethylenimine and Other Aziridines.* Academic Press, New York and London.

10. Jerne, N. K., and Nordin, A. A. (1963): Plaque formation in agar by single antibody-producing cells. *Science,* 140:404.

11. Janssen, P. A. J. (1976): The levamisole story. *Prog. Drug Res.,* 20:347–383.

12. Mackaness, G. B., Lagrange, P. H., and Ishibashi, T. (1974): The modifying effect of BCG on the immunological induction of T cells. *J. Exp. Med.,* 139:1540–1552.

13. Micksche, M., Kokoschka, E. M., Sagaster, P., and Bicker, U. (1978): Phase I study for a new immunostimulating drug, BM 06.002 in man *(This volume).*

14. Micksche, M., Kokoschka, E. M., Sagaster, P., and Bicker, U. (1977): BM 06.002: A new immunostimulating drug. *IRSC Med. Sci. (in press).*

15. Micksche, M., Kokoschka, E. M., Kokron, O., Sagaster, P., and Bicker, U. (1977): Immunostimulation in cancer patients by a new synthetic compound: BM 06.002. *Öster. Z. für Onkologie (in press).*

16. Von Ardenne, M., and Reitnauer, P. G. (1975): Nachweis krebshemmender Eigenschaften einer stark immunstimulierenden Verbindung kleiner Molekülmasse. *Arzneim. Forsch.,* 25:1369–1379.

Immune Modulation and Control of Neoplasia by Adjuvant Therapy, edited by M. A. Chirigos. Raven Press, New York, 1978.

Phase I Study for a New Immunostimulating Drug, BM 06 002, in Man

M. Micksche, *E. M. Kokoschka, **P. Sagaster, and ***U. Bicker

*Institute for Cancer Research and *II. Department of Dermatology, University of Vienna, Austria; **V. Department of Internal Medicine, Wilhelminenspital Vienna, Austria; and ***Boehringer Mannheim GmbH, Mannheim, Federal Republic of Germany*

During the last decade immunotherapy has been introduced into the strategy for treatment of malignant disease. By a variety of immunological tests it has been demonstrated that cancer patients even with localized disease show a depressed general and also tumor-specific immunity and that this unresponsiveness correlates with unfavorable prognosis (5,7,9). Therefore several attempts of immunotherapy of cancer patients have been performed. Methods used were active immunization of cancer patients with inactivated or neuraminidase-treated tumor cells or membrane extracts of these cells for induction of tumor specific immunity (6,13,16). Bacterial adjuvants like BCG or *Corynebacterium parvum* have been used for active immunostimulation in cancer patients (8,10,15). With vitamin A, used in high doses, for immunostimulation in cancer patients, a clear effect has recently been demonstrated in lung cancer patients on tumor growth and immune system (12).

A new approach was the use of synthetic immunostimulants like levamisole (16) or poly A: U (17) or glucan. These synthetic adjuvants are now investigated in clinical phase I and II trials for their usefulness in cancer therapy. Levamisole, by definition an antianergic chemotherapeutic agent, has been shown to restore cell-mediated immune reactions in immunodepressed cancer patients and to prolong the remission period and the survival time (1).

Several new substances are screened in animal models for their immune-stimulating capacity (11). One of these approaches is the synthetic compound 4-imino-1, 3-diazabicyclo (3,1,0)-hexan-2-on (BM 06 002), which is an isomere of 1-carboxamido-2-cyanaziridin. Both substances have been invented by Bicker, who has demonstrated a tumor-inhibiting effect for these compounds in transplanted methylnitrosourea-induced rat sarcoma (2). A direct cytostatic effect for these substances was never observed, and therefore it was assumed that immunological mechanisms might be responsible for the tumor inhibition. Recently it was demonstrated that the isomere (BM 06 002), which was considered to be the active substance, stimulates humoral as well as cell-mediated immune reactions in laboratory animals. Besides this, the tumor-inhibiting effect was confirmed and shown to be dependent on i mune reactions in the tumor-bearing host (3). Based on these experiments and because of the total absence of toxic side effects, a phase I study was initiated in patients with advanced noncurable cancer.

MATERIAL AND METHODS

Patients' Selection

A total number of 24 patients with histologically verified neoplastic disease has been included in this protocol. Four patients had carcinomas of the breast, four of the vulva, four of the lung, and one of the cervix. Seven patients had malignant melanoma, three seminoma, and one hypernephroma. All patients were treated previously by surgery plus chemo- or radiotherapy for recurrent disease. All patients were informed that a new form of therapy was given to them that had not yet been applied to human cases.

Drug Application

The substance BM 06 002 was supplied by Boehringer Mannheim (FRG) as a lyophilized powder in 20- and 100-mg ampules. This material was reconstituted with 10 ml of the solvent immediately before use and injected intravenously. Acute toxicity study was started with a dose of 5 mg in one patient; after no side effect was observed, another patient received 5 mg. The next higher dose of 10 mg was then given in the same way to another three patients. By this method, the dose was accelerated to 40, 80, and 100 mg in several groups of patients.

Sequential application of the compound was started again with low doses, 20 mg, and dose was increased up to 1,200 mg in the same way as for acute toxicity study.

CLINICAL AND LABORATORY INVESTIGATIONS

For clinical staging every patient was examined with X-ray and scanning before application of the drug. Presence of malignant disease was confirmed in all cases by histology and cytology.

Laboratory tests used to investigate possible side effects of therapy were the following—sedimentation rate, complete differential blood count, liver function test (GOT, GPT, LDH, bilirubin), creatinine, BUN, alcaline phosphatase, Cu, and Fe. These tests were performed before, and 1 week after, the last dose of BM 06 002 had been applied.

IMMUNOLOGICAL TESTS

Delayed Cutaneous Hypersensitivity Reactions

A battery of microbial antigens was used to investigate preexisting immunity. Antigens tested were purified tuberculin (GT 10 Hoechst-Germany), streptokinase/streptodornase (40 U/cm³, Lederle Laboratories), mumps skin test antigen (Eli Lilly Co.), *Candida* (Beecham), and toxoplasmin (Serotherapeutisches Institut Vienna). Then, 0.1 ml of the test substance was injected intradermally into the back of the patients, and reactions were read at 24 and 48 hr. A test was considered positive, when the diameter of the induration was more than 5 mm.

At the same time phytohemagglutinin (PHA p; Wellcome) was used as a parameter for lymphocyte reactivity *in vivo,* as described earlier (14). Two micrograms were applied intradermally, and a reaction was observed after 24 hr. An induration of more than 15 mm was considered positive.

Patients were also sensitized and challenged with the primary antigen dinitrochlorobenzene (DNCB; Merck, Darmstadt) according to the method of Eilber and Morton (7). The sensitization dose was 2,000 µg, and the challenge doses were 100, 50, and 25 µg. Reactions were observed after 48 hr and persistent erythema together with induration or vesiculation, or both, was graded from +2 to +4.

Keyhole-limpet hemocyanin (Schwarz/Mann, Orangeburg, N.Y.) was used also as a primary antigen, and patients were immunized with 100 µg in 0.1 ml by intracutaneous injection of this test substance and challenged after 14 days with the same dose. Maximum reaction was observed after 48 hr.

Skin tests were performed before and after application of the drug. In patients to whom one single injection was given, the interval was 1 week. Patients receiving several doses of BM 06 002 were tested in intervals of 4 to 6 weeks.

LYMPHOCYTE BLASTOGENESIS

Before skin testing, peripheral venous blood was taken for *in vitro* studies. Fifty milliliters of blood was heparinized, and lymphocytes were separated by low-speed centrifugation on a Ficol-Ronpacon® gradient (3). Lymphocytes were washed in Hank's balanced salt solution and resuspended in basal medium (Eagle) (BME; Gibco Biocult.) supplemented with antibiotics and 5% inactivated fetal calf serum. The cell concentration was adjusted to 2×10^5 lymphocytes per 0.1 ml, washed, and resuspended in RPMI medium 1640 and then distributed with a repeating dispenser to the wells of the microculture plates (micro test II culture plates, Falcom Plastics, Cal). Microcultures were set up in 6 to 12 replicates with or without addition of the appropriate concentration of mitogens, i.e., PHAP (Difco Detroit) diluted 1:10 and 1:100. Concanavalin A (Con A; Pharmacia Uppsala) in a concentration of 20 and 4 µg per ml and pokeweed mitogen (PWM) (Grand Island Biological Co., Grand Island, N.Y.) in a dilution of 10 and 100.

Incubation period was 48 hr for PHA cultures and 5 days for Con A and PWM cultures. After this incubation period in a humidified atmosphere of 5% CO_2 at 37°C, ^{3}H-thymidine was added to all cultures and plates incubated for 5 hr. Cultures were then washed 3X with saline, 2X with 5% trichloric acid, 2X with ethanol, and harvested with a multiple sample harvester device. ^{3}H-thymidine uptake was measured in a liquid scintillation counter (Beckman). Blastogenesis was then expressed as mean cpm value of replicate cultures, in net counts (mean cpm test cultures minus mean cpm control cultures). Lymphocyte blastogenesis response was investigated in the patient group receiving one single dose of BM 06 002 immediately before application of the drug and then 1 week later. In patients receiving several doses at different days, *in vitro* investigations were performed before therapy, then every other week, and then 1 week after the last injection.

RESULTS

A single dose of BM 06 002 was given to 15 patients with advanced neoplastic disease. The toxicity study was started in one patient with 5 mg intravenously (Table 1). The patient was questioned about toxic side effects immediately after injection of the substance, than after 15 min, after 1, 6, 12, 24, 48, and 72 hr.

Table 1

ACUTE TOXICITY STUDY OF BM 06 002 (SINGLE DOSE)

PATIENT	DIAGNOSIS	STAGE	AGE	PRETREATMENT	DOSE	SIDE EFFECT
1 P.Th.	Breast Ca.	III	56	Surgery, Radiotherapy	5 mg	No
2 A.K.	Vulva Ca.	III	72	Radiotherapy	5 mg	No
3 S.R.	Melanoma	III	40	Surgery	10 mg	Nausea
4 W.A.	Lung Ca.	III	73	non resectable	10 mg	No
5 K.H.	Vulva Ca.	III	68	Radiotherapy	10 mg	Headache
6 K.A.	Vulva Ca.	III	72	Radiotherapy	20 mg	No
7 H.Th.	Lung Ca.	III	78	non resectable	20 mg	No
8 B.M.	Melanoma	III	50	Immuno-, Chemotherapy	40 mg	No
9 D.F.	Lung Ca.	III	75	non resectable	40 mg	No
10 S.W.	Vulva Ca.	II	67	Radiotherapy	40 mg	No
11 B.S.	Melanoma	III	32	Immuno-, Chemotherapy	80 mg	No
12 H.K.	Lung Ca.	III	71	non resectable	80 mg	Salivation
13 D.H.	Melanoma	III	56	Immuno-, Chemotherapy	80 mg	No
14 L.H.	Seminoma	III	70	Surgery, Radioth.,Chemoth.	100 mg	No
15 B.A.	Hypernephroma	III	60	Surgery	100 mg	Vomiting

Table 2

SINGLE DOSE OF BM 06 002

PATIENT	DIAGNOSIS	BM 06 002 DOSE		Ery	WBC	PMN %	Ly %	Mono %	Fe	Cu	α_1-glob.	α_2-glob.	β-glob.	γ-glob.
1 P.Th.	Breast Ca.	5 mg	pre	4.8	4000	51	43	6	65	103	2.9	6.8	8.6	28.8
			post	4.5	4600	54	42	4	62	83	3.7	9.1	10.5	26.5
2 A.K.	Vulva Ca.	5 mg	pre	4.1	7400	81	15	4	56	/	7.2	10.9	12.0	18.9
			post	4.0	5300	82	16	2	87	/	7.6	7.5	12.6	19.6
3 S.R.	Melanoma	10 mg	pre	4.3	11300	82	16	2	71	/	/	/	/	/
			post	3.4	10700	70	20	10	92	/	/	/	/	/
4 W.A.	Lung Ca.	10 mg	pre	3.7	8700	82	7	11	59	187	4.3	10.6	11.3	16.7
			post	3.7	9450	79	19	2	86	145	4.5	12.8	13.8	20.6
5 K.H.	Vulva Ca.	10 mg	pre	4.2	6800	72	28	0	55	/	4.4	11.5	14.5	21.6
			post	4.4	5600	72	24	4	82	/	4.2	10.8	14.7	21.4
6 K.A.	Vulva Ca.	20 mg	pre	4.1	6300	73	26	1	40	/	7.2	14.1	13.3	18.2
			post	3.8	6500	73	22	5	76	/	7.2	13.7	14.7	17.4
7 H.Th.	Lung Ca.	20 mg	pre	4.5	20500	92	6	2	56	158	4.8	14.6	13.2	27.4
			post	4.3	17500	88	9	3	50	151	5.2	14.1	11.2	29.6
8 B.M.	Melanoma	40 mg	pre	4.2	3300	79	20	1	97	118	5.2	8.9	9.0	29.0
			post	3.6	3100	76	23	1	127	128	4.8	9.0	9.0	27.0
9 D.F.	Lung Ca.	40 mg	pre	4.3	5000	78	18	4	100	1C6	3.9	8.5	8.4	24.4
			post	4.3	4450	69	24	7	114	98	4.7	9.0	10.8	25.7
10 S.W.	Vulva Ca.	40 mg	pre	5.0	8000	54	44	2	70	/	6.1	11.8	4.3	12.0
			post	5.1	7900	57	40	3	/	/	7.0	11.8	4.3	12.0
11 B.S.	Melanoma	80 mg	pre	3.4	8400	87	13	0	/	/	/	/	/	/
			post	3.5	–	–	–	–	/	/	/	/	/	/
12 H.K.	Lung Ca.	80 mg	pre	3.8	9400	61	32	7	64	175	5.7	11.2	13.2	21.7
			post	3.9	9500	64	34	2	71	122	6.0	11.8	12.4	24.7
13 D.H.	Melanoma	80 mg	pre	4.6	7300	76	24	0	51	/	2.0	9.0	11.0	19.0
			post	3.9	4700	64	31	5	/	/	/	/	/	/

As no side effects were observed, another patient was injected with 5 mg BM 06 002. The next group of three patients received a single dose of 10 mg. In patient S.R. nausea was observed up to 1 hr after the application but then disappeared. The other two patients did not reveal any toxic signs when observed in the same way as the first patients. After this, the dose was increased, and two patients were injected with 20 mg, three with 40 mg, and a further three with 80 mg. In this last group a patient with nonresectable lung cancer claimed increase of salivation from 6 to 12 hr after the injection. Then two patients received 100 mg. From this group, patient B.A. with hypernephroma experienced vomiting 4 hr after the drug had been given.

The effect of this single dose on several laboratory parameters, like peripheral blood count (erythrocytes and white blood cells), Fe, Cu, and serum globulins, bilirubin, GOT, GPT, LDH, alcaline phosphatase, BUN, and creatinine, was observed. These investigations were performed immediately before application of the drug and then at least 1 week afterward. No negative effect on any of these parameters was observed (Tables 2 and 3). A slight depression in erythrocyte count but no change in peripheral white blood cell count was detected.

Eleven of these patients who received a single dose of BM 06 002 were investigated for delayed cutaneous hypersensitivity reactions before and also 1 week after the injection of the drug (Table 4). A change was considered to have occurred when the mean diameter increased by 50%. A change in reaction to recall antigens was observed in two patients to tuberculin, in four patients to streptokinase/streptodornase, in three patients to toxoplasmin, and in one patient to candidin. DNCB reactivity was investigated before and after therapy in seven

Table 3

SINGLE DOSE OF BM 06 002

PATIENTS	DIAGNOSIS	BM 06 002 DOSE		BILIRUBIN	GOT	GPT	LDH	PH.alc.	BUN	KREAT.
1 P.Th.	Breast Ca.	5 mg	pre	1.1	3	3	137	26	14	0.9
			post	1.0	3	5	162	30	15	0.8
2 A.K.	Vulva Ca.	5 mg	pre	0.5	/	/	384	53	45	1.4
			post	0.5	10	8	339	45	24	1.0
3 S.R.	Melanoma	10 mg	pre	1.0	26	9	425	1123	10	0.6
			post	1.0	18	10	348	1297	7	0.6
4 W.A.	Lung Ca.	10 mg	pre	0.5	19	14	137	68	11	0.9
			post	0.6	3	11	157	60	15	1.1
5 K.H.	Vulva Ca.	10 mg	pre	0.4	16	13	242	210	13	0.7
			post	0.3	17	12	289	192	17	0.8
6 K.A.	Vulva Ca.	20 mg	pre	0.5	/	9	283	94	10	0.6
			post	0.3	/	10	268	85	8	1.0
7 H.T.	Lung Ca.	20 mg	pre	0.5	6	7	120	92	15	0.9
			post	0.5	3	5	147	92	17	1.0
8 B.M.	Melanoma	40 mg	pre	0.7	13	6	206	/	6	0.6
			post	0.5	23	18	156	/	11	0.4
9 D.F.	Lung Ca.	40 mg	pre	1.1	7	3	368	58	8	1.2
			post	0.9	3	3	447	57	17	2.0
10 S.W.	Vulva Ca.	40 mg	pre	0.4	19	16	226	58	23	0.8
			post	0.5	14	17	304	68	14	0.8
11 B.S.	Melanoma	80 mg	pre	/	/	/	/	/	11	/
			post	/	/	/	/	/	/	/
12 H.K.	Lung Ca.	80 mg	pre	0.6	11	4	241	80	12	1.2
			post	0.9	12	4	284	76	11	1.6
13 D.H.	Melanoma	80 mg	pre	0.7	11	14	144	112	19	0.8
			post	0.4	9	6	168	/	19	0.8

Table 4

SINGLE DOSE OF BM 06 002: INFLUENCE ON DELAYED CUTANEOUS HYPERSENSITIVITY REACTIONS [*]

PATIENT	DIAGNOSIS	DOSE	TUBERCULIN	VARIDASE	TOXOPLASMIN	CANDIDIN	DNCB 100 μg	DNCB 50 μg	KLH	PHA
A.K.	Vulva Ca.	5 mg	2[a]	12	2	4	n.t.	n.t.	n.t.	15
			2[b]	15	6	5	+2	+2	10	25
K.H.	Vulva Ca.	10 mg	0	0	12	0	n.t.	n.t.	n.t.	15
			2	10	10	5	+2	+2	15	16
S.R.	Melanoma	10 mg	0	6	0	0	+1	0	n.t.	8
			0	8	0	0	+2	+1	5	10
K.A.	Vulva Ca.	20 mg	0	0	17	4	n.t.	n.t.	n.t.	16
			0	5	15	5	+3	+3	20	18
H.Th.	Lung Ca.	20 mg	0	10	8	8	+2	+2	22	32
			15	12	5	8	+3	+3	10	30
F.Th.	Breast Ca.	20 mg	0	10	12	2	+1	+1	6	18
			0	7	9	0	+2	+1	5	15
P.E.	Breast Ca.	20 mg	2	2	9	5	+1	+1	0	20
			0	6	8	8	+2	+2	20	20
S.W.	Vulva Ca.	40 mg	3	35	20	n.t.	n.t.	n.t.	n.t.	32
			2	35	15	n.t.	+3	+3	25	32
D.F.	Lung Ca.	40 mg	25	10	5	2	+1	0	7	20
			10	10	n.t.	n.t.	+2	+2	10	n.t.
H.K.	Lung Ca.	80 mg	17	7	4	n.t.	+2	+2	n.t.	30
			20	12	10	3	+2	+2	5	18
D.H.	Melanoma	80 mg	8	65	12	0	+2	+1	6	20
			21	76	26	2	+3	+2	12	27

[*] mean diameter of indurations 48 hrs after administration of the test substances (mm)

ab before (a) and after (b) administration of the drug

DNCB (0 and +1 = negative; +2 to +4 = positive)

patients. Of these, six showed an increase in reaction to 100 μg and 5 to 50 μg. A conversion from ±1, which is considered negative to plus 2 or 3, which is positive, was observed in four patients. Changes to Keyhole limpet hemocyanin (KLH) skin tests were found in one patient, and to PHA also in one patient.

Lymphocyte blastogenesis response to PHA, Con A, and PWM was investigated in six patients before and 1 week after application of BM 06 002 (Table 5). An increase of spontaneous ^{3}H-thymidine uptake was found in three patients. PHA response increased in five patients and decreased in one patient with 1:10 concentration; and in one patient increased and one decreased with the diluted PHA. Reactions to Con A (konz.) increased in two patients, reduced in one patient, and increased in three cases with diluted Con A. PWM reactions were stimulated in four patients and reduced in two. With the diluted mitogen only one patient showed an increase.

Long-term toxicity study was started again with a low dose of BM 06 002. One patient received 2 × 20 mg in 2 weeks. After no side effects were observed (Table 6), the dose was increased, and the next patient was injected with 3 × 20 mg in 2 weeks and another with 5 × 20 mg in 4 weeks. Higher doses were then given 3 × a week, i.e., 100 mg. Another patient was injected at first with 4 × 20 mg and subsequently with another course of 5 × 100 mg. Each time this patient developed a mild nausea up to 3 hr after injection of the single dose.

Again doses were increased; one patient was injected with a total dose of 800 mg in 3 weeks, and three further patients received 12 × 100 mg BM 06 002 intravenously in 4 weeks. In patient S. A. vomiting occurred 1 hr after the injection of the first two doses.

Altogether, toxic side effects were very rare and not severe. No influence on laboratory parameter, blood picture, or blood pressure was observed in any of these patients under continuous BM 06 002 therapy (Table 6). The influence

Table 5

INFLUENCE OF BM 06 OC2 ON LYMPHOCYTE BLASTOGENESIS (SINGLE DOSE)

PATIENT	DIAGNOSIS	DOSE	SPONTAN*	PHA konz.	PHA dil.	CON A konz.	CON A dil.	PWM konz.	PWM dil.
1 P.E.	Breast Ca.	20 mg	9 201	9 629[a]	2 957	4 876	3 454	18 642	3 496
			915	35 420[b]	2 021	73 741	23 100	9 109	1 651
2 H.Th.	Lung Ca.	20 mg	1 830	10 241	n.t.	20 282	n.t.	9 791	251
			14 377	111 041	56 612			41 953	16 067
3 D.F.	Lung Ca.	40 mg	214	20 717	8 369	n.t.	n.t.	8 031	3 584
			282	31 482	9 464			13 410	3 584
4 H.K.	Lung Ca.	80 mg	244	33 551	3 657	n.t.	n.t.	886	3 558
			389	41 530	4 595			1 130	8 584
5 D.H.	Melanoma	80 mg	477	56 053	57 893	36 875	56 564	19 225	28 987
			5 315	29 404	46 665	66 390	66 270	7 209	8 412
6 S.A.	Breast Ca.	80 mg	1 608	2 533	9 764	33 345	35 282	27 127	81 723
			585	86 864	23 357	12 548	50 900	66 695	62 193

* mean counts of unstimulated cultures (cpm)

a,b mean counts of replicates of test cultures before (a) and after (b) administration of the drug

n.t. non tested

Table 6

LONG TIME TOXICITY OF BM 06 CO2

PATIENT	AGE	DIAGNOSIS	STAGE	PRETREATMENT	BM 06 002 DOSE	BM 06 002 FREQUENCY	BM 06 002 TOTAL DOSE	SIDE EFFECT
1 D.R.	38	Cervix Ca.	III	Radio-, Chemotherapy	20 mg	2 (1 week)	40 mg	No
2 Th.L.	60	Breast Ca.	III	Surg., Radio-, Chemoth.	20 mg	3 (2 weeks)	60 mg	No
3 P.M.	60	Melanoma	II	Surgery	20 mg	5 (4 weeks)	100 mg	No
4 H.Th.	78	Lung Ca.	III	No	100 mg	3 (1 week)	300 mg	No
5 D.H.	56	Melanoma	III	Surgery, Immunotherapy	100 mg	4 (2 weeks)	400 mg	Dizziness
6 P.E.	51	Breast Ca.	III	Surgery, Radiotherapy	20 mg 100 mg	4x(1 week) 5x(2 weeks)	580 mg	Nausea
7 S.A.	50	Melanoma	III	Surgery, Immuno-,Chemot.	100 mg	8 (3 weeks)	800 mg	No
8 O.W.	35	Seminoma	III	Chemo-,Radioth., Surg.	100 mg	12 (4 weeks)	1200 mg	No
9 W.H.	75	Melanoma	III	Surgery, Immunotherapy	100 mg	12 (4 weeks)	1200 mg	No
10 S.A.	55	Breast Ca.	III	Surgery,Radiotherapy	100 mg	12 (4 weeks)	1200 mg	Vomiting
11 T.K.	36	Seminoma	II	Radio-, Chemotherapy	100 mg	12 (4 weeks)	1200 mg	No

of sequential applications of BM 06 002 on delayed cutaneous hypersensitivity reactions was investigated in nine of these patients (Table 7). A change in reaction, an increase of more than 50%, was observed in two patients to tuberculin, in two to streptokinase/streptodornase, in two to mumps antigen, and in three to candidin. Conversion from DNCB negative to positive was observed in two patients with 100 μg and 2 to 50 μg. An increase in response to both concentrations of DNCB from +2 to +3 was found in three patients. Response to KLH increased in three cases, whereas PHA responsiveness was positively changed only in one patient.

Table 7

INFLUENCE OF SEQUENTIAL APPLICATION OF BM 06 002 ON DCHR

PATIENT	DIAGNOSIS	DOSE	TUBERCULIN[*]	VARIDASE	MUMPS	TOXOPLASMIN	CANDIDIN	DNCB 100 μg	DNCB 50 μg	KLH	PHA
1 F.T.	Breast Ca.	3x 20 mg	0[a]	10	0	12	2	+1	+1	5	18
		+ Chemoth.	0[b]	12	9	17	6	+3	+3	10	25
2 P.E.	Breast Ca.	4x 20 mg	2	2	0	9	5	+1	+1	0	20
			2	15	5	5	3	+3	+2	8	20
		5x100 mg	2	11	5	10	10	+3	+3	35	25
3 P.M.	Melanoma	5x 20 mg	0	10	n.t.	10	0	0	0	5	15
			8	12	n.t.	17	4	0	0	8	15
4 H.T.	Lung Ca.	3x100 mg	0	10	0	8	0	+2	+2	20	32
			0	7	3	5	0	+3	+3	5	20
5 S.A.	Melanoma	4x100 mg	12	9	n.t.	10	0	+4	+4	5	11
			14	9	n.t.	9	0	n.t.	+4	5	13
		+ Chemoth.	11	10	n.t.	10	0	n.t.	+4	5	15
7 W.H.	Melanoma	12x100 mg	15	15	n.t.	12	11	+2	+2	12	12
			14	19	n.t.	10	6	+3	+2	7	15
8 T.K.	Seminoma	12x100 mg	20	20	12	7	0	+3	+3	0	20
			20	25	10	7	0	+3	+3	10	20
9 S.A.	Breast Ca.	12x100 mg	5	8	5	3	6	+2	+2	25	20
			15	14	15	5	6	+3	+3	25	25

[*] diameter of induration 48 hrs after application of test substances (in mm)

[a,b] before (a) and after (b) application of the drug

DNCB (0 and +1 = negative; +2 to +4 = positive)

Table 8

INFLUENCE OF BM 06 002 ON LYMPHOCYTE BLASTOGENESIS RESPONSE

PATIENT	DIAGNOSIS	DOSE	SPONTAN*	PHA konz.	PHA dil.	CON A konz.	CON A dil.	PWM konz.	PWM dil.
F.T.	Breast	3x 20 mg	2107	6001[a]	1175	2922	n.t.	8412	11648
		+ Chemoth.	509	21129[b]	16312	21476		650	2529
P.E.	Breast	4x 20 mg	915	3926	2021	73741	23100	9109	1651
			467	118197	68982	69862	53572	10495	74906
P.M.	Melanoma	5x 20 mg	836	13610	6520	6024	4432	26941	50884
			1998	32582	n.t.	13712	6987	85127	10136
H.Th.	Lung Ca.	3x100 mg	1830	10241	n.t.	n.t.	n.t.	291	n.t.
			14377	111041	56612			16506	16067
P.E.	Breast	4x100 mg	962	87316	32477	n.t.	n.t.	23209	19107
			4087	89254	n.t.	36473	8509	89271	14951
S.A.	Breast	1x 80 mg	1608	2533	9764	33723	33345	27137	81723
		11x100 mg	833	35147	30440	37751	23871	56994	115168
O.W.	Seminoma	12x100 mg	736	194	8181	n.t.	223	n.t.	158
			1015	895	n.t.	449	2317	4431	8398
W.H.	Melanoma	12x100 mg	1016	509	14527	37203	37143	37298	39344
			985	35720	13728	59025	37619	24450	52025
T.K.	Seminoma	12x100 mg	510	63302	18326	35284	46722	34557	65121
		+Chemoth.	1283	85002	21985	36368	42442	4798	n.t.

*   mean counts of unstimulated cultures (cpm)

a b   mean counts of replicates of test cultures before (a) and after (b) administration
      of the drug

n.t. non tested

Lymphocyte blastogenesis response to mitogens was investigated in these patients before injection of the drug and also at the end of therapy. If one compares the first results, before any therapy with those 1 week after withdrawal of BM 06 002, PHA responsiveness was increased more than 50% in six patients with concentrated PHA and in three patients with diluted mitogen (Table 8). Con A response increased in three patients with konz., and in two patients with diluted mitogen. Lymphocyte blastogenesis response to PWM (konz.) was stimulated in four cases and depressed in two. An increased response to the diluted PWM was observed with the lymphocytes of three patients; a decrease, in three patients.

There is no clear-cut evidence that any of the total doses used is more effective than the others for immunostimulation.

DISCUSSION

The main purpose of this investigation was to fulfill all the requirements of a phase I study for an immunotherapeutic agent. This should include the estimation of the maximal tolerable dose, a study of acute and long-term toxicity, and also investigations of the influence of this drug on immunological parameters.

Acute toxicity was studied in 15 patients and found to be very rare, as in four cases only, mild side effects were observed that disappeared very soon. The absence of any negative effect on laboratory parameters is also very striking in the acute and long-term toxicity investigations. Higher doses up to 1,200 mg are well tolerated and without negative effects on the investigated parameters.

Immunological investigations in patients having received one or several doses of BM 06 002 have clearly demonstrated that this drug has a pronounced influence on cell-mediated immune reactions. In this present study an increase in skin test reactivity to primary and recall antigens has been observed in more than 50% of the treated patients. Besides this immunopotentiating effect, BM 06 002 seems to restore immune function as demonstrated by conversion of DNCB test reaction from negative to positive. This effect on the immune system has been shown in lymphocyte blastogenesis response to PHA, Con A, and PWM as well as in an increase of reactivity after injection of the drug in more than 50% of the patients. Besides these effects of BM 06 002 on the immune system, the clinical outcome of the patients can be considered favorable. In one patient with multiple bone metastases, no progression was observed after the initiation of therapy, although there was a very short history of the appearance of metastatic deposits (P.E., breast cancer), and one melanoma patient had a complete remission of pulmonary metastases (W.H.).

According to the results obtained in this present phase I study, BM 06 002 can be applied without risks to patients. Due to the striking influence of this drug on the immune system, further investigations should be performed for exact dosage and timing for maximal immune stimulation and clinical effectiveness.

SUMMARY

The new synthetic substance BM 06 002 has been investigated in a phase I study in 24 patients with advanced cancer. No toxic side effects have been observed by single or multiple drug applications. BM 06 002 seems, as found in this study, to potentiate cell-mediated immunity and to restore immune function after immunosuppressive therapy in cancer patients.

REFERENCES

1. Amery, W. K. (1975): Study Group for Bronchogenic Carcinoma: Immunopotentiation with levamisole in resectable bronchogenic carcinoma: A double blind trial. *Br. Med. J.*, 3:461–464.
2. Bicker, U. (1975): N-(2-cyanethylene-)urea, an asparagine analogous cytostatic compound. *Exp. Pathol. Jena*, 10:106–108.
3. Bicker, U. (1978): BM 06 002 a new immunostimulating compound *(this volume)*.
4. Bøyum, A. (1974): Separation of blood leukocytes, granulocytes and lymphocytes. *Tissue Antigens*, 4:269–274.
5. Catalona, W. J., Sample, W. F., and Chretien, P. B. (1973): Lymphocyte reactivity in cancer patients: Correlation with tumor histology and clinical stage. *Cancer*, 31:65–71.
6. Currie, G., Lejeune, F., and Hamilton Fairley, G. (1971): Immunisation with irradiated tumor cells in malignant melanoma. *Br. Med. J.*, 11:305–310.
7. Eilber, F. R., and Morton, D. L. (1970): Impaired immunologic reactivity and recurrence following cancer surgery. *Cancer*, 25:362–367.
8. Gutterman, J. V., Mavligit, G. M., and McBride, C. M. (1973): Active immunotherapy with BCG for recurrent melanoma. *Lancet*, 1:1208–1210.
9. Hersh, E. M., Whitcar, J. P., McCredie, K. B., Bodie, G. P., and Freireich, E. J. (1971):

Chemotherapy, immunocompetence, immunosuppression and prognosis in acute leukemia. *N. Engl. J. Med.,* 285:1211–1213.

10. Israel, L. (1975): Report on 414 cases of human tumors treated with corynebacteria. In: *Corynebacterium parvum,* edited by B. Halpern, pp. 389–401. Plenum Press, N.Y.

11. Manthé, G., Kamel, M., and Dezfulian, M. (1973): An experimental screening for systemic adjuvants of immunity applicable in cancer immunotherapy. *Cancer Res.,* 33:1987–1997.

12. Micksche, M., Cerni, C., Kokron, O., Titscher, R., and Wrba, H. (1977): Vitamin A, a new approach for treatment of bronchogenic cancer. *Cancer Chemotherapy Part 9 (in press).*

13. Micksche, M., Cerni, C., Kokoschka, E. M., and Wrba, H. (1975): Immunotherapy of human melanoma with autologous tumor specific antigens and/or BCG: Characterization of the antigens and immunological follow up of the patients. *Exc. Med. Intern.,* Congr. Series No. 375:337–345.

14. Micksche, M., Kokoschka, E. M., Kokron, O., and Tatra, G. (1976): Phytohaemagglutinin skin test in cancer patients. *ICRS Med. Sci.,* 4:26.

15. Morton, D. L., Eilber, F. R., Holmes, E. C., Hunt, J. S., Ketcham, M. D., Silverstein, M. J., and Sparks, F. C. (1974): BCG immunotherapy of malignant melanoma: Summary of seven years' experience. *Ann. Surg.,* 180:635–643.

16. Tripodi, D., Parks, L. C., and Brugmans, J. (1973): Drug-induced restoration of cutaneous hypersensitivity in anergic patients with cancer. *N. Engl. J. Med.,* 289:354–357.

17. Wanebo, H. J. et al.: Influence of poly(A) · poly (U) on immune response in cancer patients. *Ann. NY Acad. Sci.,* 277:288–298.

Immune Modulation and Control of Neoplasia by Adjuvant Therapy, edited by M. A. Chirigos. Raven Press, New York, 1978.

Immunopotentiation Against the L1210 Leukemia by Pyran Copolymer and Crude Tumor Antigen

Stephen J. Mohr and *Michael A. Chirigos

*Division of Urology, University of Colorado Medical Center, Denver, Colorado, 80220; and *Laboratory of RNA Tumor Viruses, National Cancer Institute, National Institutes of Health, Bethesda, Maryland, 20014*

Pyran copolymer, NSC-46015, is the polyanionic copolymer of maleic acid and divinyl ether. It has been studied for its stability to induce interferon (4), inhibit oncogenic viral replication (2), and activate macrophage-mediated cellular immunity (3,8). Because of these properties, pyran has been tested as a possible antitumor agent but has shown little activity by itself (9). However, when combined with cytoreductive chemotherapy, pyran has been found to be an effective adjuvant to antitumor therapy (6). This adjuvant activity was partially explained by the finding that pyran could strongly and specifically potentiate the antitumor immunity induced by suboptimal vaccination with radiated tumor cells (5,7). These studies revealed that this potentiating activity (a) was dependent on both pyran and tumor vaccine dose, (b) was optimal when the two treatments were given simultaneously by the intraperitoneal route, (c) was related to the molecular weight of the pyran, and (d) was specific in producing immunity only to tumor challenge by the same cell type used for vaccination.

This report confirms these earlier observations, and answers some important questions regarding this phenomenon. We herein show that the immunopotentiating property of pyran in the L1210 system is shared with glucan and Bacillus Calmette-Guérin (BCG) and that several newly synthesized preparations of divinyl ether-maleic anhydride are also active. In addition, it is demonstrated that the protection induced by pyran and tumor vaccine is effective against other routes of challenge besides the intraperitoneal one. The protection is evident as early as 24 hr following treatment and operates in syngeneic as well as hemisyngeneic murine systems against a wide range of tumor challenge doses. The therapeutic effect of pyran and vaccine against established tumor is also presented, both alone and in combination with chemotherapy. The significance of these additional findings, their application to oncology, and further areas of research are briefly discussed.

MATERIALS AND METHODS

Mice: Adult, male B6D2F1, DBA/2, and CD2F1 mice were supplied by the Mammalian Genetics and Animal Production Section, Drug Research and Development, National Cancer Institute, National Institutes of Health, Bethesda, Md. Animals were fed Purina laboratory chow and water *ad libitum* and weighed an average of 25 g at 6 to 8 weeks of age when used experimentally.

Drugs: Pyran copolymer, NSC-46015, and other preparations of divinyl ether-maleic anhydride were obtained from the Hercules Research Center, Wilmington, Del. from David Breslow. The pyrans were dissolved in sterile physiologic saline, and the pH was titrated to 7.0 with 0.1 N NaOH. BCG and *Corynebacterium parvum* were provided by Sotiros Chaparas of the Bureau of Biologics, Bethesda, Md. Polyriboinosinic acid [poly (I)], polyribocytidylic acid [poly (C)], and polyriboxanthylic acid [poly (X)] were purchased from the P-L Biochemical Co., Milwaukee, Wis., and had S20, W values greater than 9.0. Dextran sulfate (MW 20,000) and heparin (beef lung) were purchased from the Sigma Chemical Co., St. Louis, Mo. Glucan was kindly provided by Nicholas Di Luzio, Tulane University, New Orleans, La. All drugs were dissolved in sterile physiologic saline and given on a milligram-per-kilogram basis in an injection volume equal to 1.0% of the animal's body weight.

Tumor: The L1210 murine leukemia has been carried in our laboratory in the transplantable ascites form for over 100 generations in DBA/2 mice. Viability was determined by trypan blue exclusion and cells were diluted in Eagle's minimal essential medium (MEM).

Vaccine Preparation and Administration: L1210 tumor cells, 5.0×10^7 cells/ml in Eagle's MEM, were inactivated by exposure to 5,000 rads X-radiation and control animals were routinely injected with vaccine to confirm complete tumor cell inactivation. Vaccination involved the inoculation of 10^7 radiated cells and when given in conjunction with pyran copolymer or other drug, the vaccine was given approximately 30 min prior to the drug. If they were given mixed, equal amounts of drug and vaccine were physically mixed and incubated at room temperature for 30 min before inoculation.

RESULTS

Titration of L1210 Challenge Dose: Previous experiments involving the potentiation of suboptimal vaccination with radiated L1210 tumor cells by concomitant administration of pyran copolymer utilized a subsequent challenge dose of 10^4 live L1210 cells, intraperitoneally, 1 week later. To evaluate the level of resistance generated by this treatment, two different mouse strains [B6D2F1 (H-2b/d) and CD2F1 (H-2d)] were immunized in the usual fashion and challenged with varying doses of tumor cells (Table 1). The CD2F1 mice were rendered more resistant to all challenge doses than the B6D2F1 mice. There was no relationship between the number of challenge survivors and the challenge dose given. All

TABLE 1. *Effect of challenge dose on potentiation of L1210 vaccine by pyran copolymer*

L1210 challenge[a] (no. cells/mouse)	Survivors/total[b]	
	$B_6D_2F_1$ mice	CD_2F_1 mice
10^2	12/15	19/20
10^3	4/14	20/20
10^4	6/15	18/19
10^5	5/15	19/20
10^6	8/15	19/20

[a] All animals challenged on day 0 with indicated numbers of live L1210 cells, i.p.

[b] Groups scored for survival on day 70 after challenge. There were no survivors in any control groups receiving the different doses of L1210 challenge above *(not shown)*. Test groups *(shown)* received pyran 25 mg/kg and 10^7 radiated L1210 vaccine cells, i.p., on day 7.

animals that died of leukemia had significantly prolonged survival times compared to controls (not shown in table), and hence, all animals responded to the pyran-vaccine treatment with increased immunity. However, actual long-term survivors correlated with the H-2 type of the mouse rather than with the tumor load given as challenge.

Effect of Host H-2 Type: To further evaluate the effect of the murine H-2 loci on the immunity to L1210 challenge, DBA/2 (H-2d), B6D2F1 (H-2b/d), and CD2F1 (H-2d) mice were compared after pyran-vaccine treatment (Table

TABLE 2. *Effect of mouse strain on potentiation of L1210 vaccine by pyran copolymer*

L1210 vaccine (10^7 cells, i.p., day 7)	Pyran copolymer (25 mg/kg, i.p., day 7)	Survivors/ total[a]	Average survival time[b] (days ± SE)
In DBA/2 mice (H-2[d])			
−	−	0/15	10.0 ± 0.1
+	−	0/14	10.1 ± 0.1
−	+	0/14	10.0 ± 0.1
+	+	4/15	25.1 ± 1.6
In $B_6D_2F_1$ mice (H-2[b/d])			
−	−	0/20	11.8 ± 0.2
+	−	0/20	11.7 ± 0.2
−	+	0/20	12.1 ± 0.2
+	+	10/30	34.1 ± 3.6
In CD_2F_1 mice (H-2[d])			
−	−	0/15	10.3 ± 0.1
+	−	1/15	16.1 ± 0.6
−	+	0/15	11.7 ± 0.1
+	+	18/19	33.0 ± 0.0

[a] Groups scored for survival 70 days after challenge with 10^4 live L1210 cells, i.p.

[b] Calculated from individual days of death of animals dying of systemic leukemia.

2). The hemisyngeneic CD2F1 mice demonstrated the greatest resistance, confirming the results in Table 1, but all three strains responded to immunization. Significantly, the syngeneic DBA/2 mice responded quite well, demonstrating that the immunopotentiation phenomenon is not solely due to stimulation of another immunologic response known as F1 antiparent histoincompatibility (10).

Effect of Route of Challenge: Previous studies regarding pyran's potentiation of L1210 vaccine involved the intraperitoneal route for both immunization and tumor challenge. Table 3 summarizes results of studies utilizing other routes of challenge and immunization. The intraperitoneal injection of pyran and L1210 vaccine significantly protected against subsequent intraperitoneal, intravenous, or subcutaneous tumor challenge routes. In addition, the intravenous route of vaccination partially protected animals challenged intravenously and to a lesser extent intraperitoneally, but no mice were totally resistant to challenge. Hence, the protection afforded by pyran-vaccine treatment appeared to be systemic.

Rapid Appearance of Immunity: In all previous experiments, L1210 challenge was performed 7 days after vaccine and pyran treatment. To determine how rapidly immunity to challenge develops, animals were challenged at different time intervals following immunization (Table 4). Significant immunity, both in terms of complete resistance to challenge and prolonged average survival time, was present as early as 24 hr after pyran-vaccine treatment. Maximal resistance was seen 7 days after immunization, the usual challenge interval posttreatment.

Comparison of Pyran to Other Compounds: Several immunologically active compounds, namely levamisole, poly (I:C), poly (A:U), and tilorone, have been tested against pyran for similar activity and were found ineffective (5). Multiple attempts were made to find other compounds possessing immunopotentiating properties comparable to pyran. In Table 5, BCG was effective while complete Freund's adjuvant (CFA) and *C. parvum* showed no immunopotentiating activity. It should be noted that the vaccine dose was 10^6 cells and not 10^7, which clearly has been shown to be best (7), and therefore fewer animals than usual were totally resistant to L1210 challenge. In Table 6, glucan alone was effective while the polyanions heparin and dextran sulfate, as well as the homopolyribonucleotides poly (I), poly (C), and poly (X), were totally ineffective. Therefore, the ability to strongly potentiate the immunity to live tumor challenge induced by killed tumor cell vaccination was not necessarily shared with compounds possessing similar physical properties to pyran.

In Table 7, the original pyran NSC-46015 was compared to several newly synthesized preparations with a more uniform molecular weight as measured by intrinsic viscosity. All preparations were effective and the two preparations of higher intrinsic viscosity tended to be more active than the two lower ones, similar to a previous study (7). Preparation X18802-32, an older preparation of very high intrinsic viscosity, was the least effective, yet still showed considerable activity. It should not be compared to the new preparations, however, because of the hydrolysis that takes place over many years of storage. Of significance

TABLE 3. Effect of challenge route on potentiation of L1210 vaccine by pyran copolymer in $B_6D_2F_1$ mice

Group no.	L1210 vaccine (10^7 cells, i.p., day 7)	Pyran copolymer (25 mg/kg, i.p., day 7)	Mixed pyran + vaccine[a] (i.p. or i.v., day 7)	L1210 challenge 10^4 cells (i.p., i.v., or s.c. day 0)	S/T[b]	AST[c] days	AST[c] SE
1	−	−	—	i.p.	0/18	11.5	0.2
2	+	−	—	i.p.	0/15	12.7	0.7
3	−	+	—	i.p.	0/15	12.5	0.2
4	+	+	—	i.p.	4/20	30.2	1.9
5	−	−	i.p.	i.p.	7/15	39.9	7.3
6	−	−	i.p.	i.v.	2/25	18.2	2.4
7	−	−	—	i.v.	0/25	8.9	0.1
8	−	−	i.v.	i.v.	0/19	16.5	0.4
9	−	−	i.v.	i.p.	0/23	16.6	0.6
10	−	−	—	s.c.	0/12	14.8	0.4
11	+	−	—	s.c.	0/12	16.5	0.4
12	−	+	—	s.c.	0/12	15.5	0.5
13	+	+	—	s.c.	6/12	22.3	4.0

[a]Pyran (25 mg/kg) and 10^7 radiated L1210 vaccine cells given mixed in total volume of 0.5 ml/mouse.
[b]Group scored for survival 70 days following challenge with live L1210 cells. S/T, survivors/total.
[c]AST, average survival time, average of days of death of those animals dying from systemic leukemia.

TABLE 4. *Effect of time of L1210 challenge on potentiation of L1210 vaccine by pyran copolymer*

Day of L1210 challenge (10^4 cells, i.p.)	Treatment groups[a]			
	Control (S/T AST ± SE)[c]	Pyran (S/T AST ± SE)[b]	Vaccine (S/T AST ± SE)	Pyran & vaccine (S/T AST ± SE)
Day 1	0/12 11.7 ± 0.2	0/12 12.3 ± 0.1	0/12 9.4 ± 0.2	3/20 18.9 ± 0.4
Day 2	0/12 11.4 ± 0.2	0/12 11.6 ± 0.2	0/12 9.1 ± 0.1	4/20 27.7 ± 0.4
Day 5	0/12 11.0 ± 0.2	0/12 12.5 ± 0.2	0/12 9.9 ± 0.2	8/20 34.2 ± 1.2
Day 7	0/12 10.8 ± 0.2	0/12 15.2 ± 0.4	0/12 10.7 ± 0.4	15/20 35.6 ± 1.1
Day 9	0/12 10.5 ± 0.3	0/12 13.0 ± 0.3	0/12 13.5 ± 1.2	14/20 24.2 ± 1.4

[a] Treatment consisted of pyran 25 mg/kg, i.p., on day 0 or 10^7 radiated L1210 vaccine cells, i.p., day 0, or both.

[b] S/T, survivors/total; scored 60 days after L1210 challenge in $B_6D_2F_1$ mice.

[c] AST ± SE, average survival time ± standard error; calculated from individual days of death of those animals dying of systemic leukemia.

TABLE 5. *Comparison of pyran NSC-46015 to biological stimulators*

Stimulator (i.p., day 7)[a]	L1210 vaccine (10^6 cells/mouse, i.p., day 7)	Survivors/ total[b]	Average survival time[c] (days ± SE)
None	—	0/15	9.5 ± 0.3
	+	0/15	11.5 ± 0.6
Pyran (NSC-46015)	—	0/14	12.1 ± 0.4
25 mg/kg	+	2/20	20.6 ± 1.6
BCG	—	1/15	12.4 ± 0.2
(2×10^8/mouse)	+	1/20	22.8 ± 2.0
CFA	—	0/15	9.3 ± 0.1
(0.2 mg/mouse)	+	0/20	10.6 ± 0.3
C. parvum	—	0/15	11.2 ± 0.3
(0.2 mg/mouse)	+	0/20	12.4 ± 0.4

[a] CFA, complete Freund's adjuvant.
[b] Scored 70 days after challenge of $B_6D_2F_1$ mice with 1×10^4 live L1210 cells, i.p.
[c] Calculated from the individual days of death of animals dying from systemic leukemia

is the fact that the new preparations being considered for clinical use were as effective as the old NSC-46015, no longer made, which was a mixture of polymers of varying size.

Effect of Pyran-Vaccine Against Established Tumor: To see if the strong protective effect produced by immunization with pyran and killed tumor antigen could be effective as therapy against established L1210 leukemia, animals were treated

TABLE 6. *Comparison of pyran (NSC-46015) to other biochemical polymers*

Stimulator (i.p., day 7)[a]	L1210 vaccine (10^7 cells/mouse i.p., day 7)	Survivors/ total[b]	Average survival time (days ± SE)[c]	
None	—	0/12	10.8	0.3
	+	0/12	11.2	0.5
Pyran (NSC-46015)	—	0/12	12.2	0.3
25 mg/kg	+	6/11	26.8	6.2
Glucan	—	0/12	11.2	0.2
200 mg/kg	+	9/12	17.0	1.7
Dextran SO_4	—	0/11	11.4	0.3
50 mg/kg	+	0/11	12.6	1.0
Heparin	—	0/11	11.8	0.2
25 mg/kg	+	0/11	12.4	0.5
Poly (I)	—	0/20	14.2	0.2
200 µg/mouse	+	0/20	13.2	0.2
Poly (C)	—	0/20	11.4	0.3
200 µg/mouse	+	0/20	13.6	0.2
Poly (X)	—	0/19	13.4	0.3
200 µg/mouse	+	0/20	14.6	0.2

[a] Poly (I), polyriboinosinic acid; poly (C), polyribocytidylic acid; poly (X), polyriboxanthylic acid.
[b] Scored 70 days after challenge of B_6D_2F, mice with 1×10^4 live L1210 cells, i.p.
[c] Calculated from the individual days of death of animals dying from systemic leukemia

TABLE 7. *Comparison of new pyran of uniform molecular weight against NSC-46015 ($B_6D_2F_1$ mice)*

Pyran preparation (25 mg/kg, i.p., day 7)	Intrinsic viscosity [η]	L1210 vaccine (10^7 cells/mouse, i.p., day 7)	Survivors/ total[a]	Average survival time[b] (days ± SE)	
Control	—	—	0/20	10.9	0.2
Control	—	+	0/20	11.2	0.4
NSC-46015	~0.76	—	0/19	12.0	0.2
NSC-46015	0.76	+	15/20	24.8	1.6
x19910–4	0.201	—	0/20	12.0	0.2
x19910–4	0.201	+	11/20	26.2	2.1
x20439–56	0.305	—	0/20	11.9	0.3
x20439–56	0.305	+	12/20	24.6	2.5
x20439–43	0.460	—	0/20	12.5	0.3
x20439–43	0.460	+	15/20	32.4	4.7
x20439–50	0.757	—	0/20	11.6	0.2
x20439–50	0.757	+	14/20	32.5	4.2
x18802–32	1.580	—	0/20	12.0	0.2
x18802–32	1.580	+	10/19	30.9	3.3

[a] Evaluated 70 days after all groups were challenged with 1.0×10^4 cells, i.p.
[b] Calculated from the individual days of death of animals dying from systemic leukemia.

4 days after inoculation with live L1210 with pyran, vaccine, or both (Fig. 1). No animals were cured, and the average survival times among groups differed little, although the pyran alone and pyran-vaccine groups tended to live longer at all tumor doses. Hence, although pyran is a strong immunopotentiator, it was only weakly therapeutic in this setting. It should be noted that all mice had systemic leukemia by day 4 after live tumor cell inoculation.

Pyran-Vaccine as Adjuvant to Chemotherapy of L1210: Pyran has already

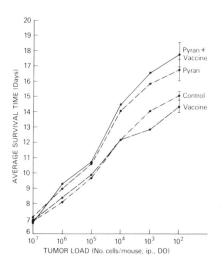

FIG. 1. Effect of pyran and vaccine against established L1210 leukemia. $B_6D_2F_1$ mice were injected intraperitoneally on day 0 with varying doses of live L1210 tumor cells. On day 4, following tumor inoculation, pyran, 25 mg/kg, L1210 tumor vaccine, 10^7 radiated cells/mouse, or both, were given intraperitoneally to the mice. The average survival times of the various groups are shown on the ordinate. The standard error of the mean for the average survival times at the 10^2 tumor cell inoculum is shown by the brackets.

TABLE 8. *Pyran potentiation of response of L1210 leukemia to cyclophosphamide chemotherapy*

L1210 (10⁴ cells, i.p., day 0)	Cyclophosphamide (200 mg/kg, i.p., day 6)	L1210 vaccine (10⁷ cells, i.p., day 9)	Pyran copolymer (25 mg/kg, i.p., day 9)	Average survival time (days ± SE)[a]
+	−	−	−	11.1 ± 0.2
+	+	−	−	16.9 ± 0.2
+	+	+	−	16.3 ± 0.4
+	+	+	+	21.9 ± 0.5
+	+	−	+	21.7 ± 0.6

[a]There were 15 animals per group and no long-term survivors.

been shown to be an effective adjuvant to chemotherapy of an established leukemia (6). The effect of the addition of tumor antigen to pyran adjuvant therapy following cytoreductive chemotherapy of established L1210 is shown in Table 8. There were no long-term survivors in this study. Chemotherapy significantly prolonged the average survival time by 5.8 days. Pyran-vaccine treatment given 3 days after the chemotherapy increased the survival time by another 25%. Pyran alone also produced the same effect if given without the tumor antigen. This study then confirms the previously demonstrated adjuvant effect of pyran to chemotherapy of established tumor. The chemotherapy serves two purposes: (a) cytoreduction and (b) production of inactivated tumor antigen for interaction with pyran. The addition of further killed antigen in the form of vaccine is unnecessary if chemotherapy is used.

DISCUSSION

This report extends the earlier observation that pyran can strongly and specifically potentiate antitumor immunity stimulated by vaccination with radiated tumor cells. Whereas initial experiments described the requirements for immunopotentiation to occur, this study examines the limits of the immunity generated by combined pyran and tumor antigen treatment. The results in Table 1 show that this immunity was strong enough to resist a wide range of tumor challenge doses. However, the challenge dose had little effect on the number of survivors, which seemed to be determined more by the H-2 type of the mouse strain used. Possibly, higher challenge doses would demonstrate the expected dose-response result. The data seem to indicate that the effect of pyran and vaccine was an all-or-nothing phenomenon, but this was not the case since the animals that died of the challenge dose had a significantly prolonged survival time (not shown in the results). Therefore, all the animals exhibited some degree of immunity.

The relationship of immunity to H-2 type was examined in Table 2, and the results obtained in DBA/2 mice confirm our initial impression that the immunopotentiating effect of pyran is directed primarily against the tumor-specific transplant antigens (TSTA) rather than histocompatibility antigens, however minor they might be. If pyran is to be useful in a clinical setting, it must stimulate immunity to autologous tumor cells and their antigens. The excellent response of the CD2F1 mice to treatment may reflect a more immunocompetent mouse strain or an additional F1 antiparent histoincompatibility response. Further work in this area is necessary to establish the actual role of H-2 in the response to pyran, but we have preliminary *in vitro* results that indicate that pyran can indeed stimulate the F1 antiparent response *(unpublished results).*

A further requirement for the usefulness of the immunity generated by pyran is that it be systemic. Previously reported experiments utilized the intraperitoneal compartment, but results in Table 3 show that the immunity was systemic in that intraperitoneal immunization could protect against subcutaneous and intravenous tumor challenges. In addition, immunity could be produced by the intravenous route of vaccination, in contrast to similar studies using BCG or *C. parvum* (1,11).

Within 24 hr of pyran-L1210 vaccine treatment, significant immunity to L1210 challenge could be detected (Table 4). This finding is in contrast to earlier reports that pyran causes an early depression of phagocytosis with an absence of macrophage activity for 3 days (3). Although we have not as yet shown that the vaccine potentiation phenomenon is related to macrophage stimulation, early *in vitro* results in our lab indicate that the macrophage plays a central role in the response *(unpublished results).* The surprisingly rapid appearance of immunity implies that pyran reduces the normal time course for sensitization.

Similar studies regarding vaccine potentiation have been reported for BCG and *C. parvum* (1,11). We could duplicate the activity of BCG in our system but not *C. parvum* (Table 5). Possibly, the *C. parvum* should have been given subcutaneously as was done in the prior study. Both of these drugs are known macrophage stimulators and we found that another macrophage stimulator, glucan, was also quite active as an immunopotentiator (Table 6). Thus, it seems that the combination of a strong stimulator of the reticuloendothelial system and killed tumor antigen causes the appearance of strong, specific antitumor immunity, provided the host is immunocompetent.

This strong antitumor immunity was not observed in the presence of an actively growing tumor (Fig. 1), implying that the immunoresponsiveness of the host animal was impaired. It is well known that actively growing tumor can be immunosuppressive to the host, but with the addition of chemotherapy the suppressive effect may be temporarily halted, while at the same time producing killed antigen to interact with the pyran (Table 8). In a clinical setting, the same principle should be followed in that combinations of surgery, chemotherapy, and radiation should be used to reduce the tumor burden as much as possible before attempts at immunostimulation are made. The use of these kinds of agents in terminal patients is bound to be unsuccessful because of the overwhelming immunosuppression caused by uncontrolled tumor growth. In addition, inactivated antigen should be made available for compounds like pyran to be effective. We recognize, of course, that conventional antitumor therapy is immunosuppressive itself.

Although the strong activity of pyran in modulating host immunity has been well established in the foregoing studies, the mechanism of action is poorly understood. We have been engaged in studies designed to isolate the responding components of the immune system when stimulated by pyran and tumor antigen. The peritoneal macrophage seems to be most important so far, but this may reflect the inadequacy of *in vitro* testing for cellular and humoral immunity. The L1210 model allows testing of various antigen extracts from the intact tumor cells for their ability to replace the killed tumor cell vaccine. If the specific antigens that interact with pyran to produce immunity could be extracted, the pyran-vaccine treatment could be applied to a wide variety of tumors. Further insight regarding pyran's mechanism of action may be found in results soon to be published from our lab indicating that pyran is capable of interacting with isolated cellular nuclei to stimulate DNA synthesis *(unpublished results)*. Certainly, the L1210 model system warrants further study because it may provide clues to a manner by which host immune defenses may eventually be directed against established autologous tumor, eradicating it and producing cures rather than remissions. It was reassuring to find that the newly synthesized pyran compounds were equally effective as the old NSC-46015, which has limited availability (Table 7). These newer, more uniform, molecular weight compounds should provide other investigators with the opportunity to study pyran's immune effects both on *in vitro* and *in vivo* levels and in clinical and nonclinical settings.

SUMMARY

Using a L1210 tumor vaccine model, pyran copolymer (NSC-46015) has been shown to be a strong stimulator of antitumor immunity. In this report, initial observations regarding pyran's immunopotentiation of vaccine have been extended to show: (a) animals were protected against intravenous and subcutaneous tumor challenge routes as well as intraperitoneal; (b) protection was apparent in syngeneic as well as hemisyngeneic host-tumor systems; (c) immunity was present within 24 hr of combined pyran-L1210 vaccination; (d) this immunity was capable of protecting against a wide range of tumor challenge doses; and (e) this potentiating property was not limited to pyran alone but was seen with other immunoadjuvants such as BCG and glucan and also with all of the newly synthesized preparations of divinyl ether-maleic anhydride. In addition, pyran and vaccine were used in trial studies as therapy against established L1210 tumor. These preliminary studies were encouraging, but showed a marked reduction in beneficial activity when pyran and vaccine were used therapeutically as opposed to prophylactically against the L1210 leukemia.

REFERENCES

1. Hawrylko, E. (1975): Immunopotentiation with BCG: Dimensions of a specific antitumor response. *J. Natl. Cancer Inst.,* 54:1189–1197.
2. Hirsch, M. S., Black, P. H., Wood, M. L., and Monaco, A. P. (1972): Effects of pyran copolymer on oncogenic virus infections in immunosuppressed hosts. *J. Immunol.,* 108:1312–1318.
3. Kaplan, A. M., Morahan, P. S., and Regelson, W. (1974): Induction of macrophage-mediated tumor-cell cytotoxicity by pyran copolymer. *J. Natl. Cancer Inst.,* 52:1919–1923.
4. Merigan, T. C. (1967): Induction of circulating interferon by synthetic anionic polymers of known composition. *Nature,* 214:416–417.
5. Mohr, S. J., and Chirigos, M. A. (1977): Potentiation of a tumor cell vaccine by pyran copolymer. In: *Control of Neoplasia by Modulation of the Immune System (Progress in Cancer Research and Therapy, Vol. 2),* edited by M. A. Chirigos, pp. 421–435. Raven Press, New York.
6. Mohr, S. J., Chirigos, M. A., Fuhrman, F. S., and Pryor, J. W. (1975): Pyran copolymer found to be an effective adjuvant to chemotherapy against a murine leukemia and solid tumor. *Cancer Res.,* 35:3750–3754.
7. Mohr, S. J., Chirigos, M. A., Smith, G. T., and Fuhrman, F. S. (1976): Specific potentiation of L1210 vaccine by pyran copolymer. *Cancer Res.,* 36:2035–2039.
8. Morahan, P. S., and Kaplan, A. M. (1976): Macrophage activation and antitumor activity of biologic and synthetic agents. *Int. J. Cancer,* 17:82–89.
9. Morahan, P. S., Munson, J. A., Baird, L. G., Kaplan, A. M., and Regelson, W. (1974): Antitumor action of pyran copolymer and tilorone against Lewis lung carcinoma and B-16 melanoma. *Cancer Res.,* 34:506–511.
10. Shearer, G. M., and Cudkowicz, G. (1975): Induction of F1 hybrid antiparent cytotoxic effector cells: An *in vitro* model for hemopoietic histoincompatibility. *Science,* 190:890–893.
11. Scott, M. T. (1975): Potentiation of the tumor-specific immune response by *Corynebacterium parvum. J. Natl. Cancer Inst.,* 55:65–72.

Immune Modulation and Control of Neoplasia by Adjuvant Therapy, edited by M. A. Chirigos. Raven Press, New York, 1978.

Effect of Dose, Route, and Timing of Pyran Copolymer Therapy Against the Madison Lung Carcinoma

Joseph D. Papamatheakis, Michael A. Chirigos, and Richard M. Schultz

Lab of RNA Tumor Viruses, National Cancer Institute, National Institutes of Health, Bethesda, Maryland 20014

Nonspecific macrophage stimulants such as pyran copolymer appear to be valuable adjuncts to conventional means of treating neoplastic disease. We have shown that pyran enhances host resistance against the Madison lung carcinoma (M109) (12). Pyran therapy resulted in: (a) enhanced macrophage inhibition of M109 DNA synthesis, (b) heavy accumulation and infiltration of histiocytes and macrophages at the tumor site, and (c) the *in vivo* association of macrophages with degenerate-appearing tumor cells. Although pyran copolymer has been shown to be an effective adjuvant in treating various other murine solid tumors (3,5–8,10,15), no in-depth studies have been conducted to determine the most effective regimen of pyran treatment. This chapter deals with the effect of timing, route, and dose of pyran on survival of BALB/c mice bearing the syngeneic M109 lung carcinoma. Furthermore, intraperitoneal pyran treatment is shown to retard the growth of artificially induced pulmonary metastases.

MATERIALS AND METHODS

Mice

Male BALB/c mice, 6 to 8 weeks old, were furnished by the Mammalian Genetics and Animal Production Section, Drug Research and Development, National Institutes of Health, Bethesda, Md. All animals weighed at least 23 g before they were used for experimentation.

Pyran Copolymer

Pyran (NSC-46015) was kindly supplied by David Breslow of Hercules Research Center, Wilmington, Del. Pyran was dissolved in 0.9% NaCl solution, adjusted to pH 7.0 by the addition of 1 N NaOH, and given i.p. at 1% body weight.

Tumor Testing

The Madison lung carcinoma (M109), a transplantable line derived from a spontaneous neoplasm in a BALB/c mouse, was kindly supplied by Ruth I. Geran, Drug Research and Development, National Cancer Institute, NIH, in its 110th passage generation. The line was subsequently adapted to tissue culture (14). For adjuvant studies, 5×10^5 viable M109 cells, suspended in serum-free RPMI-1640, were injected subcutaneously into the right inguinal region of each mouse. Deaths of mice were recorded daily, and mean survival times were calculated. The percentage increase in life-span of test groups (T) over control groups (C) inoculated with tumor alone was calculated by $(T/C-1) \times 100$. The mean survivals of pyran-treated groups in comparison to those of groups receiving 0.9% NaCl solution were evaluated statistically by Student's t-test.

Inhibition of Artificially Induced Lung Metastases

M109 cells grown *in vitro* were harvested during their exponential growth phase by gentle trypsinization, washed twice, and resuspended in serum-free RPMI-1640. The number of single viable cells was determined and adjusted to 5×10^5 cells/ml medium. Tumor cells were injected intravenously into the tail vein of normal BALB/c mice. Inoculum volume per mouse was 0.2 ml (10^5 cells). After 24 hr, the mice were randomly divided into two cages and injected intraperitoneally with either 0.9% NaCl solution or pyran copolymer at 25 mg/kg. The mice were sacrificed on day 15, and the number of pulmonary metastases was determined by inflation with India ink according to the method of Wexler (16).

RESULTS

Effects of Timing and Frequency of Pyran Treatment on Antitumor Activity

Pyran copolymer at 25 mg/kg significantly prolonged the mean survival time in all treated groups of mice bearing the M109 lung carcinoma (Table 1). A minimum increase in life-span of 41% over 0.9% NaCl solution-treated controls was achieved regardless of the time of treatment initiation or whether a single or multiple treatment regimen was employed. A single treatment late in the course of disease (day 14) was the least effective therapeutic regimen at increasing life-span ($p < 0.02$), whereas all other schedules were highly significant ($p < 0.001$). Multiple treatments were not statistically better than single treatments. Since pyran therapy at day 7 produced the best antitumor response of the single treatment groups, this timing was chosen to determine the most efficacious dose and route of pyran therapy.

TABLE 1. *Effect of single versus multiple treatments of pyran against the M109 lung carcinoma*

Days of pyran treatment (25 mg/kg/day, i.p.)	Mean survival time ± SE[a] (days)	% Increase in life-span
1. —	28.1 ± 1.73	—
2. D-3	41.2 ± 0.92**[c]	47
3. D0	43.6 ± 3.18**	55
4. D7	45.8 ± 3.09**	63
5. D14	39.7 ± 3.28*	41
6. D0(q7d × 5)[b]	53.4 ± 4.13**	90
7. D7(q7d × 4)	49.0 ± 3.02**	74
8. D14(q7d × 3)	46.6 ± 3.00**	66
9. D0(q3d × 9)	47.6 ± 3.91**	69
10. D7(q3d × 7)	45.2 ± 2.25**	61
11. D14(q3d × 5)	49.1 ± 3.90**	75

[a] 5×10^5 tumor cells were inoculated s.c. into BALB/c mice on day 0.

[b] q7d, every 7th day; q3d, every 3rd day. D, day.

[c] Probabilities that the differences are statistically different from placebo-tested controls are indicated thus: $* = p < 0.02$; $** = p < 0.001$.

Effect of Dose of Pyran Administration

To test the dose-dependency of pyran treatment, BALB/c mice were inoculated intraperitoneally with pyran at doses ranging from 100 to 0.1 mg/kg on day 7 after M109 tumor implantation. These drug doses caused no lethality. Although there was some tendency for a biphasic curve of antitumor activity (Fig. 1), significant increases in life-span were afforded over a 100-fold range of concentrations (1 to 100 mg/kg).

Effect of Route of Pyran Administration

A large group of mice were inoculated on day 0 with 5×10^5 M109 cells as previously described. On day 7, specific groups of 10 mice each were inoculated with 25 mg/kg of pyran by the subcutaneous, oral, intralesional, intravenous, or intraperitoneal routes. Systemic (intraperitoneal or intravenous) routes were

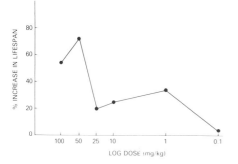

FIG. 1. Dose-response of pyran therapy against the M109 murine carcinoma. Mice were inoculated subcutaneously with 5×10^5 M109 cells. Groups of 10 mice each were given varying doses of pyran intraperitoneally on day 7 after tumor inoculation. Percentage increase in life-span was calculated by comparing mean survival times of pyran-treated mice with those receiving 0.9% NaCl solution.

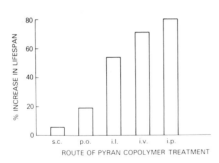

FIG. 2. Route-dependency of pyran administration against the M109 lung carcinoma. Mice were inoculated subcutaneously on day 0 with 5×10^5 M109 cells. Groups of 10 mice each received pyran at 25 mg/kg either by the subcutaneous (s.c.), oral (p.o.), intralesional (i.l.), intravenous (i.v.), or intraperitoneal (i.p.) route. The subcutaneous drug inoculation was given contralateral to the tumor site. Percentage increase in lifespan was calculated by comparing mean survival times of pyran-treated mice with those of mice receiving 0.9% NaCl solution.

TABLE 2. *Inhibition of artificially induced lung metastases of M109 lung carcinoma in BALB/c mice*

Drug treatment day 1	Mean no. lesions/lung[a]		T/T[b]
	Experiment #1	Experiment #2	
Saline	15.0, $N = 10$	18.2, $N = 5$	15/15
Pyran copolymer at 25 mg/kg	0.7, $N = 10$	0.4, $N = 5$	5/15

[a] One $\times 10^5$ M109 cells were injected intravenously on day 0. Lung lesions were identified on day 15 by inflation with India ink.

[b] T/T, mice with lung tumors/total number of mice.

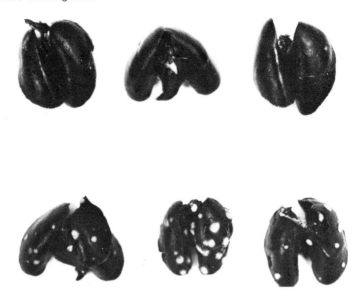

FIG. 3. Influence of pyran copolymer treatment on artificially induced M109 metastases. Mice were given 1×10^5 M109 cells intravenously on day 0 and inoculated with pyran or placebo intraperitoneally on day 1. The upper figure shows India ink-inflated lungs from pyran-treated animals. The lungs are free of identifiable tumor nodules at day 15. In contrast, the lower figure shows lungs from 0.9% NaCl solution-treated mice. Numerous tumor lesions are visualized by India ink treatment.

the most effective at increasing life-span (Fig. 2). Intralesional treatment was also capable of increasing survival time, whereas subcutaneous and oral therapy were without significant effect.

Effect of Pyran on Artificially Induced Pulmonary Metastasis

Pyran therapy has previously been shown to induce a histiocytic reaction at the primary tumor site and to inhibit tumor infiltration and growth (12). To determine if pyran were similarly effective against pulmonary metastases, pyran or 0.9% NaCl solution was administered intraperitoneally 24 hr after intravenous tumor inoculation. Mice were sacrificed on day 15, and lungs were inflated with India ink in order to visualize tumor nodules. Pyran strikingly reduced the number of pulmonary lesions in two separate experiments (Table 2). These lesions were identified histologically as the M109 carcinoma. In contrast to multiple tumors in the lungs of placebo-treated mice, many lungs from pyran-treated mice remained tumor free at day 15 (Fig. 3).

DISCUSSION

Pyran copolymer was used in several time courses and doses to test the ability of the drug to enhance host resistance against a transplantable, poorly differentiated lung carcinoma. Prolonged survival was accomplished (41 to 90% increase in life-span) regardless of the time of treatment initiation or whether a single or multiple treatment regimen was used. It appears that pyran toxicity can be minimized while retaining good activity since single treatments were as effective as multiple treatments and since pyran was active over a large range of doses (1 to 100 mg/kg). In addition, the route of pyran administration was not a severe limitation, since intraperitoneal, intravenous, and intralesional inoculations at 25 mg/kg were all effective.

Nonspecific potentiation of macrophage function appears to be a very promising approach in the treatment of malignant disease. Activated macrophages are able to discriminate and selectively destroy cells with abnormal growth properties (4). We have recently demonstrated the correlation that exists between agents having the ability to enhance host resistance against neoplasia and the capacity to induce macrophage-mediated cytotoxicity (13). Of the chemicals tested, pyran was the most active at producing tumoricidal macrophages. Although pyran therapy markedly enhanced host resistance against the syngeneic M109 carcinoma, pyran was not directly toxic for M109 cells *in vitro* (12). Suppression of tumor growth resulted via a histiocytic reaction at the tumor site.

The presence of large numbers of histiocytes in several untreated animal tumors has been associated with tumor rejection and the lessened likelihood of metastasis (1). Hanna et al. (2) showed that induction of a histiocytic granuloma with Bacillus Calmette-Guerin (BCG) at the tumor site was required for the rejection of a transplantable hepatocarcinoma in guinea pigs. Intimate contact between macrophage and target cell was a requirement for tumor cell destruction. The major limitation of the macrophage effector arm of the immune response appears to be cell concentration at the primary or disseminated tumor site. It is tempting to compare pyran copolymer with BCG, since pyran therapy provoked a marked histiocytic reaction around the subcutaneously transplanted M109 lung carcinoma in BALB/c mice (12) and since both agents activate macrophages *in vivo* (13). However, there was no granuloma development as would be seen with BCG. Pyran appears to have several distinct advantages over BCG. Macrophage activation by BCG requires functional T cells (9), whereas activation by pyran is direct (11) and does not require an immunocompetent host. Moreover, BCG requires intralesional therapy to produce a migration of histiocytes into the tumor (2), whereas intraperitoneal pyran treatment produces histiocytosis at the subcutaneous tumor site (12,15).

Pyran therapy also strikingly reduced the number of pulmonary lesions that developed after the intravenous inoculation of M109 tumor cells. Snodgrass et al. (15) have shown that a small number of macrophages, presumably of hematogenous origin, accumulated in the pulmonary interstitium of pyran-treated animals. There were regions where macrophage accumulations formed nodules that disrupted much of the normal architecture. It is tempting to speculate that these pyran-activated macrophages have a surveillance function in inhibiting or controlling metastatic cell growth.

Pyran deserves further study as an adjuvant to conventional treatment modalities in treating cancer. Pyran was effective in modulating host immunological factors even in an advanced tumor system (12). Pyran has been shown to produce a high number of "cures" against the Lewis lung carcinoma and LSTRA leukemia when combined with remission-inducing chemotherapy (6). It appears that pyran's toxicity can be minimized while retaining good antitumor activity.

SUMMARY

Pyran copolymer (NSC 46015) therapy markedly enhanced BALB/c resistance to a syngeneic M109 lung carcinoma implanted subcutaneously. Multiple dose schedules at 25 mg/kg/day were not significantly better than single doses at increasing life-span. A single intraperitoneal treatment of pyran on day 7 after tumor inoculation was effective over a dose range of 1 to 100 mg/kg. Both systemic and intralesional routes of pyran administration were effective at increasing the survival times of M109 tumor-bearing mice. Using an artificially induced metastasis system, intraperitoneal pyran therapy greatly retarded the development of pulmonary lesions.

REFERENCES

1. Eccles, S. A., and Alexander, P. (1974): Macrophage content of tumors in relation to metastatic spread and host immune reaction. *Nature,* 250:667–669.
2. Hanna, M. G., Zbar, B., and Rapp, H. J. (1972): Histopathology of tumor regression after

intralesional injection of *Mycobacterium bovis*. 1. Tumor growth and metastasis. *J. Natl. Cancer Inst.,* 48:1441–1455.

3. Harmel, R. P., and Zbar, B. (1975): Tumor suppression by pyran copolymer: Correlation with production of cytotoxic macrophages. *J. Natl. Cancer Inst.,* 54:989–992.

4. Hibbs, J. B. (1974): Discrimination between neoplastic and nonneoplastic cells *in vitro* by activated macrophages. *J. Natl. Cancer Inst.,* 53:1487–1492.

5. Kapila, K., Smith, C., and Rubin, A. A. (1971): Effect of pyran copolymer on phagocytosis and tumor growth. *RES J. Reticuloendothel. Soc.,* 9:447–450.

6. Mohr, S. J., Chirigos, M. A., Fuhrman, F. S., and Pryor, J. W. (1975): Pyran copolymer as an effective adjuvant to chemotherapy against a murine leukemia and solid tumor. *Cancer Res.,* 35:3750–3754.

7. Morahan, P. S., and Kaplan, A. M. (1976): Macrophage activation and antitumor activity of biologic and synthetic agents. *Int. J. Cancer,* 17:82–89.

8. Morahan, P. S., Munson, J. A., Baird, L. G., Kaplan, A. M., and Regelson, W. (1974): Antitumor action of pyran copolymer and tilorone against Lewis lung carcinoma and B-16 melanoma. *Cancer Res.,* 34:506–511.

9. North, R. J. (1974): T-cell dependence of macrophage activation and mobilization during infection with *Mycobacterium tuberculosis. Infect. Immun.,* 10:66–71.

10. Sandberg, J., and Goldin, A. (1971): Use of first generation transplants of a slow growing solid tumor for the evaluation of new cancer chemotherapeutic agents. *Cancer Chemother. Rep.,* 55:233–238.

11. Schultz, R. M., Papamatheakis, J. D., and Chirigos, M. A. (1977): Direct activation *in vitro* of mouse peritoneal macrophages by pyran copolymer (NSC 46015). *Cell. Immunol. (in press).*

12. Schultz, R. M., Papamatheakis, J. D., Luetzeler, J., Ruiz, P., and Chirigos, M. A. (1977): Macrophage involvement in the protective effect of pyran copolymer against the Madison lung carcinoma (M109). *Cancer Res.,* 37:358–364.

13. Schultz, R. M., Papamatheakis, J. D., Stylos, W. A., and Chirigos, M. A. (1976): Augmentation of specific macrophage-mediated cytotoxicity: Correlation with agents which enhance antitumor resistance. *Cell. Immunol.,* 25:309–316.

14. Schultz, R. M., Ruiz, P., Chirigos, M. A., Heine, U., and Nelson-Rees, W. (1977): Establishment and characterization of a cell line derived from a spontaneous murine lung carcinoma (M109). *In Vitro (in press).*

15. Snodgrass, M. J., Morahan, P. S., and Kaplan, A. M. (1975): Histopathology of the host response to Lewis lung carcinoma: Modulation by pyran. *J. Natl. Cancer Inst.,* 55:455–462.

16. Wexler, H. (1966): Accurate identification of experimental pulmonary metastases. *J. Natl. Cancer Inst.,* 36:641–645.

Immune Modulation and Control of Neoplasia by Adjuvant Therapy, edited by M. A. Chirigos. Raven Press, New York, 1978.

Immunoregulatory Macrophages from Pyran-Treated Mice

Lynn G. Baird and Alan M. Kaplan

Departments of Microbiology and Surgery, MCV/VCU Cancer Center, Medical College of Virginia, Virginia Commonwealth University, Richmond, Virginia 23298

Recent evidence suggests that macrophages have a regulatory function on both normal and tumor cell proliferation. Macrophages from animals treated with biologic or synthetic immunomodulators have been demonstrated to be selectively cytotoxic or cytostatic, or both, for tumor cells *in vitro,* while demonstrating quantitatively less cytotoxicity for normal cells (5,6,7,11). Macrophages have also been shown to regulate tumor cell (10,19,25) and fibroblast (16) proliferation *in vivo*. In addition, exogenously added macrophages have been shown either to inhibit (2–4,12,22) or to enhance (29,31) lymphocyte proliferation *in vitro* depending on the macrophage-to-lymphocyte ratio in culture (12,31).

Several lines of evidence suggest that macrophages similarly regulate lymphoproliferation *in vivo*. Adherent spleen cells from mice bearing primary Moloney sarcoma virus-induced tumors (13–15), from mice undergoing a graft-versus-host response (28), or from mice treated with *Corynebacterium parvum* (28) have been shown to inhibit the *in vitro* blastogenic response of normal spleen cells to T-cell mitogens. Furthermore, addition of spleen cells from mice subjected to a graft-versus-host reaction to normal spleen cells resulted in a marked inhibition of the antibody response of normal cells to thymic independent and dependent antigens (30). This inhibition was abolished after removal of phagocytic cells from the graft-versus-host spleen cell population (30).

Pyran copolymer is a synthetic immunomodulator shown to stimulate the reticuloendothelial system as evidenced by hepato- and splenomegaly in mice (23,24) and enhanced phagocytic activity measured by vascular clearance of colloidal carbon (20,24). In addition, pyran induces a significant increase in esterase-positive cells in the spleens of mice 5 and 10 days after a single i.v. injection (1). This investigation was undertaken to characterize further the inhibitory effect of pyran treatment on the mitogen-induced blastogenic responses of spleen cells and to determine which cell(s) was responsible for this inhibitory effect.

MATERIALS AND METHODS

Mice

Adult $(C57B1/6 \times DBA/2)F_1$ female mice were used in all experiments. Within a single experiment, mice were matched for age.

Pyran Copolymer

The clinical pyran preparation (NSC 46015), average MW of 23,000, used in these studies was obtained from the Drug Development Branch of the National Cancer Institute. The drug was suspended in saline to 90% of the desired volume. The pH of the solution was adjusted to 7 with 2N NaOH and made up to the desired volume with saline.

Spleen Cell Suspensions

Mice were sacrificed by cervical dislocation and spleens removed. Cell suspensions were prepared by forcing the spleens through 200-mesh stainless steel screens. Cells were washed three times in RPMI 1640, counted, and suspended to the desired concentration.

Peritoneal Exudate Cells

Cells were obtained from the peritoneal cavities of untreated, glycogen-treated, or pyran-treated mice by washing two times with 4 ml of RPMI. Normal peritoneal exudate cells (PEC) were obtained from either untreated mice or mice treated with glycogen (0.5 ml/mouse i.p. of a 2.5% solution, type II from oyster, Sigma G-8751) 5 days previously, a regimen that has been found to increase cell numbers without activating macrophages (18). In the experiments discussed in this report, PEC obtained from either untreated or glycogen-treated mice responded identically and are both referred to here as normal PEC (1,4,12). Activated macrophages are defined as macrophages that are cytotoxic *in vitro* to tumor cells but not to normal cells (11). Activated PEC were obtained from mice given a single injection of 25 mg pyran/kg i.p. 6 to 8 days prior to the experiment. Histologic examination of esterase-stained smears from normal or pyran-treated mice revealed that the peritoneal exudate (PE) from normal mice contained approximately 60% macrophages and 40% small lymphocytes, whereas that from pyran-treated mice contained approximately 70% macrophages and 30% small lymphocytes (1).

Blastogenic Assay

The assay for *in vitro* lymphocyte blastogenesis using ^{3}H-thymidine incorporation into DNA has been described in detail elsewhere (2–4). Briefly, a microtiter assay system was used to measure ^{3}H-thymidine incorporation into DNA after stimulation by mitogens. The T- and B-cell blastogenic responses of spleen cells were determined using phytohemagglutinin (PHA; Burroughs Wellcome) and lipopolysaccharide (LPS; Difco; *Escherichia coli* lipopolysaccharide, 0111:B4), respectively. Cultures were incubated in RPMI 1640 supplemented with 9% fresh frozen human plasma in an atmosphere of 5% CO_2 and 95% air for 48 hr, at which time 2 μCi of ^{3}H-thymidine (Schwarz-Mann, sp. act. 1.9 Ci/mmole) was added and incubation was continued for an additional 24 hr. The cultures were then harvested, and samples were counted in a liquid scintillation counter.

Data were evaluated as either (a) peak response in counts per minute (cpm) or (b) stimulation ratios, SR, where SR = (cpm with mitogen)/(cpm without mitogen).

RESULTS

To determine the effect of *in vivo* administration of pyran on the *in vitro* blastogenic response of T and B lymphocytes, mice were given a single i.v. injection of 25 mg pyran/kg at various time intervals 2 to 14 days before the spleens were assayed *in vitro* for blastogenesis. At all times, but most markedly at day 5, the mitogen-independent incorporation of ^{3}H-thymidine was significantly greater in spleen cells from pyran-treated mice compared to untreated controls (Table 1).

Using peak cpm as a measure of blastogenesis, pyran inhibited T-cell blastogenesis to PHA on days 2, 8, and 14 after *in vivo* administration (2). In contrast, on day 5, cpm in cultures from mice treated with pyran were greater than controls. However, when SR was used as a measure of blastogenesis, pyran caused depression of the response at all time intervals between 2 and 14 days after drug administration.

The specific B-cell blastogenic response of the same spleen cells to LPS, as measured by cpm, was similarly depressed on days 2, 8, and 11, was approxi-

TABLE 1. *Effect of pyran administration on mitogen-independent incorporation*

Day after pyran administration [a]	Mitogen-independent ^{3}H-thymidine incorporation (cpm ± SE)
—	90 ± 14
2	425 ± 64
5	2,269 ± 311
8	545 ± 72
11	332 ± 82
14	284 ± 17

[a] BDF$_1$ injected with 25 mg pyran/kg i.v. at the indicated time prior to removal of spleens.

mately equal to controls on day 5, and increased on day 14 (1). SR were depressed at all time intervals assayed, similar to the results obtained with PHA.

To determine the effect of i.v. administration of pyran on lymph node lymphocyte blastogenesis, mice were injected with 50 mg pyran/kg 3 days prior to the assay. Day 3 was chosen because it had previously been shown to be a time of peak inhibition of spleen cell blastogenesis. Lymph nodes were removed and pooled. Similar to the results obtained using spleen cells, pyran treatment was demonstrated to depress the blastogenic response of lymph node T lymphocytes stimulated with PHA compared to the response of normal cells (Fig. 1A and B).

In contrast to the effects of pyran on the lymph node cell response to PHA, no inhibition of the response to LPS was detected with respect to either cpm or SR *(data not presented)*. It should be noted that the LPS response of normal lymph node lymphocytes was significantly lower than that of normal spleen cells, in contrast to what was seen for the PHA response. This difference reflected the lower percentage of LPS-reactive B cells present in lymph nodes compared to spleens (9).

To determine whether the pyran-induced inhibition of mitogen-induced blastogenesis was related to the dose of pyran administered, mice were injected with i.v. doses of pyran varying between 0.2 and 75 mg/kg. Three different times of pyran administration were investigated—days −2, −5, and −10. These times were chosen from the results of the earlier time course experiments. These experiments had established that the blastogenic response of spleen cells from pyran-treated animals was maximally inhibited at day 2. By 5 days after pyran administration, the spleen cell blastogenic response was enhanced compared to controls, due to the increase in mitogen-independent incorporation. The blastogenic response of spleen cells assayed 10 days after pyran treatment was inhibited

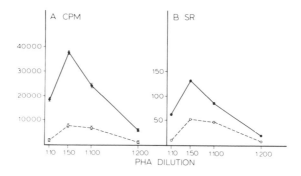

FIG. 1. The effect of pyran administration on lymph node cell blastogenesis as measured by cpm and SR. The blastogenic responses of pooled lymph nodes from untreated and pyran-treated mice were determined. Mice received 50 mg pyran/kg i.v. three days prior to assay; untreated mice were used as controls. Cells were cultured with various dilutions of PHA for 48 hr, pulsed with ³H-thymidine, and harvested 24 hr later. **A:** The PHA responses of normal and pyran-treated mice measured as cpm. **B:** The PHA responses of normal and pyran-treated mice measured as SR. ○, Mice treated with pyran; ●, untreated controls.

less than at the earlier time intervals and appeared to be beginning to return to normal. A dose-dependent increase in mitogen-independent incorporation in cells from pyran-treated animals compared to untreated controls was evident at the three times assayed (1). The effect of treatment with varying doses of pyran on the mitogen-induced blastogenic responses was then investigated. Treatment with 0.2 mg pyran/kg had no effect on the blastogenic response to PHA regardless of the time interval between drug administration and assay (Fig. 2A). Doses of pyran between 5 and 75 mg/kg given 2 days prior to assay resulted in a dose-dependent inhibition of the peak PHA response. In contrast, when pyran was administered on day -5, the peak incorporation of ^{3}H-thymidine by PHA-stimulated cultures was enhanced to 180 to 190% of the untreated control values. Furthermore, the response was insensitive to increasing doses of pyran. When pyran was injected 10 days prior to assay, peak incorporation at 5 and 25 mg pyran/kg was the same as controls, whereas doses of 50 and 75 mg/kg caused a slight enhancement. Using SR as a measure of blastogenesis, a dose-related increase in inhibition was seen with increasing doses of pyran administered at each of the three time intervals (Fig. 2B). Values for SR as percent control ranged between 70 and 90% at 0.2 mg pyran/kg and 1 to 5% at a dose of 75 mg pyran/kg.

The dose-response effect of pyran in LPS-stimulated cultures differed slightly from PHA-stimulated cultures. The inhibition of the response, as measured by ^{3}H-thymidine incorporation, was less than that seen in the response to PHA

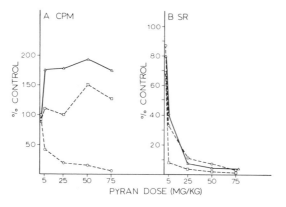

FIG. 2. The effect of varying doses of pyran on the blastogenic response of spleen cells stimulated with PHA. Mice were given a single i.v. injection of pyran between 0.2 and 75 mg/kg. The time of administration of pyran was either 2, 5, or 10 days prior to assay. Untreated mice were used as controls. Individual spleen cell suspensions were cultured with one of four dilutions of PHA (1:10, 1:50, 1:100, or 1:200) for 48 hr, pulsed with ^{3}H-thymidine, and harvested 24 hr later. Values are presented as percent control values of either cpm or SR. **A:** Blastogenic response expressed as cpm. **B:** Blastogenic response expressed as SR. ○---○, Pyran injected 2 days prior to assay; △——△, pyran injected 5 days prior to assay; □---□, pyran 10 days prior to assay. Each point represents the mean of three individually assayed spleens.

(Fig. 3A). No inhibition was seen at any time interval with pyran doses of 0.2 and 5 mg/kg. Spleen cells removed 2 days after pryan treatment were again the most inhibited, day 5 the least inhibited, and day 10 intermediate. At all times tested, a decrease in incorporation compared to controls was evident with increasing doses of pyran. Similarly, spleen cells assayed at all three times showed a dose-related depression of SR with increasing doses of the immunomodulator (Fig. 3B). The curves obtained for days 5 and 10 were quite comparable to those seen in the PHA response. Although treatment with pyran 2 days prior to assay of blastogenesis resulted in inhibition of the SR in LPS-stimulated cultures, the inhibition was less than that demonstrated when pyran was given 5 or 10 days previously.

In summary, a dose-related inhibition of mitogen-induced ^{3}H-thymidine incorporation into B and T lymphocytes was demonstrated in cultures of spleen cells obtained from mice treated 2 days previously with doses ranging from 5 to 75 mg pyran/kg. When assayed at 10 days after treatment with the high doses of pyran (50 and 75 mg/kg), the blastogenic response of B lymphocytes was inhibited as measured by ^{3}H-thymidine incorporation; T lymphocytes were not similarly inhibited. No inhibition of the blastogenic response of T and B

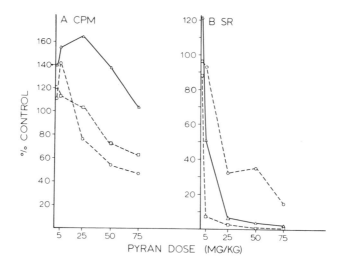

FIG. 3. The effect of varying doses of pyran on the blastogenic response of spleen cells stimulated with LPS. Mice were given a single i.v. injection of pyran between 0.2 and 75 mg/kg. The time of administration of pyran was either 2, 5, or 10 days prior to assay. Untreated mice were used as controls. Individual spleen cell suspensions were cultured with one of four dilutions of LPS (1, 5, 30, or 60 μg/culture) for 48 hr, pulsed with ^{3}H-thymidine, and harvested 24 hr later. Values are presented as percent control values of either cpm or SR. **A:** Blastogenic response expressed as cpm. **B:** Blastogenic response expressed as SR. ○---○, Pyran injected 2 days prior to assay; △—△, pyran 5 days prior to assay; □---□, pyran 10 days prior to assay. Each point represents the mean of three individually assayed spleens.

TABLE 2. *Effect of removal of adherent spleen cells on blastogenesis*

Cell population[a]	Peak PHA response[b] (Δ cpm)[c]	Peak LPS response[b] (Δ cpm)[c]
Normal spleen	36,774	78,004
Normal nonadherent[d]	94,573	130,000
Pyran spleen[e]	−24,203	11,323
Pyran nonadherent[d]	35,856	121,120

[a]5×10^5 Cells of the designated population plated per well.

[b]Values determined for the peak response of the entire dose response curve of mitogen.

[c]Δ Cpm = cpm in cultures with mitogen − cpm in cultures without mitogen.

[d]Nonadherent cells obtained after plating spleen cells in Petri dishes 3 times for 30 min at 37°C.

[e]Spleens obtained from mice treated with 50 mg/kg pyran i.v. 2 days prior to the experiment.

lymphocytes, as measured by ^{3}H-thymidine incorporation, was demonstrated when pyran was given 5 days prior to assay. Due to the enhanced background incorporation of ^{3}H-thymidine resulting from the *in vivo* mitogenic activity of pyran, the SR were suppressed throughout the assay period of 2 to 10 days post pyran treatment at all drug doses except 0.2 mg pyran/kg.

Since Scott (28) had shown that the inhibition of the PHA response in spleen cell suspensions from *C. parvum*-treated mice was mediated by macrophages, it was felt that macrophages might be similarly involved in the pyran-induced inhibition. Moreover, esterase staining of spleen cell suspensions indicated an increase in the number of macrophages in the spleens of pyran-treated animals as compared to normal controls (1). The macrophage content of normal spleens and spleens from pyran-treated animals 2 days after drug administration was similar, being 8.7 and 12.6%, respectively. By 5 days after pyran administration, the macrophage content of the spleens had increased to 29.0% and 10 days after treatment had increased still further to 41.7%. These experiments suggested that the quantitative change in splenic macrophage content and the change in splenic macrophage function was related to the inhibition of the blastogenic response.

To determine whether adherent cells (macrophages) were the suppressor population responsible for the inhibition of blastogenesis, spleens were obtained from pyran-treated and normal mice, and adherent cells were removed by plating in Petri dishes. The blastogenic response to both PHA and LPS was determined using normal and pyran spleen cells and normal and pyran nonadherent spleen cells (Table 2). The blastogenic responses of spleen cells from pyran-treated mice stimulated with PHA and LPS were significantly inhibited when compared to those of normal spleen cells. Removal of adherent cells from normal and pyran spleens caused an enhancement in the response to PHA, compared to the response of unseparated spleen cells. The response to LPS was similarly enhanced by removal of adherent cells, and the blastogenic responses of both normal and pyran spleen cells were comparable after adherence.

DISCUSSION

To elucidate further the cellular site of action of pyran, the effects of *in vivo* pyran administration on the specific mitogen-induced blastogenic responses of splenic B and T cells were investigated. LPS and PHA were used to investigate directly the effect of pyran treatment on B and T lymphocytes, respectively. A single intravenous injection of pyran was shown to depress significantly the *in vitro* mitogen-induced blastogenic responses of spleen cells at various times (2 to 14 days) after *in vivo* pyran administration. The pyran-mediated depression of spleen cell blastogenesis was demonstrated to be dose dependent. Furthermore, the blastogenic response of lymph node T lymphocytes, but not B lymphocytes, was shown to be depressed in pyran-treated mice. Although the reason for the differential effect of pyran treatment on B and T lymphocytes is not known, it could be due to a difference in the population of cells inhibiting T- and B-lymphocyte blastogenesis. These results were similar to observations reported by Scott (27,28) for the biologic immunopotentiator *C. parvum*. Treatment of mice with *C. parvum* resulted in a marked depression of the blastogenic response of mouse splenic and peripheral blood lymphocytes to PHA, whereas the response of lymph node cells from *C. parvum*-treated mice was similar to that of normal mice (8). In addition, treatment of mice with *C. parvum* had no effect on the blastogenic response of B lymphocytes (8,27). These results suggest that immunomodulators have different effects on the blastogenic response of various lymphocyte subpopulations. The depression of the blastogenic response after treatment with *C. parvum* was subsequently demonstrated to be mediated by *C. parvum*-activated macrophages. Similarly, we were able to demonstrate that removal of adherent cells from the spleens of pyran-treated animals resulted in an increase in blastogenic responses of both B and T lymphocytes (3). Scott (8,27), however, was unable to demonstrate any depression of the blastogenic response of B lymphocytes to pokeweed mitogen in TxBM mice or to LPS in intact mice treated with *C. parvum*. The lack of inhibition of B-lymphocyte blastogenic responses reported by Scott (8,27) contradicted experiments performed in this laboratory in which we found that the blastogenic response of both B and T lymphocytes from *C. parvum*-treated mice were depressed compared to cells from untreated mice (1). The difference between Scott's results and ours may be related to a differential sensitivity of B and T lymphocytes to macrophage-mediated inhibition. In this regard, pyran treatment was often demonstrated to produce greater inhibition of the blastogenic response of splenic T lymphocytes compared to B lymphocytes, and it is possible that a similar differential exists in *C. parvum*-treated mice. Scott's inability to demonstrate inhibition of B-lymphocyte blastogenic responses was also surprising since the results of our experiments as well as those of Lemke et al. (17) suggested that B lymphocytes were more susceptible to peritoneal exudate (PE) macrophage-mediated inhibition of blastogenesis than T lymphocytes. The difference in the sensitivities of B and T lymphocytes to inhibition of blastogenesis by splenic and PE macrophages suggested that two subpopulations of inhibitory macrophages were involved. Moreover, the fact that the blastogenic response of lymph node T, but not B lymphocytes, was depressed after pyran administration may be related to the fact that different subpopulations of macrophages are present in the spleens, lymph nodes, and peritoneal cavities of pyran-treated mice.

Although mitogen-induced ^{3}H-thymidine incorporation of both B and T lymphocytes could be shown to be depressed at various time intervals after *in vivo* pyran administration, mitogen-independent incorporation was enhanced in pyran-treated animals compared to untreated controls. The magnitude of this enhancement varied with the time after treatment with pyran and from experiment to experiment. The increase in mitogen-independent (background) incorporation of spleen cells was dose dependent in pyran-treated mice. The kinetics of the increase in mitogen-independent incorporation in cultures of spleen cells from pyran-treated mice were similar to the kinetics of development of splenomegaly after *in vivo* pyran administration (1).

Although mitogen-induced blastogenesis of spleen cells from pyran-treated mice was depressed at various time intervals after *in vivo* drug administration, it was enhanced 5 days after *in vivo* pyran treatment. As this had been shown to be the time of peak mitogenicity for pyran *in vivo,* it is possible that the enhancement of mitogen-induced blastogenesis demonstrated 5 days after *in vivo* pyran administration, resulted from a greater mitogen sensitivity of pyran-primed spleen cells at this time. Alternatively, pyran-primed spleen cells could be more resistant to the action of an inhibitory cell at this time. However, it should also be noted that pyran also increased the percent of esterase-positive cells (presumably macrophages) (1) as well as erythropoietic centers in the spleens of drug-treated animals (26).

The fact that the blastogenic responses of both T and B lymphocytes were similarly depressed after pyran treatment suggested that the inhibition is indirectly mediated by a third party cell, thus providing a common mechanism for both effects. As pyran had proved to be a potent stimulator of the reticuloendothelial system (20) and to activate macrophages to kill tumor cells *in vitro* (11), the obvious candidate for such a third party was the macrophage. In addition, the macrophage content of spleens from pyran-treated mice 5 and 10 days after drug treatment was significantly higher than that of spleens of normal mice. In subsequent experiments, macrophages were demonstrated to be the cell population responsible for the inhibition of blastogenesis (3,4). This effect was demonstrated in two ways: (a) removal of adherent cells from the spleens of pyran-treated animals resulted in enhancement of blastogenesis, and (b) addition of peritoneal-adherent cells from pyran-treated animals to cultures of normal spleen cells resulted in marked inhibition of blastogenesis. Evidence has been presented by Nathan et al. indicating that a PEC that was esterase positive, glass adherent, not phagocytic, and had IgM on the surface was responsible for *in vitro* tumor cell cytostasis (C. F. Nathan, R. Asofsky, and W. D. Terry, *personal communication,* and ref. 21). It is possible that a similar cell, rather than the macrophage, is involved in the regulation of lymphoproliferation, both *in vitro* and *in vivo*.

ACKNOWLEDGMENT

This research was supported in part by USPHS grant no. AI-11561.

REFERENCES

1. Baird, L. G. (1976): The Mechanism of Immunoadjuvant Activity of Pyran Copolymer. Ph.D. Thesis.
2. Baird, L. G., and Kaplan, A. M. (1975): Immunoadjuvant activity of pyran copolymer. I. Evidence for direct stimulation of T-lymphocytes and macrophages. *Cell. Immunol.*, 20:167–176.
3. Baird, L. G., and Kaplan, A. M. (1977): Macrophage regulation of mitogen-induced blastogenesis. I. Demonstration of inhibitory cells in the spleens and peritoneal exudates of mice. *Cell. Immunol.*, 28:22–35.
4. Baird, L. G., and Kaplan, A. M. (1977): Macrophage regulation of mitogen-induced blastogenesis. II. Mechanism of inhibition. *Cell. Immunol.*, 28:36–50.
5. Cleveland, R. P., Meltzer, M. S., and Zbar, B. (1974): Tumor cytotoxicity *in vitro* by macrophages from mice infected with *Mycobacterium bovis* strain BCG. *J. Natl. Cancer Inst.*, 52:1887–1894.
6. Hibbs, J. B., Lambert, L. H., and Remington, J. S. (1971): Resistance to murine tumors conferred by chronic infection with intracellular protozoa, *Toxoplasma gondii* and *Besnoitia jellisoni*. *J. Infect. Dis.*, 124:587–592.
7. Holterman, O. A., Klein, E., and Casale, G. P. (1973): Selective cytotoxicity of peritoneal leucocytes for neoplastic cells. *Cell. Immunol.*, 9:339–362.
8. Howard, J. G., Christie, G. H., and Scott, M. T. (1973): Biological effects of *Corynebacterium parvum*. IV. Adjuvant and inhibitory activities on B lymphocytes. *Cell. Immunol.*, 7:290–301.
9. Janossy, G., and Greaves, M. (1975): Functional analysis of murine and human B lymphocyte subsets. *Transplant. Rev.*, 24:177–236.
10. Kaplan, A. M., and Morahan, P. S. (1976): Macrophage mediated tumor cell cytotoxicity. *Ann. NY Acad. Sci.*, 276:134–145.
11. Kaplan, A. M., Morahan, P. S., and Regelson, W. (1974): Induction of macrophage-mediated tumor cell cytotoxicity by pyran copolymer. *J. Natl. Cancer Inst.*, 52:1919–1923.
12. Keller, R. (1975): Major changes in lymphocyte proliferation evoked by macrophages. *Cell. Immunol.*, 17:542–551.
13. Kirchner, H., Chused, T. M., Herberman, R. B., Holden, H. T., and Lavrin, D. H. (1974): Evidence of suppressor cell activity in spleens of mice bearing primary tumors induced by Moloney sarcoma virus. *J. Exp. Med.*, 139:1473–1486.
14. Kirchner, H., Herberman, R. B., Glaser, M., and Lavrin, D. H. (1974): Suppression of *in vitro* lymphocyte stimulation in mice bearing primary Moloney sarcoma virus-induced tumors. *Cell. Immunol.*, 13:32–40.
15. Kirchner, H., Muchmore, A. V., Chused, T. M., Holden, H. V., and Herberman, R. B. (1975): Inhibition of proliferation of lymphoma cells and T-lymphocytes by suppressor cells from tumor bearing mice. *J. Immunol.*, 114:206–210.
16. Leibovich, S. J., and Ross, R. (1975): The role of the macrophage in wound repair. *Am. J. Pathol.*, 78:71–89.
17. Lemke, H., Coutinho, A., Opitz, H. G., and Gronowicz, E. (1975): Macrophages suppress direct B-cell activation by lipopolysaccharide. *Scand. J. Immunol.*, 4:707–720.
18. Morahan, P. S., and Kaplan, A. M. (1976): Macrophage activation and antitumor activity of biologic and synthetic agents. *Int. J. Cancer*, 17:82–89.
19. Morahan, P. S., and Kaplan, A. M. (1977): Macrophage-mediated tumor resistance. In: *Control of Neoplasia by Modulation of the Immune System (Progress in Cancer Research and Therapy, Vol. 2)*, edited by M. A. Chirigos, pp. 449–459. Raven Press, New York.
20. Munson, A. E., Regelson, W., Lawrence, W., and Wooles, W. R. (1970): Biphasic response

of the reticuloendothelial system (RES) induced by pyran copolymer. *J. Reticuloendothel. Soc.,* 7:375–385.

21. Nathan, C. F., Hill, V. M., and Terry, W. D. (1976): Isolation of a subpopulation of adherent peritoneal cells with antitumor activity. *Nature,* 260:146–148.

22. Parkhouse, R. M. E., and Dutton, R. W. (1966): Inhibition of spleen cell DNA synthesis by autologous macrophages. *J. Immunol.,* 97:663–669.

23. Regelson, W. (1967): Prevention and treatment of Friend leukemia virus infection by interferon inducing synthetic polyanions. *Adv. Exp. Med. Biol.,* 1:315–332.

24. Regelson, W., Morahan, P. S., Kaplan, A. M., Baird, L. G., and Munson, J. A. (1973): Synthetic polyanions: Molecular weight, macrophage activation and immunologic response. In: *Activation of Macrophages,* edited by W. H. Wagner and H. Hahn, pp. 97–110. Excerpta Medica, Amsterdam.

25. Russell, S. W., Doe, W. F., and Cochrane, C. G. (1976): Number of macrophages and distribution of mitotic activity in regressing and progressing Moloney sarcomas. *J. Immunol.,* 116:164–166.

26. Schuller, G. B., Morahan, P. S., and Snodgrass, M. (1975): Inhibition and enhancement of Friend leukemia virus by pyran copolymer. *Cancer Res.,* 35:1915–1920.

27. Scott, M. T. (1972): Biological effects of the adjuvant *Corynebacterium parvum.* I. Inhibition of PHA, mixed lymphocyte and GVH reactivity. *Cell. Immunol.,* 5:459–468.

28. Scott, M. T. (1972): Biological effects of the adjuvant *Corynebacterium parvum.* II. Evidence for macrophage-T-cell interaction. *Cell. Immunol.,* 5:469–479.

29. Seeger, R. C., and Oppenheim, J. J. (1970): Synergistic interaction of macrophages and lymphocytes in antigen-induced transformation of lymphocytes. *J. Exp. Med.,* 132:44–65.

30. Sjoberg, O. (1972): Effect of allogeneic cell interaction on the primary immune response *in vitro.* Cell types involved in suppression and stimulation of antibody synthesis. *Clin. Exp. Immunol.,* 12:365–375.

31. Waldman, S. R., and Gottlieb, A. A. (1973): Macrophage regulation of DNA synthesis in lymphoid cells: Effects of a soluble factor from macrophages. *Cell. Immunol.,* 9:142–156.

Immune Modulation and Control of Neoplasia by Adjuvant Therapy, edited by M. A. Chirigos. Raven Press, New York, 1978.

Antiviral and Antitumor Functions of Activated Macrophages

Page S. Morahan and Alan M. Kaplan

Departments of Microbiology and Surgery, Medical College of Virginia, Virginia Commonwealth University, Richmond, Virginia 23298

The phagocytic, antibacterial, and antitumor activity of macrophages has been well established. Furthermore, it is known that certain conditions, such as infection of an animal with *Mycobacterium bovis, Corynebacterium parvum,* or *Toxoplasma gondii,* can increase the activity of macrophages in these various functions (5,8,11–13,15,30). The critical differences betwen normal and activated macrophages have not been completely defined. Karnovsky et al. (16) have suggested that metabolic functions of macrophages differ depending on whether they are "activated" by such immunomodulators as Bacillus Calmette-Guerin (BCG) or pyran, "stimulated" (elicited) by inoculation with sterile inflammatory agents such as thioglycollate or glycogen, or "normal" (unstimulated).[1] The relationship of these metabolic events, however, to the various functions of the macrophage remains obscure. For example, do activated macrophages use the same mechanisms as normal macrophages in killing intracellular microorganisms, but on a larger scale, or are new mechanisms developed? Furthermore, are the same mechanisms used in killing bacteria, killing tumor cells, inhibiting virus growth, and regulating proliferation of lymphocytes? The complexity of these questions is compounded by our increasing awareness that macrophages are heterogeneous (36).[2] Does this heterogeneity reflect various states of differentiation or discrete subpopulations with different origins? The present studies have been designed to begin to define the peritoneal cell population produced by various stimulating and activating treatments and to compare the activity of the peritoneal macrophage in regard to antiviral and antitumor activity.

---

[1] For clarity of discussion, the term "activated macrophage" is reserved for that cell population that exhibits cytotoxicity for neoplastic target cells.

[2] The term "macrophage" is used operationally to define the adherent peritoneal cell population, recognizing that this population is not completely homogeneous.

MATERIALS AND METHODS

Mice

Adult and suckling Balb/c mice were used for experiments regarding antiviral activity of peritoneal cells, and C57Bl/6 mice were used for experiments regarding the antitumor activity. In comparative experiments, no differences in antitumor activity between Balb/c and C57Bl/6 peritoneal cells were observed.

Drugs

Pyran copolymer, lot XA 124–177, was obtained from Hercules, Inc., Wilmington, Del. The drug was solubilized in 0.15 N NaCl, brought to pH 7.2, and injected i.p. at 25 mg/kg. The killed vaccine of *C. parvum* was obtained from Burroughs Wellcome, Triangle Research Park, N.C., and injected i.p. at 70 mg/kg. Glycogen (Sigma oyster glycogen II) was dissolved in 0.15 N NaCl at 2.5 mg/100 ml, and mice injected i.p. with 0.5 ml.

Viruses

Herpes simplex virus type 2 (HSV-2) was propagated in Hep-2 cells and titered by plaque formation in VERO cells, as previously described (28). Friend leukemia virus (FLV) was prepared as a 10% suspension of infected spleens, as previously described (34).

Tumor

A methylcholanthrene-induced fibrosarcoma (MCA 2182) was maintained by continuous s.c. passage of 1 mm³ fragments in mice (14).

Cell Cultures

Lewis lung carcinoma cells, mouse embryo fibroblasts, and WI-38 human embryonic lung fibroblast cells were grown and maintained by previously described methods (15). All cultures were screened periodically and found to be free of mycoplasma contamination.

Preparation of Peritoneal Cells

Mice were injected with saline, with glycogen to stimulate macrophages, or with pyran or *C. parvum* to activate macrophages. Peritoneal cells were obtained by peritoneal lavage in Hanks' balanced salt solution without fetal calf serum but containing 10 U/ml preservative-free heparin. Cells were washed once and suspended in Eagle's minimal essential medium containing Earle's balanced salt solution and 10% fetal calf serum. Macrophages were characterized by staining for nonspecific esterase activity (24), by Fc rosette formation with antibody-coated erythrocytes, and by obtaining differential counts on Wright's stained smears of peritoneal cells.

Antiviral and Antitumor Activity

To determine antiviral activity *in vitro,* peritoneal cells were adsorbed for 2 hr to mouse embryo fibroblasts infected with HSV-2, the nonadherent cells removed with three washes, and supernatant fluids obtained 3 days later for determination of the yields of cell-free virus. Two assays for antitumor activity were used in order to determine both the cytotoxic and cytostatic activity of peritoneal cells. To measure cytotoxic activity alone, target tumor and normal cells were prelabelled with ^{125}IUDR, incubated with peritoneal cells, and the release of radioactivity measured 48 hr later (13). For determination of cytostatic activity, target cells were incubated with peritoneal cells, and the uptake of ^{125}IUDR into the target cells was measured at 6, 12, and 24 hr (13). The details of the experiments dealing with antiviral and antitumor activity of peritoneal cells *in vivo* are described with the particular results.

Statistical Analysis

The Chi square test with Yates' correction factor was used to evaluate the difference in virus mortality and in tumor incidence between experimental and control groups. The Student's *t*-test was used to evaluate the difference in splenomegaly between treated and control groups.

RESULTS

Characterization of Normal, Stimulated, and Activated Peritoneal Cell Populations

Treatment of C57B1/6 mice with activating agents significantly increased the number of cells in the peritoneal cavity; there was a three- to 10-fold increase in the total number of peritoneal cells (Table 1). Although there was generally little change in the percent of macrophages in the activated as compared to the normal peritoneal cell population, the total number of macrophages present was substantially greater in the activated cell populations. The percent of cells possessing nonspecific esterase activity was consistently greater than the percent identified morphologically as macrophages/monocytes or as cells bearing Fc receptors. These differences may reflect various subpopulations of macrophages (36) or an unusual subpopulation of lymphocytes (29).

TABLE 1. *Characteristics of peritoneal exudate cells*

| Treatment | PEC/mouse (× 10⁶) | % Fc rosettes ± SE | % Esterase ± SE | Differential | | |
				Lympho.	Mono.	PMN
Normal	2.0 ± 0.6	28.3 ± 5.1	43.2 ± 1.5	81.2 ± 2.7	19.0 ± 2.7	0
Glycogen	4.4 ± 1.4	25.9 ± 2.8	32.0 ± 2.5	76.7 ± 1.8	22.7 ± 1.8	0.7 ± 0.7
C. parvum	7.3 ± 1.2	32.0 ± 5.0	45.1 ± 2.8	57.0 ± 5.2	36.6 ± 4.4	6.6 ± 1.8
Pyran	19.0 ± 11.8	38.9 ± 0.4	58.1 ± 3.1	68.7 ± 3.2	28.3 ± 3.2	3.0 ± 0.9

PEC, peritoneal exudate cells; PMN, polymorphonuclear leukocytes.

TABLE 2. *Antiviral activity of adherent peritoneal cells* in vitro

Treatment	HSV-2 yield ($\log_{10}$/ml PFU)	Reduction in yield ($\log_{10}$)
None	4.9	
Saline	4.5	0.4
Pyran	2.6	2.3
C. parvum	2.7	2.2

PFU, plaque-forming units.

Peritoneal exudate cells (2×10^6) were adsorbed for 2 hr to mouse embryo fibroblasts infected with HSV-2, the nonadherent cells removed with washing, and supernatant fluids harvested 3 days later to determine the yields of cell-free HSV-2.

Antiviral Activity of Adherent Peritoneal Cells *In Vitro*

Incubation of pyran- or *C. parvum*-activated peritoneal cells with mouse embryo fibroblasts infected with HSV-2 significantly reduced the yield of HSV-2, whereas normal peritoneal cells had no effect (Table 2). Glycogen-stimulated peritoneal cells were also relatively inactive (Table 3). Significant inhibition of virus growth required the addition of 2×10^6 activated peritoneal cells. Approximately 50% of these cells adhered, providing a 1:1 ratio of adherent peritoneal cells to infected mouse embryo fibroblasts.

Antiviral and Antitumor Activity of Peritoneal Cells *In Vivo*

In addition to activity *in vitro,* activated peritoneal populations exhibited significant activity *in vivo.* The transfer of pyran-activated peritoneal cells to mice protected them from subsequent infection with either HSV-2 or FLV (Table 4). Activated peritoneal cells also exhibited considerable antitumor activity when

TABLE 3. *Antiviral activity of stimulated and activated adherent peritoneal cells*

Treatment	PEC concentration	HSV-2 yield ($\log_{10}$ PFU/ml)	Reduction in virus yield ($\log_{10}$)
None	—	3.8	—
Pyran	2×10^6	2.0	1.8
	1×10^6	3.1	0.7
Glycogen	2×10^6	3.5	0.3
	1×10^6	3.8	0
Normal	2×10^6	3.2	0.6
	1×10^6	3.2	0.6

PEC, peritoneal exudate cells; PFU, plaque-forming units.

Peritoneal cells at the indicated concentrations were adsorbed for 2 hr to mouse embryo fibroblasts infected with HSV-2, the nonadherent cells removed with washing, and supernatant fluids harvested 3 days later to determine the yields of cell-free HSV-2.

TABLE 4. *Antiviral and antitumor activity of peritoneal cells* in vivo

	Peritoneal cells			
	None	Normal	Glycogen stimulated	Activated
Mortality after HSV-2 infection[a] No. dead/total (%)	11/21 (52%)	27/44 (61%)	15/39 (38%)	7/42 (17%)[d]
Splenomegaly after FLV infection[b] Mg ± SE (%)	796.1 ± 1.7	ND	1,064.1 ± 125.5 (133%)	259.4 ± 21.6[d] (33%)
Tumor incidence of MCA 2182[c] No. tumors/total (%)	10/10 (100%)	9/10 (90%)	ND	10/20 (50%)[d]

[a] Peritoneal cells were obtained from adult Balb/c mice injected i.p. 5 days previously with glycogen or 1 day previously with pyran (25 mg/kg), and 3×10^6 cells were transferred i.p. to suckling Balb/c mice injected i.p. with HSV-2 24 hr later.

[b] Peritoneal cells were obtained from adult Balb/c mice injected i.p. 5 days previously with glycogen or injected daily for 5 consecutive days with pyran (25 mg/kg each injection), and 3×10^7 cells were transferred i.p. to adult Balb/c mice infected i.p. with FLV 24 hr later.

[c] C57B1/6 mice were injected with 5×10^4 MCA 2182 tumor cells in the footpad, and injected in the tumor 3 days later with 1.2×10^6 adherent peritoneal cells obtained from C57B1/6 mice injected i.p. 7 days previously with *C. parvum* (70 mg/kg).

[d] $p < 0.05$ when compared to control receiving none or normal peritoneal cells.

the cells were injected into the MCA 2182 fibrosarcoma, as evidenced by a marked decrease in incidence of tumors. Similar to the results observed *in vitro,* the transfer of either normal or glycogen-stimulated peritoneal cells did not provide antiviral or antitumor activity.

Comparison of Antiviral Activity, Antitumor Activity, and Inhibition of Lymphocyte Proliferation by Peritoneal Cells

Table 5 summarizes our observations regarding the cytotoxic and cytostatic activity of adherent peritoneal cells for normal mouse embryo fibroblasts and Lewis lung carcinoma cells. Only pyran- or *C. parvum*-activated peritoneal cells caused a significant and selective release of ^{125}IUDR from tumor target cells. The activity required approximately 48 hr of incubation of peritoneal cells with target cells (13,15). The cytotoxicity appeared to be tumor specific since neither mouse embryo fibroblasts nor human WI-38 fibroblasts were affected (13,15).

In contrast to this tumor specificity and delayed activity in regard to cytotoxicity, activated peritoneal cells were cytostatic for both tumor and normal target cells, and this activity was apparent after as little as 6 hr of incubation of target cells with adherent peritoneal cells (13). Thus, activated adherent peritoneal cells were both cytostatic and cytotoxic, but only the cytotoxic activity was tumor selective. Cytostatic activity was also expressed by the ability of activated macrophages to inhibit the proliferation of lymphocytes in response

TABLE 5. *Comparison of various inhibitory functions of adherent peritoneal cells*

| Treatment | Antiviral activity | Antitumor Activity | | | | Inhibition of lymphocyte proliferation |
| | | Cytotoxicity | | Cytostasis | | |
		LL	(MEF)	LL	MEF	
Normal	—	—	—	—	—	+
Glycogen	±	—	—	—	—	+
Pyran	++	++	—	++	++	++
C. parvum	++	++	—	++	++	++

LL, Lewis lung carcinoma; MEF, mouse embryo fibroblasts.

to mitogens (1–3). Both normal and stimulated peritoneal cells exhibited some inhibitory activity, indicating that lymphocytes may be particularly sensitive to inhibition of proliferation.

In general, pyran- or *C. parvum*-activated adherent peritoneal cells showed the greatest activity in all the functions examined—antiviral, tumor cytotoxicity, and inhibition of proliferation of various cells, including lymphocytes. Normal peritoneal cells or peritoneal cells stimulated by glycogen were much less active, producing only inhibition of lymphocyte proliferation.

DISCUSSION

Macrophages, in the apparent absence of acquired immunologic mechanisms, have been shown to play a role in both innate resistance to infectious disease and resistance to tumors. Furthermore, the participation of macrophages in lymphoproliferation (1–3,19), wound healing (4,23), inhibition of viral growth (27), and regulation of tumor cell proliferation (13,17,18,20,22) suggests that macrophages play a general biologic role in the control of proliferative events. For example, macrophages have been implicated in the regression of the tadpole tail (33), and Hibbs (10) has suggested that macrophages play a role in some types of tissue remodelling that occur in normal embryogenesis.

Whether a homogeneous population of macrophages mediates these diverse events or various macrophage subpopulations each mediate selected events is unknown. Much evidence indicates that peritoneal macrophages are heterogeneous with respect to their Fc receptors (32,36), ability to mediate phagocytosis (31), ability to bind lectins (25), and cellular distribution of endocytized antigen (21). However, this functional heterogeneity may reflect various states of differentiation rather than discrete subpopulations with different origins. Functional heterogeneity is also probably related to the degree of activation of the macrophages, reflecting the varying proportion of activated or normal cells within a given population.

In the present study we have assayed the ability of normal, stimulated, or activated macrophages to inhibit viral replication, tumor cell growth, and lymphocyte proliferation or to be cytotoxic to tumor cells. Our results indicate that normal peritoneal macrophages can inhibit mitogen-induced lymphocyte proliferation, but do not inhibit viral replication or tumor cell proliferation. In contrast, macrophages activated by either pyran or *C. parvum* demonstrate tumor selective cytoxicity, inhibit viral replication and tumor cell proliferation, and are three to five times more efficient at inhibiting lymphoproliferation than are normal macrophages. Glycogen-stimulated macrophages behave as normal macrophages except for their marginal inhibition of viral proliferation, although macrophages stimulated by another inflammatory agent, thioglycollate, do inhibit viral proliferation (27).

Mechanistically, little is known about how macrophages mediate these effects. The most obvious mechanisms by which macrophages could inhibit lymphocyte blastogenesis *in vitro* are cytostasis or cytotoxicity. Baird and Kaplan (3) have previously shown that the number of viable lymphocytes per culture did not decrease in the presence of normal or activated macrophages, suggesting that cytotoxicity was not the mechanism of the inhibition of lymphoproliferation. However, the presence of blast cells could not be demonstrated in cultures incubated with macrophages, suggesting that macrophages acted by inhibiting blast formation. It has not been established whether macrophage-soluble factors are the primary mode by which lymphoproliferation is regulated, or merely an additional minor regulatory mode with cell-cell interaction being the major requirement.

The enhanced ability of pyran- or *C. parvum*-activated macrophages to inhibit lymphoproliferation has not been completely defined. The inhibitory effect of normal cells could be due to a subpopulation of activated cells within the normal population. Thus, treatment with pyran or *C. parvum* would only serve to drive a greater proportion of macrophages into the activated population. Nathan et al. (C. F. Nathan, R. Asofsky, and W. D. Terry, *personal communication*) have recently described a subpopulation of cells in peritoneal exudates of mice that are glass adherent, nonphagocytic, and esterase positive, and have IgM on their surface. These authors have shown a threefold increase in the percent of these cells present in the peritoneal cavity of mice immunized with BCG and have suggested that these cells are responsible for cytostasis against tumor cells (29). Whether or not this population of cells is also responsible for inhibition of lymphoproliferation is unknown.

Activated but not normal macrophages have been shown to inhibit tumor cell proliferation *in vitro* (13); however, we have demonstrated that normal fibroblast proliferation is similarly inhibited (13). These data must now be reevaluated in light of our increasing evidence for heterogeneity among peritoneal cell populations (36). Although activated macrophages are cytostatic to both tumor cells and normal cells, most reports indicate that they are cytotoxic only to tumor cells (10,15,26). Little is known of the relationship of the early cytostatic effects of activated macrophages on tumor cells in culture to their ultimate cytotoxic effects. Activated macrophage-mediated cytotoxicity has been shown to be a delayed event occurring between 24 and 48 hr after the introduction of macrophages to cultured tumor cells. Hibbs (10) has presented data that the killing mechanism is a result of the selective transfer of lysosomes from activated macrophages to tumor cells, after which the target tumor cells undergo heterolysis. Recent morphologic data by Hanna et al. (9) have suggested that activated macrophages interact with tumor cells via cytoplasmic extensions and that primary lysosomes, initially detected only in histiocytes, were later observed also in neoplastic target cells. However, Currie and Basham (6) have recently demonstrated that a heat labile supernatant product from endotoxin-activated rat macrophages was selectively lytic for tumor cells. In contrast, Hibbs et al. (10), Kaplan et al. (15), and Meltzer et al. (26) have suggested that macrophage-mediated tumor cell cytostasis required cell-to-cell contact. Clearly, further experimentation is required to resolve this issue.

In the present chapter we have shown that both pyran- and *C. parvum*-activated peritoneal macrophages, but not normal or glycogen-stimulated macrophages, reduced the virus yield from mouse embryo fibroblasts infected with HSV-2. Macrophage-mediated antiviral activity was nonspecific with respect to the virus (27). Morahan et al. (27) have demonstrated that antiviral activity was most pronounced against multiple cycles of viral infection initiated at a low multiplicity of infection. Single-cycle virus growth was not affected, suggesting that the major inhibition was on subsequent cycles of virus growth. If the antiviral effect was directed primarily against virus-infected cells, the effect could have occurred through a change in cell metabolism so that less virus was replicated or through destruction of virus-infected cells and regrowth of normal cells. Stott et al. (35) have recently shown that normal alveolar macrophages lysed parainfluenza virus-infected cells.

We conclude that macrophages may play a general biologic role in the control of proliferation of cells and microorganisms, as well as in tissue destruction and remodelling. Whether differences in macrophages in these various functions reflect discrete subpopulations of cells or varying states in a differentiation/maturation pathway remains unclear. It is, however, clear that activation of macrophages enhances their antiviral and antitumor activity and their ability to inhibit lymphocyte proliferation. Whether activation merely provides a driving force for differentiation or alters the proportion of subpopulations of cells remains to be established. It is clear, however, that macrophages can, under certain circumstances, control tumor growth and viral proliferation. Moreover, immunomodulators certainly have the ability to enhance these macrophage functions. Their interactions with macrophages must be deciphered, if immunomodulators are to play a rational role in either antiviral or antitumor therapy.

ACKNOWLEDGMENT

This research was supported by USPHS grants CA-16193 and CA-1537, and contract CB-43877. Page S. Morahan is a USPHS Research Career Development

Awardee, AI 70863. The authors thank J. A. Munson and S. C. Johnson for their excellent technical assistance.

REFERENCES

1. Baird, L. G., and Kaplan, A. M. (1975): Immunoadjuvant activity of pyran copolymer I. Evidence for direct stimulation of T-lymphocytes and macrophages. *Cell. Immunol.,* 26:167–176.
2. Baird, L. G., and Kaplan, A. M. (1977): Macrophage regulation of mitogen-induced blastogenesis. I. Demonstration of inhibitory cells in the spleens and peritoneal exudates of mice. *Cell. Immunol.,* 28:22–35.
3. Baird, L. G., and Kaplan, A. M. (1977): Macrophage regulation of mitogen-induced blastogenesis. II. Mechanism of inhibition. *Cell. Immunol.,* 28:36–50.
4. Clark, R. A., Stone, R. D., Leung, D. Y. K., Silver, I., Hohn, D. C., and Hunt, T. K. (1976): Role of macrophages in wound healing. *Surg. Forum,* 27:16–18.
5. Cleveland, R. P., Meltzer, M. S., and Zbar, B. (1974): Tumor cytotoxicity *in vitro* by macrophages from mice infected with *Mycobacterium bovis* strain BCG. *J. Natl. Cancer Inst.,* 52:1887–1894.
6. Currie, G. A., and Basham, C. (1975): Activated macrophages release a factor which lyses malignant cells but not normal cells. *J. Exp. Med.,* 142:1600–1605.
7. Evans, R., and Alexander, P. (1976): Mechanisms of extracellular killing of nucleated mammalian cells by macrophages. In: *Immunobiology of the Macrophage,* edited by D. S. Nelson, pp. 509–535. Academic Press, New York.
8. Ghaffar, A., Cullen, R. T., Dunbar, N., and Woodruff, M. F. A. (1974): Antitumor effect *in vitro* of lymphocytes and macrophages from mice treated with *Corynebacterium parvum. Br. J. Cancer,* 29:199–205.
9. Hanna, M. G., Bucana, C., Hibbs, B., and Fidler, I. J. (1976): Morphologic aspects of tumor cell cytotoxicity by effector cells of the macrophage-histocyte compartment: *In vitro* and *in vivo* studies in BCG-mediated tumor regression. In: *The Macrophage in Neoplasia,* edited by M. Fink, pp. 113–134. Academic Press, New York.
10. Hibbs, J. B. (1974): Heterolysis by macrophages activated by Bacillus Calmette-Guerin: Lysosome exocytosis into tumor cells. *Science,* 184:468–471.
11. Hibbs, J. B., Jr., Lambert, L. H., Jr., and Remington, J. S. (1971): Resistance to murine tumors conferred by chronic infection with intracellular protozoa, *Toxoplasma gondii* and *Besnoitia jellisoni. J. Infect. Dis.,* 124:587–592.
12. Holtermann, O. A., Klein, E., and Casale, G. P. (1973): Selective cytotoxicity of peritoneal leucocytes for neoplastic cells. *Cell. Immunol.,* 9:339–352.
13. Kaplan, A. M., Baird, L. G., and Morahan, P. S. (1977): Macrophage regulation of tumor cell growth and mitogen-induced blastogenesis. In: *Control of Neoplasia by Modulation of the Immune System (Progress in Cancer Research and Therapy, Vol. 2),* edited by M. A. Chirigos, pp. 461–474. Raven Press, New York.
14. Kaplan, A. M., and Morahan, P. S. (1976): Macrophage-mediated tumor cell cytotoxicity. *Ann. NY Acad. Sci.,* 276:134–145.
15. Kaplan, A. M., Morahan, P. S., and Regelson, W. (1974): Induction of macrophage-mediated tumor-cell cytotoxicity by pyran copolymer. *J. Natl. Cancer Inst.,* 52:1919–1921.
16. Karnovsky, M. L., Lazdins, J., Drath, D., and Harper, A. (1975): Biochemical characteristics of activated macrophages. *Ann. NY Acad. Sci.,* 256:266–274.
17. Keller, R. (1973): Cytostatic elimination of syngeneic rat tumor cells *in vitro* by nonspecifically activated macrophages. *J. Exp. Med.,* 138: 625–644.
18. Keller, R. (1974): Modulation of cell proliferation by macrophages: A possible function apart from cytotoxic tumor rejection. *Br. J. Cancer,* 30:401–415.
19. Keller, R. (1975): Major changes in lymphocyte proliferation evoked by activated macrophages. *Cell. Immunol.,* 17:542–551.
20. Keller, R. (1976): Cytostatic and cytocidal effects of activated macrophages. In: *Immunobiology of the Macrophage,* edited by D. S. Nelson, pp. 487–508. Academic Press, New York.
21. Kolsch, E., and Mitchison, N. A. (1968): Subcellular distribution of antigen in macrophages. *J. Exp. Med.,* 128:1059–1079.

22. Krahenbuhl, J. L., Lambert, L. H., and Remington, J. S. (1976): The effects of activated macrophages on tumor target cells: Escape from cytostasis. *Cell. Immunol.,* 25:279–293.
23. Leibovich, S. J., and Ross, R. (1975): The role of the macrophage in wound repair. *Am. J. Pathol.,* 78:71–91.
24. Li, C. Y., Lam, K. W., and Yam, L. T. (1973): Esterases in human leukocytes. *J. Histochem. Cytochem.,* 21:1–12.
25. Loor, F., and Roelants, G. E. (1974): The dynamic state of the macrophage plasma membrane attachment and fate of immunoglobulin, antigen and lectins. *Eur. J. Immunol.,* 7:649–660.
26. Meltzer, M. S., Tucker, R. W., Sanford, K. K., and Leonard, E. J. (1975): Interaction of BCG-activated macrophages with neoplastic and nonneoplastic cell lines *in vitro:* Quantitation of the cytotoxic reaction by release of tritiated thymidine from prelabelled target cells. *J. Natl. Cancer Inst.,* 54:1177–1184.
27. Morahan, P. S., Glasgow, L. A., Crane, J. L., Jr., and Kern, E. R. (1977): Comparison of antiviral and antitumor activity of activated macrophages. *Cell. Immunol.,* 28:404–415.
28. Morahan, P. S., and McCord, R. S. (1975): Resistance to herpes simplex type 2 virus induced by an immunopotentiator in immunosuppressed mice. *J. Immunol.,* 115:311–313.
29. Nathan, C. F., Hill, V. M., and Terry, W. D. (1976): Isolation of a subpopulation of adherent peritoneal cells with antitumor activity. *Nature,* 260:146–148.
30. Parr, I., Wheller, E., and Alexander, P. (1973): Similarities of the antitumor action of endotoxin, lipid A and double stranded RNA. *Br. J. Cancer,* 27:379–389.
31. Perkins, E. H., and Leonard, M. R. (1963): Specificity of phagocytosis as it may relate to antibody formation. *J. Immunol.,* 90:228–237.
32. Rhodes, J. R. (1975): Macrophage heterogeneity in receptor activity: The activation of macrophage Fc receptor function *in vivo* and *in vitro. J. Immunol.,* 114:976–981.
33. Saunders, J. W. (1966): Death in embryonic systems. Science, 154:604–612.
34. Schuller, G. B., Morahan, P. S., and Snodgrass, M. J. (1975): Inhibition and enhancement of Friend leukemia virus by pyran copolymer. *Cancer Res.,* 35:1915–1920.
35. Stott, E. J., Probert, M., and Thomas, L. H. (1975): Cytotoxicity of alveolar macrophages for virus-infected cells. *Nature,* 255:710.
36. Walker, W. S. (1976): Functional heterogeneity of macrophages. In: *Immunobiology of the Macrophage,* edited by P. S. Nelson, pp. 91–111. Academic Press, New York.

Immune Modulation and Control of Neoplasia by Adjuvant Therapy, edited by M. A. Chirigos. Raven Press, New York, 1978.

Correlation Between Antitumor Activity and Macrophage Activation by Polyanions

Richard M. Schultz, Joseph D. Papamatheakis, and M. A. Chirigos

Lab of RNA Tumor Viruses, National Cancer Institute, National Institutes of Health, Bethesda, Maryland 20014

Macrophages activated by a variety of biologic and synthetic agents appear to have an extremely important, if not critical, role in antineoplastic host defenses. We have recently demonstrated that nonspecific macrophage activation correlates well with the ability of adjuvants to enhance antitumor resistance (16). The rendering of normal, noncytotoxic macrophages tumoricidal is defined here as macrophage activation. There are two separate mechanisms by which resting macrophages are converted to cytotoxic effector cells (Fig. 1): (a) they may be "armed" by a product from specifically sensitized T lymphocytes and activated on subsequent exposure to the appropriate antigen, as is the case for Bacillus Calmette-Guerin (BCG) (10) and *Corynebacterium parvum* (3), and (b) macrophages may be activated by direct exposure to polyanions or lymphokines (MAFs) *in vitro* (1,4,5,14) or *in vivo* (9,16,17).

We have recently shown that pyran copolymer markedly increases resistance of BALB/c mice bearing the Madison lung carcinoma (M109) (15). Systemic treatment with pyran resulted in a prominent histiocytic infiltrate at the tumor site in which macrophages were often associated with necrobiotic tumor cells. Similarly, morphologically activated macrophages that potently arrested DNA synthesis of tumor cells *in vitro* were recovered from pyran-treated animals. The present study further demonstrates the importance of activated macrophages in adjuvant-induced resistance to the M109 lung carcinoma and compares pyran to other polyanions with regard to both systemic antitumor activity and macrophage activation.

MATERIALS AND METHODS

Mice

Male BALB/c and CD2F1 mice, 6 to 8 weeks old, were obtained from the Mammalian Genetics and Animal Production Section, National Institutes of Health, Bethesda, Md. All animals weighed at least 23 g before they were used for experimentation.

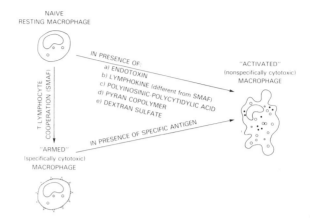

FIG. 1. Pathways whereby macrophages are converted to cytotoxic effector cells. Macrophages may be either directly activated following exposure to polyanions or lymphokine (MAF) *in vitro* or activated when "armed" macrophages encounter the relevant antigen.

Drugs

Pyran NSC-46015, a copolymer of divinyl ether and maleic anhydride, was kindly supplied by D. Breslow, Hercules Research Center, Wilmington, Del. The sodium salts of dextran sulfate and diethylaminoethyl-dextran (DEAE-dextran), each approximately 5×10^5 MW, were obtained from Pharmacia Fine Chemicals, Uppsala, Sweden. Polyinosinic-polycytidylic [poly(I) $\cdot$ poly (C)] acid was purchased from Miles Laboratories, Inc., Elkhart, Ind. The molecular structures of these compounds are given in Fig. 2. Drugs were dissolved in serum-free RPMI-1640 medium and adjusted to pH 7.2 by the addition of 1 N NaOH.

Target Cells

Established cell lines of MBL-2 (H2b[C57B1/6]) murine leukemia and M109 (H2d[BALB/c]) murine alveolar carcinoma cells were maintained in RPMI-1640 medium supplemented with 20% heat-inactivated (56°C, 30 min) fetal calf serum, 100 μg/ml gentamicin solution, 0.075% NaHCO$_3$, and 10 mM HEPES buffer (RPMI-FCS).

Peritoneal Macrophages

Noninduced peritoneal macrophages were harvested and purified by adherence as previously described (17). Representative preparations of purified adherent cells were stained with Giemsa stain; >95% of the cells observed had morphologic characteristics of macrophages. Macrophages were kept in an ice bath prior to use to prevent adherence.

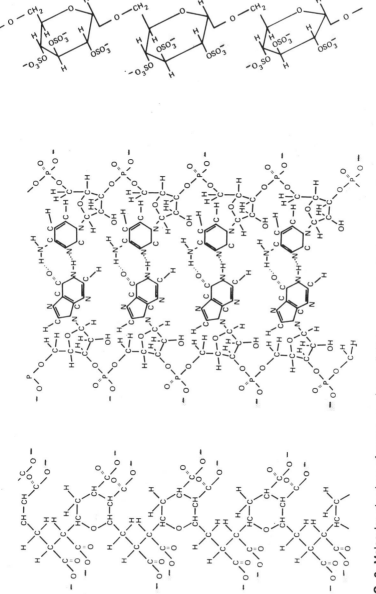

FIG. 2. Molecular structure of pyran copolymer *(left)* is compared with two other polyanions, poly(I) · poly(C) *(center)* and dextran sulfate *(right)*. Note the high density of negative charges that give these polymers their anionic nature.

Tumor Testing

The Madison lung carcinoma (M109), a transplantable line derived from a spontaneous neoplasm in a BALB/c mouse, was kindly supplied by Ruth I. Geran, Drug Research and Development, National Cancer Institute, NIH, Bethesda, Md. For adjuvant studies, 5×10^5 viable M109 cells, suspended in serum-free RPMI-1640 medium, were injected subcutaneously in the right inguinal region of each mouse. Drugs were administered intraperitoneally on day 7 after tumor inoculation. Deaths of mice were recorded daily, and median survival times were calculated. The percent increase in life-span of test groups (T) over control groups (C) inoculated with tumor alone was calculated by (T/C — 1) $\times$ 100. The mean survivals of drug-treated groups in comparison to those of groups receiving 0.9% NaCl solution were evaluated statistically by the Student's t-test.

Test for Activation of Macrophages *In Vivo*

The ability of activated macrophages to diminish target cell proliferation was measured by the inhibition-of-DNA-synthesis (IDS) assay previously described (15). Since macrophages do not proliferate and incorporate significant thymidine under our culture conditions, the IDS assay has proved advantageous in yielding reliable and reproducible results. Briefly, target cells were trypsinized from exponentially growing cultures, resuspended at 5.0×10^4 cells/ml RPMI-FCS, and 2 ml aliquots were placed in 30-mm tissue culture dishes. Purified peritoneal macrophages were adjusted to 1.0×10^6 cells/ml RPMI-FCS, and 1 ml was added to the target cell cultures. DNA synthesis of the target cells was assessed after 20 hr of incubation at 37°C. Triplicate cultures of each set of dishes as well as cultures consisting of tumor cells alone and macrophages alone were pulsed with 2.0 μCi of tritiated thymidine (sp. act. 10 Ci/mmoles) for 2 hr at 37°C. At the end of the incubation, the cells were detached with trypsin, centrifuged at $600 \times g$ for 10 min, and resuspended in 0.5 ml Dulbecco's phosphate-buffered saline. Four milliliters of chilled 10% trichloroacetic acid (TCA) was added to each tube, and precipitation was allowed to go for 30 min at 4°C. The resultant precipitate was collected on glass fiber paper and washed with cold 10% TCA. The filters were air dried and assayed for radioactivity using Aquasol solubilizer (New England Nuclear, Boston, Mass.). The percent specific inhibition of DNA synthesis was calculated by the following formula:

$$\% \text{ Specific inhibition} = \left(\frac{cpm_N - cpm_E}{cpm_N} \right) \times 100$$

where cpm_N = mean counts per min in cultures containing effector cells from normal control mice and where cpm_E = mean counts per min in cultures containing test effector cells.

Test for Direct Macrophage Activation *In Vitro*

The method used for measuring the ability of drugs to produce growth-inhibitory macrophages *in vitro* has previously been described (14). Approximately 1.0×10^6 purified peritoneal macrophages were seeded in 35-mm tissue culture dishes in 1 ml RPMI-FCS. MBL-2 target cells were then adjusted to 5×10^4 cells/ml RPMI-FCS, and 2 ml aliquots were immediately admixed with the macrophage cultures. Drugs were made up in 10X solutions, and 0.3 ml was added to the cell mixtures. Toxicity controls consisting of MBL-2 cells alone in the presence of drug were also included in each experiment. All cultures were maintained in a humidified, 5% CO_2-in-air incubator at 37°C, and viable leukemia cells were counted daily using a hemocytometer. Percent growth inhibition of MBL-2 cells due to macrophage-drug interaction was calculated by comparison to MBL-2 cells grown in the presence of normal macrophages alone.

RESULTS

Association of Antitumor Activity of Polyanions with Macrophage Activation

The synthetic polyanions were tested for systemic antitumor activity against the syngeneic M109 lung carcinoma. The polycation DEAE-dextran was incorporated in this study as a control. Pyran copolymer at 25 mg/kg on day 7 after tumor inoculation was the most significant ($p < 0.001$) at prolonging the median survival time of tumor-bearing mice (Fig. 3A). Poly(I) · poly(C) at 10 mg/kg also had significant antitumor activity ($p < 0.02$), whereas dextran sulfate (25 mg/kg) and DEAE-dextran (25 mg/kg) were without significant effect.

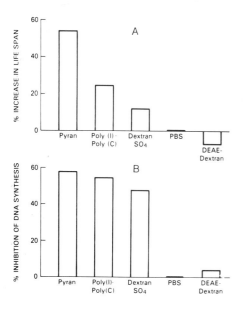

FIG. 3. A: Effect of polyanionic therapy on life-span of mice bearing the M109 lung carcinoma. Tumor cells (5×10^5) were inoculated s.c. into BALB/c mice on day 0. Drugs including pyran (25 mg/kg), poly(I) · poly(C) (10 mg/kg), dextran sulfate (25 mg/kg), and DEAE-dextran (25 mg/kg) were given i.p. on day 7. Experiments involved 10 mice/group. **B:** Effect of polyanion treatment on the cytostatic activity of BALB/c peritoneal macrophages. Drugs at the same dose levels as in **A** were inoculated intraperitoneally on day 0. Macrophages were harvested 6 days later and tested for their ability to inhibit M109 cell DNA synthesis. The values are means obtained from triplicate samples. PBS, Dulbecco's phosphate-buffered saline.

TABLE 1. *Ability of various drugs to activate murine peritoneal macrophages* in vivo

Drug	Growth inhibition at following dose (mg/kg)[a]				
	100	25	10	1	0.1
Pyran copolymer	—	+	++	—	—
Poly (I) · poly (C)	toxic	—	++	+	—
Dextran sulfate	—	+	—	—	—
DEAE-dextran	—	—	—	—	—

[a]Macrophages were harvested 6 days after i.p. drug administration and tested for ability to inhibit M109 cell proliferation. —, Growth inhibition <25%; +, growth inhibition 25–50%; ++, >50% of control value.

These agents were tested under similar conditions for the ability to produce growth-inhibitory macrophages. Peritoneal macrophages were collected 6 days after intraperitoneal administration of drugs and tested against syngeneic M109 target cells (Fig. 3B). All polyanions markedly stimulated ($p < 0.001$) BALB/c macrophages to inhibit M109 DNA synthesis. DEAE-dextran did not activate macrophages and was similarly ineffective in prolonging the life of mice bearing the M109 tumor.

Dose Response of Macrophage Activation *In Vivo* by Polyanions

Further experiments were performed to test the dose dependency of polyanion-induced macrophage activation. Drugs were administered intraperitoneally at doses ranging from 100 to 0.1 mg/kg. Macrophages were harvested on day 6. Activation by polyanions was sharply dose dependent (Table 1). Pyran copolymer and poly(I) · poly(C) treatment produced optimal macrophage stimulation at 10 mg/kg, whereas dextran sulfate required 25 mg/kg. Higher levels of drug were completely inhibitory. DEAE-dextran was without significant effect.

Dose Response of Direct Macrophage Activation *in Vitro* by Polyanions

The drugs were tested for their ability to transform normal resting macrophages into cytostatic effector cells *in vitro* (Table 2). Macrophage activation

TABLE 2. *Ability of various drugs to activate murine peritoneal macrophages* in vitro

Drug	Growth inhibition at 48 hr of (µg/ml)[a]			
	100	10	1	0.1
Pyran copolymer	+	++	—	—
Poly (I) · poly (C)	—	—	++	—
Dextran sulfate	—	+	—	—
DEAE-dextran	Toxic	—	—	—

[a]—, Growth inhibition of MBL-2 target cells <25%; +, between 25 and 50%; ++, >50% of control value.

to inhibit MBL-2 leukemia cell growth was sharply dose dependent. Neither allogeneic macrophages nor drug alone interfered with MBL-2 cell growth. A peak of cytostatic activity was observed for pyran and dextran sulfate at 10 $\mu g/ml$ and poly(I) $\cdot$ poly(C) at 1 $\mu g/ml$. Pyran and poly(I) $\cdot$ poly(C) were much more effective in optimal concentrations than dextran sulfate at producing growth-inhibitory macrophages.

DISCUSSION

Aside from their traditional roles as anticoagulants (12) and inducers of interferon (7,8), systemic polyanion treatment in mice enhances host antitumor resistance and produces multiple effects on the immune response including direct stimulation of B cells (13), enhanced circulating antibody levels (2,17), and direct macrophage activation (14). We have previously shown that systemic pyran therapy against the M109 lung carcinoma resulted in: (a) enhanced macrophage inhibition of tumor cell DNA synthesis, (b) heavy accumulation and infiltration of histiocytes and macrophages at the tumor site, and (c) the association of histiocytes with necrobiotic tumor cells (15). We have found no direct antimitotic activity of pyran for tumor cells, unless the tumor cell cultures contain macrophages. These observations support the concept that pyran enhances host resistance to neoplasia by mobilization and activation of the reticuloendothelial elements of the host's defense. Moreover, results in our laboratory show that trypan blue treatment (a selective macrophage toxin) can completely abrogate pyran's ability to enhance BALB/c resistance against the M109 tumor.

The present study was undertaken to compare pyran with other polyanions for macrophage activation and antitumor activity. The role of activated macrophages as the major effectors of the antitumor resistance induced by both synthetic and biologic immunopotentiators has become increasingly evident (9,16). The cytotoxicity expressed by activated macrophages is purported to be specific for neoplastic, as opposed to normal, cells but is immunologically nonspecific with regard to different tumor cells (6). We report here that macrophages recovered 6 days after intraperitoneal polyanion treatment effectively suppressed DNA synthesis of M109 tumor cells *in vitro;* this activity was sharply dose dependent with supraoptimal levels of drug being completely inhibitory. Moreover, purified cultures of peritoneal macrophages exposed to polyanions *in vitro* were transformed to cytostatic effector cells. This response was similarly dose dependent and allowed for macrophage activation independent of lymphokine. Pyran copolymer and poly(I) $\cdot$ poly(C) were the most effective agents at both producing growth-inhibitory macrophages *in vivo* and *in vitro* and increasing the life-span of syngeneic mice bearing the M109 carcinoma. The polycation DEAE-dextran did not significantly activate macrophages or enhance tumor resistance.

The data presented are consistent with the hypothesis that nonspecifically activated macrophages are involved in resistance to the M109 lung carcinoma by polyanions. Perhaps the most notable polyanion in macrophage activation and enhancement of host resistance to neoplasia is pyran copolymer. Pyran's effect on modulating host immunologic factors, even in an advanced tumor system (15), and its effect on inhibiting metastases (11) strongly support the potential use of pyran copolymer as an adjuvant to conventional tumor treatment modalities.

SUMMARY

Pyran copolymer (NSC-46015), poly(I) · poly(C), and dextran sulfate were studied for their ability to produce growth-inhibitory macrophages and to enhance host resistance against a transplantable, spontaneous murine lung carcinoma (M109). Morphologically activated macrophages were recovered from polyanion-treated animals that potently inhibited DNA synthesis of M109 tumor cells *in vitro*. Moreover, purified cultures of normal resting macrophages were transformed to cytostatic effector cells in the presence of drug. Pyran and poly(I) · poly(C) were the most effective drugs at enhancing macrophage function, and both *in vivo* and *in vitro* activation were highly dose dependent. Similarly, systemic pyran and poly(I) · poly(C) therapy significantly increased the life-span of mice bearing the M109 tumor. The resistance to neoplasia induced by these agents appears to result from direct activation of the reticuloendothelial elements of the host's defense.

REFERENCES

1. Alexander, P., and Evans, R. (1971): Endotoxin and double stranded RNA render macrophages cytotoxic. *Nature [New Biol.]*, 232:76–78.
2. Braun, W., Regelson, W., Yasima, Y., and Ishizuka, M. (1970): Stimulation of antibody formation by pyran copolymer. *Proc. Soc. Exp. Biol. Med.*, 133:171–175.
3. Christie, G. H., and Bomford, R. (1975): Mechanisms of macrophage activation by *Corynebacterium parvum*. 1. *In vivo* experiments. *Cell. Immunol.*, 17:141–149.
4. Churchill, W. H., Piessens, W. F., Sulis, C. A., and David, J. R. (1975): Macrophages activated as suspension cultures with lymphocyte mediators devoid of antigen become cytotoxic for tumor cells. *J. Immunol.*, 115:781–786.
5. Fidler, I. J., Darnell, J. H., and Budmen, M. B. (1976): Tumoricidal properties of mouse macrophages activated with mediators from rat lymphocytes stimulated with concanavalin A. *Cancer Res.*, 36: 3608–3615.
6. Hibbs, J. B. (1974): Discrimination between neoplastic and nonneoplastic cells *in vitro* by activated macrophages. *J. Natl. Cancer Inst.*, 53:1487–1492.
7. Merigan, T. C. (1967): Induction of circulating interferon by synthetic anionic polymers of known composition. *Nature*, 214:416–417.
8. Merigan, T. C., and Finkelstein, M. S. (1968): Interferon–stimulating and *in vivo* antiviral effects of various synthetic anionic polymers. *Virology*, 35:363–374.
9. Morahan, P. S., and Kaplan, A. M. (1976): Macrophage activation and antitumor activity of biologic and synthetic agents. *Int. J. Cancer*, 17:82–89.
10. North, R. J. (1974): T-cell dependence of macrophage activation and mobilization during infection with *Mycobacterium tuberculosis*. *Infect. Immun.*, 10:66–71.
11. Papamatheakis, J. D., Chirigos, M. A., and Schultz, R. M. (1978): Effect of dose, route, and timing of pyran copolymer therapy against the Madison lung carcinoma *(This volume)*.
12. Regelson, W. (1974): The antimitotic activity of polyanions: Heparin and heparinoids. *J. Med. (Basel)*, 5:50–68.

13. Ruhl, H., Vogt, W., Bochert, G., Schmidt, S., and Diamanstein, T. (1973): Stimulation of mouse lymphoid cells by polyanions *in vitro.* In: *Lymphocyte Recognition and Effector Mechanisms,* edited by K. Lindahl-Kiessling and D. Osoba, pp. 31–37. Academic Press, New York.

14. Schultz, R. M., Papamatheakis, J. D., and Chirigos, M. A. (1977): Direct activation *in vitro* of mouse peritoneal macrophages by pyran copolymer (NSC 46015). *Cell. Immunol.,* 29:403–409.

15. Schultz, R. M., Papamatheakis, J. D., Luetzeler, J., Ruiz, P., and Chirigos, M. A. (1977): Macrophage involvement in the protective effect of pyran copolymer against the Madison lung carcinoma (M109). *Cancer Res.,* 37:358–364.

16. Schultz, R. M., Papamatheakis, J. D., Stylos, W. A., and Chirigos, M. A. (1976): Augmentation of specific macrophage-mediated cytotoxicity: Correlation with agents which enhance antitumor resistance. *Cell. Immunol.,* 25:309–316.

17. Schultz, R. M., Woods, W. A., Mohr, S. J., and Chirigos, M. A. (1976): Immune response of BALB/c × DBA/2 F_1 mice to a tumor allograft during pyran copolymer-induced tumor enhancement. *Cancer Res.,* 36:1641–1646.

Immune Modulation and Control of Neoplasia by Adjuvant Therapy, edited by M. A. Chirigos. Raven Press, New York, 1978.

Clinical Study of the Synthetic Polyanion Pyran Copolymer (NSC 46015, Diveema) and Its Role in Future Clinical Trials

[1]W. Regelson, [2]B. I. Shnider, [3]J. Colsky, [4]K. B. Olson, [5]J. F. Holland, [1]C. L. Johnston, Jr., and [6]L. H. Dennis

[1]*Medical College of Virginia, Virginia Commonwealth University, Richmond, Virginia 23298;* [2]*Georgetown University, School of Medicine, Georgetown University Medical Division, D.C. General Hospital, Washington, D.C. 20003;* [3]*Cedars of Lebanon Hospital, Miami, Florida 33136;* [4]*810 Oak View Drive, New Smyrna Beach, Florida 32069;* [5]*Mt. Sinai Hospital, New York, New York 10029; and* [6]*831 University Boulevard, Silver Spring, Maryland 20903*

Pryan copolymer (NSC 46015, Diveema) is parenterally active against a variety of transplanted, viral, and carcinogen-induced tumors. These have included CA 755, Lewis lung (27–29,36,50,51,56,61), B16 melanoma (51), Ehrlich carcinoma (36), Friend leukemia (36,77,82–84,91), Rauscher leukemia (26,36,66), Dunning ascites leukemia (36), L1210 leukemia (47–49,90), C3H mammary tumor transplants (90), methylcholanthrene-derived transplants (32) and dimethylbenzanthracene (DMBA)-induced tumors (17), LSTRA sarcoma (66), Madison lung carcinoma (63), and prostatic adenocarcinoma in the rat (14). Pyran prevents polyoma-induced tumors and Rauscher leukemia in thymectomized mice (26) and DMBA-induced tumors in the hamster cheek pouch (17).

Pyran induces interferon in both man and mouse (40–43,77), but antitumor and antiviral activity does not correlate with interferon induction (23,76,85). Interestingly, pyran can both stimulate and inhibit host immune response (2–6, 9,31,76) and alter *in vitro* lymphoblastic response to lipopolysaccharide (LPS) or phytohemagglutinin (PHA) (2–6). Pyran inhibits the early cation dependent steps of complement activity (39,101). Pyran can prevent adjuvant-induced arthritis (31), and its effects on skin graft survival are controversial.

Toxicologically, the clinically tested pyran fraction (NSC 46015) interferes with liver microsomal enzyme hydrolysis (10,59,60,102), causes hepatosplenomegaly (76,85) and anemia, increases sensitivity to endotoxin lethality (57), and prevents fibrin formation (16,69,87,94). Clinical pyran accelerates the removal of plutonium bound to liver (24,35). Toxicology and the antiviral and immune modulating effects of pyran relate to its molecular weight. The role of molecular weight of pyran fractions has been reviewed in several articles (10,52–54,61, 62,71–76,79–81).

Pyran's antitumor action can be related to macrophage activation (2–5,27, 28,50,51,56,74,79–81) in mice, and antiviral action may be based on similar mechanisms (30,55).

Clinical samples of pyran initially inhibit phagocytic clearance of colloidal particulates followed by a later stimulation (10,52,54,56,58,61,62,71–73,75, 76,79–81,83,85,86). Pyran also enhances resistance to staphylococcal, pneumococcal, and cryptococcal infection (58,76,83,86). Resistance to cryptococcal lethality does not relate to phagocytic stimulation, whereas antibacterial resistance is only seen during the period of increased phagocytosis.

Of clinical importance is the potential adjuvant action of pyran copolymer in enhancing antiviral vaccine activity (11) and prolonged antitumor activity at nontoxic concentrations following chemotherapeutic response (47–49,66, 92,93).

In this clinical study, pyran was evaluated in a Phase I–Phase II intravenous effort to establish its tolerance and potential as an antitumor agent.

Our clinical study began in 1966 but was delayed at intervals because of supply problems related to providing similar molecular weight samples and evidence of increasing toxicity on shelf storage of the sterile hydrolyzed lyophilized salt. In 1971, a new formulation was tested in which pyran was provided in sterile ampules as the anhydride given following sterile water or saline dilution as the freshly hydrolyzed material. This proved too toxic for continued clinical trial.

Clinical study has determined that the consistent limiting toxicity of pyran is transient thrombocytopenia. However, leukopenia can accompany thrombocytopenia but is a less constant although equally reversible finding. Cytoplasmic inclusions are seen in circulating leukocytes, nucleated marrow cells, and phagocytic cells of liver and spleen after pyran administration. Although not dose limiting, fever is seen in 50% of patients despite the absence of pyrogen on rabbit test (19). In addition, fever can develop in the absence of shaking chills.

In an independent pediatric study of pyran's antiviral action against Dawson's encephalitis: hemolysis, helmet cell (schizontocyte) formation, and reversible renal failure were seen (33). Two of three patients in this study also developed transient maculopapular eruptions following a single injection, which was not seen in our more extensive study. However, hypotension, seizure activity, transient blindness and death have been seen as unpredictable side effects, particularly when pyran was given too rapidly as an intravenous push in the study reported here. More recently, this toxicity appears to be a consistent consequence of utilization of the freshly hydrolyzed anhydride rather than the earlier lyophilized hydrolyzed formulation previously used. Immediate anticoagulant effects were seen at higher dosage, but hemorrhage was never seen and was not a limiting factor in drug administration. In single dosage trial, pyran as the hydrolyzed salt was given to four adults at 18 mg/kg without toxicity despite potent anticoagulant action (16).

Significant antitumor action lasting 3 months was seen in one patient with ovarian cancer, but our study was limited to a predominantly inpatient preterminal population, and evaluation of any single tumor type was inadequate.

Pyran has some superficial resemblance to the synthetic polynucleotide poly rI:rC (1,52–54), which has shown no activity in man attributable to its rapid degradation by serum ribonucleases. Newer stabilized polynucleotides as well as glucans (15) have been clinically evaluated, and one should assume from animal data and our clinical experience with pyran that toxicity for these new reticulo-endothelial stimulating agents might be similar.

CHEMISTRY AND TOXICOLOGY

Pyran copolymer[1] is a typical anhydride which, in the presence of water, becomes hydrolyzed to the corresponding carboxylic acid. The active tumor inhibitory agent is the polycarboxylic hydrolyzed material, and in this it resembles other anionic polyelectrolytes which have shown antitumor, antiviral, and enzyme inhibitory activity (61,62,71–73).

The initial clinical as well as all the animal toxicity studies were done with the lyophilized hydrolysate of pyran. Of interest, the initial animal toxicity studies were performed with material of average 30,000 molecular weight (MW) while the clinical studies (NSC 46015) were done with pyran of average 18,000 or 23,000 MW.

Preclinical pharmacology (36) showed that the acute intraperitoneal LD_{50} in mouse and rat were 106 mg/kg and 12 mg/kg, respectively. In dogs, 64 mg/kg given i.v. at 30 min-intervals for 7 hr was necessary before death ensued. Retching, tremor, respiratory slowing, and weakness occurred immediately postinjection.

In chronic toxicity studies in dogs, the median lethal dose was estimated to be between 16 and 32 mg/kg/day. Weight loss appeared at 4 mg/kg at about the 15th day. Melena was observed at 8, 16, or 32 mg/kg/day i.v., and jaundice and emaciation were noted in all dogs studied. At 8 and 16 mg/kg, peripheral edema and ascites, accompanied by jaundice, were seen by the third week. Interestingly, none of these side effects was observed in man.

In relation to the above, the livers of dogs and monkeys receiving 4 mg/kg showed focal cloudy swelling and central necrosis. In addition, a reduction of hepatic glycogen and fatty metamorphosis was observed in the monkeys. In dogs, liver function (SGOT and BSP) was the most sensitive indicator of toxic effects, and SGOT elevations were obtained in every dog at dosages greater than 2 mg/kg. A return to normal, however, occurred in 28 days, following discontinuation of the drug. None of this was seen in man, even at a dosage as high as 18 mg/kg!

In relation to kidney changes, NPN or BUN values rose in all dogs and

---

[1] Pyran copolymer (NSC 46015), pyran-3,4 dicarboxylic anhydride, tetra-hydro-2-methyl-6-(tetrahydro 2,5-dixo,3-furyl)-polymer is provided by Hercules (Wilmington, Delaware) through the Cancer Chemotherapy National Service Center.

monkeys at 16 mg/kg. These BUN elevations fell to normal in 3/3 monkeys within 2 weeks of discontinuation of treatment. Based on this, it is not surprising that the Stanford group noted transient renal failure in one patient at 16 mg/kg (33). However, as mentioned previously, this was not seen in our study at lower dosages or in adults with single dosage as high as 18 mg/kg of the hydrolyzed lyophilized salt.

In monkeys, edema at the site of intravenous injection was seen despite evidence that no infiltration occurred. Ascites was not seen and emaciation was slower to develop as compared to the dog. Of interest, prolonged (2 hr) infusion in the dog did not significantly differ from acute intravenous injection in relation to overall toxicity, which differed from what we saw clinically. This also differs from animal toxicology with related ethylene maleic anhydride copolymers where ascites was a consistent toxicity in dogs (44).

Anemia and lymphoid involution of bone marrow and spleen occurred at 8 mg/kg or 16 mg/kg in dogs and monkeys. In dogs, leukocytosis was common, but leukopenia was seen in one of 21 dogs tested and not at all in 15 monkeys studied.

Thrombocytopenia was seen in dogs, but there was no correlation between the degrees of platelet fall and the dose of drug administered. Thrombocytopenia developed on the average of 20 days posttreatment and occurred at all dose levels.

Mice showed significant increases in liver and splenic weight following pyran administration which is associated with the loss of splenic germinal centers and increased macrophage activity in liver and spleen. Mice also showed anemia, SGOT elevation, and enhanced sensitivity to the lethal action of endotoxin, as well as inhibition of type I (hexobarbital) and type II (aminopyrene) drug metabolism (54,58–61,72,79–81,102).

Following single intraperitoneal pyran administration in mice, cytoplasmic inclusions are seen (77,86) in monocytes and polymorphonuclear leukocytes of the peripheral blood as early as 48 hr later. Similar inclusions are seen in histiocytes of liver and spleen. These inclusions are similar to those reported for tilorone and related interferon inducers, including atabrine (21,34,89,100).

CLINICAL STUDIES

In the initial Phase I study, pyran copolymer was given to advanced cancer patients no longer responsive to other treatment. For study, survival had to be estimated at 1 month, and patients had to be off other forms of chemotherapy or radiotherapy for at least 2 weeks without signs of marrow depression or active sepsis and liver disease.

For this initial study, pyran copolymer (NSC 46015) was provided in sterile 20 ml vials containing 0.1 mg of the lyophilized hydrolysate. It was stored in the refrigerator at 4–10°C until use. When reconstituted with 20 ml of water for injection, a solution resulted, with a pH of 7.7, which contained 5 mg/ml of drug. Drug was kept in the refrigerator at all times until use and was discarded if not given within 24 hr. In all cases, pyran was given as a 1-hr infusion in 100 cc of saline.

In the initial study, pyran copolymer was given for 36 courses to 29 patients. Twenty-three of these courses were given at doses below 4 mg/kg; the starting dose was 0.015 mg/kg with the highest single dose given of 16 mg/kg. Drug was given daily for up to 62 days with a median treatment period of 14 days.

The major limiting toxicity of this Phase I study was thrombocytopenia which appeared in all patients at a dose of 8 mg/kg or higher and was noted in three of eight patients at 4.0 mg/kg and in one patient at a dose as low as 0.2 mg/kg.

Thrombocytopenia could be seen as early as 24 hr postdrug, and was observed in 15 of 29 patients at all dosages used. Leukopenia between 3 to 5,000/mm^3 accompanying thrombocytopenia was seen in 5 to 36 courses with similar onset and recovery.

The median onset of thrombocytopenia was 13 days for a range of 1 to 28 days. The time of onset of thrombocytopenia was not always dose related; one patient showed thrombocytopenia at 0.2 mg/kg/day in 3 days whereas one group of 3 patients at 12 mg/kg/day showed their onset of significant platelet depression at 13, 18, and 23 days.

Platelet counts were usually done 24 hr after drug administration, but a significant platelet fall could be seen before 24 to 48 hr. This was observed in half the patients, studied at 12, 15, and 18 mg/kg following single dose (16). Platelets recovered in all patients within 24 to 48 hr following discontinuation of drug, and no serious hemorrhage was related to platelet depression. Similar results were seen by Leavitt et al. (33) in their use of pyran in children with Dawson's encephalitis at 16 mg/kg/day.

The nonlimiting toxicity seen was chills and/or fever >101°F which was observed in 10 of 13 patients at doses of 8 mg/kg or higher. Fever could reach a peak of 104°F, but subsided within 24 to 48 hr following drug discontinuation. Fever was not necessarily associated with platelet depression; however, 11 of 13 pyrexic patients at a dosage of 8 mg/kg or greater showed thrombocytopenia. The onset of fever and/or chills was within 6 hr postpyran but was also observed as early as 2 to 4 hr after drug. Fever usually occurred with the first dose given and recurred thereafter, but it could be observed for the first time as late as 9 to 13 days after administration of the first dose. In occasional patients, chills and/or fever was associated with anxiety and precardial oppression, and in one patient with a past history of angina, pyran appeared to precipitate a severe anginal attack with myocardial infarction.

Following the above initial experience, a total of 33 patients were given pyran, 12 mg/kg/day, in a Phase II study. This program included patients with measurable disease, but it was apparent from patient accrual data that essentially only preterminal patients were studied. Evaluation was further complicated by the exhaustion of the initial supply of ampuled pyran and the need for a new clinical supply from the original synthesized material. New material was also synthesized because of observations in mice that prolonged shelf storage decreased therapeutic index.

For this Phase II population, the duration of study lasted 1 to 29 days, for a median study period of 9 days. However, eight patients received pyran for 2 days or less. Of 22 patients with dates of death recorded, death occurred within 1 to 102 days postpyran for a median survival of 16 days from the onset of the pyran study. In all but one patient, death was not associated with side effects that could be related to the drug.

Of the patients studied, only three were children and all but one were above the age of 40 for a median age of 58. More than half the patients had been given single or multiple trials of chemotherapy before receiving pyran.

Among these 33 patients in the Phase II study, total dosage ranged from 350 to 33,000 mg for a median total dose of 3,000 mg. Ten of these patients showed significant platelet fall >50% of starting value with three patients showing values <120,000/mm³ but greater than 90,000/mm³ while six had platelet depression <90,000/mm³. The lowest platelet value was 5,000/mm³. Recovery of platelets following pyran's discontinuation occurred in 2 to 5 days.

Nine patients showed leukopenia with white blood cell count (WBC) <5,000/mm³. The lowest WBC seen was 1,900/mm³, while the median fall in white count was to 3,500/mm³. Leukopenia was seen in association with thrombocytopenia in 5 of 10 cases and, as was true for platelet recovery, return to normal occurred in 2 to 5 days. Not enough differentials were recorded to define the character of the leukopenia but it appeared to be a pancytopenia.

Interestingly, fever was not seen as frequently in this Phase II portion of the study, and leukopenia was not as striking during the earlier Phase I study.

An additional group of six patients received pyran twice a week (biw), while five received it on a weekly basis at dosages ranging from 600 to 9,100 mg total dose. Of those receiving pyran b.i.w., four showed a significant platelet fall, two to lows of 28,000/mm³ which, in contrast to daily administration, took 3 weeks to return to normal in one case. No patient receiving pyran on a single weekly basis had a significant platelet fall, but two of these patients at 2 and 8 weeks showed a fall in WBC to values just under 5,000/mm³.

In relation to cardiovascular toxicity, three patients on pyran showed transient hypotension immediately after infusion, and one patient with chills, tachycardia, and anxiety showed a transient "mottled cyanosis" of his lower extremities. One patient suffered an anginal episode, and another showed confusion, somnolence, and seizure activity on the 23rd day at the lower dosage of 4 mg/kg/day. Repeat treatment after 14 days, however, was without similar effect. There were five cases of more serious side effects described below, three of which were observed among seven patients in our final study using the freshly hydrolyzed anhydride formulation.

Case Reports of Severe (Acute) Toxicity

Case # 1. A 10-year-old neuroblastoma patient was treated with pyran following failure of radiation, vincristine, and cytoxan. At the time of pyran administration he showed evidence of CNS metastasis with papilledema, tinnitus, double vision, and frequent vomiting. He was on prednisone for cerebral edema and was given 12 mg/kg of pyran for a 1-hr infusion. Midway through the infusion (180 mg), however, he developed severe headache, numbness, and weakness of extremities. Pyran was discontinued and 20 min later he complained of difficulty in seeing out of his left eye and stated that his "joints hurt." Within 30 min he was feeling so much better that his initial reaction to the drug was thought to be "hysterical." However, 35 min later (65 min from drug discontinuation) tonic-clonic seizure developed with complete loss of responsiveness, a spontaneous trousseau reaction, trismus, and bilateral Babinskis followed by flaccid paralysis of all extremities. Recovery was rapid, but repeated "seizure" episodes occurred irregularly during a 1-hr period. "Seizures" were of momentary duration and decreasing severity, and the entire episode was followed by complete lucidity and recovery 1 hr after onset. The patient did not complain of visual loss and fell asleep.

The next day his visual acuity was seriously diminished bilaterally. He was unable to distinguish fingers and faces at two feet, but this gradually and completely improved spontaneously in 2 days. Despite visual loss, there were no eyeground changes accountable for the change!

Blood calcium was 17.4 mg at the time of the initial seizure episode and his platelet count was normal but fell to 27,000/mm^3 2 days later, returning to 70,000/mm^3 in 10 days. His blood calcium was normal 24 hr following the above episode.

He was subsequently treated with repeat radiation to the skull, combined with vincristine and cytoxan, and expired some 3 months later of his disease.

Case # 2. A 44-year-old male with carcinoma of the base of the tongue received pyran on a single weekly basis of 12 mg/kg for 675 mg for each dose of the freshly hydrolyzed anhydride formulation. By error, pyran was given as a 15-min saline infusion (100 ml) instead of the usual 1-hr infusion. Following this the patient complained of marked general weakness, numbness in hands and feet, and pain in his abdomen and back. These symptoms subsided within 1 to 2 hr, but his BP dropped to 60/50 and remained at these levels for 24 hr followed by spontaneous recovery.

During the hypotensive period his only complaints were somnolence and weakness. Subsequently, he was given pyran as a weekly 2 hr infusion and he no longer showed these symptoms. Of note, he also showed marked facial edema first seen at 2 hr postpyran infusion which persisted for 24 hr and was seen with each course. Pyran was discontinued after 8 weeks with no clinical improvement although the drug was initially continued, despite the initial toxicity, because of a clinical impression of a significant regression of tumor (>50%) not confirmed by subsequent measurement.

Case # 3. In a case similar to the pediatric patient with neuroblastoma, a 24-year-old male with a mesothelial sarcoma of the peritoneum was given pyran, 12 mg/kg for 960 mg of the freshly prepared anhydride. His problem was one of partial intestinal obstruction and hemorrhagic ascites related to a peritoneal tumor. Following two single daily doses of pyran, he complained of nausea, faintness, and diarrhea accompanied by a mild fever to 102°. Pyran was withheld for 1 week after which a repeat course at the same dose was given. Thirty minutes postinfusion he had a severe episode of faintness and nausea with dimming and blurring of vision. His BP showed a moderate fall to 95/65 which was not related to hemorrhage as his hemoglobin and hematocrit were stable, as were his platelets and blood calcium. His ocular fundi showed no change, and in 8 hr his vision was back to normal with full recovery from symptoms. Due to his disease, however, he died of intestinal obstruction within a week.

Case # 4. In another episode, a 47-year-old woman with a metastatic carcinoma of the liver from an unknown primary was treated with the anhydride pyran formulation following failure of 5-FU and cytoxan. One eye was missing secondary to previous trauma.

She was started on pyran with a dose of 648 mg (12 mg/kg) and the next morning awoke complaining of loss of vision in her remaining eye. This was associated with progressive hypotension and fall in hemoglobin from 10 to 6 mg but no observable change in eyegrounds or evident hemorrhage or jaundice. She expired in shock 29 hr after her single dose of pyran.

Her platelets the day of death were 87,000/mm^3 from the previous day's value of 137,000/mm^3. Again, there was no gross evidence of bleeding although prothrombin concentration was 20%. Transfusions were unable to maintain effective circulating blood volume, and this patient has to be considered a drug death. Unfortunately, an autopsy was not obtained.

Other toxic changes after pyran administration have been seen in two patients who developed soreness of the mouth, cheilosis, and depapillation of the tongue at 9 and 40 days after starting the drug in the earlier Phase I study. Lymphocytosis was seen in one 2-year-old child with neuroblastoma who during 21 days of pyran administration at 6 mg/kg showed a lymphocyte differential increase from 30 to 97% with no significant change in the total WBC. Thrombocytopenia, 5.0 to 34,000/mm^3 was present at the onset of study secondary to marrow replacement, but no hemorrhage was seen during the treatment period. Similarly, a patient with chronic myelocytic leukemia, in an acute blastic crisis, who received pyran at 6 mg/kg with platelets 50,000/mm^3 at onset of study had no bleeding or significant effect on a rising WBC. One patient with acute myeloblastic leukemia showed nuclear inclusions in her myeloblasts in addition to the usual cytoplasmic basophilic inclusions following one dose of pyran, but no significant changes in status occurred and death ensued after 6 days. These inclusions are similar to what has been seen most recently in astrocytes following heat trauma to the skull during tilorone administration (33).

Where looked for, cytoplasmic inclusions could be found within 2 weeks of drug administration in the peripheral white blood cells of all patients receiving 8 mg/kg day or higher.

A selected number of patients under treatment with pyran copolymer had bone marrow examination as part of a blind study. Bone marrow specimens were sent to clinical pathology without specification of patient's treatment. It was noted that there was increased histiocytic (marrow macrophage) activity. This was not quantified but, in comparative study, was greater than: 1. in bone marrow of the same patients prior to pyran treatment, 2. in patients with known metastatic tumor not receiving such treatment, and 3. in material from patients whose marrows were examined for nontumor conditions. This increased histiocytic activity was manifested by increased phagocytosis of both nucleated and nonnucleated hematopoietic cells. However, the striking feature was the presence of large amounts of reddish-purple basophilic or metachromatically appearing material in the cytoplasm of all nucleated marrow elements. These cytoplasmic inclusions were spherical or globular in form. The typical intracellular appearance is illustrated by Figs. 1–4 obtained from two patients, one with poorly differentiated squamous cell carcinoma of the lung and the other with an acute myelocytic luekemia.

Phagocytized material was easily seen in macrophages in both low and high power views, and the basophilic or metachromatic material bears superficial resemblance to mucopolysaccharide but was not identified by more extensive cytochemical staining.

In summary, combining both Phase I and Phase II studies, 39 patients received more than two doses of pyran at 12 mg/kg. Their cancers included: 11 epidermoid carcinoma of the lung, 8 head and neck epidermoid tumors, 7 sarcomas (undifferentiated 3), 2 stomach adenocarcinomas, 2 neuroblastomas, and one each of ovary, uterus, cervix, colon, esophagus, and parotid. Included among these 39 patients are seven who received the more recent anhydride rather than the earlier hydrolysate lyophilized formulation.

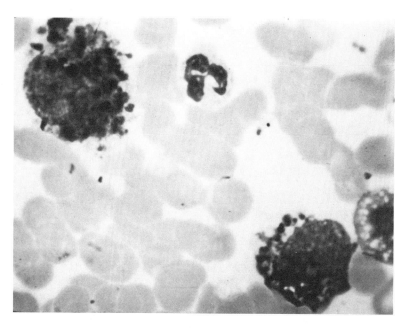

FIG. 1. Cancer of the lung patient. Marrow sample showing clumping cell "debris" and basophilic inclusions.

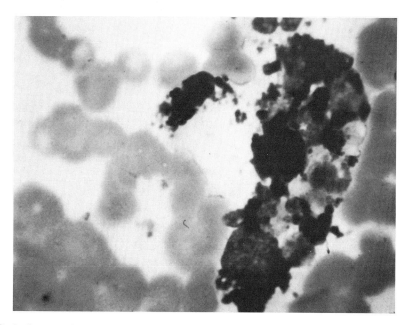

FIG. 2. Cancer of the lung patient showing clumped cells surrounded by extruded debris that may make up the material found in the cytoplasm of isolated cells.

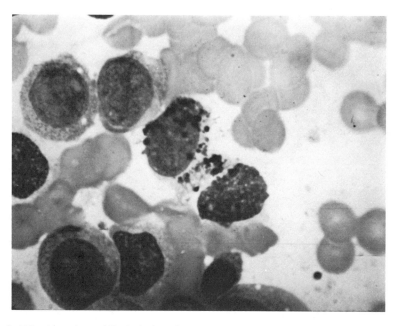

FIG. 3. This shows basophilic inclusions in marrow of acute myelocytic leukemia. One can make a case for its nuclear origin.

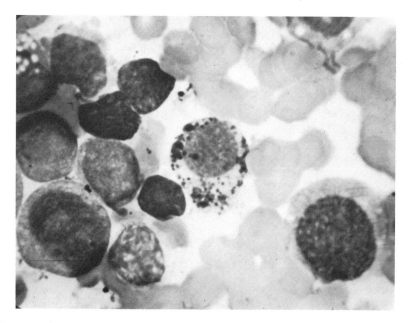

FIG. 4. This shows changes found in acute myeloblastic leukemic marrow that suggest cytoplastic inclusions might derive from the nucleus.

The newer formulation of pyran was used in the last seven patients in our series where pyran was prepared and stored in sterile ampules as the anhydride rather than the hydrolyzed salt. The anhydride was dissolved in saline and utilized immediately, given as with the other preparation in 100 cc of saline. Before dilution, the pH of this preparation is 2.4, but despite the low pH no pain was seen on i.v. administration. Sclerosis appears to be a problem on repeated administration of this preparation. Buffering in sodium bicarbonate and plasma has been tried and may be an alternative way to give it, but acute toxic reactions in two of seven patients precluded further testing. We are concerned about pyran's administration in human plasma. When pyran was given to mice in their own serum, its toxicity was significantly increased. In clinicial trial with this freshly hydrolyzed preparation, three of seven patients (Case #2–4) showed serious hypotension as reported. In two of these, hypotension occurred before visual loss was seen.

In relation to antitumor response, only one patient had clear improvement of subjective and objective disease related to pyran administration.

Case Report of Tumor Response

Case #5. This was a 53-year-old white female with a pseudomyxomatous carcinoma of the ovary.

One year following palliative resection, partial obstruction and ascites developed with failure of sequential systemic trials of 5-fluorouracil, methotrexate, and mitomycin C, as well as local thiotepa and atabrine into recurrent ascites. The patient suffered from hematemesis and had complete intestinal obstruction. She was considered preterminal and maintained on hyperalimentation via inferior vena caval catheter. A trial of the new clinical supply of pyran as the freshly hydrolyzed anhydride was given. She received a test dose of 400 mg followed by 600 mg (12 mg/kg), given b.i.w., which she received for 1 month with marked clinical improvement indicated by a decrease in ascites and in the volume of her abdominal masses. Within 1 month she was able to take fluids by mouth for the first time and no longer required transfusions and hyperalimentation. From a completely bed-fast existence, she was able to sit in a chair, watch television, and return home on weekend passes.

However, after the first month, further treatment was curtailed because of sclerosis of blood vessels, and we were cautious about continuing further trial because acute hypotension and visual losses had been seen in other patients.

She died with respiratory infection and reappearance of abdominal obstruction 4 months after the onset of pyran treatment. In summary, 1 month after b.i.w. pyran as the freshly administered hydrolysate, there was subjective and objective improvement in this ovarian cancer patient, but this was limited to 3 months of her remaining existence.

CLOTTING STUDIES

Patients selected were those with advanced cancer not demonstrating significant liver involvement and exhibiting a normal coagulation profile which included normal prothrombin time, activated partial thromboplastin time, normal thrombin time, bleeding time, and platelet counts.

Pyran was given to the same patient on three successive days in increasing doses where tolerated. Doses of 12, 15, and 18 mg/kg were administered over 30 to 60 min in saline infusions as outlined in the original clinical protocol. Base-line coagulation studies included prothrombin time (Quick), activated partial thromboplastin time (Landgell), thrombin time (Dennis and Conrad), platelet count (Brecher and Cronkite), and bleeding time (Ivy). Platelet count, euglobulin lysis time, and other clotting studies were obtained immediately prior to and at 30 and 180 min after pyran infusion.

Nine patients were studied at 12 mg/kg, seven at 15 mg/kg, and four at 18 mg/kg. These studies revealed that acutely following the intravenous infusion, there was a marked prolongation of the one-stage prothrombin time, the activated partial thromboplastin time, and thrombin time. One patient showed shortened euglobulin lysis time 180 min after pyran administration. Changes occurred in bleeding time, platelet count, and thrombin time of patients receiving 12 and 15 mg/kg of pyran copolymer.

This study suggested that pyran was able to interfere with all three stages of blood coagulation including the formation of thromboplastin, the activation of thrombin, and the interaction of thrombin and fibrinogen to form fibrin. As mentioned earlier, significant thrombocytopenia ($<50\%$ of initial platelet level) was noted during these rapid serial determinations, but no clinical bleeding was encountered with pyran administration despite a mild increase in bleeding time.

In one patient an attempt was made to see if *in vitro* anticoagulant effects could correlate with *in vivo* action. *In vitro* anticoagulant activity of the patient's blood was titrated with increasing quantities of pyran. This was contrasted to *in vivo* coagulation studies where following preinfusion base-line studies, 600 mg of pyran (12 mg/kg of the lyophilized hydrolyzed material) was given in a 2-hr infusion, and clotting (Lee-White) and prothrombin time (Quick) was

TABLE 1. *Titration of pyran clotting effects in man*

Results			
In vitro titration			
mg NSC 46015/ml blood			Clotting time (min)
0			5.5
0.08			7.0
0.16			9.5
0.24			16.8
0.32			27.5
0.40			∞
In vivo anticoagulant			
	Clotting time	Prothrombin time	mg 46015[a]/ml blood
Preinfusion	5.5	13.3	0
Postinfusion	9.5	19.2	0.2

[a] Estimated.
Approximately 3,000 ml blood volume.
600 mg of 46015 infused.

TABLE 2. In vitro and in vivo study of pyran on clotting and blood parameters in the dog[a]

mg XA124-177/ml blood	Lee-White clotting time
0.	6.5
0.05	8.5
0.10	12.5
0.20	13.5
0.30	20.5
0.50	33.0
1.00	∞

Time	ml/inf[b]	mg/inf[b]	mg/inf/kg[b]	mg/ml blood	Sed. rate (mm/hr)	Lee-White clot time	Prothrombin time (sec)	HCT	WBC mm³	Hb g%
0	0	0	0	0	21	6.5	8.2	42	7,350	12.8
15	11.5	115	11.5	0.16	8	7.5	8.3	44	7,400	13.2
30	22.9	229	22.9	0.32	9	7.5	8.2	44	4,500	12.4
45	34.3	343	34.3	0.47	9	8.0	7.6	50	3,050	13.6
60	45.8	458	45.8	0.63	10	8.5	7.9	51	2,550	14.0
90	68.8	688	68.8	0.95	8	8.5	8.0	50	4,300	14.7
120	91.7	917	91.7	1.26	8	9.0	8.6	50	3,400	14.2

[a] Dog XA-124-177 #1, 10 kg, Beagle.
[b] Rate of infusion was 0.764 ml/min of 10 mg/ml.

TABLE 3. Effect of pyran copolymers on blood clotting time in DBA2 female mice

Polymer number	Clotting time (min) [a,b]
Control (8)	3.4 ± 0.2
XA124–177 (5)	
25 mg/kg i.v.	3.7 ± 0.3
X17525–67–1 (8)	
100 mg/kg i.v.	3.8 ± 0.2

[a] Mean ± SE of clotting times in mice given either 0.2 ml of 0.15 M NaCl or the pyran copolymer 5 min before clotting time determination.

[b] Blood collected by cardiac puncture and clotting time determined on 0.5 ml of blood.

determined before and after pyran administration. The patient weighed 45 kg and had an estimated 3 liters of blood.

Table 1 shows *in vitro* and *in vivo* results of this study. Based on this comparison, it was estimated that approximately 0.2 mg/ml of pyran was present in blood following 2 hr of pyran infusion to a total dose of 600 mg. There was an approximate doubling of *in vivo* clotting time during this period (see Table 1).

Interestingly, two dogs studied in similar fashion did not show the same correlation between intravenous infusion and *in vitro* effects (Table 2). Further, despite more rapid (stat intravenous) infusion of pyran at higher dosage to both mouse and dogs as compared to what was done clinically in man, mice clotting time showed absolutely no effect despite infusion of 25 mg/kg and 100 mg/kg of two different fractions of pyran of similar MW to the NSC 46015 clinical material (Table 3).

Of additional interest (see Table 2) was pyran copolymer's distinct effect on the sedimentation rate in both dogs studied, with decreases from 43 to 9 in one dog and 21 to 8 in another. Unfortunately, this interesting observation was not studied in man.

Other physiologic parameters studied in the dog included hematocrit, hemoglobin, and white count determination. Heart rate and blood pressure were also monitored with no visible change, although it had been observed in dog rnodels that prolonged administration of the polyanion polyethylene sulfonate (PES) had a hypotensive effect.

DISCUSSION

Pyran copolymer had been administered to 62 patients with cancer, 39 patients receiving two doses or more at 12 mg/kg. An additional 10 patients were involved in clotting studies and received up to 18 mg/kg in daily, single infusions. The major limiting side effects have been thrombocytopenia and leukopenia seen in one-third of patients. The fall in platelet and white counts occurred within

2 days to 3 weeks but was usually maximal at 5 days after treatment, with recovery in 2–5 days. A relative platelet fall could be observed in 30 to 180 days postpyran in most patients but was not consistent and may be distinct from that seen on chronic administration. Pyrexia >101° was also seen in 50% of patients but was not a debilitating contraindication.

The major limiting toxicity has been vascular in nature associated with the unpredictable development of hypotension in six cases (mottled cyanosis in one of these), seizure in two patients, and impairment of vision in three, with complete loss of vision in one case who expired in shock (Case #4). Vision returned within 2 hr to 2 days in the other two patients. Other significantly toxic side effects have included facial edema, onset of angina with mycardial infarction in one other patient, and confusion and somnolence in 3 patients.

Our experience with pyran copolymer is not surprising in view of our past clinical trial with the related polyanion PES (78). Certain dextrans behave similarly (97).

Recent data (S. Chien, *personal communication*) have shown heparin to produce red cell aggregation which may explain vascular and platelet effects of polyanions.

Discussion of platelet and vascular toxicity of heparin and heparinoids has been elaborated on in past review (70). Polyanions produce what has been defined as a "macromolecular syndrome" (70) resembling anaphylactic or anaphylactoid responses seen in the days of arsephenamine use (8,25,67,68).

The presence of basophilic inclusions in the cytoplasm of histiocytes and white blood cells of bone marrow and peripheral blood of patients (Figs. 1 to 4) and in the phagocytes of liver and spleen in mice are characteristic for both pyran copolymer and PES. The mechanism for the formulation of these basophilic inclusions is not clear, but both pyran and PES cause swelling of the nucleus with extrusion of DNA and histone (7,13,38,45,46,71,73,98). This is accompanied by an associated increase in nucleolar size and the turning on of RNA and protein synthesis in resting cells (7,45). *In vitro* pyran and related polyanions cause tremendous swelling of cell surface in tissue culture. This is particularly true of the macrophage (22,96).

Pertinent to the above, cytoplasmic inclusions produced by polyanions also are similar to what has been seen for tilorone and related congenors as well as atabrine and other small MW interferon inducers (21,34,95,100). All of these compounds which induce the cytoplasmic inclusions have antiviral activity and, in similar fashion to pyran copolymer, tilorone and related compounds inhibit both DNA polymerase and reverse transcriptase (64,65).

The transient blindness is probably vascular in origin in contrast to inclusions produced by atabrine, tilorone (21,34,95,100) or poly I:C (37).

The following can be said for our clinical experience with pyran copolymer and its place in future clinical trial.

1. The clinical formulation (the lyophilized hydrolyzed salt and the freshly hydrolyzed anhydride) of pyran copolymer (MW average 18 to 23,000) (NSC

46015) is too toxic for continued intravenous trial at 12 mg/kg/day because of episodes of unpredictable hypotension, blindness, and sclerosis of blood vessels with the anhydride formulation.

2. Pyrexia, thrombocytopenia, leukopenia, and anticoagulant effects are not seriously limiting toxicities.

3. Decreasing dosage of the clinically current material (NSC 46015), while warranted for adjuvant study, is a questionable procedure in view of laboratory animal evidence of improved therapeutic antitumor index of lower (<15,000 MW) pyran which should be made clinically available.

4. Basophilic cytoplasmic inclusions are found in leukocytes, and occasional *p*-aminosalicylic acid-positive intranuclear inclusions are seen in similar fashion to what has subsequently been observed for tilorone (Figs. 1–4).

5. In adults, intravenous NSC 46015 at 12 mg/kg/day or single dose up to 18 mg/kg/day did not produce evident hemolysis. Schizontocyte ("helmet") cells and renal toxicity have not been seen at this dosage in contrast to reported pediatric experience (33).

Further study of pyran's action during endogenous virus infection is warranted in view of persistent fever and maculopapular eruptions produced by pyran in two of three pediatric patients with Dawson's encephalitis and evidence that the presence of virus can influence action (20).

6. Although NSC 46015 produces liver and renal damage and inhibits drug-metabolizing enzymes in mice and dogs, and in preclinical toxicity studies, this was not a clinical problem, nor was it observed at autopsy at the dosage studied. This is important to further study, as polyanions apparently have unique species-related toxicology, and pyran is less toxic in man in contrast to dogs and monkeys!

Polyanions can block aldosterone action which was not studied but is of physiologic interest (12).

7. Intravenous pyran reduces BAME and TAME splenic esterase activity, while intraperitoneal pyran stimulates esterase activity and this correlates with resistance to Friend leukemia and mouse strain viral suspectibility (88,91). Thus, the route of pyran administration is critical to its biologic action.

Following pyran, poly I:C, or tilorone administration, the presence of C virus particles in tumors can accelerate tumor growth (20).

8. Pyran has a dose-related *in vitro* and *in vivo* anticoagulant effect, but prolonged anticoagulant activity was not associated with clinical hemorrhage. Mice and dogs do not show the same sensitivity to the anticoagulant action of pyran as does man (Tables 1–3).

9. In view of pyran's action in mobilizing plutonium from liver binding (24,35), its clinical use with chelators could be warranted in plutonium poisoning. Additional uses are seen in effects on serum oxygenation (18) and mobilizing lymphocytes (99).

10. Significant antitumor activity with objective and subjective improvement was seen in one patient with myxomatous ovarian cancer, Case #5, in this

study. However, a sufficient number of patients were not treated in any tumor category, and almost all patients in Phase II study were in the preterminal phases of their disease with treatment limited to a median of 9 to 14 days.

11. Future clinical study should involve:

    a. Development of low MW clinical material of improved therapeutic index.

    b. Adjuvant use at lower dosage on a weekly or biweekly schedule.

    c. Regional or intratumoral use in subcutaneous, intrapleural disease.

    d. Pyran should be looked at as an adjuvant to the development of effective antitumor and/or antiviral vaccines in view of the experience of Campbell and Richmond in the hoof and mouth disease model (11) and in view of the experience of the Chirigos group (47–49,63,66) with pyran's effect on prolonging remission following chemotherapeutic response to BCNU with and without the simultaneous administration of radiated tumor cells.

    e. Pyran should be examined for anticomplement or complement-activating activity in view of *in vitro* inhibiting effects and clinical similarities to endotoxin action (39,101).

Finally, it should be repeatedly emphasized that while toxicity of the current clinical formulation precludes further broad-based intravenous clinical testing, it should stimulate renewed interest in the formulation of less toxic fractions and their use in adjuvant antitumor and antiviral programs.

ACKNOWLEDGMENTS

This research was supported by U.S.P.H.S., N.C.I., Eastern Cooperative Oncology Group Programs CA 10572, CA 02824, CA 02822, CA 06594, and the Hercules Company, Wilmington, Delaware.

REFERENCES

1. Adamson, R. H., Fabro, S., Homan, E. R., O'Gara, R. W., and Zendzian, R. P. (1969): Pharmacology of polyriboinosinic: polyribocytidylic acid, a new antiviral and antitumor agent. *Antimicrob. Agents Chemother.,* 9:148–152.
2. Baird, L. G., and Kaplan, A. M. (1976): Immunoadjuvant activity of pyran copolymer. II. Macrophage regulation of T and B cell blastogenesis. *Submitted for publication.*
3. Baird, L. G., and Kaplan, A. M. (1976): Macrophage mediated inhibition of lymphocyte blastogenesis. In: *Proc. 10th Leukocyte Culture Conf.,* Academic Press, N.Y. *(in press).*
4. Baird, L. G., and Kaplan, A. M. (1975): Immunoadjuvant activity of pyran copolymer. I. Evidence for direct stimulation of T-lymphocytes and macrophages. *Cell Immunol.,* 20:167–176.
5. Baird, L. G. (1976): The mechanisms of immunoadjuvant activity of pyran copolymer. Ph.D. Thesis, Dept. of Microbiology, Medical College of Va., Va. Commonwealth University, Richmond 23298.
6. Baird, L. G. (1978): Immunoregulatory macrophages from pyran-treated mice *(this volume).*
7. Berezney, R., and Coffey, D. S. (1976): The nuclear protein matrix: Isolation, structure and functions. In: *Adv. in Enzyme Regulation* 14, edited by G. Weber, pp. 63–100. Pergamon Press, Oxford.

8. Black, D. R., Eckstein, F., DeClercq, Q. E., and Merigan, T. C. (1973): Studies on the toxicity and antiviral activity of various polynucleotides. *Antimicrob. Agents Chemother.,* 3:198–206.

9. Braun, W., Regelson, W., Yajima, Y., and Ishizuka, M. (1970): Stimulation of antibody formation by pyran copolymer. *Proc. Soc. Exp. Biol. Med.,* 133:171–175.

10. Breslow, D. S., Edwards, E. I., and Newburg, N. R. (1973): Divinyl ether-maleic anhydride (pyran) copolyner used to demonstrate the effect of molecular weight of biological activity. *Nature,* 246:160–162.

11. Campbell, C. H., and Richmond, J. Y. (1973): Enhancement by two carboxylic acid interferon inducers of resistance stimulated in mice by foot and mouth disease vaccine. *Infect. Immunol.,* 7:199–204.

12. Chremos, A. N., Laidlaw, J. C., and Ruse, J. L. (1969): Effect of sulfated mucopolysaccharide (R01–8307) on the zona glomerulosa of regenerating rat adrenal glands and intact glands in sodium deprived rats. *Endocrinology,* 85:337–341.

13. Coffey, D. S., Barrack, E. R., and Heston, W. D. (1973): The regulation of nuclear DNA template restrictions by acidic polymers. *Brady Research Monograph II.* Johns Hopkins Univ. School of Med., Baltimore.

14. Coffey, I. S. (1976): *Personal communication.*

15. DiLuzio, N. R., Cook, J. A., Cohen, C., Rodrigue, J., Kokoshis, P., and McNamee, R. B. (1978): Enhancement of the inhibitory effect of cyclophosphamide on experimental acute myelogenous leukemia by glucan immunopotentiation and response of serum lysozyme *(this volume).*

16. Dennis, L. H., Angeles, A., Baig, M., and Shnider, B. I. (1969): The effect of pyran polymer on the hemostatic mechanism. *Proc. Soc. Clin. Pharmacol.*

17. Elzay, R., and Regelson, W. (1976): Effect of pyran copolymer on DMBA experimental oral carcinogenesis with golden Syrian hamster. Research annotation. *J. Dent. Res.,* 55(6):1138.

18. Evans, J. C. (1975): *Personal communication.*

19. Gander, G. W., and Goodale, F. (1973): Studies on the endogenous pyrogen released in response to poly I:poly C. *The Pharmacology of Thermoregulation Symp.,* San Francisco, 1972, pp. 255–263. Karger, Basel.

20. Gazdar, A. F., Steinberg, A. D., Spahn, G. F., and Baron, S. (1972): Interferon inducers: Enhancement of viral oncogenesis in mice and rats. *Proc. Soc. Exp. Biol. Med.,* 139:1132–1137.

21. Glaz, E. T., Talas, M. (1975): Comparison of the activity of small molecular interferon inducers: Tilorone and acridine drugs. *Arch. Virol.,* 48:375–384.

22. Goodell, E. M., Munson, A. E., and Carchman, R. A. (1976): Growth and phagocytosis characteristics of P388Di cells in tissue culture. *Reticuloendothel. Soc.,* 20:35A.

23. Gresser, I. (1976): Antitumor effects of interferon. In: *Cancer: A Comprehensive Treatise,* edited by F. Becker *(in press).*

24. Guilmette, R. A., and Lindenbaum, A. (1975): Progress in the use of pyran copolymers for decorporation of polymeric plutonium. *Proc. Workshop on Biological Effects and Toxicity of Pu-239 and Ra-226,* Sun Valley, Idaho, October *(in press).*

25. Hamilton, L. (1972): *Personal communication.*

26. Hirsch, M. S., Block, P. H., Wood, M. L., and Monaco, A. P. (1972): Effects of pyran copolymer on oncogeneic virus infections in immunosuppressed hosts. *J. Immunol.,* 108(5):1312–1318.

27. Kaplan, A. M., Baird, L. G., and Morahan, P. S. (1977): Macrophage regulation of tumor cell growth and mitogen induced blastogenesis. In: *Control of Neoplasia by Modulation of the Immune System (Progress in Cancer Research and Therapy, Vol. 2),* edited by M. A. Chirigos, pp. 461–474. Raven Press, New York.

28. Kaplan, A. M., and Morahan, P. S. (1976): Macrophage mediated tumor cell cytotoxicity. *Ann. N. Y. Acad. Sci.,* 276:134–145.

29. Kaplan, A. M., Walker, P. L., and Morahan, P. S. (1977): Tumor cell cytotoxicity versus cytostasis of pyran activated macrophages. In: *Modulation of Host Immune Resistance in the Prevention or Treatment of Induced Neoplasias,* edited by M. A. Chirigos. Fogarty Intl. Center Proc. No. 28, pp. 277–286. HEW Publ. No. (NIH) 77–893. U.S. Government Printing Office, Washington, D.C.

30. Kaplan, A. M., and Morahan, P. S. (1976): Macrophage activity against viruses and tumor cells and in regulation of lymphoproliferation. *J. Reticuloendothel. Soc.,* 20(60):31A.

31. Kapusta, M. A., and Mendelson, J. (1969): The inhibition of adjuvant disease in rats by interferon inducing agent pyran copolymer. *Arthritis Rheum.,* 12(5):463–471.

32. Kopila, K., Smith, C., and Rubin, A. A. (1971): Methylcholanthrene transplants. *J. Reticuloendothel. Soc.,* 9:447–450.

33. Leavitt, T. J., Merigan, T. C., and Freeman, J. M. (1971): Hemolytic-uremic-like syndrome following polycarboxylate interferon induction. Treatment of Dawson's inclusion-body encephalitis. *Am. J. Dis. Child.,* 121:43–47.

34. Levine, S., Sowinski, R., and Hoenig, E. M. (1975): Nuclear bodies produced in astrocytes by tilorone. *Am. J. Pathol.,* 78:319–330.

35. Lindenbaum, A., Rosenthal, M. W., and Guilmette, R. A. (1975): Retention of polymeric plutonium in mouse tissues as affected by antiviral compounds and their analogs. In: *Proc. I.A.E.A. Symp. on Diagnosis and Treatment of Internally Deposited Radionucleotides.* Vienna, Austria, December IAEA-SR-6/22.

36. Little, A. P. *Preclinical Toxicology of NSC 46015 Hydrolysate Report to Cancer Chemotherapy National Service Center,* March 5, 1964, Contract #SA-43-ph-3789. Little, Brown, Boston, Mass.

37. Mathé, G. (1973): *Personal communication.*

38. Matyasova, J., Skalka, M., and Cejkova, M. (1974): The importance of molecular weight of inorganic polyphosphates for their interaction with deoxyribonucleoprotein of animal tissue. *Folia Biol. (Praha),* 20:193–204.

39. McKenzie, D. (1976): *Personal communication.* Also: Colsky, J., McKenzie, D., and Hettrick, D. L. Complement reactivity of cancer patients measurements by immune lysis and immune adherents. *Cancer Res.,* 27:2386–2394.

40. Merigan, T. C. (1967): Induction of circulating interferon by synthetic anionic polymers of known composition. *Nature (Lond.),* 214:416–417.

41. Merigan, T. C. (1967): *Discussion, Ciba Foundation Symposium on Interferon,* edited by G. E. W. Wolstenholme and M. O'Connor, pp. 50–60. J. A. Churchill, London, England.

42. Merigan, T. C., and Finklestein, M. S. (1968): Interferon-stimulating and *in vivo* antiviral effects of various synthetic anionic polymers. *Virology,* 35:363–374.

43. Merigan, T. C., and Regelson, W. (1967): Interferon induction in man by a synthetic polyanion of defined composition. *New Engl. J. Med.,* 277:1283–1287.

44. Mihich, E., Simpson, C. L., Regelson, W., and Mulhern, P. I. (1960): Pharmacological study of ammoniated ethylene maleic polymer, M.W. 20,000–30,000 (AEMA 20–30). *Fed. Proc.,* 19:142A.

45. Miller, G., Berlowitz, L., and Regelson, W. (1971): Chromatin and histones in mealy bug cell explants: Activation and decondensation of facultative heterochromatin by a synthetic polyanion. *Chromasoma,* 32:251–261.

46. Miller, G. J., Berlowitz, L., and Regelson, W. (1972): Chromatin and histones in hen erythrocyte nuclei: Morphologic change induced by selective binding of histones with a synthetic polyanion. *Exp. Cell Res.,* 71:409–421.

47. Mohr, S. J., and Chirigos, M.A. (1978): Immunopotentiation against the L1210 leukemia by pyran copolymer and crude tumor antigen *(this volume).*

48. Mohr, S. J., and Chirigos, M. A. (1977): Potentiation of a tumor cell vaccine by pyran copolymer. In: *Control of Neoplasia by Modulation of the Immune System (Progress in Cancer Research and Therapy, Vol. 2),* edited by M. A. Chirigos, pp. 421–439. Raven Press, New York.

49. Mohr, S. J., Chirigos, M. A., Fuhrman, F. S., and Pryor, J. W. (1975): Pyran copolymer found to be effective adjuvant to chemotherapy against a murine leukemia and solid tumor. *Cancer Res.,* 35:3750–3754.

50. Morahan, P. S., and Kaplan, A. M. (1977): Macrophage-mediated tumor resistance. In: *Control of Neoplasia by Modulation of the Immune System (Progress in Cancer Research and Therapy, Vol. 2),* edited by M. A. Chirigos, pp. 449–459. Raven Press, New York.

51. Morahan, P. S., Munson, J. A., Baird, L. G., Kaplan, A. M., and Regelson, W. (1974): Antitumor action of pyran copolymer and tilorone against Lewis lung carcinoma and B-16 melanoma. *Cancer Res.,* 34:506–511.

52. Morahan, P. S., Munson, A. E., Regelson, W., Commerford, S. L., and Hamilton, L. D. (1972): Antiviral activity and side effects of polyriboinosinic cytidylic acid complexes as effected by molecular size. *Proc. Natl. Acad. Sci. USA,* 69:842–846.

53. Morahan, P. S., Munson, A. E., Regelson, W., and Hamilton, L. D. (1971): Pyran and polynucleotides: Comparison of biologic activities. International Colloquium on Interferon and Interferon inducers, Leuven, Belgium, September.

54. Morahan, P. S., Regelson, W., and Munson, A. E. (1972): Pyran and polyribonucleotides: Differences in biological activities. *Antimicrob. Agents Chemother.,* 2:16–22.

55. Morahan, P. S. (1978): Antiviral and antitumor functions of activated macrophages *(this volume).*

56. Morahan, P. S., and Kaplan, A. M. (1976): Host cells associated with Lewis lung carcinoma. *J. Reticuloendothel. Soc.,* 20(71):36A.

57. Munson, A. E., and Regelson, W. (1971): Sensitization to endotoxin by pyran copolymer. *Proc. Soc. Exp. Biol. Med.,* 137(2):553–557.

58. Munson, A. E., Regelson, W., Lawrence, W., Jr., and Wooles, W. R. (1970): The biphasic response of the reticuloendothelial system (RES) produced by pyran copolymer and its relation to immunologic response. *J. Reticuloendothel. Soc.,* 7:375–385.

59. Munson, A. E., Regelson, W., and Munson, J. A. (1972): Effect of 4 antiviral agents on hepatic microsomal mixed functional oxidase enzymes. *Toxicol. Appl. Pharmacol.,* 22:299–300.

60. Munson, A. E., and Wooles, W. R. (1969): The relationship between hexobarbital metabolism and reticuloendothelial (RE) activity. *The Pharmacologist,* 11(174):261.

61. Ottenbrite, R. M., Regelson, W., Kaplan, A. M., Morahan, P. S., and Munson, A. E. (1976): Biological activity of anionic polymers. *Am. Chem. Soc. Polymer Preprints,* New Orleans.

62. Ottenbrite, R. M., and Regelson, W. (1976): Biological activity of water soluble polymers. In: *Encyclopedia of Polymer Sciences and Technology,* edited by H. M. Bikales *(in press).*

63. Papamatheakis, J., Chirigos, M. A., and Schultz, R. M. (1978): Effect of dose, route, and timing of pyran copolymer therapy against the Madison lung carcinoma *(this volume).*

64. Papas, T. S., Woods, W. A., and Chirigos, M. A. (1975): Active site probes and the selective inhibition of RNA tumor viral DNA polymerases: In: *Modulation of Host Immune Resistance in the Prevention or Treatment of Induced Neoplasias,* edited by M. A. Chirigos. Fogarty Intl. Center Proc. No. 28, pp. 369–375. HEW Publ. No. (NIH) 77–893. U.S. Government Printing Office, Washington, D.C.

65. Papas, T. S., Pry, T. W., and Chirigos, M. A. (1974): Inhibition of RNA-dependent DNA polymerase of Avian myeloblastosis virus by pyran copolymer. *Proc. Natl. Acad. Sci. USA,* 7:367–370.

66. Pearson, J. W., Gibson, W. T., and Chirigos, M. A. (1970): Use of a murine sarcoma virus in an *in vivo* assay for anti-viral and anti-tumor agents. *Cancer Res.,* 30:2024–2028.

67. Phillips, B. M., Hartnagel, R. E., Kraus, P. J., Tamako, R. P., Fronesca, E. C., and Kowlaski, R. L. (1971): Systemic toxicity of polyinosinic acid: Polycytidylic acid in rodents and dogs. *Toxicol. Appl. Pharmacol.,* 18:220–239.

68. Philips, F. S., Fleisher, M., Hamilton, L. D., Schwartz, M. K., and Sternberg, S. S. (1971): Polyinosinic-polycytidylic acid toxicity. In: *Biological Effects of Polynucleotides,* edited by R. F. Beers and W. Braun, Springer-Verlag, New York, pp. 259–273.

69. Qureshi, G. D., Roberts, P., and Regelson, W. (1976): *In preparation.*

70. Regelson, W. (1968): Thrombocytopenic and related physiologic effects of heparin and heparinoids: A macromolecular-induced syndrome? *Hematol. Rev.,* 1:193.

71. Regelson, W. (1968): The growth regulating activity of polyanions. In: *Advances in Cancer Res.,* pp. 237–287. Academic Press, New York.

72. Regelson, W. (1973): The biologic activity of water-soluble polymers. In: *Water Soluble Polymers II,* edited by N. M. Bikales, pp. 161–177. Plenum Press, New York.

73. Regelson, W. (1968): Anionic polyelectrolytes as antimitotic agents. *Adv. Chemother.,* 3:303–371.

74. Regelson, W. (1974): The antimitotic activity of polyanions: Heparin and heparinoids. *J. Med.,* 5:50–68.

75. Regelson, W. (1973): Host modulation of resistance to infection and neoplasia. *Med. Chem.* 8, 17:160–172.

76. Regelson, W. (1970): Part I: The biologic activity of polyanions: A brief review of antitumor, antiviral, antibacterial action and some theories in regard to mechanism. *L'Interferon,* 6:353–379.

77. Regelson, W. (1967): Prevention and treatment of Friend leukemia virus infection by interferon

inducing synthetic polyanions. The reticuloendothelial system and artherosclerosis. *Adv. Exp. Med. Biol.,* 1:315–332.

78. Regelson, W., and Holland, J. F. (1962): The effect of an anionic polyelectrolyte (polyethylene sulfonate) in patients with cancer. The clinical pharmacology of a macromolecule. *Clin. Pharmacol. Ther.,* 3:730–749.

79. Regelson, W., Morahan, P. S., Kaplan, A. M., Baird, L. G., and Munson, J. A. (1974): Synthetic polyanions: Molecular weight, macrophage activation and immunologic response. In: *Activation of Macrophages,* edited by W. H. Wagner and H. Hahn, pp. 98–110. Excerpta Medica, Amsterdam—American Elsevier, New York.

80. Regelson, W., Morahan, P., and Kaplan, A. M. (1975): The role of molecular weight in pharmacologic and biologic activity of synthetic polyanions. In: *Polyelectrolytes and Their Application,* edited by A. Rembaum and E. Seligny, pp. 131–144, Reidel Publ., Dordrecht, Holland.

81. Regelson, W., Roberts, P., Morahan, P., and Kaplan, A. M. (1976): The biologic activity of polyanions (synthetic polyanions and heparinoids). In: *Seminars in Thrombosis and Hemostasis, Suppl. 1 (in press).*

82. Regelson, W., Munson, A. E., and Merigan, T. C. (1967): The control of susceptibility to leukemia virus infection and tumor induction by synthetic polyanions and other compounds which induce or block interferon production: Their possible relation to the reticuloendothelial system. *Abs. Vth Int. Cong. on Chemotherapy,* V. Weiner Med. Akad., p. 407.

83. Regelson W., and Munson, A. E. (1970): The reticuloendothelial effects of interferon inducers: Polyanionic and non-polyanionic phylaxis against microorganisms. *Ann. N.Y. Acad. Sci.* 173:831–841.

84. Regelson, W., Munson, A. E., and the Eastern Oncology Study Group (Silver Spring, Maryland) (1970): Polyanions as anti-tumor agents: The biologic activity and reticuloendothelial activity of pyran copolymer and poly:inosinic and cytidylic acid (Poly rI:rC). In: *Xth Int. Cancer Cong.,* Houston, Texas, May.

85. Regelson, W., Munson, A. E., Wooles, W. R., Lawrence, W., Jr., and Levy, H. (1970): Part II: Reticuloendothelial action of interferon inducers: The biphasic action of pyran copolymer and polynucleotides on phagocytic and immunologic response. *L'Interferon,* 6:381–395.

86. Regelson, W., Munson, A. E., and Wooles, W. (1970): The biologic activity of synthetic polymers: Interferon inducers and reticuloendothelial response: Polyanions. *Interferon Symp. Series Immunobiol. Standard.,* 14:227–236.

87. Roberts, P. S., Regelson, W., and Kingsbury, B. (1973): Determination of fibrinogen in normal plasma in the presence and absence of anticoagulants. *J. Lab. Clin. Med.,* 2:822–828.

88. Roberts, P. S., and Regelson, W. (1976): *Personal communication.*

89. Rehovsky, M. W., Newberne, J. W., and Gibson, J. P. (1970): Effects of an oral interferon-inducer on the hematopoietic and reticuloendothelial system. *Toxicol. Appl. Pharmacol.,* 17:556–558.

90. Sandberg, J., and Goldin, A. (1971): Use of first generation transplants of a slow growing solid tumor for the evaluation of new cancer chemotherapeutic agents. *Cancer Chemother. Reports,* 55(1):233–238.

91. Schuller, G. B., Morahan, P. S., and Snodgrass, M. (1975): Inhibition and enhancement of Friend leukemia virus by pyran copolymer. *Cancer Res.,* 35:1915–1920.

92. Schultz, R. M., Papamatheakis, J. D., and Chirigos, M. A. (1978): Correlation between antitumor activity and macrophage activation by polyanions *(this volume).*

93. Schultz, R. M., Papamatheakis, J. D., and Chirigos, M. A. (1976): Correlation between polyanion induced macrophage activation and anti-tumor activity. *J. Reticuloendothel. Soc.,* 20(71):xx–xx.

94. Shamash, Y., and Alexander, B. (1969): Coagulation studies with linear copolymers of aliphatic hydrocarbons and maleic acid: New ideas of anticoagulants. *Biochim. Biophys. Acta.,* 194:449–461.

95. Siminoff, P., Bernard, A. M., Hursky, V. S., and Price, K. E. (1973): BL-20803 a new low molecular weight interferon inducer. *Antimicrob. Agents Chemother.,* 3:742–743.

96. Snodgrass, M. J., Kaplan, A. M., and Harris, T. M. (1976): Macrophage mobility in response to carcinoma cells and their soluble by products. *J. Reticuloendothel. Soc.,* 20(113):57A.

97. Spector, J. I., Lang, E., and Crosby, W. H. (1975): Coagulation changes in baboons during acute experimental hemoglobinemia and dextran infusion. *Am. J. Pathol.,* 78(3):469–476.

98. Tunis, M., and Regelson, W. (1965): The interaction of nucleated cells with anionic polyelectrolytes and inhibition of the interaction by pancreatic deoxyribonuclease. *Exp. Cell Res.,* 40:383–395.
99. Von Bekkum, D. W. (1972): *Personal communication.*
100. Wampler, G. L., Kuperminc, M., and Regelson, W. (1973): Tilorone (DEAE-Fluorenone) hydrochloride phase I study of a non-marrow depressing antitumor agent. *Cancer Chemother. Rep.,* 57(2):209–217.
101. White, G. S. (1970): *Personal communication.* Dept. of Hypersensitivity, Diseases Research, Upjohn Co., Kalamazoo, Michigan.
102. Wooles, W., and Munson, A. E. (1971): The effect of stimulants and depressants of reticuloendothelial activity on drug metabolism. *J. Reticuloendothel. Soc.,* 9:108–119.

Subject Index

Abscess, cold, 263
Accidental infections, levamisole and, 53–54
Actinomycin D
  dosage, 120
  and levamisole in refractory malignant melanoma, 119–128
  survival with, 124–125f
Adenocarcinoma
  agranulocytosis in, 161–162
  glucan and, 172
Adenosine
  -inhibited RFC, 66, 69f, 70, 71
  monophosphate, cyclic, see AMP, cyclic
Adjuvant
  mechanism, immunological, 386
  therapeutic setting, 94
Adriamycin, 51, 131–138
  congestive heart failure and, 132
Agammaglobulinemia, 321
Agranulocytosis with levamisole, 160–162
AHS, see Serum, activated human
Albumin, 143
AmB, see Amphotericin B
AME, see Amphotericin methyl ester
Aminophylline, 324t, 325t, 328
AMP, cyclic
  DB, 320, 323–329
  -inhibited RFC, 66, 69f, 70, 71
  levamisole and, 7
  levels in lymphocytes treated with levamisole, 23–27
  thymosin fraction 5 and, 285–286, 289
Amphotericin
  B (AmB)
    properties of, 381–387
    strain-specific effects of, 385
  methyl ester (AME), 383–386
Anergy, 148–150
  defined, 158
  levamisole and, 4, 5
Animal studies, levamisole in, 2, 3t
Antiantibody systems, 148–150
Antibodies, lymphocytotoxic, 56–57
Anticytoplasmic antibodies, 148
  increase in, 151–153
Anti-Y-globulins, 149
Antiidiotypic antibodies, 149
Antimembrane antibodies, 148
  increase in, 151–153
Antitumor
  action of glucan, 183–193

immunity, 153
Aphthous ulceration, recurrent, levamisole and, 3
Apoferritin, 141–143
Apoptotic bodies, 263
Arthritis, rheumatoid, levamisole and, 3
Ataxia telangiectasia (AT), 165, 167t, 168
  thymosin and, 336, 338–339, 343
Augmentation index, IgG, 385
Autoantibodies, lymphocytotoxic, 57
Azathioprine, E-rosette test and, 66, 68–70
Aziridines, 389

B cell
  hyperactivity, levamisole and, 6
  mitogens, 295–298
B cells
  eliminating adherent, 260–261
  stimulation of, 465
B-lymphocyte response, splenic, 217
B lymphocytes, see also Lymphocytes
  defined, 320
  effect of pyran on, 442
  glucan and, 256
Bach thymic factor, 313
Bacillus Calmette-Guérin (BCG), 119
  breast cancer and, 131–138, 163–164
  comparison with glucan and levamisole, 221–231
  CY and, 178–179
  glucan and, 246
  histiocytic granuloma and, 431–432
  immunostimulant effects of, 385–387
  immunotherapy with levamisole, tumor vaccines, and, 147–155
  macrophages and, 192
  pyran and, 418, 421t
  side effects, 221
  in stage 3B melanoma, 357–370
BCG, see Bacillus Calmette-Guérin
BCNU (1,3-bis(2-chloroethyl)-1-nitrosourea), 381
  thymosin and, 305–310
Blast cells, 454
Blastogenesis
  inhibition of, 443
  lymph node cell, 438
  lymphocyte, see Lymphocyte blastogenesis
  spleen cell, 438–443
Blood
  cell counts, white, 55t

Blood *(contd.)*
  clotting and pyran copolymer, 479–482
  sedimentation rate and pyran copolymer,
    482
BM 06 002, 389–400
  phase I study for, 403–412
  toxicity study of, 406–411
Body weight, CY and glucan influence on,
  174
Bone marrow
  acceptance, glucan and, 207
  cellularity, glucan and, 196t
  depression, levamisole and, 59–60
  examination, pyran copolymer and, 476
  transplantation candidates, levamisole
    and, 58
Bovine serum albumin (BSA) gradient fractionation, 320, 325–327t
Breast cancer
  cell-mediated immunity and, 137–138
  immunocompetence of advanced, 131
  levamisole and, 100–102, 131–138, 162–
    163
  metastatic sites in, 133t
  stage IV
    response rate, 134t
    survival, 135f
  survival rate with levamisole in, 101f
Brinase, 157
Bromosulfophthalein (BSP) retention
  studies and glucan, 309–310, 313t
Brucellosis, 157, 160
Bruton disease, 165, 168
BSA, *see* Bovine serum albumin
BSP, *see* Bromosulfophthalein
Burden, tumor, *see* Tumor load

cAMP, *see* AMP, cyclic
Cancer
  breast, *see* Breast cancer
  immunotherapy studies, variables in, 94t
  lung, *see* Lung cancer
  patients, thymosin and, 347–355
  radiosensitive, 100
  studies, levamisole in, 93–104
Candida albicans, 96, 398, 399f
Candidiasis, mucocutaneous, thymosin and,
  338t, 339t, 341–342
Carcinoma
  bronchiogenic, 49
  Ehrlich ascites, 394, 395f
  squamous cell (SCC)
    agranulocytosis in, 160
    cyclic AMP in lymphocytes from
      patients with, 23–27
    prostaglandin $F_{2\alpha}$ levels with, 26
Carcinosarcoma, Walker, 394–395

Cell
  chimerism, 342
  -mediated immunity
    breast cancer and, 137–138
    defective, 107, 373
    effector cells in, 273
    glucan and, 171
    levamisole and, 85–92
    in lung cancer, 107–118
    measurement of, 108
    thymus gland and, 281
  -to-cell contact, 273, 455
CFA, *see* Freund's adjuvant, complete
CFU-C, *see* Granulocyte-monocyte
  progenitors
Chemoimmunoadjuvant effect with
  thymosin, 308
Chemotactic activity, defined, 31t
Chemotaxis
  assays, 30
  monocyte, *see* Monocyte chemotaxis,
    human
  produced by influenza, 29
Chemotherapy
  levamisole and, 51, 59
  regimens, prior, 127–128
Chlorambucil, 51
1,3-bis(2-Chloroethyl)-1-nitrosourea, *see*
  BCNU
CLL, *see* Leukemia, chronic lymphocytic
Clotting
  studies of pyran copolymer, 479–482
  time and pyran copolymer, 480–482
Colony
  -forming efficiency, lung, 368
  -stimulating activity (CSA), 196–199
Concanavalin A (Con A)
  BM 06 002 and, 409
  glucan and, 186–187, 256, 259–261
  levamisole and, 166t, 167t
  lung cancer and, 109, 112–114
  response in lymph node cells, 295–298
  thymosin and, 296–298
    in 3B melanoma, 358, 362, 264–367
    in thymocyte-mitogen bioassay,
      313–317
Congenital immunodeficiencies, levamisole
  and, 165–169
Corynebacterium parvum
  breast cancer and, 131, 138
  CY and, 178–179
  fibrosarcoma and, 191–192
  glucan and, 246
    compared, 235–240
  macrophages and, 454
  pyran and, 418, 421t, 442
  side effects, 221

Corynebacterium parvum (contd.)
  spleen weights with, 237
  thymosin and, 368
CR, *see* Remission, complete
^{51}Cr
  labeling, 88f, 89
  release test for macrophage-mediated
    cytotoxicity, 242–243
CSA, *see* Colony-stimulating activity
Cutaneous delayed hypersensitivity, *see*
  Hypersensitivity
Cyclophosphamide (CY), 51,131–138
  in acute myelogenous leukemia, 171–181
  BM 06 002 and, 393–396
  hemorrhagic cystitis and, 132
  pyran and, 423t
  thymosin and, 305–307
Cystitis, hemorrhagic, *see* Hemmorrhagic
  cystitis
Cytostasis
  macrophage-mediated, 243
    glucan and, 244–245
  tumor cell, 455
  of tumor cell proliferation, 189–190
Cytostatics, 389–390
Cytotoxicity
  lymphocyte, *see* Lymphocyte
    cytotoxicity
  lymphocyte-mediated, 88–91
  lymphoproliferation and, 454
  macrophage-mediated
    ^{51}Cr release test for, 242–243
    glucan and, 243–244
  percent, 86–87

DCH, *see* Hypersensitivity, delayed
  cutaneous
DEAE-dextran, *see* Diethylaminoethyl-
  dextran
Death rates in levamisole study, 100t
Delayed cutaneous hypersensitivity, *see*
  Hypersensitivity
Dependence, dose, 229–231
Dermatophytin skin test response, 364–367
Dextran sulfate
  molecular structure of, 461f
  pyran and, 418, 421t
Diethylaminoethyl-dextran (DEAE-
  dextran), 460, 463, 464
DiGeorge syndrome, thymosin with, 336–
  341, 343–344
Dimethyl triazeno imidazole carboxamide
  (DTIC), 119
  in stage 3B melanoma, 357–370
2, 4-Dinitrochlorobenzene (DNCB), 85, 96,
  405
  sensitization, 108

skin tests, 109–110
  evaluation of, 116–117
Disease
  -free interval of stage 3B melanoma, 362–
    365f
  progressive, defined, 120
  stable (S), defined, 120
Dissemination, levamisole inhibiting
  hematogenous, 102
Diveema, *see* Pyran copolymer
DNA synthesis
  inhibition of, 243–245
  assay, 362
  levamisole and, 75–76
DNCB, *see* 2, 4-Dinitrochlorobenzene
DNP$_5$-thymosin, 299, 300t, 302
Dosage
  actinomycin D, 120
  glucan, 250–251
  levamisole, 94, 95f, 97, 102, 104, 120
  thymosin, 362–363, 366, 367
Dose dependence, 229–231
  of glucan, 244f, 258
  of pyran, 429
Doubling time of tumor, 104
DTIC, *see* Dimethyl triazeno imidazole carboxamide

E-rosette
  counts, 55t
  formation
    in T lymphocytes, 65–71
    thymosin and, 289t
    trypsinization and, 66–67
  -forming cells (ERFC)
    defined, 335
    in Hodgkin's disease, 141–144
    levamisole and, 51–52
    thymosin and, 366–367
  -forming lymphocytes, 319–329
  test, 65
E-rosettes
  azathioprine and, 66, 68–70
  glucan and mitogens and, 260
  thymosin and, 377, 378t
EAC, *see* Erythrocyte-antibody complement
Effector cells in cell-mediated immunity,
  273
Ehrlich ascites carcinoma, 394, 395f
Electron microscopy of macrophages, 257,
  264–271
Embryo fibroblast cultures, 85–86
Emperipolesis, 263
EMT6 tumor, 11–19
Encephalitis, herpesvirus, 75

Endotoxin, 317–318; *see also* Lipopolysaccharide
ERFC, *see* E-rosette-forming cells
Erythrocyte-antibody complement (EAC), 320
Erythrocytes, sheep, preparation of, 391–392
Erythroleukemia cells, 202
Escherichia coli lipopolysaccharide, 296–298
Esterase-positive cells, 443
Exacerbation of underlying infections with levamisole, 160
Exocytosis, 274

F(ab')₂ fragments, 149
FAC therapy, 131–138
FACOM therapy, 163f
Fc receptor, 320
Ferritin, 141–144
Fetuin, 143
Fibroblast cultures, embryo, 85–86
Fibrosarcoma
    Corynebacterium parvum and, 191–192
    model, glucan and *Corynebacterium parvum* compared in, 235–240
    regression of, glucan and, 238
Filopodia attachments, 204
5-Fluorouracil, 131–138
    gastrointestinal toxicity and, 132
Freund's adjuvant, 2t, 3t
    complete (CFA), pyran and, 418, 421t
Friend
    leukemia cells, 202
    virus leukemia, 391, 394, 395t

Gastrointestinal toxicity, 5-fluorouracil and, 132
Glucan, 171
    action of, 255–256
    -activated macrophages, 201–205
    antitumor action of, 183–193
    bone marrow cellularity and, 196t
    cell-mediated immunity and, 171
    clinical experiences with, 255–276
    compared with *Corynebacterium parvum*, 235–240
    compared with BCG and levamisole, 221–231
    death due to, 236–237
    dosage, 250–251
    dose dependency of, 244f, 258
    fibrosarcoma regression by, 238
    granuloma, 180–181
    hepatic metastases suppressed by, 207–217
    immunopotentiation in acute myelogenous leukemia, 171–181

increased granulopoiesis and macrophage production and, 195–199
    -induced tumor regression, morphology of, 261–271
    intralesional, metastatic tumors with, 249–254
    intraperitoneal administration of, 258
    macrophage cell length and, 202–204
    macrophage-mediated
        antitumor action of, 178
        cytostasis and, 244–245
        cytotoxicity and, 243–244
    macrophages, peritoneal, and, 197t
    mitogens and, 259–261
    phagocytic activity and, 189
    preparation of, 239
    pyran and, 418, 421t
    reticuloendothelial system and, 207, 241
    side effects, 252
    spleen
        cells and, 186–187
        cellularity and, 197t
        weights and, 237
    thymus independence and, 245–246
    topical application of, 251
    tumor
        growth delay and, 237–240
        load, increased, and, 213
    tumoricidal effect of peritoneal macrophages and, 241–247
Glutaraldehyde-treated tumor cells, 213–214
Glycogen, 447, 454
Glycoprotein α-acid, 143
Glucosamine incorporation, levamisole and, 44
GMP, cyclic
    8 Br, thymosin and, 320, 323–328
    levamisole and, 7–8
    thymosin fraction 5 and, 285–286, 289
Graft-versus-host (GVH) reaction, 435
    amphotericin B and, 384–385
    glucan and, 171, 207
Granulocyte-monocyte progenitors (CFU-C), 196–198
Granulocytopenia, 50
    transient, levamisole and, 7
Granuloma
    glucan, 180–181
    histiocytic, BCG and, 431–432
Granulopoiesis, increased, 195–199
Guanosine 3'5' cyclic monophosphate, *see* GMP, cyclic
GVH, *see* Graft-versus-host

H-2 antigens, 87
³H-proline labeling, 88f, 89
HD, *see* Hodgkin's disease

Heart failure, congestive, adriamycin and,
132
Helper T cells, 230
Hemolysin response, 207
Hemorrhagic cystitis, cyclophosphamide
and, 132
Heparin
polyanions and, 483
pyran and, 418, 421t
Hepatic metastases, glucan suppression of,
207–217
Herpes infections, recurrent, levamisole
and, 5
Herpesvirus encephalitis, 75
Heterocytolysis, 274
Hexose monophosphate shunt (HMPS),
activity of, 81–82
Histamine, 247
Histiocytic granuloma and BCG, 431–432
Histocompatibility antigen, 424
H-2^k, 87
HMPS, *see* Hexose monophosphate shunt
Hodgkin's disease (HD), 107
and levamisole, 50–55, 59–60
unblocking effect, 141–144
MOPP chemotherapy and, 160
Host defense, tumor cell quantity and, 19
Hypersensitivity
cutaneous delayed (CDH), 54
delayed cutaneous (DCH), 107
with MB 06 002, 405
MacKanes' delayed, 391–392
Hypogammaglobulinemia
acquired, thymosin and, 338t, 339t, 342–
343
variable, 165, 166t

IDS, *see* Inhibition-of-DNA-synthesis assay
IgG
antibodies, 147–148
augmentation index, 385
IgM to, antibody production switch, 384
IgM to IgG antibody production switch, 384
Immune
complex disease, 148–150
regulation, deranged, in melanoma, 147–
151
response
idiotypic, 149
levamisole and, 2t
Immunity, antitumor, 153
Immunocompetence
of advanced breast cancer patients, 131
impaired, 23
thymosin dose and, 366
Immunodeficiencies, congenital, levamisole
in, 165–169
Immunodeficiency disease
combined, 321

primary, thymosin and, 333–344
severe combined (SCID), 165, 168
thymosin and, 337, 338t, 339t, 342
Immunological deficiency, levamisole and,
6
Immunology-prognosis link-up, 96–97
Immunomodulators
combined with irradiated tumor cells,
226–231
macrophages and, 455
Immunoreactivity, levamisole and, 19
Immunoregulatory α-globulin (IRA), 103
Immunostimulant action of transfer factor,
169
Immunosuppressive disease, lung cancer as,
111
Immunotherapy
combination, with levamisole, BCG, and
tumor vaccines, 147–155
studies, cancer, variables, in, 94t
tumor enhancement by, 103–104
Infection, incidence of, 137
Infections, accidental, levamisole and, 53–
54
Influenza
acute, levamisole effect with, 24, 25t
chemotaxis produced by, 29
infection, levamisole and, 4
Inhibition-of-DNA-synthesis (IDS) assay,
362
Interferon induction, 469
IRA, *see* Immunoregulatory α-globulin
Isoproterenol, 322, 324t, 328

Jerne's plaque test, 398, 399f

Keyhole limpet hemocyanin (KLH), 405,
409
KHT fibrosarcoma, 11–13, 15, 18–20

L1210 leukemia
challenge dose, 416–420
pyran copolymer and, 415–425
Lamellipodia, adherent, 204
LCFU, *see* Leukemia colony-forming unit
LDCF, *see* Lymphocyte-derived
chemotactic factor
Lentinan, 183, 191, 242–246
Leprosy, levamisole and, 3
Leukemia
cells, 381
syngeneic, 201–205
chronic lymphocytic (CLL), levamisole
and, 50–55, 59–60
colony-forming unit (LCFU), 382t
glucan in, 179
myelogenous, cyclophosphamide and
glucan and, 171–181
myeloid, levamisole and, 99–100

Leukocyte
  counts, 55t
  polymorphonuclear (PMN), chemotaxis, 30
Leukopenia
  BM 06 002 and, 395
  pyran copolymer and, 474
Levamisole (LMS)
  and actinomycin D in refractory malignant melanoma, 119–128
  acute influenza and, 34, 35t
  animal studies with, 2, 3t
  in breast cancer, 131–138, 162–163
  in cancer studies, 93–104
  and cell-mediated immunity, 85–92
    in lung cancer, 107–118
  chemotherapy and, 51, 59
  comparison with glucan and BCG, 221–231
  in congenital immunodeficiencies, 165–169
  cyclic AMP in lymphocytes treated with, 23–27
  death rates with, 100t
  DNA synthesis and, 75–76
  dosage, 94, 95f, 97, 102, 104, 120
  E-rosette formation in T lymphocytes and, 65–71
  effect of, 2t
  exacerbation of underlying infections with, 160
  experimental cancers of mice and, 95f
  glucosamine incorporation and, 44
  human
    malignant lymphoma and, 49–60
    monocyte chemotaxis and, 29–36
    mononuclear phagocytes and, 39–45
  immune response and, 2t
  immunoreactivity and, 19
  immunotherapy with BCG, tumor vaccines, and, 147–155
  intensive alternate-day, 126
  lymphocyte proliferation and, 43–44
  metastasis formation and, 97–99
  migratory response of human monocytes and, 29
  monotherapy, 95f, 96
  nausea with, 159
  phagocytosis and, 41–45
  pyran and, 418
  with radiotherapy in murine tumor growth, 11, 14–21
  rash with, 159–160
  side effects, 7t, 57–58, 121–122
    management of, 157–164
  suckling rat spleen cells and, 75–83
  survival with, 124–125f
  T cells and, 1
  thymosin and, 368

  toxicity, 136t
  treatment, 1–9
    evaluation of, 103–104
    tritiated, 77–80
    tritiated thymidine and uridine incorporation and, 78t, 79f
    unblocking effect of, on T lymphocytes, 141–144
    vomiting with, 159
Lewis lung tumor, 391, 397t
Lipid emulsion, RE test, see RE test lipid emulsion
Lipopolysaccharide (LPS), see also Endotoxin
  Escherichia coli, 296–298
  pyran and, 437–442
Liver
  function, glucan and, 210
  metastases, glucan and, 211, 212f, 214f, 216f
  weight, 190
    CY and glucan influence on, 174, 176t
LMS, see Levamisole
Load, tumor, see Tumor load
LPS, see Lipopolysaccharide
Lung
  cancer
    as immunosuppressive disease, 111
    levamisole effect on cell-mediated immunity in, 107–118
    T-cell levels in, 117
  metastases, 98–99
    glucan and, 210–211, 213f, 215f
  weight, CY and glucan influence on, 174, 176t
Ly phenotypes, differentiation of T lymphocytes into, 301t, 302
Lymph node
  cell blastogenesis, 438
  cells, Con A response in, 295–298
Lymphadenopathy, immunoblastic, 97
Lymphocyte
  blastogenesis, 109
    BM 06 002 and, 405–406, 411
  counts, 55t
    low, 158–159
  culture, mixed (MLC), 108, 109, 112–115
    assay, 321
    reaction, thymosin and, 334
  cytotoxicity, 148
    increase in, 151–153
    to melanoma, 25f
  -derived chemotactic factor (LDCF), 31
  -mediated cytotoxicity, 88–91
  proliferation, levamisole and, 43–44
  reactivity
    in vitro, 110–117
    mixed (MLR), thymosin and, 289t
    to phytohemagglutinin, 97

Lymphocyte *(contd.)*
  response to thymosin, 347–355
  responses, *in vitro,* 321
Lymphocytes, *see also* B lymphocytes; T
    lymphocytes
  cyclic AMP in, treated with levamisole,
    23–27
  E-rosette forming, 319–329
  glucan action and, 183–193
  levamisole and, 2t, 80, 82–84
  macrophages versus, 246
  mature (T_2), 379
  mitomycin C-treated allogeneic, 109
  peripheral blood, 358–359
  prostaglandins and, 27
Lymphocytotoxic
  antibodies, 56–57
  autoantibodies, 57
Lymphocytotoxins, 274
Lymphokines, 45, 460f, 465
Lymphoma
  agranulocytosis in, 160
  human malignant, levamisole with, 49–60
  non-Hodgkin's malignant (NHL), le-
    vamisole and, 50–55, 59–60
Lymphoproliferation
  cytotoxicity and, 454
  regulation of, 435–444
Lymphotoxin, thymosin and, 289t
Lysis, contact, versus phagocytosis, 216
Lysosome system, 274–275
Lysosomes, primary, 455
Lysozyme, serum
  in acute myelogenous leukemia, 171–181
  concentration, 177–181

M109, *see* Madison lung carcinoma
Macroglobulin, *see* Pregnancy-associated α-
    macroglobulin
Macromolecular syndrome, 483
Macrophage
  -activating factors (MAF), 460f
  activation, 459
    polyanions and, 463–466
  adherence, percent, 202
  cell length, glucan and, 202–204
  -mediated
    antitumor action of glucan, 178
    cytostasis, *see* Cytostasis, macrophage-
      mediated
    cytotoxicity, *see* Cytotoxicity,
      macrophage-mediated
  production, increased, 195–199
  regulation, levamisole and, 75–83
Macrophages, 29, 435, 453
  activated
    antiviral and antitumor functions of,
      447–455
    polyanions and, 459–466

BCG and, 192
  defined, 447
  glucan
    action and, 183–193
    -activated, 201–205
  immunomodulators and, 455
  immunoregulatory, pyran and, 435–444
  levamisole and, 80, 82–84
  lymphocytes versus, 246
  peritoneal, 453–455
    glucan and, 197t
    tumoricidal effect of, 241–247
  resting, 44
  soluble factors synthesized by, 275
  transmission electron microscopy of, 257,
    264–271
Madison lung carcinoma (M109), 459
  pyran copolymer and, 427–432
MAF, *see* Macrophage-activating factors
Mannan, 255
Measles, levamisole and, 5
Melanoma
  antiantibody systems in, 149
  cyclic AMP in lymphocytes from patients
    with, 23–27
  glucan and, 172
  human, 147
  lymphocyte cytotoxicity to, 25f
  malignant, 103
  melanotic, 96
  prostaglandin $F_{2\alpha}$ levels with, 26
  recurrence of, 27
  refractory malignant, levamisole and
    actinomycin D and, 119–128
  stage 3B, 357–370
    disease-free interval of, 362–365f
  T-cell levels and, 350
Melphalan, 51
MEM, *see* Minimum essential medium
Membrane antibodies, 148
MER, *see* Methanol extraction residue
Metastases
  blood-borne, 153
  hepatic, glucan suppression of, 207–217
  lung, 98–99
  predicted number of, 224
  pulmonary
    pyran and, 431
    remission of, 412
Metastasis formation, levamisole treatment
    and, 97–99
Metastatic
  sites in breast cancer, 133t
  tumors and intralesional glucan, 249–254
Methanol extraction residue (MER), 192
Methotrexate, 132
Micrometastases, 96, 357
Migration inhibitory factor (MIF) produc-
    tion, thymosin and, 286, 287f, 289t

Migratory response of human monocytes, 29
Minimum essential medium (MEM), 222
Mitochondria, *Tetrahymena,* 81
Mitogens
    B-cell, 295–298
    glucan added to, 259–261
Mitomycin C
    toxicity, 179
    -treated allogeneic lymphocytes, 109
MLC, *see* Lymphocyte culture, mixed
MLR, *see* Lymphocyte reactivity, mixed
MM, *see* Myeloma, multiple
Monoamine oxidase inhibitor
    tranylcypromine sulphate, 160
Monocyte chemotaxis
    assay, 30
    human, levamisole and, 29–36
Monocytes, defined, 321–322
Monocytopoiesis, 199
MOPP chemotherapy, Hodgkin's disease and, 160
MST, *see* Survival time, median
Multiple sclerosis, agranulocytosis in, 160
Murine tumor growth, levamisole with radioactivity in, 11, 14–21
Myeloma, multiple (MM), levamisole and, 50–55, 59–60
Myelosuppression, 122
    degree of, 137

Nausea with levamisole, 159
NBP, *see* Nitrobenzylpyridine
Neutropenia, 136
    cyclic, levamisole and, 60
Neutrophil immigration, 261–262
Nezelof's syndrome, thymosin and, 336–339
NHL, *see* Lymphomas, non-Hodgkin's malignant
Nitrobenzylpyridine (NBP) determinations, 393–394
NSC 46015, *see* Pyran copolymer
Null cells
    circulating, 329
    defined, 321

Osteosarcoma, Ridgeway, 394

PAM, *see* Pregnancy-associated α-macroglobulin
PBL, *see* Lymphocytes, peripheral blood
PEC, *see* Peritoneal exudate cells
Peripolesis, 263, 269f, 273
Peritoneal
    cell population, 447
    cells
        in vivo, 451–452

preparation of, 448–449
    exudate cells (PEC), 436, 442–443, 450t
Peroxidase activity, spleen cell, 82
PES, *see* Polyethylene sulfonate
PFC, *see* Plaque-forming cells
$PGF_{2\alpha}$, *see* Prostaglandin $F_{2\alpha}$
PHA, *see* Phytohemagglutinin
Phagocyte functions, levamisole and, 6
Phagocytes
    human mononuclear
        glucan effects on, 261
        levamisole effects on, 39–45
        obtaining, 39
    isolated, levamisole and, 2t
Phagocytic activity, glucan and, 189
Phagocytosis
    contact lysis versus, 216
    levamisole effects on, 41–45
    piecemeal, 274
    of whole tumor cells, 263
Phytohemagglutinin (PHA), 109, 112–115, 141
    BM 06 002 and, 398f, 409
    glucan and, 256, 259–261
    lymphocyte reactivity to, 97
    pyran and, 437–442
    response in lymph node cells, 296–298
    thymosin and, 319–323
        in 3B melanoma, 358, 362, 364–369
Plaque
    -forming cells (PFC), 383
    test, Jerne's, 398, 399f
Platelet counts and pyran, 473–474
Plutonium poisoning and pyran, 484
PMN, *see* Leukocyte, polymorphonuclear
Pokeweed mitogen (PWM), 109, 112–115, 166t, 167t
    BM 06 002 and, 409
    glucan and, 256, 259–261
Poly (A:U), 403
    pyran and, 418
Poly (C) and pyran, 418, 421t
Poly (I) and pyran, 418, 421t
Poly (I:C)
    macrophage activation and, 463–466
    molecular structure of, 461f
    pyran and, 418
    thymosin and, 295
Poly (X) and pyran, 418, 421t
Polyanions, macrophage activation by, 459–466
Polyethylene sulfonate (PES), 482, 483
Polyriboinosinic-polyribocytidylic acid, *see* Poly (I:C)
PPD, *see* Purified protein derivative
PR, *see* Remission, partial
Prednisone, 51
Pregnancy-associated α-macroglobulin (PAM), 103

Prognosis
  clinical evaluations of, 97
  -immunology link-up, 96–97
Progression, defined, 133
Proline labeling, 88f, 89
Prostaglandin $F_{2\alpha}$ ($PGF_{2\alpha}$), 24
  levels with melanoma and SCC, 26
Prostaglandins, lymphocytes and, 27
Prothrombin time and pyran copolymer,
    480–482
Psoriasis with levamisole, 160
Purified protein derivative (PPD), 109, 112–
    115, 166t, 167t
  thymosin and, 286
PWM, *see* Pokeweed mitogen
Pyran copolymer (NSC 46015, Diveema),
    415, 469–472
  antitumor effect of, 192
  bone marrow examination and, 476
  clinical study of, 472–479
  clotting studies of, 479–482
  dose-dependency of, 429
  L1210 leukemia and, 415–425
  L1210 vaccine and, 214–215
  macrophage activation and, 242–246,
    463–466
  macrophages and, 454
    immunoregulatory, 435–444
  Madison lung carcinoma and, 427–432
  molecular structure of, 461f
  polyanions and, 459–466
  pyrexia and, 483
  route-dependency of, 429–431
  sedimentation rate and, 482
  toxicity, case reports of severe, 475–479
  toxicology, 471–472
  transient thrombocytopenia and, 470, 473
Pyrexia and pyran copolymer, 483

Radiation
  dose to cure mouse tumors, 14f
  portal and T-cell levels, 351–353
Radiosensitive cancers and levamisole, 100
Radiotherapy
  and levamisole, 103
  in murine tumor growth, 11, 14–21
Rash with levamisole, 159–160
Rat, suckling, spleen cells, levamisole and,
    75–83
RE, *see* Reticuloendothelial
Regressions, tumor, levamisole and, 17–18,
    19, 20
Remission
  complete (CR), 119
    in breast cancer, 133
  duration, 133
  partial (PR), 119
    in breast cancer, 133
    defined, 120

RES, *see* Reticuloendothelial system
Respiratory tract infections, levamisole and,
    5
Response rate in stage IV breast cancer,
    134t
Reticuloendothelial (RE)
  stimulants, 201
  -stimulating agent, 171
  system (RES)
    glucan and, 207, 241
    glucan effect on phagocytic activity of,
    189
  test lipid emulsion, 173–176, 185
RFC (rosette-forming cells), *see* E-rosette-
    forming cells
Rheumatoid factors, polyclonal, 149
Ridgeway osteosarcoma, 394
Rosette-forming cells (RFC), *see* E-rosette-
    forming cells
Route-dependency of pyran, 429–431

S, *see* Disease, stable
Sarcomas, soft tissue (STS), levamisole
    and, 50–53, 59
SCC, *see* Carcinoma, squamous cell
SCID, *see* Immunodeficiency disease,
    severe combined
Scleroglucan, 241–246
Sedimentation rate and pyran copolymer,
    482
Serotonin, 247
Serum
  activated human (AHS), 31
  antibodies, 147–148
Severe combined immunodeficiency
    disease, *see* Immunodeficiency disease,
    severe combined
Sheep red blood
  cell rosettes, *see* E-rosettes
  cells (SRBC), 375
SI, *see* Stimulation index
Side effects, *see* Toxicity
Skin
  disease, chronic fungal, thymosin and,
    338–339t, 341–342
  infections, pyogenic and mycotic, le-
    vamisole and, 5
  tests
    delayed hypersensitivity, 375
    DNCB, 109–110
    new positive, 376
SKSD, *see* Streptokinase-streptodornase
Soluble factors synthesized by
    macrophages, 275
Spleen
  cell
    blastogenesis, 438–443
    peroxidase activity, 82

Spleen *(contd.)*
  cells
    Con A response in, 295
    glucan and, 186–187
    suckling rat, levamisole and, 75–83
  cellularity, glucan and, 197t
  fraction 5, 286
  weight, 190, 237
    CY and glucan influence on, 174, 176t
Splenectomy, 302
SR, *see* Stimulation ratio
SRBC, *see* Sheep red blood cells
Staphylococcus aureus, 75
Stimulation
  index (SI), 358
    thymosin, 315–319
  ratio (SR), pyran and, 437–441
Strain-specific effects of amphotericin B, 385
Streptokinase, 157
  -streptodornase (SKSD), 166t, 167t, 410
STS, *see* Sarcomas, soft tissue
Suppressor
  effect on helper T cells, 230
  T-cell activity, 260
  T cells, 272
Survival
  with actinomycin D and levamisole, 124–125f
  rate in breast cancer, 101f
  in stage IV breast cancer, 135f
  time, median (MST)
    pyran copolymer and, 463
    thymosin and, 306–310

T_2, *see* Lymphocytes, mature
T-cell
  differentiation
    in vitro induction of, 319–329
    levamisole and, 8
  functions, levamisole and, 6
  levels
    in lung cancer, 117
    melanoma and, 350
    radiation portal and, 351–353
    thymosin and, 347–355
  markers, 319
  maturation, 293–302
  rosette formation, 335
  surface markers, maturation of, 299, 302
T cells (thymus-derived cells), 281
  enrichment of, 260–261
  glucan and, 256
  helper, 230
  levamisole and, 1
  maturation of, thymosin and, 293–302
  suppressor, *see* Suppressor T cells
  thymosin and, 334

T-lymphocyte
  function, thymosin and, 333–344
  response, splenic, 217
T lymphocytes, *see also* Lymphocytes
  defined, 320
  differentiation of, into Ly phenotypes, 301t, 302
  levamisole unblocking effect on, 141–144
  peripheral human, E-rosette formation in, 65–71
  pyran and, 442
  trypsin and, 66–67
T/C ratio, 462
  thymosin, 315–319
TEM, *see* Transmission electron microscopy
Tetrahymena pyriformis, 80–82
Tetramisole, 29–30, 31–35t, 85
Thioglycollate, 447, 454
Thrombin time and pyran copolymer, 480–482
Thrombocytopenia, transient, pyran and, 470, 473
Thymectomy, 286–288, 369, 373
Thymic humoral factor, 313
Thymidine, tritiated, 109, 112–115, 186
  BM 06 002 and, 409
  incorporation, 76
    levamisole and, 78t, 79f
    pyran and, 437–441
Thymin, *see* Thymopoietin
Thymocyte-mitogen (TM) bioassay for thymosin, 313–318
Thymopoietin, 8, 71, 313, 319
Thymosin, 373
  α_1, 284, 287t, 289t
  α_2, 286, 287t
  chemistry and biology of, 281–290
  disseminated solid tumors and, 373–379
  DNP$_5$-, 299, 300t, 302
  dosage, 362–363, 366, 367
  dose, immunocompetence and, 366
  fraction 5, 281–290, 293, 336
  in vitro and *in vivo* studies with, 305–311
  levamisole and, 368
  polypeptides, nomenclature for, 282–285
  in stage 3B melanoma, 357–370
  T-lymphocyte function and, 333–344
  thymocyte-mitogen bioassay for, 313–318
  toxicity, 378–379
  tumor enhancement and, 368–369
Thymus
  -derived cells, *see* T cells
  gland, 333
    cell-mediated immunity and, 281
  independence, glucan and, 245–246
Tilorone and pyran, 418
Tiredness with levamisole, 157

TM, *see* Thymocyte-mitogen
Toxicity
  glucan, 258
  hematologic, 122
    in stage IV breast cancer, 135t
  levamisole, 136t
  nonhematologic, 121–122
    in stage IV breast cancer, 135t
  study of BM 06 002, 406–411
Toxicology, pyran copolymer, 471–472
Transfer factor, immunostimulant action of, 169
Transfusion requirements, repeated, levamisole and, 58
Transmission electron microscopy (TEM) of macrophages, 257, 264–271
Transplantation antigen, H-2^b, 87
Tranylcypromine sulphate, monoamine oxidase inhibitor, 160
Trichophyton, diffuse cutaneous, thymosin and 338–339t, 342
Trypsinization and E-rosette formation, 66–67
TSTA, *see* Tumor-specific transplant antigen
Tumor
  burden, *see* Tumor load
  cell
    cytostasis, 455
    proliferation, cytostasis of, 189–190
  cells
    actinomycin D-resistant, 381
    effects of irradiated, 225
    glutaraldehyde-treated, 213–214
    irradiated, combined with immunomodulators, 226–231
    number of, host defense and, 19
    whole, phagocytosis of, 263
  enhancement
    by immunotherapy, 103–104
    thymosin and, 368–369
  growth delay, glucan and, 237–240
  load, 110–111

heavier, levamisole and, 97, 102
  increased, glucan and, 213
  thymosin and, 308–310
  regression
    levamisole and, 17–18, 19, 20
    morphology of glucan-induced, 261–271
  -specific transplant antigen (TSTA), 424
  vaccines
    immunotherapy with levamisole, BCG, and 147–155
    pyran and, 415
  weight, 190
Tumoricidal effect of peritoneal macrophages, 241–247
Tumors
  disseminated solid, 374
    thymosin and, 373–379
  doubling time of, 104
  metastatic, *see* Metastatic tumors
  murine, *see* Murine tumor growth
  radiation dose to cure mouse, 14f
  slow-growing, 94, 95f

Upper respiratory tract infections, levamisole and, 4
Uridine incorporation, levamisole and, 78t

Vaccine-induced antitumor immunity, 153–154
Vaccines, tumor, *see* vaccines
Vitamin A, 403
Vomiting and levamisole, 159

Walker carcinosarcoma, 394–395
Warfarin, 163–164
Weight changes, CY and glucan influence on, 174, 176t
White blood cell (WBC) counts, 55t
Wiskott-Aldrich syndrome, 165, 166t, 168
  thymosin with, 336, 338–339, 343–344

Zymosan, 179, 195